BLADDER CANCER – FROM BASIC SCIENCE TO ROBOTIC SURGERY

Edited by **Abdullah Erdem Canda**

Bladder Cancer – From Basic Science to Robotic Surgery
Edited by Abdullah Erdem Canda

Published by InTech

Janeza Trdine 9, 51000 Rijeka, Croatia

Publishing Process Manager Tajana Jevtic

Technical Editor Teodora Smiljanic

Cover Designer InTech Design Team

Additional hard copies can be obtained from orders@intechopen.com

Bladder Cancer – From Basic Science to Robotic Surgery, Edited by Abdullah Erdem Canda
p. cm.
ISBN 978-953-307-839-7

For EU product safety concerns:
IN TECH d.o.o., Prolaz Marije Krucifikse Kozulić 3, 51000 Rijeka, Croatia,
info@intechopen.com or visit our website at intechopen.com.

Meet the editor

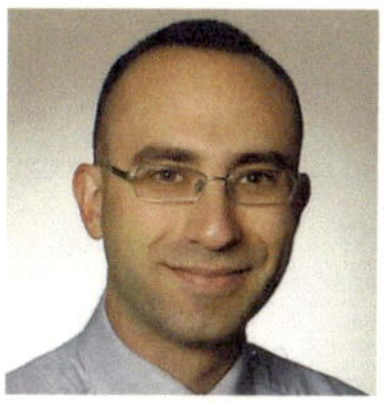

Dr Canda has graduated from Hacettepe University, School of Medicine in Ankara, Turkey in 1997, and completed his urology residency between 1998-2003 at Dokuz Eylul University, School of Medicine in Izmir, Turkey. From 2004 to 2005 he undertook research and clinical fellowships at The University of Sheffield, Department of Biomedical Sciences and Royal Hallamshire Hospital, Department of Urology in Sheffield and Southmead Hospital, Bristol Urological Institute, United Kingdom. Dr Canda also did laparoscopy urology fellowship at The University of Heidelberg, SLK Kliniken Heilbronn, Germany in 2007. His main areas of interest are robotic and laparoscopic urology, uro-oncology, reconstructive urology, endourology, uro-pharmacology, and basic science research. He has been working at Ankara Ataturk Training and Research Hospital, 1st Urology Clinic in Ankara and one of the leading robotic urology institutions in Turkey, since 2008. In 2011, he has been appointed as an associate professor of urology.

Contents

Preface

Bladder cancer is an malignant disease affecting many patients worldwide. This book includes chapters related to tumor biology, epidemiology, biomarkers, prognostic factors, clinical presentation and diagnosis of bladder cancer, treatment of bladder cancer including surgery, chemotherapy, radiation therapy, and immunotherapy. I would like to thank all the authors and co-authors who have contributed to this book, as well as the InTech Open Access Publisher team, and particularly Ms.Tajana Jevtic, who has been very helpful as a process manager during the preparation of the book. Hopefully this book will be beneficial and useful for colleagues who are interested in bladder cancer.

Dr. Abdullah Erdem Canda
Associate Professor of Urology
Ankara Atatürk Training and Research Hospital
1st Urology Clinic
Ankara,
Turkey

Part 1

Tumor Biology and Bladder Cancer

1

Bladder Cancer Biology

Susanne Fuessel, Doreen Kunze and Manfred P. Wirth
Department of Urology, Technical University of Dresden
Germany

1. Introduction

At present, bladder cancer (BCa) is worldwide the 9th most common tumor; in men it represents the 7th and in women 17th most common malignancy (Ploeg et al., 2009). In the European Union approximately 104,400 newly diagnosed BCa and 36,500 BCa-related deaths were estimated for the year 2006 (Ferlay et al., 2007). In the United States, approximately 70,530 new cases and 14,680 BCa-related deaths were expected for 2010 (Jemal et al., 2010). Men are three to four times more frequently affected than women (Ferlay et al., 2007; Jemal et al., 2010).

Detection of BCa is hampered due to lately emerging symptoms, such as hematuria, and the lack of specific tumor markers. Treatment options, particularly for the advanced disease, appear currently insufficient, leading together with the BCa-inherent high recurrence and progression rates to the relatively high BCa-related mortality (Ferlay et al., 2007). For the development of more specific and efficient diagnostic tools and therapeutic approaches a profound understanding of the onset and course of this disease is indispensable.

Molecular alterations that presumably lead to malignant transformation of the bladder urothelium belong to specified pathways involved in regulation of cellular homeostasis. As consequence of genetic and epigenetic alterations as well as of changes in subsequent regulatory mechanisms several major cellular processes are influenced in a manner that results in tumor development and progression. Regulation of the cell cycle, cell death and cell growth belong to these processes as well as the control of signal transduction and gene regulation. Particularly important for tumor cell spread and metastasis are changes in the regulation of interactions with stromal cells and extracellular components, of tumor cell migration and invasion and of angiogenesis (Mitra & Cote, 2009).

Interestingly, numerous associations between risk factors for the development of BCa and the affected cellular processes were identified (Mitra & Cote, 2009). For tobacco smoking or the occupational exposure to aromatic amines, polycyclic aromatic hydrocarbons and aniline dyes – the major environmental risk factors that contribute to BCa genesis – strong associations with alterations in cell cycle regulation have been reported (Bosetti et al., 2007; Golka et al., 2004; Mitra & Cote, 2009; Strope & Montie, 2008). Other factors such as use of hair dyes, several noxious substances and drugs, dietary components and urological pathologies influence with more or less evidence the control of cell cycle and the regulation of gene expression or signal transduction (Golka et al., 2004; Kelsh et al., 2008; Michaud, 2007; Mitra & Cote, 2009; Shiff et al., 2009).

Not only environmental risk factors determine the risk of BCa development, but also strong correlations with a genetic predisposition or polymorphisms in detoxification or repair genes leading to alterations in gene expression and regulation have been described (Bellmunt et al., 2007; Dong et al., 2008; Franekova et al., 2008; Garcia-Closas et al., 2006; Horikawa et al., 2008a; Kellen et al., 2007; Mitra & Cote, 2009; Sanderson et al., 2007).
Several genome-wide association studies revealed the association of different single nucleotide polymorphisms (SNPs) with an altered risk of BCa. Strong associations of SNPs on the chromosomes 3q28, 4p16.3, 8q24.21 and 8q24.3 with the risk of BCa development were observed (Kiemeney et al., 2008, 2010; Rothman et al., 2010; X. Wu et al., 2009). Rothman *et al.* identified also new chromosomal regions on 2q37.1, 19q12 and 22q13.1, which are related to the susceptibility for BCa (Rothman et al., 2010).

2. Different clinical behavior due to varying genetic & molecular pathways

Clinical behavior and outcome of superficial, non muscle-invasive BCa doubtless differ from muscle-invasive BCa what is the result of varying molecular pathways characteristic for each subtype [Fig.1]. The more frequently diagnosed non muscle-invasive BCa comprise papillary Ta tumors confined to the mucosa and T1 tumors spread into submucosal layers of the bladder. In dependence on tumor grade, stage and size, the presence of concomitant *carcinoma in situ* (*CIS*), the occurrence of multifocal lesions and the prior recurrence rate the risk of recurrence of non muscle-invasive Ta/T1 BCa and the risk of progression to muscle-invasive BCa differ considerably (Babjuk et al., 2011; Sylvester et al., 2006). In principle, flat *CIS* lesions also belong to the group of non muscle-invasive BCa but are associated with a higher aggressiveness due to a completely different tumor biological behavior rather resembling muscle-invasive BCa (Kitamura & Tsukamoto, 2006; Pashos et al., 2002).
It appears meaningful to regard the different types of non muscle-invasive BCa separately due to dissimilar phenotype-specific alterations in molecular and cellular pathways, which are also reflected by the varying clinical behavior. Ta tumors, which account for approximately 70% of non muscle-invasive BCa, bear a relatively high risk of local recurrence but rarely become muscle-invasive BCa (Kitamura & Tsukamoto, 2006; Pashos et al., 2002; Van Rhijn et al., 2009; Wu, 2005). The remaining non-muscle invasive BCa consist of 20% T1 tumors and about 10% primary *CIS* (Kitamura & Tsukamoto, 2006; Van Rhijn et al., 2009). Particularly, high grade T1 tumors (previously T1G3) have an increased propensity to progress compared to low grade T1 and Ta tumors (Emiliozzi et al., 2008; Kitamura & Tsukamoto, 2006). In contrast, *CIS* lesions are rather characterized by molecular alterations that are also observed in muscle-invasive BCa. Therefore, a high risk of progression of these *CIS* tumors seems to be implicated and leads to a poor outcome similar to that of muscle-invasive BCa (Knowles, 2008; Wu, 2005).
In low-grade papillary tumors a constitutively activated receptor tyrosine kinase/RAS pathway in consequence of activating mutations in the genes FGFR3 (*fibroblast growth factor receptor 3*) or HRAS (*Harvey rat sarcoma viral oncogene homolog*) was described (Jebar et al., 2005; Knowles, 2008; Wu, 2005). The rate of FGFR3 mutations of about 70% in Ta and in low-grade tumors is much higher than in invasive BCa with a rate of 10-20% (Bakkar et al., 2003; Billerey et al., 2001; Rieger-Christ et al., 2003; Serizawa et al., 2011).
Activating HRAS mutations are detected with an estimated overall frequency of 10-15% without a clear association with tumor grade or stage (Jebar et al., 2005; Knowles, 2008; Kompier et al., 2010a; Oxford & Theodorescu, 2003; Serizawa et al., 2011). Interestingly,

mutations in FGFR3 and in RAS genes are mutually exclusive events and therefore suggested to represent alternative means to activate the MAPK (*mitogen-activated protein kinase*) pathway resulting in the same phenotype (Jebar et al., 2005; Kompier et al., 2010a).
Furthermore, deletions of chromosome 9 belong to the most common genetic alterations in Ta tumors with a frequency of 36-66% (Knowles, 2008). Several putative tumor suppressor genes (TSG) located on this chromosome are affected by such deletions in combination with loss of heterozygosity (LOH) events, mutations or promoter hypermethylation (Knowles, 2008). Amongst others, the CDKN2A locus on 9p21 encoding the TSG $p16^{INK4A}$ and $p14^{ARF}$ is altered as well as PTCH1 (9q22.3), DBC1 (9q32-33) and TSC1 (9q34) located on the long arm of chromosome 9 (Aboulkassim et al., 2003; Berggren et al., 2003; Cairns et al., 1995; Chapman et al., 2005; Knowles, 2003, 2008; Lopez-Beltran et al., 2008; S.V. Williams et al., 2002; Williamson et al., 1995). LOH events in these chromosomal regions are associated with a high tumor grade and an elevated risk of recurrence of Ta and T1 tumors (Simoneau et al., 2000).

In principle, T1 tumors belong to the group of non-muscle-invasive BCa but obviously differ in their clinical behavior from Ta tumors since they show a higher potential for invasive growth and risk to progression. Nevertheless, dedifferentiation reflected by the tumor grade is a crucial factor for the determination of the phenotype resulting from differing molecular alterations (Kitamura & Tsukamoto, 2006). High-grade Ta tumors (TaG3) display a FGFR3 mutation frequency of 34% ranging between that of TaG1 (58-82%) and T1G3 tumors (17%) paralleling the phenotype and clinical behavior (Hernandez et al., 2005; Herr, 2000; Junker et al., 2008; Kitamura & Tsukamoto, 2006; Van Oers et al., 2007). Additionally, a high rate of homozygous deletions of the CDKN2A/INK4A gene, which was associated with an increased relative risk of recurrence, was observed in high-grade Ta tumors (Orlow et al., 1999).

Deletions or promoter hypermethylation of the CDKN2A/INK4A gene affect the expression of its gene products $p14^{ARF}$ and $p16^{INK4A}$ finally leading to deregulation in the p53 and RB1 (*retinoblastoma 1*) pathways. Alterations in these pathways are in fact molecular characteristics for *CIS* lesions and muscle-invasive BCa but can also be found in papillary tumors progressed to an invasive stage (Kitamura & Tsukamoto, 2006; Mitra & Cote, 2009; Orlow et al., 1999). Inactivation of p53 in muscle-invasive BCa is predominantly the consequence of allelic loss and mutations in this gene or of the homozygous deletion of its regulator $p14^{ARF}$ (Mitra & Cote, 2009). Disturbed expression or uninhibited hyperphosphorylation of the tumor suppressor RB1 result in its inactivation (Mitra & Cote, 2009). Simultaneous dysfunction of p53 and RB1, the two central regulators of the cell cycle and apoptosis, is observed in more than 50% of high grade T1 tumors and in the majority of muscle-invasive BCa (Kitamura & Tsukamoto, 2006; Knowles, 2008). Furthermore, two other alterations affecting the p53 pathway are characteristic for muscle-invasive BCa: the lack of $p21^{Waf1}$, the *cyclin-dependent kinase inhibitor 1A* (CDKN1A), and overexpression of the p53-regulator MDM2 (*Mdm2 p53 binding protein homolog (mouse)*) (Mitra & Cote, 2009).

Muscle-invasive BCa display a high number and variety of chromosomal alterations such as loss of 5q, 6q, 8p, 9p, 9q, 10q, 11p, 11q, 17p and Y or gains of 1q, 3q, 5p, 6p, 7p, 8q, 17q, 20p and 20q (Blaveri et al., 2005; Heidenblad et al., 2008; Knowles, 2008; Richter et al., 1998; Simon et al., 2000).

The frequency of specific genomic alterations increases with tumor stage and is associated with a worse outcome (Blaveri et al., 2005; Richter et al., 1998). Several genes putatively relevant for tumor proliferation and progression are located in these altered chromosomal regions such as the transcription factors E2F3 and SOX4 on 6p22 or the supposed oncogene YWHAZ (14-3-3-zeta) on 8q22 (Heidenblad et al., 2008). Interestingly, amplification of 6p22 containing E2F3, which is involved in cell cycle regulation, and the frequently occurring homozygous deletions of CDKN2A and CDKN2B on 9p21 exist mutually exclusive indicating that they possibly play complementary roles (Feber et al., 2004; Heidenblad et al., 2008; Hurst et al., 2008; Oeggerli et al., 2004, 2006; Olsson et al., 2007).

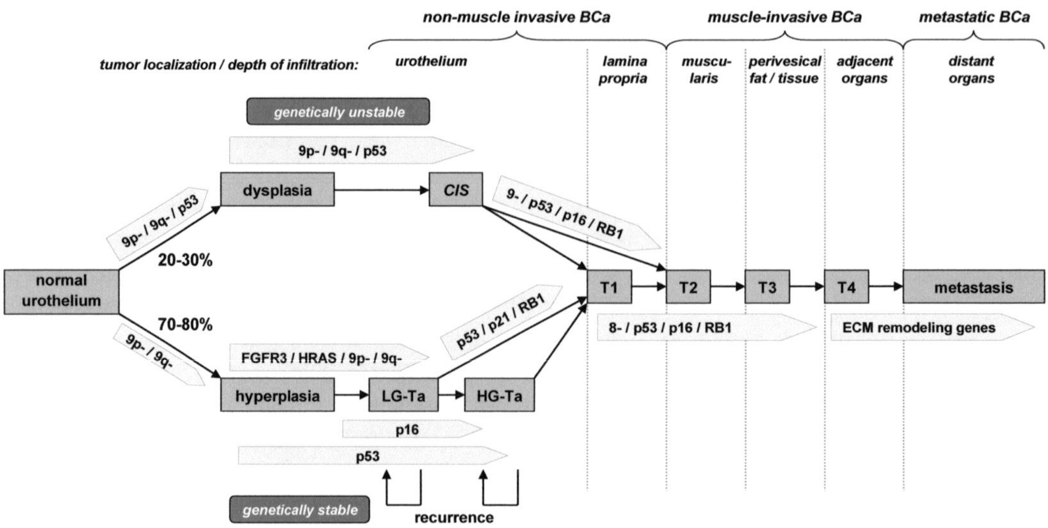

Fig. 1. Molecular pathways of BCa development and progression
Non-muscle invasive and muscle-invasive BCa fundamentally differ in their geno- and phenotypes. Varying genetic aberrations as well as the occurrence of p53 mutations in the normal urothelium are of crucial importance, which route of tumor progression will be followed. *Carcinoma in situ* (*CIS*) or muscle-invasive BCa, which may emerge from dysplasia of the urothelium, possess generally a high risk of progression. Papillary, non-muscle invasive Ta tumors, which are characterized by a high risk of recurrence and a lower risk of progression, rather develop from hyperplasia of the urothelium.
Abbreviations: 9p- / 9q- - loss of the short / long arm of chromosome 9, BCa - bladder cancer, *CIS* - *Carcinoma in situ*, ECM - extracellular matrix, HG-Ta - high grade Ta tumor, LG-Ta - low grade Ta tumor, T1 to T4 - tumor stages 1 to 4.

During progression and metastasis profound changes of regulatory networks involving the extracellular matrix (ECM), cell adhesion and migration, attraction of blood vessels and neovascularization occur, which characterize advanced tumor stages (Mitra & Cote, 2009). These processes comprise alterations in the regulation of cadherins, which are responsible for epithelial cell-cell adhesion, and *matrix metalloproteinases* (MMPs), which play an important role in the ECM-degradation as prerequisite for tumor cell migration (Mitra & Cote, 2009; Slaton et al., 2004; Wallard et al., 2006). Angiogenesis is driven by angiogenic factors such as the *vascular endothelial growth factor* (VEGF), one of the key factors responsible for tumor progression (Crew, 1999a).

3. Alterations in cell cycle regulation

Correct course of cell cycle is controlled by the p53 and RB1 pathways that are tightly linked with each other and influence regulation of apoptosis, signal transduction and gene expression [Fig.2]. The TSG p53, the central regulator of these processes, is located on chromosome 17p13.1, a region that is affected by allelic loss more frequently in BCa of higher stage and grade (Knowles, 2008; Olumi et al., 1990). Parallel to the loss of one 17p allele, frequently occurring mutations lead to the inactivation of the tumor suppressor p53 (Cordon-Cardo et al., 1994; Dalbagni et al., 1993; Sidransky et al., 1991). Mutated p53 becomes resistant to degradation and due to this longer stability detectable in the nucleus by immunohistochemistry (Dalbagni et al., 1993; Esrig et al., 1993). Such mutations were observed with a high frequency in BCa of higher stage and grade (Dalbagni et al., 1993; Esrig et al., 1993; Fujimoto et al., 1992; Puzio-Kuter et al., 2009; Serizawa et al., 2011; Sidransky et al., 1991). Therefore, the assessment of the nuclear immunoreactivity of altered p53 facilitates prognostic conclusions (Esrig et al., 1993; Kuczyk et al., 1995; Sarkis et al., 1993, 1995; Serth et al., 1995). Particularly for invasive, but still organ-confined BCa without metastasis (T1-2b N0 M0) and also for advanced BCa p53 is of prognostic importance with regard to the prediction of recurrence and cancer-specific mortality after radical cystectomy (Shariat et al., 2009a, 2009b). Nevertheless, nuclear accumulation and mutations of p53 provide differing contribution to the prediction of the outcome. Mutations and altered protein stability of p53 lead to worst prognosis compared to patients with one of these events and to patients with wild-type p53 and unchanged protein stability, who showed a more favorable outcome (George et al., 2007).

Interestingly, a study on BCa patients without evidence of distant metastases suggested that tumors harboring p53 mutations are more susceptible to adjuvant chemotherapy containing DNA-damaging agents such as e.g. cisplatin and doxorubicin (Cote et al., 1997). Possibly, these chemotherapeutics induce apoptosis in p53-mutated cells by uncoupling of the S and M cell cycle phases (Waldman et al., 1996). These observations built the basis for a large international multicenter clinical trial dealing with the assessment of response rates of high-risk patients with organ-confined invasive BCa to a chemotherapy containing DNA-damaging agents (Mitra et al., 2007). However, first data analysis did not confirm the predictive value of p53 immunohistochemistry (Stadler, 2009).

Wild-type p53 controls cell cycle progression at G1-S transition by transcriptional activation of $p21^{WAF1}$ (CDKN1A), a cyclin-dependent kinase inhibitor (CDKI) that additionally can be regulated by p53-independent mechanisms (El-Deiry et al., 1993; Michieli et al., 1994; Parker et al., 1995; Stein et al., 1998). As potent CDKI, $p21^{Waf1}$ inhibits the activity of cyclin-CDK2 or -CDK4 complexes, and thus functions as a regulator of cell cycle progression at G1 (Mitra et al., 2007). Loss or under-expression of $p21^{Waf1}$ appears to have impact on tumor progression and consequently on the outcome of the patients (Stein et al., 1998). Patients with wild-type p53 and $p21^{Waf1}$ positivity had the best prognosis whereas patients with altered p53 and maintained $p21^{Waf1}$ expression displayed worse outcome and patients with altered p53 and lack of $p21^{Waf1}$ showed the highest rate of recurrence and worst survival (Stein et al., 1998).

MDM2, located on chromosome 12q14.3-q15, is another component involved in the regulatory network of p53 and an indispensable factor for the feedback control of p53 stability. Transcription of MDM2 is induced by p53. In the form of an autoregulatory loop, MDM2 can build a complex with p53 and transports it to the proteasome for degradation (Mitra & Cote, 2009; Wu et al., 1993, 2005).

Degraded p53 in turn causes reduction in MDM2 levels, but this can be bypassed by MDM2 gene amplification, which is observed approximately in 5% of the BCa with an increased frequency in tumors of higher stage and grade (Simon et al., 2002). Additionally, MDM2 overexpression is a common event in BCa in strong association with p53 nuclear immunoreactivity (Lianes et al., 1994; Lu et al., 2002; Pfister et al., 1999, 2000). A combined assessment of alterations of p53, $p21^{Waf1}$ and MDM2 revealed that patients with mutant p53 and/or p53 nuclear overexpression, loss of $p21^{Waf1}$ and MDM2 nuclear overexpression exhibited the worst outcome (Lu et al., 2002). Furthermore, a specific SNP at nucleotide position 309 in the MDM2 promoter region was evaluated for prognostic and predictive purposes. It can predict a poor outcome particularly in conjunction with the mutation and SNP status of p53 (Horikawa et al., 2008b; Sanchez-Carbayo et al., 2007; Shinohara et al., 2009).

The chromosomal region 9q21, which is frequently lost in non-muscle invasive and in muscle-invasive BCa, harbors the gene locus CDKN2A (*cyclin-dependent kinase inhibitor 2A*) whose transcription results in two different splice variants, $p14^{ARF}$ and $p16^{INK4A}$ (Knowles, 2008; Quelle et al., 1995; S.G. Williams & Stein, 2004). Normally, $p14^{ARF}$ is induced by the transcription factor E2F and can inhibit transcription of MDM2 thereby blocking the MDM2-induced p53 degradation (S.G. Williams & Stein, 2004). Thus, $p14^{ARF}$ builds a link between the p53 and the RB1 pathways. The expression of the splice variant $p14^{ARF}$ is predominantly reduced by homozygous deletions and also by promoter hypermethylation in BCa (Chang et al., 2003; Dominguez et al., 2003; Kawamoto et al., 2006; W.J. Kim & Quan, 2005).

The gene product of the other splice variant, $p16^{INK4A}$, normally functions as CDKI by blocking the cyclin D-CDK4/6-mediated phosphorylation of the RB1 protein thereby maintaining it in its active hypophosphorylated state and preventing exit from the G1 phase (Quelle et al., 1995; Serrano et al., 1993). In a study on BCa of all stages and grades homozygous deletion of $p16^{INK4A}$ was observed in a lower frequency than of $p14^{ARF}$ (Chang et al., 2003). In another study on non-muscle invasive BCa a higher risk of recurrence was found for homozygous deletion of the CDKN2A gene where loss of both splice variants $p14^{ARF}$ and $p16^{INK4A}$ correlated with clinicopathological parameters of a worse prognosis due to the potential deregulation of both the p53 and RB1 pathways (Orlow et al., 1999).

Additionally, hypermethylation in the promoter region of $p16^{INK4A}$ was reported for BCa in a range of 6-60% (Chang et al., 2003; Chapman et al., 2005; Dominguez et al., 2003; Kawamoto et al., 2006; W.J. Kim & Quan, 2005; Orlow et al., 1999). Loss of $p16^{INK4A}$ protein expression in T1 tumors correlated significantly with a reduced progression-free survival and was an independent predictor of tumor progression (Kruger et al., 2005). In another study, aberrant $p16^{INK4A}$ protein expression was found to be an adverse prognostic factor only in T3-T4 tumors whereas abnormal immunoreactivity of p53 and $p16^{INK4A}$ was identified as an independent predictor of reduced survival for all muscle-invasive BCa (Korkolopoulou et al., 2001).

Concluding data on BCa, homozygous deletions in the CDKN2A gene were not associated with tumor stage or grade supporting the hypothesis that chromosomal alteration of 9p21 is an early event in bladder carcinogenesis (Berggren et al., 2003). Nevertheless, aberrant methylation of $p14^{ARF}$ and $p16^{INK4A}$ occurs more frequently in muscle-invasive than in non-muscle invasive BCa and seems to be associated with adverse clincopathological parameters as well as with a poor outcome (Dominguez et al., 2003; Kawamoto et al., 2006).

The CDKN2B gene located adjacent to CDKN2A on 9p21 encodes the CDKI p15^{INK4B}, which inhibits cyclin D1-CDK4/6 complexes similar to p16^{INK4A} (Orlow et al., 1995). In contrast to p16^{INK4A} no association was observed between the expression and promoter methylation status of p15^{INK4B} whereas the rate of chromosomal alterations was comparable (M.W. Chan et al., 2002; Gonzalez-Zulueta et al., 1995; Le Frere-Belda et al., 2004; Orlow et al., 1995). Decreased p15^{INK4B} mRNA expression was only observed in non-muscle invasive BCa; in muscle invasive BCa p15^{INK4B} expression varied widely (Le Frere-Belda et al., 2001). The authors concluded that decreased p15^{INK4B} expression might be an important step in early neoplastic transformation of the urothelium and could be caused by other mechanisms than deletion or promoter hypermethylation (Le Frere-Belda et al., 2001).

The potential TSG p27^{Kip1} (CDKN1B) is located on chromosome 12p13.1-p12 and belongs to the Kip1 family of CDKIs. It inhibits cyclin D-CDK4/6 and cyclin E/A-CDK2 complexes consequently preventing RB1 hyperphosphorylation (Coats et al., 1996; Polyak et al., 1994). The prognostic value of p27^{Kip1} was analyzed in several immunohistochemistry studies on non-muscle and muscle-invasive BCa which revealed that this factor is preferentially expressed in early stage BCa (Franke et al., 2000; Korkolopoulou et al., 2000; Rabbani et al., 2007). In non-muscle invasive BCa expression of p27^{Kip1} decreased significantly with increasing grade and a significant correlation between low p27^{Kip1} expression and shorter disease-free survival and overall survival was observed, facts that support the hypothesis that loss of p27^{Kip1} confers a selective growth advantage to tumor cells (Kamai et al., 2001; Korkolopoulou et al., 2000; Migaldi et al., 2000; Sgambato et al., 1999). However, some studies on non-muscle invasive and/or muscle-invasive BCa did not reveal a significant association between the loss of p27^{Kip1} and outcome (Doganay et al., 2003; Franke et al., 2000; Kuczyk et al., 1999), whereas other reports showed that a decreased expression of p27^{Kip1} significantly correlated with worse prognosis (Kamai et al., 2001; Rabbani & Cordon-Cardo, 2000).

Another central pathway influencing cell cycle progression is the regulatory network around the nuclear phosphoprotein RB1, a TSG located on chromosome 13q14 (Cairns et al., 1991; Mitra et al., 2007; Takahashi et al., 1991; S.G. Williams & Stein, 2004). RB1 in its physiological active, hypophosphorylated form inhibits cell cycle progression at the G1-S checkpoint by sequestering transcription factors of the E2F family (Chellappan et al., 1991; Fung et al., 1987; Hiebert et al., 1992; Mihara et al., 1989). Hyperphosphorylation of RB1 abolishes its cell cycle-inhibitory activity by the release of E2F transcription factors leading to transcription of genes involved in DNA synthesis and progression through mitosis (Degregori et al., 1995; Hernando et al., 2004; Mitra et al., 2007). RB1 becomes hyperphosphorylated by different cyclin-CDK complexes, such as cyclin D1-CDK4/6 and cyclin E-CDK2, which in turn can be inhibited by specific CDKIs, such as p16^{INK4A}, p21^{Waf1} and p27^{Kip1}. The phosphorylation-mediated inactivation of RB1 can be the consequence of the already described loss of different CDKIs (Mitra et al., 2007).

In addition, mutations and LOH events in the RB1 gene can also lead to loss of RB1 expression and consequently to unregulated cellular proliferation (Miyamoto et al., 1995; Wada et al., 2000; Xu et al., 1993). Therefore, both aberrant RB1 down-regulation and dominance of the hyperphosphorylated inactive RB1 can be associated with tumor progression (Cote et al., 1998). For BCa, the proportion of RB1 alterations due to loss or inactivation was reported to increase with tumor stage and grade (Cairns et al., 1991; Ishikawa et al., 1991; Wada et al., 2000; Xu et al., 1993).

Particularly muscle-invasive, advanced BCa with an altered RB1 expression had a more aggressive behavior reflected by significantly decreased survival (Cordon-Cardo et al., 1992; Cote et al., 1998; Logothetis et al., 1992).
Regarding both p53 and RB1 – the key players of cell cycle regulation – as well as the other components of this regulatory network, a combined analysis of multiple factors seems to be reasonable. Therefore, a multitude of comprehensive immunohistochemical analyses of different cell cycle regulators such as p53, RB1, MDM2, cyclin D1 and E, $p14^{ARF}$, $p16^{INK4A}$, $p21^{Waf1}$, $p27^{Kip1}$, Ki67 and PCNA (*proliferating cell nuclear antigen*) were performed on tissue specimens originating from non-muscle invasive and muscle-invasive BCa (Brunner et al., 2008; Cordon-Cardo et al., 1997; Cote et al., 1998; Grossman et al., 1998; Hitchings et al., 2004; Kamai et al., 2001; Korkolopoulou et al., 2000; Lu et al., 2002; Migaldi et al., 2000; Niehans et al., 1999; Pfister et al., 1999, 2000; Sarkar et al., 2000; Shariat et al., 2004, 2006, 2007a, 2007b, 2007c; 2007d, 2009a; Tut et al., 2001).

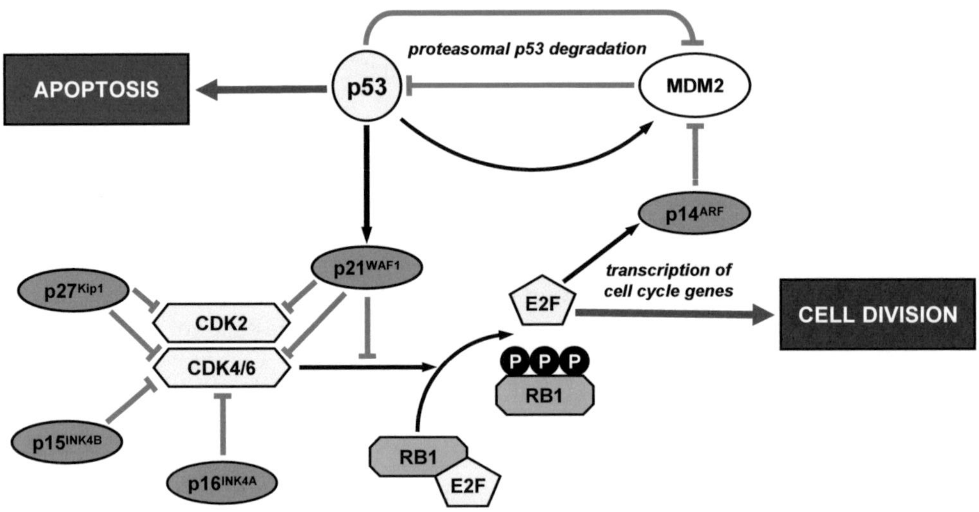

Fig. 2. Simplified illustration of the interactive network between the p53 & RB1 pathways Transcription of MDM2 is induced by p53. In the form of an autoregulatory loop, MDM2 conveys p53 by ubiquitination to proteasomal degradation. Degraded p53 in turn causes reduction in MDM2 levels. Wild-type p53 can induce transcription of the CDKI $p21^{WAF1}$, which inhibits the activity of cyclin-CDK2 or -CDK4 complexes similar to the CDKI $p15^{INK4B}$, $p16^{INK4A}$ and $p27^{Kip1}$. When RB1 gets hyperphosphorylated by different cyclin-CDK complexes bound E2F transcription factors are released leading to the induction of cell cycle-promoting genes, but also to transcription of $p14^{ARF}$, which can inhibit MDM2. Abbreviations: CDK - cyclin-dependent kinase, CDKI - cyclin-dependent kinase inhibitor, E2F - E2F transcription factors, MDM2 - *Mdm2 p53 binding protein homolog (mouse)*, $p14^{ARF}$ and p16 ^{INK4A} - splice variants of the *cyclin-dependent kinase inhibitor 2A* gene, $p15^{INK4B}$ – *cyclin-dependent kinase inhibitor 2B*, $p27^{Kip1}$ – *cyclin-dependent kinase inhibitor 1B*, RB1 – *retinoblastoma 1*.

The bottom line of most of these studies is that changes in gene expression, which can be caused by chromosomal alterations, promoter hypermethylation or altered regulation of transcriptional induction, as well as alterations of stability, modification and activity of the different involved factors contribute to deregulation of the complex processes during cell cycle progression. The number of altered components correlates with the severity of dysfunction and deregulation finally leading to increased aggressiveness of the tumor and to worse prognosis. Most promising candidates, when analyzed in parallel with regard to prediction of the outcome of BCa patients, seem to be p53, RB1, $p16^{INK4A}$, $p21^{Waf1}$, $p27^{Kip1}$ and the proliferation marker Ki67. This prognostic information can support the stratification of the tumors according to their aggressiveness and the selection of adapted treatment options (Grossman et al., 1998).

4. Deregulation of cell death pathways

Course of development, cell differentiation and homeostasis is normally regulated by the tight control of cell death pathways [Fig.3]. This programmed cell death, the apoptosis, is usually induced by a variety of extra- and intracellular stimuli and is mediated by a complex arrangement of sensors, regulators and effectors whose interactions are frequently perturbed in tumor cells. Failure of apoptosis permits mutated cells to continue progression through the cell cycle, to accumulate mutations and to increase molecular deregulations. The resulting unrestricted propagation of active oncogenes and defective TSG finally leads to the uncontrolled proliferation and spread of these abnormal cells (Bryan et al., 2005a; Duggan et al., 2001; Mcknight et al., 2005). Defects and deregulation in the extrinsic and in the intrinsic apoptotic pathways contribute to development and progression of many tumors including BCa and are also the main reason for therapeutic failure. Particularly, defective p53 fails as detector of DNA damage and main inductor of apoptosis, when DNA repair was not achieved (Duggan et al., 2001).

The extrinsic apoptotic pathway is induced through the stimulation of cell surface death receptors by their corresponding ligands while the intrinsic pathway is switched on by the disruption of mitochondrial membranes. There is a cross-talk between both routes that finally lead to the cleavage of cellular proteins by caspases and subsequently to the degradation of the cells by gradual destruction of cellular components (Mcknight et al., 2005).

Transmembrane death receptors, such as FAS (CD95, APO-1), TNFR1, TRAILR1 or TRAILR2, belong to the *tumor necrosis factor* (TNF) receptor superfamily and contain an intracellular death domain. After binding of the respective ligands, such as FAS ligand, TNFα or TRAIL, extracellular death signals are transmitted via these domains by formation of a death-inducing signaling complex that activates the initiator caspases 8 and 10 (Mcknight et al., 2005; Mitra & Cote, 2009). Impairment of this processes was reported in BCa e.g. for FAS-mediated apoptosis that might be caused by mutation or decreased expression of FAS, which is associated with disease progression and poor outcome (Lee et al., 1999; Mcknight et al., 2005; Yamana et al., 2005). An alternative splice variant of FAS results in circulating soluble FAS that can capture the respective ligands and consequently prevent the normal death signal transduction. Soluble FAS, which was detected in serum and also in urine samples from BCa patients, could serve as predictor of recurrence and progression of BCa (Mizutani et al., 2001; Svatek et al., 2006).

The intrinsic or mitochondrial induced apoptotic pathway can be initiated by DNA damage or different cellular stress signals (Mcknight et al., 2005). The BCL2 (*B-cell CLL/lymphoma 2*) family, which plays a crucial role in the intrinsic apoptotic pathway, consists of anti-apoptotic members, such as BCL2 and BCLXL (*BCL2-like 1*), as well as of pro-apoptotic members, such as BAX (*BCL2-associated X protein*), BID (*BH3 interacting domain death agonist*) and BAD (*BCL2-associated agonist of cell death*). BCL2 is an integral protein of the outer mitochondrial membrane that is involved in the control of ion channels, inhibition of cytochrome c release from the mitochondria or modulation of caspase activation (Mcknight et al., 2005; Mitra & Cote, 2009).

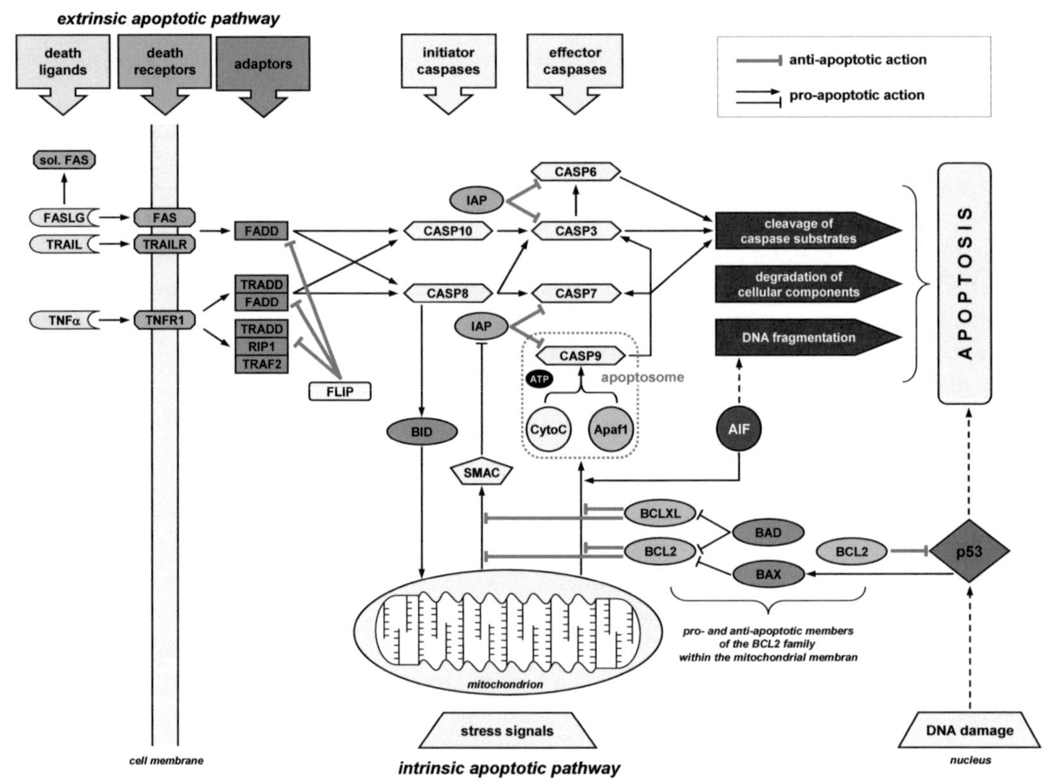

Fig. 3. Simplified illustration of the apoptotic cell death pathways
The extrinsic apoptotic pathway is induced through stimulation of cell surface death receptors by their corresponding ligands. The intrinsic mitochondrial route of apoptosis is initiated by DNA damage and cellular stress signals. Both pathways are interconnected and lead to the caspase-mediated cleavage of cellular proteins and consequently to the gradual degradation of further cellular components and cellular destruction.
Abbreviations: AIF – *apoptosis-inducing factor*, APAF1 – *apoptotic peptidase activating factor 1*, ATP – adenosine-5'-triphosphate, BAD – *BCL2-associated agonist of cell death*, BAX – *BCL2-associated X protein*, BCL2 – *B-cell CLL/lymphoma 2*, BCLXL – *BCL2-like 1*, BID – *BH3 interacting domain death agonist*, CASP – caspase, Cyto C – cytochrome c, DNA – deoxyribonucleic acid, FADD – *Fas-associated via death domain*, FAS – *Fas (TNF receptor superfamily, member 6)*, FASLG – *Fas ligand*, FLIP – *FLICE-inhibitory protein*, IAP – inhibitors of apoptosis, RIP1 – *receptor interacting protein 1*, SMAC – *second mitochondria-derived activator of caspase*, TNFR – *tumor necrosis factor receptor*, TRADD – *TNFR1-associated death domain protein*, TRAF2 – *TNF receptor-associated factor 2*, TRAIL – *TNF-related apoptosis inducing ligand*.

The export of cytochrome c into the cytoplasm and its binding to APAF1 (*apoptotic peptidase activating factor 1*) together with ATP induces the formation of apoptosomes that can cleave and activate pro-caspase 9. Subsequently, caspase 9 activates the effector caspases 3 and 7, which can be alternatively activated in the extrinsic pathway by the initiator caspases 8 and 10 as mentioned above. This caspase cascade finally commits the cell to apoptosis by gradual degradation of cellular proteins (Mcknight et al., 2005; Mitra & Cote, 2009).

BCL2 can block the apoptotic death and thereby trigger tumor recurrence and progression as well as mediate resistance to chemotherapy and radiation (Duggan et al., 2001). Different studies on non-muscle invasive and muscle-invasive BCa showed, that BCL2 was up-regulated in a varying number of the analyzed cases ranging from 41 to 63% (Cooke et al., 2000; Korkolopoulou et al., 2002; Liukkonen et al., 1997; Maluf et al., 2006; Ong et al., 2001). This BCL2 up-regulation correlated only partially with tumor stage and grade, but was frequently indicative for patients with poor prognosis after chemo- and/or radiotherapy (Cooke et al., 2000; Hussain et al., 2003; Ong et al., 2001; Pollack et al., 1997). Expression analyses of BCL2 together with other prognostic markers such as p53 and MDM2 revealed their usefulness as complementary predictors of survival of patients with non-muscle invasive and muscle-invasive BCa (Gonzalez-Campora et al., 2007; Maluf et al., 2006; Ong et al., 2001; Wolf et al., 2001).

Furthermore, the ratio between the anti-apoptotic factor BCL2 and the pro-apoptotic factor BAX seems to act as a cellular rheostat that might be predictive for a cell's response toward life or death after an apoptotic stimulus (Gazzaniga et al., 1996). BAX can be activated by BID that in turn can be induced by the initiator caspase 8. BAX forms a heterodimer with BCL2 and functions as an apoptotic activator by increasing the opening of the mitochondrial *voltage-dependent anion channel* (VDAC), which leads to the loss in membrane potential and the release of cytochrome c. The predominant expression of BCL2 over that of BAX correlated with a worse outcome and shorter time to relapse in low grade and non-muscle invasive BCa (Gazzaniga et al., 1996, 2003).

Apoptotic cell death can also be hampered by members of the IAP (inhibitor of apoptosis proteins) family that are also known as *baculoviral IAP repeat-containing* (BIRC) proteins. With regard to BCa, survivin (BIRC5) is the most interesting IAP since it can serve as diagnostic, prognostic and predictive marker (Margulis et al., 2008). Survivin inhibits apoptosis, promotes cell proliferation and enhances angiogenesis leading to its prominent role for tumor onset and progression in general and in particular for BCa (Margulis et al., 2008). For this tumor entity, high survivin expression at mRNA and protein levels is associated with advanced tumor grade and stage as well as with affection of lymph nodes (Karam et al., 2007a; I.J. Schultz et al., 2003; Shariat et al., 2007a; Swana et al., 1999; Weikert et al., 2005a). Survivin may serve either alone or together with other markers, such as p53, BCL2 and caspase 3, as a significant predictor of disease recurrence, progression and/or mortality after transurethral resection or radical cystectomy (Gonzalez et al., 2008; Karam et al., 2007a; 2007b; Ku et al., 2004; Shariat et al., 2007a). Response to chemo- and radiotherapy could also be estimated by the use of survivin as a predictive marker in BCa patients (Hausladen et al., 2003; Weiss et al., 2009).

For XIAP (*X-linked inhibitor of apoptosis* / BIRC4), which can directly inhibit the action of caspase 3, 7 and 9 and also interfere with the TNFR-associated cell death signaling, an up-regulation and association with an earlier recurrence was described in non-muscle invasive BCa (Dubrez-Daloz et al., 2008; Li et al., 2007).

Another IAP - cIAP2 (BIRC3) - that regulates apoptosis by binding to the TNFR-associated factors TRAF1 and TRAF2, has been shown to provoke chemoresistance when overexpressed in BCa cell lines (Jonsson et al., 2003). In expression analyses of livin (BIRC7) in tissue specimens from non-muscle invasive BCa only its anti-apoptotic isoform α was detected which was significantly associated with BCa relapse (Gazzaniga et al., 2003; Liu et al., 2009).

5. Immortalization of tumor cells – importance of the human telomerase

Activation of the human telomerase represents a very early event during the development of malignant tumors that leads to immortalization and as a consequence to the capability for unlimited division of tumor cells (Hiyama & Hiyama, 2002). Telomeres, the ends of eukaryotic chromosomes, normally get truncated during each cell division until they reach a critical length. This results in a severe impairment of the division capability leading to senescence of the cells (Harley, 1991). This senescence and the consequential cell death can be bypassed through activation of the telomerase ribonucleoprotein complex, since its catalytic subunit TERT (*telomerase reverse transcriptase*) supports the continuous prolongation of telomeres (Blackburn, 2005). Most of the differentiated somatic cells do not possess telomerase activity, whereas germline and stem cells as well as tumor cells frequently are telomerase-positive (Hiyama & Hiyama, 2002; N.W. Kim et al., 1994).

Several studies proved that TERT as well as the *telomerase RNA component* (TERC) represent essential subunits of the telomerase complex, but only TERT is specifically induced in cancer and functions as limiting factor of the enzymatic telomerase activity (Ito et al., 1998; Meyerson et al., 1997). Nevertheless, TERT protects the chromosomal ends also independently from its catalytic activity through its so-called capping function thereby providing tumor cells with further survival benefit (Blackburn, 2005; Blasco, 2002; S.W. Chan & Blackburn, 2002).

For most tumors it remains unclear whether TERT expression originates from telomerase-positive tumor stem cells or from the activation of the gene during tumorigenesis. A number of transcription factors, tumor suppressors, cell cycle inhibitors, hormones, cytokines and oncogenes have been implicated in the control of TERT expression but without providing a clear explanation for the tumor-specific TERT activity so far (Ducrest et al., 2002; Kyo et al., 2008).

Definitely, a tumor-specific activation of the telomerase complex is detectable in the majority of BCa. In contrast to telomerase-negative normal urothelium cells, > 90% of the analyzed BCa tissue specimens displayed a high expression and activity of telomerase (de Kok et al., 2000a; Heine et al., 1998; Hiyama & Hiyama, 2002; Ito et al., 1998; Lin et al., 1996; Muller, 2002). Therefore, the detection of TERT expression or the determination of telomerase activity in tissue or urine samples from patients suspected of having BCa is very useful for tumor detection (Alvarez & Lokeshwar, 2007; Glas et al., 2003; Muller, 2002; Weikert et al., 2005b). Possibly, quantitative determination of the TERT transcript levels in urine or bladder washings can support the prediction of recurrent BCa (Brems-Eskildsen et al., 2010; de Kok et al., 2000b).

6. Alterations in cell growth signaling

Cell growth signaling is transduced from the cell surface to the nucleus by different signaling cascades which can be altered and disturbed in tumor cells at different levels leading to uncontrolled cell growth and proliferation [Fig.4]. In principle, peptide growth factors bind to their corresponding growth factor receptors on the cell surface leading to receptor activation and via several signal transduction events to the activation of downstream factors (RAS and RAF1). Through the subsequent activation of the MAPK pathway several transcription factors, such as MYC (*v-myc myelocytomatosis viral oncogene homolog (avian)*) or ELK1 (*ETS-like transcription factor 1*), are induced, which finally regulate the expression of growth-promoting genes. Transmission of extracellular growth signals can be altered in tumor cells at different levels of these cascades, e.g. by an abnormally increased supply of growth factors or by amplification, mutation or alternative up-regulation of the growth factor receptors leading to their constitutive, excessive and uncontrolled activity (Hanahan & Weinberg, 2000). Mutations or other regulatory alterations affecting downstream targets, such as members of the RAS family, can additionally provide tumor cells with an increased growth potential (Jebar et al., 2005; Knowles, 2008).

FGFR3, one of the four members of the FGFR family, is constitutively activated by different mutations, which are found in approximately 70% of low-grade Ta and to a much lower extent of 10-20% in muscle-invasive BCa (Bakkar et al., 2003; Billerey et al., 2001; Hernandez et al., 2006; Jebar et al., 2005; Junker et al., 2008; Knowles, 2008; Kompier et al., 2010a; Rieger-Christ et al., 2003; Van Oers et al., 2007; Van Rhijn et al., 2004). The most frequent mutations lead to amino acid substitutions to cysteine residues which can build covalent disulfide bonds mimicking dimerization and thereby activation of the receptor (Kompier et al., 2010b). Mutated FGFR3 correlates with favorable disease parameters and improved survival (Kompier et al., 2010b; Van Oers et al., 2007, 2009; Van Rhijn et al., 2001, 2004, 2010). In a recent multicenter study, the so called molecular grade, a combination of the FGFR3 mutation status and the proliferation marker Ki67, could improve the predictive accuracy of the EORTC (European Organisation for Research and Treatment of Cancer) risk scores for progression (Van Rhijn et al., 2010).

Mutated FGFR3 leads to the activation of the RAS-MAPK-pathway and consequently to an augmented transduction of growth signals. RAS mutations are found in BCa with an overall frequency of approximately 10-15% and do not depend on tumor grade or stage, (Jebar et al., 2005; Knowles, 2008; Kompier et al., 2010a; Oxford & Theodorescu, 2003; Serizawa et al., 2011). Such mutations occur in all three RAS genes (HRAS, NRAS and KRAS) whereby HRAS is affected most frequently (Jebar et al., 2005). Interestingly, simultaneous mutations in FGFR3 and RAS, both resulting in the activation of the same pathway, are very uncommon and rather occur mutually exclusive (Jebar et al., 2005). Thus, low grade and Ta tumors harbor mutations either of FGFR3 or HRAS in more than 80% of the cases reflecting the necessity of constitutive activation of the MAPK pathway for non muscle-invasive BCa (Jebar et al., 2005; Knowles, 2008).

Additionally, the up-regulation of FGFs can contribute to the pathogenesis of cancer (Bryan et al., 2005a). Levels of FGF1 (acidic FGF) in urine samples correlated with tumor stage (Chopin et al., 1993). An association with an increased tumor stage and early local recurrence was shown for the expression of FGF2 (basic FGF) (Bryan et al., 2005a; Gazzaniga et al., 1999).

The *epidermal growth factor* (EGF) receptor family comprising EGFR (ERBB1), ERBB2 (HER-2/neu), ERBB3 (HER3) and ERBB4 (HER4) represents another tyrosine kinase receptor family involved in growth signaling in BCa cells that can also transduce extracelluar growth signals via the RAS-MAPK pathway or alternatively via the *phosphatidylinositol 3-kinase* (PIK3)-Akt pathway (Bryan et al., 2005a; Mitra & Cote, 2009). Expression at mRNA and protein level of all members of the EGFR family was observed in BCa specimens but with varying patterns of coexpression and differing prognostic impact, possibly depending on the size and composition of the patients cohorts and the detection techniques used in the different studies (Amsellem-Ouazana et al., 2006; Chow et al., 2001; Chow et al., 1997b; Forster et al., 2011; Junttila et al., 2003; Kassouf et al., 2008; Memon et al., 2006; Rotterud et al., 2005). Increased expression of EGFR and ERBB2 has been observed in a number of studies (Black & Dinney, 2008; Mitra & Cote, 2009). Many of these analyses revealed a correlation between increased levels of these two receptors and parameters of high risk tumors or of a poor prognosis for BCa patients (Black & Dinney, 2008; Mitra & Cote, 2009).

Several studies analyzed the BCa-related impact of growth factors activating EGFR, which comprise EGF, TGFα (*transforming growth factor alpha*), HB-EGF (*heparin-binding EGF-like growth factor*), epiregulin and others. Levels of TGFα in tissue samples and urine specimens from BCa patients correlated strongly with poor prognosis (Gazzaniga et al., 1998; Ravery et al., 1997; Thogersen et al., 2001; Turkeri et al., 1998). An association with tumor recurrence was also observed for EGF in BCa tissues, but not for urinary EGF (Chow et al., 1997a; Turkeri et al., 1998). Further studies revealed also an inverse correlation between the expression of epiregulin or nuclear HB-EGF and the survival of BCa patients (Adam et al., 2003; Kramer et al., 2007; Thogersen et al., 2001).

Another growth signaling pathway profoundly altered in many tumor entities including BCa is that of VEGF. This pathway is predominantly involved in the regulation of angiogenesis through the attraction and direction of blood vessels to the tumor by VEGF, which is secreted by tumor cells (Sato et al., 1998). Additionally, an autocrine function of VEGF in direct activation of the tumor cells themselves is assumed due to the observed up-regulation of different VEGF receptors such as FLT1 (VEGFR1) and KDR (VEGFR2 = FLK1) in BCa (Black & Dinney, 2008; Sato et al., 1998; Xia et al., 2006). An increased expression of KDR in BCa patients correlated with higher disease stage, muscle invasion and lymph node metastasis (Mitra et al., 2006; Xia et al., 2006).

PIK3CA (*phosphoinositide-3-kinase catalytic subunit alpha*) is part of the Akt signaling pathway and in this way also involved in the transformation of extracellular growth signals into an increased potential of cell proliferation and survival. PIK3CA mutations with an overall frequency of 13-25% seem to be a common event that occurs early in bladder carcinogenesis (Kompier et al., 2010a; Lopez-Knowles et al., 2006; Platt et al., 2009; Serizawa et al., 2011). A correlation with low stage and grade was observed in several studies (Lopez-Knowles et al., 2006; Serizawa et al., 2011). Interestingly, PIK3CA mutations were shown to be strongly associated with FGFR3 mutations possibly indicating cooperative oncogenic effects (Castillo-Martin et al., 2010; Kompier et al., 2010a; Lopez-Knowles et al., 2006; Serizawa et al., 2011). However, PIK3CA mutations showed no correlation with progression or disease-specific survival (Kompier et al., 2010a).

PTEN (*phosphatase and tensin homolog*), which is a phosphatidylinositol-3,4,5-trisphosphate 3-phosphatase and as such a negative regulator of the PIK3/Akt signaling pathway, acts by this way as a TSG. The PTEN gene located on 10q23.3 is frequently inactivated by chromosomal loss and mutations in a number of malignant tumors including BCa (Aveyard et al., 1999; Cairns et al., 1998; Knowles et al., 2009; Platt et al., 2009; Teng et al., 1997). The rate of LOH events and allelic imbalances in a chromosomal region including the PTEN gene is with 23-32% in muscle-invasive BCa notably higher than in non-muscle invasive BCa (Aveyard et al., 1999; Cappellen et al., 1997; Knowles et al., 2009). Nevertheless, mutations in the retained PTEN allele or homozygous deletions do not occur very frequently indicating the existence of further mechanisms of PTEN inactivation (Aveyard et al., 1999; Cairns et al., 1998; Platt et al., 2009). A reduction in PTEN protein levels in BCa tissue specimens was observed in several studies and correlated with higher grade and/or higher stage (Harris et al., 2008; Platt et al., 2009; Puzio-Kuter et al., 2009; L. Schultz et al., 2010; Sun et al., 2011; Tsuruta et al., 2006). Interestingly, a reduced PTEN expression was related to poor outcome in BCa patients, particularly in those displaying alterations of p53 and PTEN (Puzio-Kuter et al., 2009).

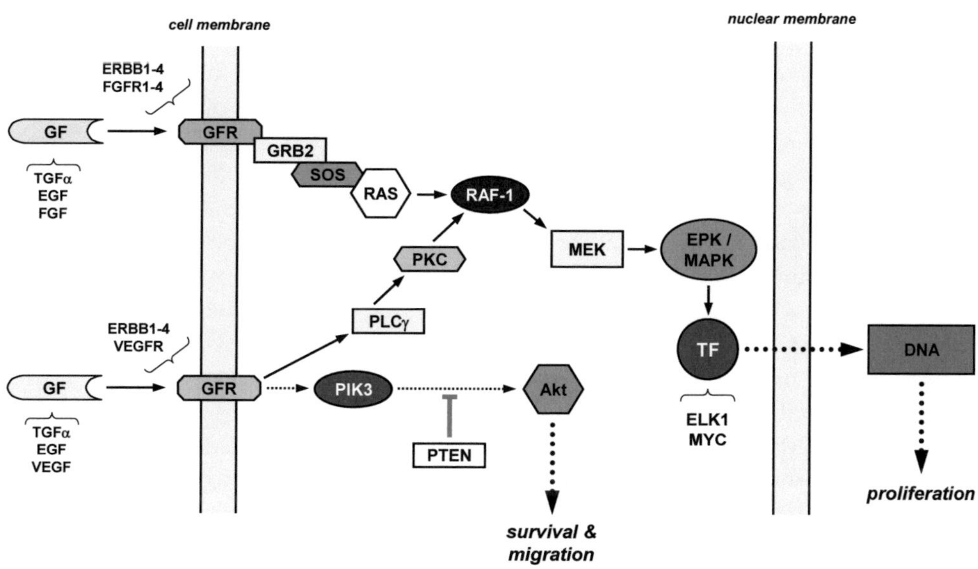

Fig. 4. Simplified illustration of the principles of growth factor signaling
Growth factors bind to their corresponding receptors at the cell surface thereby starting signaling cascades which transduce the signal through cytoplasmatic factors into the nucleus. There, genes supporting survival, proliferation and migration of the tumor cells are induced as final consequence. For BCa, the RAS/RAF/MEK/ERK- and the PIK3/AKT-pathways are of particular importance.
Abbreviations: Akt - *v-akt murine thymoma viral oncogene homolog 1*, DNA - deoxyribonucleic acid, EGF - *epidermal growth factor*, ELK - *member of ETS oncogene family*, ERBB - EGF receptor family member, ERK = MAPK1 - *mitogen-activated protein kinase 1*, FGF - *fibroblast growth factor*, FGFR - FGF receptor family member, GF - growth factor, GFR - growth factor receptor, GRB2 - *growth factor receptor-bound protein 2*, MEK - *mitogen-activated protein kinase kinase*, MYC - *v-myc myelocytomatosis viral oncogene homolog*, PIK3 - *phosphoinositide-3-kinase*, PKC - *protein kinase C*, PLCγ - *phospholipase C gamma*,
PTEN - *phosphatase and tensin homolog*, RAF-1 - *v-raf-1 murine leukemia viral oncogene homolog 1*, RAS - *rat sarcoma viral oncogene homolog*, SOS - *son of sevenless homolog*,
TF - transcription factor, VEGF - *vascular endothelial growth factor*, VEGFR - VEGF receptor family member.

The activation of the PIK3 pathway leads to transmission of extracellular growth signals via the phosphorylation of the serine-threonine protein kinase Akt (*v-akt murine thymoma viral oncogene homolog 1*) to the activation of several downstream signaling routes resulting in an increased proliferation, survival or migration of tumor cells (Wu et al., 2004). Elevated levels of phosphorylated Akt (pAkt) compared to normal bladder tissue were observed in different immunohistochemical studies on BCa tissue specimens (L. Schultz et al., 2010; Wu et al., 2004). Increased detection rates of pAkt correlated significantly with high-grade and advanced stage BCa as well as with a poor clinical outcome and survival (Sun et al., 2011). Furthermore, Askham *et al.* reported the detection of a transforming Akt mutation (G49A / E17K) in 2.7% of 184 analyzed BCa samples (Askham et al., 2010).

7. Tumor angiogenesis and metastasis

Angiogenesis comprises the recruitment and accelerated formation of new blood vessels from the surrounding vasculature. After proteolytic degradation of the adjacent ECM activated endothelial cells become able to migrate and invade as well as to maturate to coalescent, water-tight blood tubules (S.G. Williams & Stein, 2004). This essential physiologic process that occurs during development, reproduction and repair is tightly controlled by stimulatory and inhibitory regulators. During tumor genesis and progression this balance is disturbed by the up-regulation of angiogenic inducers and/or loss of anti-angiogenic factors which can be secreted by the tumor cells themselves, by neighboring tumor-associated stromal cells or by tumor-infiltrating inflammatory cells (S.G. Williams & Stein, 2004). Newly formed blood vessels provide the tumor cells with oxygen and nutrients, which is an essential prerequisite for rapid tumor growth and also for tumor cell spread during metastasis (Mitra & Cote, 2009). A high microvessel density (MVD) in the tumor as reflector of angiogenic processes is a strong predictor of a poor outcome of BCa patients (Bochner et al., 1995; Canoglu et al., 2004; Chaudhary et al., 1999; Dickinson et al., 1994; Hawke et al., 1998; Jaeger et al., 1995; Philp et al., 1996).

Hypoxia, which is frequently occurring in growing tumors, results in elevated levels of the hypoxia-inducible transcription factors HIF-1 and HIF-2. Stability of the HIF-1 subunit α is regulated by the cellular oxygen concentration via the inhibition of its oxygen-dependent degradation. HIF-1α (HIF1A) can induce transcription of VEGF which in turn stimulates tumor vascularization (Mitra & Cote, 2009). In BCa specimens, a significant positive correlation between HIF-1α, VEGF and MVD was observed (Chai et al., 2008; Theodoropoulos et al., 2004). Similar to MVD and VEGF, HIF-1α can serve as indicator of a high recurrence rate and short survival of patients with non-muscle invasive and muscle-invasive BCa (Chai et al., 2008; Palit et al., 2005; Theodoropoulos et al., 2004). Focused on non-muscle invasive BCa, HIF-1α overexpression combined with aberrant nuclear p53 accumulation seemed to indicate an aggressive phenotype with a high risk of progression (Theodoropoulos et al., 2005).

High mRNA expression of VEGF in non-muscle invasive BCa correlated with high recurrence and progression rates, particularly in combination with aberrant p53 staining (Crew et al., 1997). Elevated VEGF protein levels in urine samples from patients with non-muscle invasive BCa showed a significant association with tumor recurrence (Crew et al., 1999b).

Elevated VEGF serum levels were observed in BCa patients with high tumor grade and stage, with vascular invasion, *CIS* tumors or distant metastases and correlated with a shorter disease-free survival (Bernardini et al., 2001). Furthermore, VEGF expression and MVD in biopsy specimens taken prior to therapy were significant predictors of recurrence of muscle-invasive BCa after neoadjuvant chemotherapy and radical cystectomy (Inoue et al., 2000). Increased VEGF levels in tissue samples from patients with locally advanced BCa treated by radical cystectomy and chemotherapy (MVAC) were strongly related to poor disease-specific survival (Slaton et al., 2004).

Thrombospondin-1 (TSP-1) is an ECM component glycoprotein that functions as potent inhibitor of angiogenesis. Expression analyses of this putative tumor suppressor in tissue specimens from patients with muscle-invasive BCa who underwent radical cystectomy revealed a significant association between low TSP-1 levels and increased recurrence rates as well as with a decreased overall survival (Grossfeld et al., 1997). In non-muscle invasive BCa a reduced perivascular TSP-1 staining served as independent predictor of progression to muscle-invasive or metastatic disease (Goddard et al., 2002). Furthermore, expression of *angiopoietin 2* (ANG-2), an angiogenic modulator that potentiates angiogenesis in presence of VEGF, was identified as a strong and independent predictor of tumor recurrence of non-muscle invasive BCa (Szarvas et al., 2008).

The scaffolding ECM serves to maintain endothelial cell function and its degradation is mediated amongst others by MMPs. Additionally, MMPs activate the basic and acidic FGF (FGF1 and FGF2) as well as the *scatter factor* (SF; identical to HGF = *hepatocyte growth factor*) – all regulators which promote migration and invasion of endothelial cells as well as of tumor cells thereby supporting angiogenesis and metastasis (Mitra & Cote, 2009). These factors are also stimulated by plasmin that is proteolytically generated by the *urokinase-type plasminogen activator* (uPA = PLAU = *plasminogen activator, urokinase*). uPA, which can be induced by VEGF, as well as its receptor uPAR (PLAUR= *plasminogen activator, urokinase receptor*) are also involved in ECM degradation, adhesion and migration of tumor cells (Mitra & Cote, 2009).

Determination of the FGF1 and FGF2 levels in urine samples of patients with BCa revealed their prognostic value as indicators of increased disease stage and high rates of local recurrence (Chopin et al., 1993; Gazzaniga et al., 1999; Gravas et al., 2004; Nguyen et al., 1993). SF/HGF levels in urine and serum samples were elevated in BCa patients and related particularly to higher tumor stages as well as to metastasis and worse survival (Gohji et al., 2000; Joseph et al., 1995; Rosen et al., 1997; Wang et al., 2007). The receptor of SF/HFG, the *met proto-oncogene* (MET), was also detected in BCa tissue specimens. Its up-regulation correlated with disease progression and poor long-term survival (Cheng et al., 2002, 2005; Joseph et al., 1995; Miyata et al., 2009).

A significant association between the expression of uPA and uPAR was observed in BCa tissues; both factors were higher in muscle-invasive than in non-muscle invasive BCa and correlated with a worse outcome (Champelovier et al., 2002; Hasui et al., 1994; Seddighzadeh et al., 2002). Elevated levels of uPA and uPAR were also detected in urine and plasma samples from BCa patients compared to controls without BCa (Casella et al., 2002; Shariat et al., 2003). Furthermore, increased preoperative uPA plasma levels in BCa patients were shown to be indicators of a poor outcome after radical cystectomy (Shariat et al., 2003).

Metastasis is initiated by the ability of the tumor to degrade the ECM and to invade the basement membrane followed by the invasion of tumor cells into blood and lymphatic vessels, the path for tumor cell to spread into regional lymph nodes and secondary organs (Gontero et al., 2004; Mitra & Cote, 2009). Several key mediators are involved in metastatic spread such as cadherins which are located at adherens junctions and desmosomes between neighboring cells. Particularly, E-cadherin plays an important role in epithelial cell-cell contacts which is mediated by homodimerization and anchoring to the actin cytoskeleton via binding to catenins (Bryan et al., 2005b). In BCa patients, a reduced expression of E-cadherin was associated with an increased aggressiveness and a higher risk of tumor recurrence and progression as well as with a shorter survival (Bringuier et al., 1993; Byrne et al., 2001; Mahnken et al., 2005; Mhawech-Fauceglia et al., 2006; Nakopoulou et al., 2000; Popov et al., 2000). Immunohistochemical analyses of E-cadherin, α- and β-catenin revealed that loss of these factors can indicate a poor survival of BCa patients (Clairotte et al., 2006; Garcia Del Muro et al., 2000; Kashibuchi et al., 2007; Mialhe et al., 1997; Shimazui et al., 1996).

In addition, integrins are involved in the regulation of processes linked to tumor cell invasion and migration consequently leading to metastasis. Integrins are heterodimeric transmembrane glycoproteins on the surface of tumor cells that function as receptors of ECM proteins such as laminin and collagen. Thereby, integrins serve as molecular links between the ECM and the intracellular actin cytoskeleton and are in this way involved in the maintenance of normal tissue architecture (Gontero et al., 2004). Among the numerous members of the integrin family $\alpha6\beta4$ integrin, which closely interacts with collagen VII and laminin thereby restricting cell migration, is one of the best studied integrins in BCa patients (Gontero et al., 2004). Altered expression of $\alpha6\beta4$ integrin was observed in superficial BCa; in muscle-invasive BCa loss of $\alpha6\beta4$ integrin and/or collagen VII or lack of their co-localization was reported (Liebert et al., 1994). BCa patients with weak $\alpha6\beta4$ integrin immunoreactivity showed a better outcome than those with either no or strong expression (Grossman et al., 2000).

MMPs and members of the uPA system are proteases involved not only in invasion processes of endothelial cells, they are also key factors triggering the invasion of tumor cells by degradation of ECM and the basement membrane (Gontero et al., 2004). MMPs are frequently overexpressed and secreted in human tumors (Bryan et al., 2005b; Wallard et al., 2006). Additionally, members of the ADAM (*a disintegrin and metalloproteinase domain*) family have been implicated in cancer progression (Frohlich et al., 2006). An imbalance between MMPs and their natural counterparts, the *tissue inhibitors of metalloproteases* (TIMPs), which is frequently observed in tumors, is also assumed to support tumor cell invasion and metastasis (Gontero et al., 2004). TIMPs might be paradoxically up-regulated in response to the elevation of MMPs levels (Gontero et al., 2004).

For BCa, MMP-2 and MMP-9 are of particular prognostic importance since increase in their tissue levels correlated with higher tumor grade and/or stage (Davies et al., 1993; Kanayama et al., 1998; Papathoma et al., 2000). Overexpression of MMP-2 and MMP-9 in BCa tissues was associated with disease progression and poor survival (Durkan et al., 2003; Vasala et al., 2003). The ratio of the MMP-9 to E-cadherin levels in BCa tissue specimens was also useful for prediction of the disease-specific survival of patients with locally advanced BCa (Slaton et al., 2004).

Additionally, poor outcome was reported for BCa patients with high levels of TIMP-2 in tumor and/or stromal cells and for patients with increased tissue expression of MMP-2 and TIMP-2 or MMP-9 and TIMP-2 (Gakiopoulou et al., 2003; Grignon et al., 1996; Hara et al., 2001; Kanayama et al., 1998).

Higher recurrence rates and poor prognosis were observed in BCa patients with high serum levels of MMP-2, MMP-3 or with high ratios of the serum levels of MMP-2 to TIMP-2 (Gohji et al., 1996a, 1996b, 1998). MMP-1, MMP-2, MMP-9 and TIMP-1 were also detectable in urine samples from BCa patients and correlated with increasing grade and/or stage (Durkan et al., 2003; Durkan et al., 2001; Gerhards et al., 2001; Nutt et al., 1998, 2003; Sier et al., 2000). Urinary MMP-1 was associated with higher rates of disease progression and death from cancer (Durkan et al., 2001).

ADAM12, a disintegrin and metalloproteinase, that was shown to be up-regulated in BCa tissues in association with disease stage, could also be detected in urine samples, where it might serve as biomarker reflecting presence of BCa (Frohlich et al., 2006).

8. Conclusion

On the basis of specific genetic and molecular patterns two clearly distinguishable types of BCa can be defined, which differ in their phenotype and clinical behavior. They mainly diverge in the genetic stability and in the presence of alterations in the genes p53 and FGFR3. The knowledge of BCa-related genetic and molecular processes provides the basis for the development of new diagnostic and therapeutic approaches. Molecular-diagnostic assays can be designed for BCa subtypes, e.g. for low grade and low stage tumors, which are poorly detectable by the currently used techniques. Furthermore, new BCa subtype-selective therapeutics will provide more specific and effective treatment options leading to the reduction of tumor recurrence and progression. After successful implementation, both aspects will improve clinical outcome of BCa patients and save costs for diagnosis and therapy for this tumor type, which are huge compared to other tumor entities.

9. References

Aboulkassim, T.O.; LaRue, H.; Lemieux, P.; Rousseau, F. & Fradet, Y. (2003). Alteration of the PATCHED locus in superficial bladder cancer. *Oncogene*, Vol.22, No.19, pp. 2967-2971

Adam, R.M.; Danciu, T.; McLellan, D.L.; Borer, J.G.; Lin, J.; Zurakowski, D.; Weinstein, M.H.; Rajjayabun, P.H.; Mellon, J.K. & Freeman, M.R. (2003). A nuclear form of the heparin-binding epidermal growth factor-like growth factor precursor is a feature of aggressive transitional cell carcinoma. *Cancer Res*, Vol.63, No.2, pp. 484-490

Alvarez, A. & Lokeshwar, V.B. (2007). Bladder cancer biomarkers: current developments and future implementation. *Curr Opin Urol*, Vol.17, No.5, pp. 341-346

Amsellem-Ouazana, D.; Bieche, I.; Tozlu, S.; Botto, H.; Debre, B. & Lidereau, R. (2006). Gene expression profiling of ERBB receptors and ligands in human transitional cell carcinoma of the bladder. *J Urol*, Vol.175, No.3 Pt 1, pp. 1127-1132

Askham, J.M.; Platt, F.; Chambers, P.A.; Snowden, H.; Taylor, C.F. & Knowles, M.A. (2010). AKT1 mutations in bladder cancer: identification of a novel oncogenic mutation that can co-operate with E17K. *Oncogene*, Vol.29, No.1, pp. 150-155

Aveyard, J.S.; Skilleter, A.; Habuchi, T. & Knowles, M.A. (1999). Somatic mutation of PTEN in bladder carcinoma. *Br J Cancer*, Vol.80, No.5-6, pp. 904-908

Babjuk, M.; Oosterlinck, W.; Sylvester, R.; Kaasinen, E.; Bohle, A.; Palou-Redorta, J. & Roupret, M. (2011). EAU guidelines on non-muscle-invasive urothelial carcinoma of the bladder, the 2011 update. *Eur Urol*, Vol.59, No.6, pp. 997-1008

Bakkar, A.A.; Wallerand, H.; Radvanyi, F.; Lahaye, J.B.; Pissard, S.; Lecerf, L.; Kouyoumdjian, J.C.; Abbou, C.C.; Pairon, J.C.; Jaurand, M.C.; Thiery, J.P.; Chopin, D.K. & de Medina, S.G. (2003). FGFR3 and TP53 gene mutations define two distinct pathways in urothelial cell carcinoma of the bladder. *Cancer Res*, Vol.63, No.23, pp. 8108-8112

Bellmunt, J.; Paz-Ares, L.; Cuello, M.; Cecere, F.L.; Albiol, S.; Guillem, V.; Gallardo, E.; Carles, J.; Mendez, P.; de la Cruz, J.J.; Taron, M.; Rosell, R. & Baselga, J. (2007). Gene expression of ERCC1 as a novel prognostic marker in advanced bladder cancer patients receiving cisplatin-based chemotherapy. *Ann Oncol*, Vol.18, No.3, pp. 522-528

Berggren, P.; Kumar, R.; Sakano, S.; Hemminki, L.; Wada, T.; Steineck, G.; Adolfsson, J.; Larsson, P.; Norming, U.; Wijkstrom, H. & Hemminki, K. (2003). Detecting homozygous deletions in the CDKN2A(p16(INK4a))/ARF(p14(ARF)) gene in urinary bladder cancer using real-time quantitative PCR. *Clin Cancer Res*, Vol.9, No.1, pp. 235-242

Bernardini, S.; Fauconnet, S.; Chabannes, E.; Henry, P.C.; Adessi, G. & Bittard, H. (2001). Serum levels of vascular endothelial growth factor as a prognostic factor in bladder cancer. *J Urol*, Vol.166, No.4, pp. 1275-1279

Billerey, C.; Chopin, D.; Aubriot-Lorton, M.H.; Ricol, D.; Gil Diez de Medina, S.; Van Rhijn, B.; Bralet, M.P.; Lefrere-Belda, M.A.; Lahaye, J.B.; Abbou, C.C.; Bonaventure, J.; Zafrani, E.S.; van der Kwast, T.; Thiery, J.P. & Radvanyi, F. (2001). Frequent FGFR3 mutations in papillary non-invasive bladder (pTa) tumors. *Am J Pathol*, Vol.158, No.6, pp. 1955-1959

Black, P.C. & Dinney, C.P. (2008). Growth factors and receptors as prognostic markers in urothelial carcinoma. *Curr Urol Rep*, Vol.9, No.1, pp. 55-61

Blackburn, E.H. (2005). Telomeres and telomerase: their mechanisms of action and the effects of altering their functions. *FEBS Lett*, Vol.579, No.4, pp. 859-862

Blasco, M.A. (2002). Telomerase beyond telomeres. *Nat Rev Cancer*, Vol.2, No.8, pp. 627-633

Blaveri, E.; Brewer, J.L.; Roydasgupta, R.; Fridlyand, J.; DeVries, S.; Koppie, T.; Pejavar, S.; Mehta, K.; Carroll, P.; Simko, J.P. & Waldman, F.M. (2005). Bladder cancer stage and outcome by array-based comparative genomic hybridization. *Clin Cancer Res*, Vol.11, No.19 Pt 1, pp. 7012-7022

Bochner, B.H.; Cote, R.J.; Weidner, N.; Groshen, S.; Chen, S.C.; Skinner, D.G. & Nichols, P.W. (1995). Angiogenesis in bladder cancer: relationship between microvessel density and tumor prognosis. *J Natl Cancer Inst*, Vol.87, No.21, pp. 1603-1612

Bosetti, C.; Boffetta, P. & La Vecchia, C. (2007). Occupational exposures to polycyclic aromatic hydrocarbons, and respiratory and urinary tract cancers: a quantitative review to 2005. *Ann Oncol*, Vol.18, No.3, pp. 431-446

Brems-Eskildsen, A.S.; Zieger, K.; Toldbod, H.; Holcomb, C.; Higuchi, R.; Mansilla, F.; Munksgaard, P.P.; Borre, M.; Orntoft, T.F. & Dyrskjot, L. (2010). Prediction and diagnosis of bladder cancer recurrence based on urinary content of hTERT, SENP1, PPP1CA, and MCM5 transcripts. *BMC Cancer*, Vol.10, pp. 646

Bringuier, P.P.; Umbas, R.; Schaafsma, H.E.; Karthaus, H.F.; Debruyne, F.M. & Schalken, J.A. (1993). Decreased E-cadherin immunoreactivity correlates with poor survival in patients with bladder tumors. *Cancer Res*, Vol.53, No.14, pp. 3241-3245

Brunner, A.; Verdorfer, I.; Prelog, M.; Mayerl, C.; Mikuz, G. & Tzankov, A. (2008). Large-scale analysis of cell cycle regulators in urothelial bladder cancer identifies p16 and p27 as potentially useful prognostic markers. *Pathobiology*, Vol.75, No.1, pp. 25-33

Bryan, R.T.; Hussain, S.A.; James, N.D.; Jankowski, J.A. & Wallace, D.M. (2005a). Molecular pathways in bladder cancer: part 1. *BJU Int*, Vol.95, No.4, pp. 485-490

Bryan, R.T.; Hussain, S.A.; James, N.D.; Jankowski, J.A. & Wallace, D.M. (2005b). Molecular pathways in bladder cancer: part 2. *BJU Int*, Vol.95, No.4, pp. 491-496

Byrne, R.R.; Shariat, S.F.; Brown, R.; Kattan, M.W.; Morton, R.J.; Wheeler, T.M. & Lerner, S.P. (2001). E-cadherin immunostaining of bladder transitional cell carcinoma, carcinoma in situ and lymph node metastases with long-term followup. *J Urol*, Vol.165, No.5, pp. 1473-1479

Cairns, P.; Proctor, A.J. & Knowles, M.A. (1991). Loss of heterozygosity at the RB locus is frequent and correlates with muscle invasion in bladder carcinoma. *Oncogene*, Vol.6, No.12, pp. 2305-2309

Cairns, P.; Polascik, T.J.; Eby, Y.; Tokino, K.; Califano, J.; Merlo, A.; Mao, L.; Herath, J.; Jenkins, R.; Westra, W. & et al. (1995). Frequency of homozygous deletion at p16/CDKN2 in primary human tumours. *Nat Genet*, Vol.11, No.2, pp. 210-212

Cairns, P.; Evron, E.; Okami, K.; Halachmi, N.; Esteller, M.; Herman, J.G.; Bose, S.; Wang, S.I.; Parsons, R. & Sidransky, D. (1998). Point mutation and homozygous deletion of PTEN/MMAC1 in primary bladder cancers. *Oncogene*, Vol.16, No.24, pp. 3215-3218

Canoglu, A.; Gogus, C.; Beduk, Y.; Orhan, D.; Tulunay, O. & Baltaci, S. (2004). Microvessel density as a prognostic marker in bladder carcinoma: correlation with tumor grade, stage and prognosis. *Int Urol Nephrol*, Vol.36, No.3, pp. 401-405

Cappellen, D.; Gil Diez de Medina, S.; Chopin, D.; Thiery, J.P. & Radvanyi, F. (1997). Frequent loss of heterozygosity on chromosome 10q in muscle-invasive transitional cell carcinomas of the bladder. *Oncogene*, Vol.14, No.25, pp. 3059-3066

Casella, R.; Shariat, S.F.; Monoski, M.A. & Lerner, S.P. (2002). Urinary levels of urokinase-type plasminogen activator and its receptor in the detection of bladder carcinoma. *Cancer*, Vol.95, No.12, pp. 2494-2499

Castillo-Martin, M.; Domingo-Domenech, J.; Karni-Schmidt, O.; Matos, T. & Cordon-Cardo, C. (2010). Molecular pathways of urothelial development and bladder tumorigenesis. *Urol Oncol*, Vol.28, No.4, pp. 401-408

Chai, C.Y.; Chen, W.T.; Hung, W.C.; Kang, W.Y.; Huang, Y.C.; Su, Y.C. & Yang, C.H. (2008). Hypoxia-inducible factor-1alpha expression correlates with focal macrophage infiltration, angiogenesis and unfavourable prognosis in urothelial carcinoma. *J Clin Pathol*, Vol.61, No.5, pp. 658-664

Champelovier, P.; Boucard, N.; Levacher, G.; Simon, A.; Seigneurin, D. & Praloran, V. (2002). Plasminogen- and colony-stimulating factor-1-associated markers in bladder carcinoma: diagnostic value of urokinase plasminogen activator receptor and plasminogen activator inhibitor type-2 using immunocytochemical analysis. *Urol Res*, Vol.30, No.5, pp. 301-309

Chan, M.W.; Chan, L.W.; Tang, N.L.; Tong, J.H.; Lo, K.W.; Lee, T.L.; Cheung, H.Y.; Wong, W.S.; Chan, P.S.; Lai, F.M. & To, K.F. (2002). Hypermethylation of multiple genes in tumor tissues and voided urine in urinary bladder cancer patients. *Clin Cancer Res*, Vol.8, No.2, pp. 464-470

Chan, S.W. & Blackburn, E.H. (2002). New ways not to make ends meet: telomerase, DNA damage proteins and heterochromatin. *Oncogene*, Vol.21, No.4, pp. 553-563

Chang, L.L.; Yeh, W.T.; Yang, S.Y.; Wu, W.J. & Huang, C.H. (2003). Genetic alterations of p16INK4a and p14ARF genes in human bladder cancer. *J Urol*, Vol.170, No.2 Pt 1, pp. 595-600

Chapman, E.J.; Harnden, P.; Chambers, P.; Johnston, C. & Knowles, M.A. (2005). Comprehensive analysis of CDKN2A status in microdissected urothelial cell carcinoma reveals potential haploinsufficiency, a high frequency of homozygous co-deletion and associations with clinical phenotype. *Clin Cancer Res*, Vol.11, No.16, pp. 5740-5747

Chaudhary, R.; Bromley, M.; Clarke, N.W.; Betts, C.D.; Barnard, R.J.; Ryder, W.D. & Kumar, S. (1999). Prognostic relevance of micro-vessel density in cancer of the urinary bladder. *Anticancer Res*, Vol.19, No.4C, pp. 3479-3484

Chellappan, S.P.; Hiebert, S.; Mudryj, M.; Horowitz, J.M. & Nevins, J.R. (1991). The E2F transcription factor is a cellular target for the RB protein. *Cell*, Vol.65, No.6, pp. 1053-1061

Cheng, H.L.; Trink, B.; Tzai, T.S.; Liu, H.S.; Chan, S.H.; Ho, C.L.; Sidransky, D. & Chow, N.H. (2002). Overexpression of c-met as a prognostic indicator for transitional cell carcinoma of the urinary bladder: a comparison with p53 nuclear accumulation. *J Clin Oncol*, Vol.20, No.6, pp. 1544-1550

Cheng, H.L.; Liu, H.S.; Lin, Y.J.; Chen, H.H.; Hsu, P.Y.; Chang, T.Y.; Ho, C.L.; Tzai, T.S. & Chow, N.H. (2005). Co-expression of RON and MET is a prognostic indicator for patients with transitional-cell carcinoma of the bladder. *Br J Cancer*, Vol.92, No.10, pp. 1906-1914

Chopin, D.K.; Caruelle, J.P.; Colombel, M.; Palcy, S.; Ravery, V.; Caruelle, D.; Abbou, C.C. & Barritault, D. (1993). Increased immunodetection of acidic fibroblast growth factor in bladder cancer, detectable in urine. *J Urol*, Vol.150, No.4, pp. 1126-1130

Chow, N.H.; Liu, H.S.; Lee, E.I.; Chang, C.J.; Chan, S.H.; Cheng, H.L.; Tzai, T.S. & Lin, J.S. (1997a). Significance of urinary epidermal growth factor and its receptor expression in human bladder cancer. *Anticancer Res*, Vol.17, No.2B, pp. 1293-1296

Chow, N.H.; Liu, H.S.; Yang, H.B.; Chan, S.H. & Su, I.J. (1997b). Expression patterns of erbB receptor family in normal urothelium and transitional cell carcinoma. An immunohistochemical study. *Virchows Arch*, Vol.430, No.6, pp. 461-466

Chow, N.H.; Chan, S.H.; Tzai, T.S.; Ho, C.L. & Liu, H.S. (2001). Expression profiles of ErbB family receptors and prognosis in primary transitional cell carcinoma of the urinary bladder. *Clin Cancer Res*, Vol.7, No.7, pp. 1957-1962

Clairotte, A.; Lascombe, I.; Fauconnet, S.; Mauny, F.; Felix, S.; Algros, M.P.; Bittard, H. & Kantelip, B. (2006). Expression of E-cadherin and alpha-, beta-, gamma-catenins in patients with bladder cancer: identification of gamma-catenin as a new prognostic marker of neoplastic progression in T1 superficial urothelial tumors. *Am J Clin Pathol*, Vol.125, No.1, pp. 119-126

Coats, S.; Flanagan, W.M.; Nourse, J. & Roberts, J.M. (1996). Requirement of p27Kip1 for restriction point control of the fibroblast cell cycle. *Science*, Vol.272, No.5263, pp. 877-880

Cooke, P.W.; James, N.D.; Ganesan, R.; Burton, A.; Young, L.S. & Wallace, D.M. (2000). Bcl-2 expression identifies patients with advanced bladder cancer treated by radiotherapy who benefit from neoadjuvant chemotherapy. *BJU Int*, Vol.85, No.7, pp. 829-835

Cordon-Cardo, C.; Wartinger, D.; Petrylak, D.; Dalbagni, G.; Fair, W.R.; Fuks, Z. & Reuter, V.E. (1992). Altered expression of the retinoblastoma gene product: prognostic indicator in bladder cancer. *J Natl Cancer Inst*, Vol.84, No.16, pp. 1251-1256

Cordon-Cardo, C.; Dalbagni, G.; Saez, G.T.; Oliva, M.R.; Zhang, Z.F.; Rosai, J.; Reuter, V.E. & Pellicer, A. (1994). p53 mutations in human bladder cancer: genotypic versus phenotypic patterns. *Int J Cancer*, Vol.56, No.3, pp. 347-353

Cordon-Cardo, C.; Zhang, Z.F.; Dalbagni, G.; Drobnjak, M.; Charytonowicz, E.; Hu, S.X.; Xu, H.J.; Reuter, V.E. & Benedict, W.F. (1997). Cooperative effects of p53 and pRB alterations in primary superficial bladder tumors. *Cancer Res*, Vol.57, No.7, pp. 1217-1221

Cote, R.J.; Esrig, D.; Groshen, S.; Jones, P.A. & Skinner, D.G. (1997). p53 and treatment of bladder cancer. *Nature*, Vol.385, No.6612, pp. 123-125

Cote, R.J.; Dunn, M.D.; Chatterjee, S.J.; Stein, J.P.; Shi, S.R.; Tran, Q.C.; Hu, S.X.; Xu, H.J.; Groshen, S.; Taylor, C.R.; Skinner, D.G. & Benedict, W.F. (1998). Elevated and absent pRb expression is associated with bladder cancer progression and has cooperative effects with p53. *Cancer Res*, Vol.58, No.6, pp. 1090-1094

Crew, J.P.; O'Brien, T.; Bradburn, M.; Fuggle, S.; Bicknell, R.; Cranston, D. & Harris, A.L. (1997). Vascular endothelial growth factor is a predictor of relapse and stage progression in superficial bladder cancer. *Cancer Res*, Vol.57, No.23, pp. 5281-5285

Crew, J.P. (1999a). Vascular endothelial growth factor: an important angiogenic mediator in bladder cancer. *Eur Urol*, Vol.35, No.1, pp. 2-8

Crew, J.P.; O'Brien, T.; Bicknell, R.; Fuggle, S.; Cranston, D. & Harris, A.L. (1999b). Urinary vascular endothelial growth factor and its correlation with bladder cancer recurrence rates. *J Urol*, Vol.161, No.3, pp. 799-804

Dalbagni, G.; Presti, J.C., Jr.; Reuter, V.E.; Zhang, Z.F.; Sarkis, A.S.; Fair, W.R. & Cordon-Cardo, C. (1993). Molecular genetic alterations of chromosome 17 and p53 nuclear overexpression in human bladder cancer. *Diagn Mol Pathol*, Vol.2, No.1, pp. 4-13

Davies, B.; Waxman, J.; Wasan, H.; Abel, P.; Williams, G.; Krausz, T.; Neal, D.; Thomas, D.; Hanby, A. & Balkwill, F. (1993). Levels of matrix metalloproteases in bladder cancer correlate with tumor grade and invasion. *Cancer Res*, Vol.53, No.22, pp. 5365-5369

de Kok, J.B.; Schalken, J.A.; Aalders, T.W.; Ruers, T.J.; Willems, H.L. & Swinkels, D.W. (2000a). Quantitative measurement of telomerase reverse transcriptase (hTERT) mRNA in urothelial cell carcinomas. *Int J Cancer*, Vol.87, No.2, pp. 217-220

de Kok, J.B.; van Balken, M.R.; Roelofs, R.W.; van Aarssen, Y.A.; Swinkels, D.W. & Klein Gunnewiek, J.M. (2000b). Quantification of hTERT mRNA and telomerase activity in bladder washings of patients with recurrent urothelial cell carcinomas. *Clin Chem*, Vol.46, No.12, pp. 2003-2007

DeGregori, J.; Kowalik, T. & Nevins, J.R. (1995). Cellular targets for activation by the E2F1 transcription factor include DNA synthesis- and G1/S-regulatory genes. *Mol Cell Biol*, Vol.15, No.8, pp. 4215-4224

Dickinson, A.J.; Fox, S.B.; Persad, R.A.; Hollyer, J.; Sibley, G.N. & Harris, A.L. (1994). Quantification of angiogenesis as an independent predictor of prognosis in invasive bladder carcinomas. *Br J Urol*, Vol.74, No.6, pp. 762-766

Doganay, L.; Altaner, S.; Bilgi, S.; Kaya, E.; Ekuklu, G. & Kutlu, K. (2003). Expression of the cyclin-dependent kinase inhibitor p27 in transitional cell bladder cancers: is it a good predictor for tumor behavior? *Int Urol Nephrol*, Vol.35, No.2, pp. 181-188

Dominguez, G.; Silva, J.; Garcia, J.M.; Silva, J.M.; Rodriguez, R.; Munoz, C.; Chacon, I.; Sanchez, R.; Carballido, J.; Colas, A.; Espana, P. & Bonilla, F. (2003). Prevalence of aberrant methylation of p14ARF over p16INK4a in some human primary tumors. *Mutat Res*, Vol.530, No.1-2, pp. 9-17

Dong, L.M.; Potter, J.D.; White, E.; Ulrich, C.M.; Cardon, L.R. & Peters, U. (2008). Genetic susceptibility to cancer: the role of polymorphisms in candidate genes. *Jama*, Vol.299, No.20, pp. 2423-2436

Dubrez-Daloz, L.; Dupoux, A. & Cartier, J. (2008). IAPs: more than just inhibitors of apoptosis proteins. *Cell Cycle*, Vol.7, No.8, pp. 1036-1046

Ducrest, A.L.; Szutorisz, H.; Lingner, J. & Nabholz, M. (2002). Regulation of the human telomerase reverse transcriptase gene. *Oncogene*, Vol.21, No.4, pp. 541-552

Duggan, B.J.; Kelly, J.D.; Keane, P.F. & Johnston, S.R. (2001). Molecular targets for the therapeutic manipulation of apoptosis in bladder cancer. *J Urol*, Vol.165, No.3, pp. 946-954

Durkan, G.C.; Nutt, J.E.; Rajjayabun, P.H.; Neal, D.E.; Lunec, J. & Mellon, J.K. (2001). Prognostic significance of matrix metalloproteinase-1 and tissue inhibitor of metalloproteinase-1 in voided urine samples from patients with transitional cell carcinoma of the bladder. *Clin Cancer Res*, Vol.7, No.11, pp. 3450-3456

Durkan, G.C.; Nutt, J.E.; Marsh, C.; Rajjayabun, P.H.; Robinson, M.C.; Neal, D.E.; Lunec, J. & Mellon, J.K. (2003). Alteration in urinary matrix metalloproteinase-9 to tissue inhibitor of metalloproteinase-1 ratio predicts recurrence in nonmuscle-invasive bladder cancer. *Clin Cancer Res*, Vol.9, No.7, pp. 2576-2582

el-Deiry, W.S.; Tokino, T.; Velculescu, V.E.; Levy, D.B.; Parsons, R.; Trent, J.M.; Lin, D.; Mercer, W.E.; Kinzler, K.W. & Vogelstein, B. (1993). WAF1, a potential mediator of p53 tumor suppression. *Cell*, Vol.75, No.4, pp. 817-825

Emiliozzi, P.; Pansadoro, A. & Pansadoro, V. (2008). The optimal management of T1G3 bladder cancer. *BJU Int*, Vol.102, No.9 Pt B, pp. 1265-1273

Esrig, D.; Spruck, C.H., 3rd; Nichols, P.W.; Chaiwun, B.; Steven, K.; Groshen, S.; Chen, S.C.; Skinner, D.G.; Jones, P.A. & Cote, R.J. (1993). p53 nuclear protein accumulation correlates with mutations in the p53 gene, tumor grade, and stage in bladder cancer. *Am J Pathol*, Vol.143, No.5, pp. 1389-1397

Feber, A.; Clark, J.; Goodwin, G.; Dodson, A.R.; Smith, P.H.; Fletcher, A.; Edwards, S.; Flohr, P.; Falconer, A.; Roe, T.; Kovacs, G.; Dennis, N.; Fisher, C.; Wooster, R.; Huddart, R.; Foster, C.S. & Cooper, C.S. (2004). Amplification and overexpression of E2F3 in human bladder cancer. *Oncogene*, Vol.23, No.8, pp. 1627-1630

Ferlay, J.; Autier, P.; Boniol, M.; Heanue, M.; Colombet, M. & Boyle, P. (2007). Estimates of the cancer incidence and mortality in Europe in 2006. *Ann Oncol*, Vol.18, No.3, pp. 581-592

Forster, J.A.; Paul, A.B.; Harnden, P. & Knowles, M.A. (2011). Expression of NRG1 and its receptors in human bladder cancer. *Br J Cancer*, Vol.104, No.7, pp. 1135-1143

Franekova, M.; Halasova, E.; Bukovska, E.; Luptak, J. & Dobrota, D. (2008). Gene polymorphisms in bladder cancer. *Urol Oncol*, Vol.26, No.1, pp. 1-8

Franke, K.H.; Miklosi, M.; Goebell, P.; Clasen, S.; Steinhoff, C.; Anastasiadis, A.G.; Gerharz, C. & Schulz, W.A. (2000). Cyclin-dependent kinase inhibitor P27(KIP1) is expressed preferentially in early stages of urothelial carcinoma. *Urology*, Vol.56, No.4, pp. 689-695

Frohlich, C.; Albrechtsen, R.; Dyrskjot, L.; Rudkjaer, L.; Orntoft, T.F. & Wewer, U.M. (2006). Molecular profiling of ADAM12 in human bladder cancer. *Clin Cancer Res*, Vol.12, No.24, pp. 7359-7368

Fujimoto, K.; Yamada, Y.; Okajima, E.; Kakizoe, T.; Sasaki, H.; Sugimura, T. & Terada, M. (1992). Frequent association of p53 gene mutation in invasive bladder cancer. *Cancer Res*, Vol.52, No.6, pp. 1393-1398

Fung, Y.K.; Murphree, A.L.; T'Ang, A.; Qian, J.; Hinrichs, S.H. & Benedict, W.F. (1987). Structural evidence for the authenticity of the human retinoblastoma gene. *Science*, Vol.236, No.4809, pp. 1657-1661

Gakiopoulou, H.; Nakopoulou, L.; Siatelis, A.; Mavrommatis, I.; Panayotopoulou, E.G.; Tsirmpa, I.; Stravodimos, C. & Giannopoulos, A. (2003). Tissue inhibitor of metalloproteinase-2 as a multifunctional molecule of which the expression is associated with adverse prognosis of patients with urothelial bladder carcinomas. *Clin Cancer Res*, Vol.9, No.15, pp. 5573-5581

Garcia-Closas, M.; Malats, N.; Real, F.X.; Welch, R.; Kogevinas, M.; Chatterjee, N.; Pfeiffer, R.; Silverman, D.; Dosemeci, M.; Tardon, A.; Serra, C.; Carrato, A.; Garcia-Closas, R.; Castano-Vinyals, G.; Chanock, S.; Yeager, M. & Rothman, N. (2006). Genetic variation in the nucleotide excision repair pathway and bladder cancer risk. *Cancer Epidemiol Biomarkers Prev*, Vol.15, No.3, pp. 536-542

Garcia del Muro, X.; Torregrosa, A.; Munoz, J.; Castellsague, X.; Condom, E.; Vigues, F.; Arance, A.; Fabra, A. & Germa, J.R. (2000). Prognostic value of the expression of E-cadherin and beta-catenin in bladder cancer. *Eur J Cancer*, Vol.36, No.3, pp. 357-362

Gazzaniga, P.; Gradilone, A.; Vercillo, R.; Gandini, O.; Silvestri, I.; Napolitano, M.; Albonici, L.; Vincenzoni, A.; Gallucci, M.; Frati, L. & Agliano, A.M. (1996). Bcl-2/bax mRNA expression ratio as prognostic factor in low-grade urinary bladder cancer. *Int J Cancer*, Vol.69, No.2, pp. 100-104

Gazzaniga, P.; Gradilone, A.; Silvestri, I.; Gandini, O.; Napolitano, M.; Vercillo, R.; Vincenzoni, A.; Gallucci, M.; Frati, L. & Agliano, A.M. (1998). High levels of transforming growth factor-alpha (TGF-alpha) mRNA may predict local relapses in early stage urinary bladder cancer. *Eur J Cancer*, Vol.34, No.6, pp. 934-936

Gazzaniga, P.; Gandini, O.; Gradilone, A.; Silvestri, I.; Giuliani, L.; Magnanti, M.; Gallucci, M.; Saccani, G.; Frati, L. & Agliano, A.M. (1999). Detection of basic fibroblast growth factor mRNA in urinary bladder cancer: correlation with local relapses. *Int J Oncol*, Vol.14, No.6, pp. 1123-1127

Gazzaniga, P.; Gradilone, A.; Giuliani, L.; Gandini, O.; Silvestri, I.; Nofroni, I.; Saccani, G.; Frati, L. & Agliano, A.M. (2003). Expression and prognostic significance of LIVIN, SURVIVIN and other apoptosis-related genes in the progression of superficial bladder cancer. *Ann Oncol*, Vol.14, No.1, pp. 85-90

George, B.; Datar, R.H.; Wu, L.; Cai, J.; Patten, N.; Beil, S.J.; Groshen, S.; Stein, J.; Skinner, D.; Jones, P.A. & Cote, R.J. (2007). p53 gene and protein status: the role of p53 alterations in predicting outcome in patients with bladder cancer. *J Clin Oncol*, Vol.25, No.34, pp. 5352-5358

Gerhards, S.; Jung, K.; Koenig, F.; Daniltchenko, D.; Hauptmann, S.; Schnorr, D. & Loening, S.A. (2001). Excretion of matrix metalloproteinases 2 and 9 in urine is associated with a high stage and grade of bladder carcinoma. *Urology*, Vol.57, No.4, pp. 675-679

Glas, A.S.; Roos, D.; Deutekom, M.; Zwinderman, A.H.; Bossuyt, P.M. & Kurth, K.H. (2003). Tumor markers in the diagnosis of primary bladder cancer. A systematic review. *J Urol*, Vol.169, No.6, pp. 1975-1982

Goddard, J.C.; Sutton, C.D.; Jones, J.L.; O'Byrne, K.J. & Kockelbergh, R.C. (2002). Reduced thrombospondin-1 at presentation predicts disease progression in superficial bladder cancer. *Eur Urol*, Vol.42, No.5, pp. 464-468

Gohji, K.; Fujimoto, N.; Fujii, A.; Komiyama, T.; Okawa, J. & Nakajima, M. (1996a). Prognostic significance of circulating matrix metalloproteinase-2 to tissue inhibitor of metalloproteinases-2 ratio in recurrence of urothelial cancer after complete resection. *Cancer Res*, Vol.56, No.14, pp. 3196-3198

Gohji, K.; Fujimoto, N.; Komiyama, T.; Fujii, A.; Ohkawa, J.; Kamidono, S. & Nakajima, M. (1996b). Elevation of serum levels of matrix metalloproteinase-2 and -3 as new predictors of recurrence in patients with urothelial carcinoma. *Cancer*, Vol.78, No.11, pp. 2379-2387

Gohji, K.; Fujimoto, N.; Ohkawa, J.; Fujii, A. & Nakajima, M. (1998). Imbalance between serum matrix metalloproteinase-2 and its inhibitor as a predictor of recurrence of urothelial cancer. *Br J Cancer*, Vol.77, No.4, pp. 650-655

Gohji, K.; Nomi, M.; Niitani, Y.; Kitazawa, S.; Fujii, A.; Katsuoka, Y. & Nakajima, M. (2000). Independent prognostic value of serum hepatocyte growth factor in bladder cancer. *J Clin Oncol*, Vol.18, No.16, pp. 2963-2971

Golka, K.; Wiese, A.; Assennato, G. & Bolt, H.M. (2004). Occupational exposure and urological cancer. *World J Urol*, Vol.21, No.6, pp. 382-391

Gontero, P.; Banisadr, S.; Frea, B. & Brausi, M. (2004). Metastasis markers in bladder cancer: a review of the literature and clinical considerations. *Eur Urol*, Vol.46, No.3, pp. 296-311

Gonzalez-Campora, R.; Davalos-Casanova, G.; Beato-Moreno, A.; Garcia-Escudero, A.; Pareja Megia, M.J.; Montironi, R. & Lopez-Beltran, A. (2007). BCL-2, TP53 and BAX protein expression in superficial urothelial bladder carcinoma. *Cancer Lett*, Vol.250, No.2, pp. 292-299

Gonzalez-Zulueta, M.; Bender, C.M.; Yang, A.S.; Nguyen, T.; Beart, R.W.; Van Tornout, J.M. & Jones, P.A. (1995). Methylation of the 5' CpG island of the p16/CDKN2 tumor suppressor gene in normal and transformed human tissues correlates with gene silencing. *Cancer Res*, Vol.55, No.20, pp. 4531-4535

Gonzalez, S.; Aubert, S.; Kerdraon, O.; Haddad, O.; Fantoni, J.C.; Biserte, J. & Leroy, X. (2008). Prognostic value of combined p53 and survivin in pT1G3 urothelial carcinoma of the bladder. *Am J Clin Pathol*, Vol.129, No.2, pp. 232-237

Gravas, S.; Bosinakou, I.; Kehayas, P. & Giannopoulos, A. (2004). Urinary basic fibroblast growth factor in bladder cancer patients. Histopathological correlation and clinical potential. *Urol Int*, Vol.73, No.2, pp. 173-177

Grignon, D.J.; Sakr, W.; Toth, M.; Ravery, V.; Angulo, J.; Shamsa, F.; Pontes, J.E.; Crissman, J.C. & Fridman, R. (1996). High levels of tissue inhibitor of metalloproteinase-2 (TIMP-2) expression are associated with poor outcome in invasive bladder cancer. *Cancer Res*, Vol.56, No.7, pp. 1654-1659

Grossfeld, G.D.; Ginsberg, D.A.; Stein, J.P.; Bochner, B.H.; Esrig, D.; Groshen, S.; Dunn, M.; Nichols, P.W.; Taylor, C.R.; Skinner, D.G. & Cote, R.J. (1997). Thrombospondin-1 expression in bladder cancer: association with p53 alterations, tumor angiogenesis, and tumor progression. *J Natl Cancer Inst*, Vol.89, No.3, pp. 219-227

Grossman, H.B.; Liebert, M.; Antelo, M.; Dinney, C.P.; Hu, S.X.; Palmer, J.L. & Benedict, W.F. (1998). p53 and RB expression predict progression in T1 bladder cancer. *Clin Cancer Res*, Vol.4, No.4, pp. 829-834

Grossman, H.B.; Lee, C.; Bromberg, J. & Liebert, M. (2000). Expression of the alpha6beta4 integrin provides prognostic information in bladder cancer. *Oncol Rep*, Vol.7, No.1, pp. 13-16

Hanahan, D. & Weinberg, R.A. (2000). The hallmarks of cancer. *Cell*, Vol.100, No.1, pp. 57-70

Hara, I.; Miyake, H.; Hara, S.; Arakawa, S. & Kamidono, S. (2001). Significance of matrix metalloproteinases and tissue inhibitors of metalloproteinase expression in the recurrence of superficial transitional cell carcinoma of the bladder. *J Urol*, Vol.165, No.5, pp. 1769-1772

Harley, C.B. (1991). Telomere loss: mitotic clock or genetic time bomb? *Mutat Res*, Vol.256, No.2-6, pp. 271-282

Harris, L.D.; De La Cerda, J.; Tuziak, T.; Rosen, D.; Xiao, L.; Shen, Y.; Sabichi, A.L.; Czerniak, B. & Grossman, H.B. (2008). Analysis of the expression of biomarkers in urinary bladder cancer using a tissue microarray. *Mol Carcinog*, Vol.47, No.9, pp. 678-685

Hasui, Y.; Marutsuka, K.; Nishi, S.; Kitada, S.; Osada, Y. & Sumiyoshi, A. (1994). The content of urokinase-type plasminogen activator and tumor recurrence in superficial bladder cancer. *J Urol*, Vol.151, No.1, pp. 16-19;

Hausladen, D.A.; Wheeler, M.A.; Altieri, D.C.; Colberg, J.W. & Weiss, R.M. (2003). Effect of intravesical treatment of transitional cell carcinoma with bacillus Calmette-Guerin and mitomycin C on urinary survivin levels and outcome. *J Urol*, Vol.170, No.1, pp. 230-234

Hawke, C.K.; Delahunt, B. & Davidson, P.J. (1998). Microvessel density as a prognostic marker for transitional cell carcinoma of the bladder. *Br J Urol*, Vol.81, No.4, pp. 585-590

Heidenblad, M.; Lindgren, D.; Jonson, T.; Liedberg, F.; Veerla, S.; Chebil, G.; Gudjonsson, S.; Borg, A.; Mansson, W. & Hoglund, M. (2008). Tiling resolution array CGH and high density expression profiling of urothelial carcinomas delineate genomic amplicons and candidate target genes specific for advanced tumors. *BMC Med Genomics*, Vol.1, pp. 3

Heine, B.; Hummel, M.; Muller, M.; Heicappell, R.; Miller, K. & Stein, H. (1998). Non-radioactive measurement of telomerase activity in human bladder cancer, bladder washings, and in urine. *J Pathol*, Vol.184, No.1, pp. 71-76

Hernandez, S.; Lopez-Knowles, E.; Lloreta, J.; Kogevinas, M.; Jaramillo, R.; Amoros, A.; Tardon, A.; Garcia-Closas, R.; Serra, C.; Carrato, A.; Malats, N. & Real, F.X. (2005). FGFR3 and Tp53 mutations in T1G3 transitional bladder carcinomas: independent distribution and lack of association with prognosis. *Clin Cancer Res*, Vol.11, No.15, pp. 5444-5450

Hernandez, S.; Lopez-Knowles, E.; Lloreta, J.; Kogevinas, M.; Amoros, A.; Tardon, A.; Carrato, A.; Serra, C.; Malats, N. & Real, F.X. (2006). Prospective study of FGFR3 mutations as a prognostic factor in nonmuscle invasive urothelial bladder carcinomas. *J Clin Oncol*, Vol.24, No.22, pp. 3664-3671

Hernando, E.; Nahle, Z.; Juan, G.; Diaz-Rodriguez, E.; Alaminos, M.; Hemann, M.; Michel, L.; Mittal, V.; Gerald, W.; Benezra, R.; Lowe, S.W. & Cordon-Cardo, C. (2004). Rb inactivation promotes genomic instability by uncoupling cell cycle progression from mitotic control. *Nature*, Vol.430, No.7001, pp. 797-802

Herr, H.W. (2000). Tumor progression and survival of patients with high grade, noninvasive papillary (TaG3) bladder tumors: 15-year outcome. *J Urol*, Vol.163, No.1, pp. 60-61;

Hiebert, S.W.; Chellappan, S.P.; Horowitz, J.M. & Nevins, J.R. (1992). The interaction of RB with E2F coincides with an inhibition of the transcriptional activity of E2F. *Genes Dev*, Vol.6, No.2, pp. 177-185

Hitchings, A.W.; Kumar, M.; Jordan, S.; Nargund, V.; Martin, J. & Berney, D.M. (2004). Prediction of progression in pTa and pT1 bladder carcinomas with p53, p16 and pRb. *Br J Cancer*, Vol.91, No.3, pp. 552-557

Hiyama, E. & Hiyama, K. (2002). Clinical utility of telomerase in cancer. *Oncogene*, Vol.21, No.4, pp. 643-649

Horikawa, Y.; Gu, J. & Wu, X. (2008a). Genetic susceptibility to bladder cancer with an emphasis on gene-gene and gene-environmental interactions. *Curr Opin Urol*, Vol.18, No.5, pp. 493-498

Horikawa, Y.; Nadaoka, J.; Saito, M.; Kumazawa, T.; Inoue, T.; Yuasa, T.; Tsuchiya, N.; Nishiyama, H.; Ogawa, O. & Habuchi, T. (2008b). Clinical implications of the MDM2 SNP309 and p53 Arg72Pro polymorphisms in transitional cell carcinoma of the bladder. *Oncol Rep*, Vol.20, No.1, pp. 49-55

Hurst, C.D.; Tomlinson, D.C.; Williams, S.V.; Platt, F.M. & Knowles, M.A. (2008). Inactivation of the Rb pathway and overexpression of both isoforms of E2F3 are obligate events in bladder tumours with 6p22 amplification. *Oncogene*, Vol.27, No.19, pp. 2716-2727

Hussain, S.A.; Ganesan, R.; Hiller, L.; Cooke, P.W.; Murray, P.; Young, L.S. & James, N.D. (2003). BCL2 expression predicts survival in patients receiving synchronous chemoradiotherapy in advanced transitional cell carcinoma of the bladder. *Oncol Rep*, Vol.10, No.3, pp. 571-576

Inoue, K.; Slaton, J.W.; Karashima, T.; Yoshikawa, C.; Shuin, T.; Sweeney, P.; Millikan, R. & Dinney, C.P. (2000). The prognostic value of angiogenesis factor expression for predicting recurrence and metastasis of bladder cancer after neoadjuvant chemotherapy and radical cystectomy. *Clin Cancer Res*, Vol.6, No.12, pp. 4866-4873

Ishikawa, J.; Xu, H.J.; Hu, S.X.; Yandell, D.W.; Maeda, S.; Kamidono, S.; Benedict, W.F. & Takahashi, R. (1991). Inactivation of the retinoblastoma gene in human bladder and renal cell carcinomas. *Cancer Res*, Vol.51, No.20, pp. 5736-5743

Ito, H.; Kyo, S.; Kanaya, T.; Takakura, M.; Inoue, M. & Namiki, M. (1998). Expression of human telomerase subunits and correlation with telomerase activity in urothelial cancer. *Clin Cancer Res*, Vol.4, No.7, pp. 1603-1608

Jaeger, T.M.; Weidner, N.; Chew, K.; Moore, D.H.; Kerschmann, R.L.; Waldman, F.M. & Carroll, P.R. (1995). Tumor angiogenesis correlates with lymph node metastases in invasive bladder cancer. *J Urol*, Vol.154, No.1, pp. 69-71

Jebar, A.H.; Hurst, C.D.; Tomlinson, D.C.; Johnston, C.; Taylor, C.F. & Knowles, M.A. (2005). FGFR3 and Ras gene mutations are mutually exclusive genetic events in urothelial cell carcinoma. *Oncogene*, Vol.24, No.33, pp. 5218-5225

Jemal, A.; Siegel, R.; Xu, J. & Ward, E. (2010). Cancer statistics, 2010. *CA Cancer J Clin*, Vol.60, No.5, pp. 277-300

Jonsson, G.; Paulie, S. & Grandien, A. (2003). cIAP-2 block apoptotic events in bladder cancer cells. *Anticancer Res*, Vol.23, No.4, pp. 3311-3316

Joseph, A.; Weiss, G.H.; Jin, L.; Fuchs, A.; Chowdhury, S.; O'Shaugnessy, P.; Goldberg, I.D. & Rosen, E.M. (1995). Expression of scatter factor in human bladder carcinoma. *J Natl Cancer Inst*, Vol.87, No.5, pp. 372-377

Junker, K.; van Oers, J.M.; Zwarthoff, E.C.; Kania, I.; Schubert, J. & Hartmann, A. (2008). Fibroblast growth factor receptor 3 mutations in bladder tumors correlate with low frequency of chromosome alterations. *Neoplasia*, Vol.10, No.1, pp. 1-7

Junttila, T.T.; Laato, M.; Vahlberg, T.; Soderstrom, K.O.; Visakorpi, T.; Isola, J. & Elenius, K. (2003). Identification of patients with transitional cell carcinoma of the bladder overexpressing ErbB2, ErbB3, or specific ErbB4 isoforms: real-time reverse transcription-PCR analysis in estimation of ErbB receptor status from cancer patients. *Clin Cancer Res*, Vol.9, No.14, pp. 5346-5357

Kamai, T.; Takagi, K.; Asami, H.; Ito, Y.; Oshima, H. & Yoshida, K.I. (2001). Decreasing of p27(Kip1)and cyclin E protein levels is associated with progression from superficial into invasive bladder cancer. *Br J Cancer*, Vol.84, No.9, pp. 1242-1251

Kanayama, H.; Yokota, K.; Kurokawa, Y.; Murakami, Y.; Nishitani, M. & Kagawa, S. (1998). Prognostic values of matrix metalloproteinase-2 and tissue inhibitor of metalloproteinase-2 expression in bladder cancer. *Cancer*, Vol.82, No.7, pp. 1359-1366

Karam, J.A.; Lotan, Y.; Ashfaq, R.; Sagalowsky, A.I. & Shariat, S.F. (2007a). Survivin expression in patients with non-muscle-invasive urothelial cell carcinoma of the bladder. *Urology*, Vol.70, No.3, pp. 482-486

Karam, J.A.; Lotan, Y.; Karakiewicz, P.I.; Ashfaq, R.; Sagalowsky, A.I.; Roehrborn, C.G. & Shariat, S.F. (2007b). Use of combined apoptosis biomarkers for prediction of bladder cancer recurrence and mortality after radical cystectomy. *Lancet Oncol*, Vol.8, No.2, pp. 128-136

Kashibuchi, K.; Tomita, K.; Schalken, J.A.; Kume, H.; Takeuchi, T. & Kitamura, T. (2007). The prognostic value of E-cadherin, alpha-, beta- and gamma-catenin in bladder cancer patients who underwent radical cystectomy. *Int J Urol*, Vol.14, No.9, pp. 789-794

Kassouf, W.; Black, P.C.; Tuziak, T.; Bondaruk, J.; Lee, S.; Brown, G.A.; Adam, L.; Wei, C.; Baggerly, K.; Bar-Eli, M.; McConkey, D.; Czerniak, B. & Dinney, C.P. (2008). Distinctive expression pattern of ErbB family receptors signifies an aggressive variant of bladder cancer. *J Urol*, Vol.179, No.1, pp. 353-358

Kawamoto, K.; Enokida, H.; Gotanda, T.; Kubo, H.; Nishiyama, K.; Kawahara, M. & Nakagawa, M. (2006). p16INK4a and p14ARF methylation as a potential biomarker for human bladder cancer. *Biochem Biophys Res Commun*, Vol.339, No.3, pp. 790-796

Kellen, E.; Hemelt, M.; Broberg, K.; Golka, K.; Kristensen, V.N.; Hung, R.J.; Matullo, G.; Mittal, R.D.; Porru, S.; Povey, A.; Schulz, W.A.; Shen, J.; Buntinx, F.; Zeegers, M.P. & Taioli, E. (2007). Pooled analysis and meta-analysis of the glutathione S-transferase P1 Ile 105Val polymorphism and bladder cancer: a HuGE-GSEC review. *Am J Epidemiol*, Vol.165, No.11, pp. 1221-1230

Kelsh, M.A.; Alexander, D.D.; Kalmes, R.M. & Buffler, P.A. (2008). Personal use of hair dyes and risk of bladder cancer: a meta-analysis of epidemiologic data. *Cancer Causes Control*, Vol.19, No.6, pp. 549-558

Kiemeney, L.A.; Thorlacius, S.; Sulem, P.; Geller, F.; Aben, K.K.; Stacey, S.N.; Gudmundsson, J.; Jakobsdottir, M.; Bergthorsson, J.T.; Sigurdsson, A.; Blondal, T.; Witjes, J.A.; Vermeulen, S.H.; Hulsbergen-van de Kaa, C.A.; Swinkels, D.W.; Ploeg, M.; Cornel, E.B.; Vergunst, H.; Thorgeirsson, T.E.; Gudbjartsson, D.; Gudjonsson, S.A.;

Thorleifsson, G.; Kristinsson, K.T.; Mouy, M.; Snorradottir, S.; Placidi, D.; Campagna, M.; Arici, C.; Koppova, K.; Gurzau, E.; Rudnai, P.; Kellen, E.; Polidoro, S.; Guarrera, S.; Sacerdote, C.; Sanchez, M.; Saez, B.; Valdivia, G.; Ryk, C.; de Verdier, P.; Lindblom, A.; Golka, K.; Bishop, D.T.; Knowles, M.A.; Nikulasson, S.; Petursdottir, V.; Jonsson, E.; Geirsson, G.; Kristjansson, B.; Mayordomo, J.I.; Steineck, G.; Porru, S.; Buntinx, F.; Zeegers, M.P.; Fletcher, T.; Kumar, R.; Matullo, G.; Vineis, P.; Kiltie, A.E.; Gulcher, J.R.; Thorsteinsdottir, U.; Kong, A.; Rafnar, T. & Stefansson, K. (2008). Sequence variant on 8q24 confers susceptibility to urinary bladder cancer. *Nat Genet*, Vol.40, No.11, pp. 1307-1312

Kiemeney, L.A.; Sulem, P.; Besenbacher, S.; Vermeulen, S.H.; Sigurdsson, A.; Thorleifsson, G.; Gudbjartsson, D.F.; Stacey, S.N.; Gudmundsson, J.; Zanon, C.; Kostic, J.; Masson, G.; Bjarnason, H.; Palsson, S.T.; Skarphedinsson, O.B.; Gudjonsson, S.A.; Witjes, J.A.; Grotenhuis, A.J.; Verhaegh, G.W.; Bishop, D.T.; Sak, S.C.; Choudhury, A.; Elliott, F.; Barrett, J.H.; Hurst, C.D.; de Verdier, P.J.; Ryk, C.; Rudnai, P.; Gurzau, E.; Koppova, K.; Vineis, P.; Polidoro, S.; Guarrera, S.; Sacerdote, C.; Campagna, M.; Placidi, D.; Arici, C.; Zeegers, M.P.; Kellen, E.; Gutierrez, B.S.; Sanz-Velez, J.I.; Sanchez-Zalabardo, M.; Valdivia, G.; Garcia-Prats, M.D.; Hengstler, J.G.; Blaszkewicz, M.; Dietrich, H.; Ophoff, R.A.; van den Berg, L.H.; Alexiusdottir, K.; Kristjansson, K.; Geirsson, G.; Nikulasson, S.; Petursdottir, V.; Kong, A.; Thorgeirsson, T.; Mungan, N.A.; Lindblom, A.; van Es, M.A.; Porru, S.; Buntinx, F.; Golka, K.; Mayordomo, J.I.; Kumar, R.; Matullo, G.; Steineck, G.; Kiltie, A.E.; Aben, K.K.; Jonsson, E.; Thorsteinsdottir, U.; Knowles, M.A.; Rafnar, T. & Stefansson, K. (2010). A sequence variant at 4p16.3 confers susceptibility to urinary bladder cancer. *Nat Genet*, Vol.42, No.5, pp. 415-419

Kim, N.W.; Piatyszek, M.A.; Prowse, K.R.; Harley, C.B.; West, M.D.; Ho, P.L.; Coviello, G.M.; Wright, W.E.; Weinrich, S.L. & Shay, J.W. (1994). Specific association of human telomerase activity with immortal cells and cancer. *Science*, Vol.266, No.5193, pp. 2011-2015

Kim, W.J. & Quan, C. (2005). Genetic and epigenetic aspects of bladder cancer. *J Cell Biochem*, Vol.95, No.1, pp. 24-33

Kitamura, H. & Tsukamoto, T. (2006). Early bladder cancer: concept, diagnosis, and management. *Int J Clin Oncol*, Vol.11, No.1, pp. 28-37

Knowles, M.A.; Habuchi, T.; Kennedy, W. & Cuthbert-Heavens, D. (2003). Mutation spectrum of the 9q34 tuberous sclerosis gene TSC1 in transitional cell carcinoma of the bladder. *Cancer Res*, Vol.63, No.22, pp. 7652-7656

Knowles, M.A. (2008). Molecular pathogenesis of bladder cancer. *Int J Clin Oncol*, Vol.13, No.4, pp. 287-297

Knowles, M.A.; Platt, F.M.; Ross, R.L. & Hurst, C.D. (2009). Phosphatidylinositol 3-kinase (PI3K) pathway activation in bladder cancer. *Cancer Metastasis Rev*, Vol.28, No.3-4, pp. 305-316

Kompier, L.C.; Lurkin, I.; van der Aa, M.N.; van Rhijn, B.W.; van der Kwast, T.H. & Zwarthoff, E.C. (2010a). FGFR3, HRAS, KRAS, NRAS and PIK3CA mutations in bladder cancer and their potential as biomarkers for surveillance and therapy. *PLoS One*, Vol.5, No.11, pp. e13821

Kompier, L.C.; van Tilborg, A.A. & Zwarthoff, E.C. (2010b). Bladder cancer: novel molecular characteristics, diagnostic, and therapeutic implications. *Urol Oncol*, Vol.28, No.1, pp. 91-96

Korkolopoulou, P.; Christodoulou, P.; Konstantinidou, A.E.; Thomas-Tsagli, E.; Kapralos, P. & Davaris, P. (2000). Cell cycle regulators in bladder cancer: a multivariate survival study with emphasis on p27Kip1. *Hum Pathol*, Vol.31, No.6, pp. 751-760

Korkolopoulou, P.; Christodoulou, P.; Lazaris, A.; Thomas-Tsagli, E.; Kapralos, P.; Papanikolaou, A.; Kalliteraki, I. & Davaris, P. (2001). Prognostic implications of aberrations in p16/pRb pathway in urothelial bladder carcinomas: a multivariate analysis including p53 expression and proliferation markers. *Eur Urol*, Vol.39, No.2, pp. 167-177

Korkolopoulou, P.; Lazaris, A.; Konstantinidou, A.E.; Kavantzas, N.; Patsouris, E.; Christodoulou, P.; Thomas-Tsagli, E. & Davaris, P. (2002). Differential expression of bcl-2 family proteins in bladder carcinomas. Relationship with apoptotic rate and survival. *Eur Urol*, Vol.41, No.3, pp. 274-283

Kramer, C.; Klasmeyer, K.; Bojar, H.; Schulz, W.A.; Ackermann, R. & Grimm, M.O. (2007). Heparin-binding epidermal growth factor-like growth factor isoforms and epidermal growth factor receptor/ErbB1 expression in bladder cancer and their relation to clinical outcome. *Cancer*, Vol.109, No.10, pp. 2016-2024

Kruger, S.; Mahnken, A.; Kausch, I. & Feller, A.C. (2005). P16 immunoreactivity is an independent predictor of tumor progression in minimally invasive urothelial bladder carcinoma. *Eur Urol*, Vol.47, No.4, pp. 463-467

Ku, J.H.; Kwak, C.; Lee, H.S.; Park, H.K.; Lee, E. & Lee, S.E. (2004). Expression of survivin, a novel inhibitor of apoptosis, in superficial transitional cell carcinoma of the bladder. *J Urol*, Vol.171, No.2 Pt 1, pp. 631-635

Kuczyk, M.A.; Bokemeyer, C.; Serth, J.; Hervatin, C.; Oelke, M.; Hofner, K.; Tan, H.K. & Jonas, U. (1995). p53 overexpression as a prognostic factor for advanced stage bladder cancer. *Eur J Cancer*, Vol.31A, No.13-14, pp. 2243-2247

Kuczyk, M.A.; Machtens, S.; Bokemeyer, C.; Hradil, K.; Macheel, I.; Jetscho, V.; Hartmann, J.; Thon, W.F.; Jonas, U. & Serth, J. (1999). Prognostic value of p27Kip1 and p21WAF/Cip protein expression in muscle invasive bladder cancer. *Oncol Rep*, Vol.6, No.3, pp. 687-693

Kyo, S.; Takakura, M.; Fujiwara, T. & Inoue, M. (2008). Understanding and exploiting hTERT promoter regulation for diagnosis and treatment of human cancers. *Cancer Sci*, Vol.99, No.8, pp. 1528-1538

Le Frere-Belda, M.A.; Cappellen, D.; Daher, A.; Gil-Diez-de-Medina, S.; Besse, F.; Abbou, C.C.; Thiery, J.P.; Zafrani, E.S.; Chopin, D.K. & Radvanyi, F. (2001). p15(INK4b) in bladder carcinomas: decreased expression in superficial tumours. *Br J Cancer*, Vol.85, No.10, pp. 1515-1521

Le Frere-Belda, M.A.; Gil Diez de Medina, S.; Daher, A.; Martin, N.; Albaud, B.; Heudes, D.; Abbou, C.C.; Thiery, J.P.; Zafrani, E.S.; Radvanyi, F. & Chopin, D. (2004). Profiles of the 2 INK4a gene products, p16 and p14ARF, in human reference urothelium and bladder carcinomas, according to pRb and p53 protein status. *Hum Pathol*, Vol.35, No.7, pp. 817-824

Lee, S.H.; Shin, M.S.; Park, W.S.; Kim, S.Y.; Dong, S.M.; Pi, J.H.; Lee, H.K.; Kim, H.S.; Jang, J.J.; Kim, C.S.; Kim, S.H.; Lee, J.Y. & Yoo, N.J. (1999). Alterations of Fas (APO-1/CD95) gene in transitional cell carcinomas of urinary bladder. *Cancer Res*, Vol.59, No.13, pp. 3068-3072

Li, M.; Song, T.; Yin, Z.F. & Na, Y.Q. (2007). XIAP as a prognostic marker of early recurrence of nonmuscular invasive bladder cancer. *Chin Med J (Engl)*, Vol.120, No.6, pp. 469-473

Lianes, P.; Orlow, I.; Zhang, Z.F.; Oliva, M.R.; Sarkis, A.S.; Reuter, V.E. & Cordon-Cardo, C. (1994). Altered patterns of MDM2 and TP53 expression in human bladder cancer. *J Natl Cancer Inst*, Vol.86, No.17, pp. 1325-1330

Liebert, M.; Washington, R.; Wedemeyer, G.; Carey, T.E. & Grossman, H.B. (1994). Loss of co-localization of alpha 6 beta 4 integrin and collagen VII in bladder cancer. *Am J Pathol*, Vol.144, No.4, pp. 787-795

Lin, Y.; Miyamoto, H.; Fujinami, K.; Uemura, H.; Hosaka, M.; Iwasaki, Y. & Kubota, Y. (1996). Telomerase activity in human bladder cancer. *Clin Cancer Res*, Vol.2, No.6, pp. 929-932

Liu, H.B.; Kong, C.Z.; Zeng, Y.; Liu, X.K.; Bi, J.B.; Jiang, Y.J. & Han, S. (2009). Livin may serve as a marker for prognosis of bladder cancer relapse and a target of bladder cancer treatment. *Urol Oncol*, Vol.27, No.3, pp. 277-283

Liukkonen, T.J.; Lipponen, P.K.; Helle, M. & Jauhiainen, K.E. (1997). Immunoreactivity of bcl-2, p53 and EGFr is associated with tumor stage, grade and cell proliferation in superficial bladder cancer. Finnbladder III Group. *Urol Res*, Vol.25, No.1, pp. 1-7

Logothetis, C.J.; Xu, H.J.; Ro, J.Y.; Hu, S.X.; Sahin, A.; Ordonez, N. & Benedict, W.F. (1992). Altered expression of retinoblastoma protein and known prognostic variables in locally advanced bladder cancer. *J Natl Cancer Inst*, Vol.84, No.16, pp. 1256-1261

Lopez-Beltran, A.; Alvarez-Kindelan, J.; Luque, R.J.; Blanca, A.; Quintero, A.; Montironi, R.; Cheng, L.; Gonzalez-Campora, R. & Requena, M.J. (2008). Loss of heterozygosity at 9q32-33 (DBC1 locus) in primary non-invasive papillary urothelial neoplasm of low malignant potential and low-grade urothelial carcinoma of the bladder and their associated normal urothelium. *J Pathol*, Vol.215, No.3, pp. 263-272

Lopez-Knowles, E.; Hernandez, S.; Malats, N.; Kogevinas, M.; Lloreta, J.; Carrato, A.; Tardon, A.; Serra, C. & Real, F.X. (2006). PIK3CA mutations are an early genetic alteration associated with FGFR3 mutations in superficial papillary bladder tumors. *Cancer Res*, Vol.66, No.15, pp. 7401-7404

Lu, M.L.; Wikman, F.; Orntoft, T.F.; Charytonowicz, E.; Rabbani, F.; Zhang, Z.; Dalbagni, G.; Pohar, K.S.; Yu, G. & Cordon-Cardo, C. (2002). Impact of alterations affecting the p53 pathway in bladder cancer on clinical outcome, assessed by conventional and array-based methods. *Clin Cancer Res*, Vol.8, No.1, pp. 171-179

Mahnken, A.; Kausch, I.; Feller, A.C. & Kruger, S. (2005). E-cadherin immunoreactivity correlates with recurrence and progression of minimally invasive transitional cell carcinomas of the urinary bladder. *Oncol Rep*, Vol.14, No.4, pp. 1065-1070

Maluf, F.C.; Cordon-Cardo, C.; Verbel, D.A.; Satagopan, J.M.; Boyle, M.G.; Herr, H. & Bajorin, D.F. (2006). Assessing interactions between mdm-2, p53, and bcl-2 as prognostic variables in muscle-invasive bladder cancer treated with neo-adjuvant chemotherapy followed by locoregional surgical treatment. *Ann Oncol*, Vol.17, No.11, pp. 1677-1686

Margulis, V.; Lotan, Y. & Shariat, S.F. (2008). Survivin: a promising biomarker for detection and prognosis of bladder cancer. *World J Urol*, Vol.26, No.1, pp. 59-65

McKnight, J.J.; Gray, S.B.; O'Kane, H.F.; Johnston, S.R. & Williamson, K.E. (2005). Apoptosis and chemotherapy for bladder cancer. *J Urol*, Vol.173, No.3, pp. 683-690

Memon, A.A.; Sorensen, B.S.; Meldgaard, P.; Fokdal, L.; Thykjaer, T. & Nexo, E. (2006). The relation between survival and expression of HER1 and HER2 depends on the expression of HER3 and HER4: a study in bladder cancer patients. *Br J Cancer*, Vol.94, No.11, pp. 1703-1709

Meyerson, M.; Counter, C.M.; Eaton, E.N.; Ellisen, L.W.; Steiner, P.; Caddle, S.D.; Ziaugra, L.; Beijersbergen, R.L.; Davidoff, M.J.; Liu, Q.; Bacchetti, S.; Haber, D.A. & Weinberg, R.A. (1997). hEST2, the putative human telomerase catalytic subunit gene, is up-regulated in tumor cells and during immortalization. *Cell*, Vol.90, No.4, pp. 785-795

Mhawech-Fauceglia, P.; Cheney, R.T. & Schwaller, J. (2006). Genetic alterations in urothelial bladder carcinoma: an updated review. *Cancer*, Vol.106, No.6, pp. 1205-1216

Mialhe, A.; Louis, J.; Montlevier, S.; Peoch, M.; Pasquier, D.; Bosson, J.L.; Rambeaud, J.J. & Seigneurin, D. (1997). Expression of E-cadherin and alpha-,beta- and gamma-catenins in human bladder carcinomas: are they good prognostic factors? *Invasion Metastasis*, Vol.17, No.3, pp. 124-137

Michaud, D.S. (2007). Chronic inflammation and bladder cancer. *Urol Oncol*, Vol.25, No.3, pp. 260-268

Michieli, P.; Chedid, M.; Lin, D.; Pierce, J.H.; Mercer, W.E. & Givol, D. (1994). Induction of WAF1/CIP1 by a p53-independent pathway. *Cancer Res*, Vol.54, No.13, pp. 3391-3395

Migaldi, M.; Sgambato, A.; Garagnani, L.; Ardito, R.; Ferrari, P.; De Gaetani, C.; Cittadini, A. & Trentini, G.P. (2000). Loss of p21Waf1 expression is a strong predictor of reduced survival in primary superficial bladder cancers. *Clin Cancer Res*, Vol.6, No.8, pp. 3131-3138

Mihara, K.; Cao, X.R.; Yen, A.; Chandler, S.; Driscoll, B.; Murphree, A.L.; T'Ang, A. & Fung, Y.K. (1989). Cell cycle-dependent regulation of phosphorylation of the human retinoblastoma gene product. *Science*, Vol.246, No.4935, pp. 1300-1303

Mitra, A.P.; Datar, R.H. & Cote, R.J. (2006). Molecular pathways in invasive bladder cancer: new insights into mechanisms, progression, and target identification. *J Clin Oncol*, Vol.24, No.35, pp. 5552-5564

Mitra, A.P.; Birkhahn, M. & Cote, R.J. (2007). p53 and retinoblastoma pathways in bladder cancer. *World J Urol*, Vol.25, No.6, pp. 563-571

Mitra, A.P. & Cote, R.J. (2009). Molecular pathogenesis and diagnostics of bladder cancer. *Annu Rev Pathol*, Vol.4, pp. 251-285

Miyamoto, H.; Shuin, T.; Torigoe, S.; Iwasaki, Y. & Kubota, Y. (1995). Retinoblastoma gene mutations in primary human bladder cancer. *Br J Cancer*, Vol.71, No.4, pp. 831-835

Miyata, Y.; Sagara, Y.; Kanda, S.; Hayashi, T. & Kanetake, H. (2009). Phosphorylated hepatocyte growth factor receptor/c-Met is associated with tumor growth and prognosis in patients with bladder cancer: correlation with matrix metalloproteinase-2 and -7 and E-cadherin. *Hum Pathol*, Vol.40, No.4, pp. 496-504

Mizutani, Y.; Hongo, F.; Sato, N.; Ogawa, O.; Yoshida, O. & Miki, T. (2001). Significance of serum soluble Fas ligand in patients with bladder carcinoma. *Cancer*, Vol.92, No.2, pp. 287-293

Muller, M. (2002). Telomerase: its clinical relevance in the diagnosis of bladder cancer. *Oncogene*, Vol.21, No.4, pp. 650-655

Nakopoulou, L.; Zervas, A.; Gakiopoulou-Givalou, H.; Constantinides, C.; Doumanis, G.; Davaris, P. & Dimopoulos, C. (2000). Prognostic value of E-cadherin, beta-catenin,

P120ctn in patients with transitional cell bladder cancer. *Anticancer Res*, Vol.20, No.6B, pp. 4571-4578

Nguyen, M.; Watanabe, H.; Budson, A.E.; Richie, J.P. & Folkman, J. (1993). Elevated levels of the angiogenic peptide basic fibroblast growth factor in urine of bladder cancer patients. *J Natl Cancer Inst*, Vol.85, No.3, pp. 241-242

Niehans, G.A.; Kratzke, R.A.; Froberg, M.K.; Aeppli, D.M.; Nguyen, P.L. & Geradts, J. (1999). G1 checkpoint protein and p53 abnormalities occur in most invasive transitional cell carcinomas of the urinary bladder. *Br J Cancer*, Vol.80, No.8, pp. 1175-1184

Nutt, J.E.; Mellon, J.K.; Qureshi, K. & Lunec, J. (1998). Matrix metalloproteinase-1 is induced by epidermal growth factor in human bladder tumour cell lines and is detectable in urine of patients with bladder tumours. *Br J Cancer*, Vol.78, No.2, pp. 215-220

Nutt, J.E.; Durkan, G.C.; Mellon, J.K. & Lunec, J. (2003). Matrix metalloproteinases (MMPs) in bladder cancer: the induction of MMP9 by epidermal growth factor and its detection in urine. *BJU Int*, Vol.91, No.1, pp. 99-104

Oeggerli, M.; Tomovska, S.; Schraml, P.; Calvano-Forte, D.; Schafroth, S.; Simon, R.; Gasser, T.; Mihatsch, M.J. & Sauter, G. (2004). E2F3 amplification and overexpression is associated with invasive tumor growth and rapid tumor cell proliferation in urinary bladder cancer. *Oncogene*, Vol.23, No.33, pp. 5616-5623

Oeggerli, M.; Schraml, P.; Ruiz, C.; Bloch, M.; Novotny, H.; Mirlacher, M.; Sauter, G. & Simon, R. (2006). E2F3 is the main target gene of the 6p22 amplicon with high specificity for human bladder cancer. *Oncogene*, Vol.25, No.49, pp. 6538-6543

Olsson, A.Y.; Feber, A.; Edwards, S.; Te Poele, R.; Giddings, I.; Merson, S. & Cooper, C.S. (2007). Role of E2F3 expression in modulating cellular proliferation rate in human bladder and prostate cancer cells. *Oncogene*, Vol.26, No.7, pp. 1028-1037

Olumi, A.F.; Tsai, Y.C.; Nichols, P.W.; Skinner, D.G.; Cain, D.R.; Bender, L.I. & Jones, P.A. (1990). Allelic loss of chromosome 17p distinguishes high grade from low grade transitional cell carcinomas of the bladder. *Cancer Res*, Vol.50, No.21, pp. 7081-7083

Ong, F.; Moonen, L.M.; Gallee, M.P.; ten Bosch, C.; Zerp, S.F.; Hart, A.A.; Bartelink, H. & Verheij, M. (2001). Prognostic factors in transitional cell cancer of the bladder: an emerging role for Bcl-2 and p53. *Radiother Oncol*, Vol.61, No.2, pp. 169-175

Orlow, I.; Lacombe, L.; Hannon, G.J.; Serrano, M.; Pellicer, I.; Dalbagni, G.; Reuter, V.E.; Zhang, Z.F.; Beach, D. & Cordon-Cardo, C. (1995). Deletion of the p16 and p15 genes in human bladder tumors. *J Natl Cancer Inst*, Vol.87, No.20, pp. 1524-1529

Orlow, I.; LaRue, H.; Osman, I.; Lacombe, L.; Moore, L.; Rabbani, F.; Meyer, F.; Fradet, Y. & Cordon-Cardo, C. (1999). Deletions of the INK4A gene in superficial bladder tumors. Association with recurrence. *Am J Pathol*, Vol.155, No.1, pp. 105-113

Oxford, G. & Theodorescu, D. (2003). The role of Ras superfamily proteins in bladder cancer progression. *J Urol*, Vol.170, No.5, pp. 1987-1993

Palit, V.; Phillips, R.M.; Puri, R.; Shah, T. & Bibby, M.C. (2005). Expression of HIF-1alpha and Glut-1 in human bladder cancer. *Oncol Rep*, Vol.14, No.4, pp. 909-913

Papathoma, A.S.; Petraki, C.; Grigorakis, A.; Papakonstantinou, H.; Karavana, V.; Stefanakis, S.; Sotsiou, F. & Pintzas, A. (2000). Prognostic significance of matrix metalloproteinases 2 and 9 in bladder cancer. *Anticancer Res*, Vol.20, No.3B, pp. 2009-2013

Parker, S.B.; Eichele, G.; Zhang, P.; Rawls, A.; Sands, A.T.; Bradley, A.; Olson, E.N.; Harper, J.W. & Elledge, S.J. (1995). p53-independent expression of p21Cip1 in muscle and other terminally differentiating cells. *Science*, Vol.267, No.5200, pp. 1024-1027

Pashos, C.L.; Botteman, M.F.; Laskin, B.L. & Redaelli, A. (2002). Bladder cancer: epidemiology, diagnosis, and management. *Cancer Pract*, Vol.10, No.6, pp. 311-322

Pfister, C.; Moore, L.; Allard, P.; Larue, H.; Lacombe, L.; Tetu, B.; Meyer, F. & Fradet, Y. (1999). Predictive value of cell cycle markers p53, MDM2, p21, and Ki-67 in superficial bladder tumor recurrence. *Clin Cancer Res*, Vol.5, No.12, pp. 4079-4084

Pfister, C.; Larue, H.; Moore, L.; Lacombe, L.; Veilleux, C.; Tetu, B.; Meyer, F. & Fradet, Y. (2000). Tumorigenic pathways in low-stage bladder cancer based on p53, MDM2 and p21 phenotypes. *Int J Cancer*, Vol.89, No.1, pp. 100-104

Philp, E.A.; Stephenson, T.J. & Reed, M.W. (1996). Prognostic significance of angiogenesis in transitional cell carcinoma of the human urinary bladder. *Br J Urol*, Vol.77, No.3, pp. 352-357

Platt, F.M.; Hurst, C.D.; Taylor, C.F.; Gregory, W.M.; Harnden, P. & Knowles, M.A. (2009). Spectrum of phosphatidylinositol 3-kinase pathway gene alterations in bladder cancer. *Clin Cancer Res*, Vol.15, No.19, pp. 6008-6017

Ploeg, M.; Aben, K.K. & Kiemeney, L.A. (2009). The present and future burden of urinary bladder cancer in the world. *World J Urol*, Vol.27, No.3, pp. 289-293

Pollack, A.; Wu, C.S.; Czerniak, B.; Zagars, G.K.; Benedict, W.F. & McDonnell, T.J. (1997). Abnormal bcl-2 and pRb expression are independent correlates of radiation response in muscle-invasive bladder cancer. *Clin Cancer Res*, Vol.3, No.10, pp. 1823-1829

Polyak, K.; Lee, M.H.; Erdjument-Bromage, H.; Koff, A.; Roberts, J.M.; Tempst, P. & Massague, J. (1994). Cloning of p27Kip1, a cyclin-dependent kinase inhibitor and a potential mediator of extracellular antimitogenic signals. *Cell*, Vol.78, No.1, pp. 59-66

Popov, Z.; Gil-Diez de Medina, S.; Lefrere-Belda, M.A.; Hoznek, A.; Bastuji-Garin, S.; Abbou, C.C.; Thiery, J.P.; Radvanyi, F. & Chopin, D.K. (2000). Low E-cadherin expression in bladder cancer at the transcriptional and protein level provides prognostic information. *Br J Cancer*, Vol.83, No.2, pp. 209-214

Puzio-Kuter, A.M.; Castillo-Martin, M.; Kinkade, C.W.; Wang, X.; Shen, T.H.; Matos, T.; Shen, M.M.; Cordon-Cardo, C. & Abate-Shen, C. (2009). Inactivation of p53 and Pten promotes invasive bladder cancer. *Genes Dev*, Vol.23, No.6, pp. 675-680

Quelle, D.E.; Zindy, F.; Ashmun, R.A. & Sherr, C.J. (1995). Alternative reading frames of the INK4a tumor suppressor gene encode two unrelated proteins capable of inducing cell cycle arrest. *Cell*, Vol.83, No.6, pp. 993-1000

Rabbani, F. & Cordon-Cardo, C. (2000). Mutation of cell cycle regulators and their impact on superficial bladder cancer. *Urol Clin North Am*, Vol.27, No.1, pp. 83-102,

Rabbani, F.; Koppie, T.M.; Charytonowicz, E.; Drobnjak, M.; Bochner, B.H. & Cordon-Cardo, C. (2007). Prognostic significance of p27Kip1 expression in bladder cancer. *BJU Int*, Vol.100, No.2, pp. 259-263

Ravery, V.; Grignon, D.; Angulo, J.; Pontes, E.; Montie, J.; Crissman, J. & Chopin, D. (1997). Evaluation of epidermal growth factor receptor, transforming growth factor alpha, epidermal growth factor and c-erbB2 in the progression of invasive bladder cancer. *Urol Res*, Vol.25, No.1, pp. 9-17

Richter, J.; Beffa, L.; Wagner, U.; Schraml, P.; Gasser, T.C.; Moch, H.; Mihatsch, M.J. & Sauter, G. (1998). Patterns of chromosomal imbalances in advanced urinary bladder cancer detected by comparative genomic hybridization. *Am J Pathol*, Vol.153, No.5, pp. 1615-1621

Rieger-Christ, K.M.; Mourtzinos, A.; Lee, P.J.; Zagha, R.M.; Cain, J.; Silverman, M.; Libertino, J.A. & Summerhayes, I.C. (2003). Identification of fibroblast growth factor receptor 3 mutations in urine sediment DNA samples complements cytology in bladder tumor detection. *Cancer*, Vol.98, No.4, pp. 737-744

Rosen, E.M.; Joseph, A.; Jin, L.; Yao, Y.; Chau, M.H.; Fuchs, A.; Gomella, L.; Hastings, H.; Goldberg, I.D. & Weiss, G.H. (1997). Urinary and tissue levels of scatter factor in transitional cell carcinoma of bladder. *J Urol*, Vol.157, No.1, pp. 72-78

Rothman, N.; Garcia-Closas, M.; Chatterjee, N.; Malats, N.; Wu, X.; Figueroa, J.D.; Real, F.X.; Van Den Berg, D.; Matullo, G.; Baris, D.; Thun, M.; Kiemeney, L.A.; Vineis, P.; De Vivo, I.; Albanes, D.; Purdue, M.P.; Rafnar, T.; Hildebrandt, M.A.; Kiltie, A.E.; Cussenot, O.; Golka, K.; Kumar, R.; Taylor, J.A.; Mayordomo, J.I.; Jacobs, K.B.; Kogevinas, M.; Hutchinson, A.; Wang, Z.; Fu, Y.P.; Prokunina-Olsson, L.; Burdett, L.; Yeager, M.; Wheeler, W.; Tardon, A.; Serra, C.; Carrato, A.; Garcia-Closas, R.; Lloreta, J.; Johnson, A.; Schwenn, M.; Karagas, M.R.; Schned, A.; Andriole, G., Jr.; Grubb, R., 3rd; Black, A.; Jacobs, E.J.; Diver, W.R.; Gapstur, S.M.; Weinstein, S.J.; Virtamo, J.; Cortessis, V.K.; Gago-Dominguez, M.; Pike, M.C.; Stern, M.C.; Yuan, J.M.; Hunter, D.J.; McGrath, M.; Dinney, C.P.; Czerniak, B.; Chen, M.; Yang, H.; Vermeulen, S.H.; Aben, K.K.; Witjes, J.A.; Makkinje, R.R.; Sulem, P.; Besenbacher, S.; Stefansson, K.; Riboli, E.; Brennan, P.; Panico, S.; Navarro, C.; Allen, N.E.; Bueno-de-Mesquita, H.B.; Trichopoulos, D.; Caporaso, N.; Landi, M.T.; Canzian, F.; Ljungberg, B.; Tjonneland, A.; Clavel-Chapelon, F.; Bishop, D.T.; Teo, M.T.; Knowles, M.A.; Guarrera, S.; Polidoro, S.; Ricceri, F.; Sacerdote, C.; Allione, A.; Cancel-Tassin, G.; Selinski, S.; Hengstler, J.G.; Dietrich, H.; Fletcher, T.; Rudnai, P.; Gurzau, E.; Koppova, K.; Bolick, S.C.; Godfrey, A.; Xu, Z.; Sanz-Velez, J.I.; M, D.G.-P.; Sanchez, M.; Valdivia, G.; Porru, S.; Benhamou, S.; Hoover, R.N.; Fraumeni, J.F., Jr.; Silverman, D.T. & Chanock, S.J. (2010). A multi-stage genome-wide association study of bladder cancer identifies multiple susceptibility loci. *Nat Genet*, Vol.42, No.11, pp. 978-984

Rotterud, R.; Nesland, J.M.; Berner, A. & Fossa, S.D. (2005). Expression of the epidermal growth factor receptor family in normal and malignant urothelium. *BJU Int*, Vol.95, No.9, pp. 1344-1350

Sanchez-Carbayo, M.; Socci, N.D.; Kirchoff, T.; Erill, N.; Offit, K.; Bochner, B.H. & Cordon-Cardo, C. (2007). A polymorphism in HDM2 (SNP309) associates with early onset in superficial tumors, TP53 mutations, and poor outcome in invasive bladder cancer. *Clin Cancer Res*, Vol.13, No.11, pp. 3215-3220

Sanderson, S.; Salanti, G. & Higgins, J. (2007). Joint effects of the N-acetyltransferase 1 and 2 (NAT1 and NAT2) genes and smoking on bladder carcinogenesis: a literature-based systematic HuGE review and evidence synthesis. *Am J Epidemiol*, Vol.166, No.7, pp. 741-751

Sarkar, S.; Julicher, K.P.; Burger, M.S.; Della Valle, V.; Larsen, C.J.; Yeager, T.R.; Grossman, T.B.; Nickells, R.W.; Protzel, C.; Jarrard, D.F. & Reznikoff, C.A. (2000). Different combinations of genetic/epigenetic alterations inactivate the p53 and pRb pathways in invasive human bladder cancers. *Cancer Res*, Vol.60, No.14, pp. 3862-3871

Sarkis, A.S.; Dalbagni, G.; Cordon-Cardo, C.; Zhang, Z.F.; Sheinfeld, J.; Fair, W.R.; Herr, H.W. & Reuter, V.E. (1993). Nuclear overexpression of p53 protein in transitional cell bladder carcinoma: a marker for disease progression. *J Natl Cancer Inst*, Vol.85, No.1, pp. 53-59

Sarkis, A.S.; Bajorin, D.F.; Reuter, V.E.; Herr, H.W.; Netto, G.; Zhang, Z.F.; Schultz, P.K.; Cordon-Cardo, C. & Scher, H.I. (1995). Prognostic value of p53 nuclear overexpression in patients with invasive bladder cancer treated with neoadjuvant MVAC. *J Clin Oncol*, Vol.13, No.6, pp. 1384-1390

Sato, K.; Sasaki, R.; Ogura, Y.; Shimoda, N.; Togashi, H.; Terada, K.; Sugiyama, T.; Kakinuma, H.; Ogawa, O. & Kato, T. (1998). Expression of vascular endothelial growth factor gene and its receptor (flt-1) gene in urinary bladder cancer. *Tohoku J Exp Med*, Vol.185, No.3, pp. 173-184

Schultz, I.J.; Kiemeney, L.A.; Witjes, J.A.; Schalken, J.A.; Willems, J.L.; Swinkels, D.W. & de Kok, J.B. (2003). Survivin mRNA expression is elevated in malignant urothelial cell carcinomas and predicts time to recurrence. *Anticancer Res*, Vol.23, No.4, pp. 3327-3331

Schultz, L.; Albadine, R.; Hicks, J.; Jadallah, S.; DeMarzo, A.M.; Chen, Y.B.; Neilsen, M.E.; Gonzalgo, M.L.; Sidransky, D.; Schoenberg, M. & Netto, G.J. (2010). Expression status and prognostic significance of mammalian target of rapamycin pathway members in urothelial carcinoma of urinary bladder after cystectomy. *Cancer*, Vol.116, No.23, pp. 5517-5526

Seddighzadeh, M.; Steineck, G.; Larsson, P.; Wijkstrom, H.; Norming, U.; Onelov, E. & Linder, S. (2002). Expression of UPA and UPAR is associated with the clinical course of urinary bladder neoplasms. *Int J Cancer*, Vol.99, No.5, pp. 721-726

Serizawa, R.R.; Ralfkiaer, U.; Steven, K.; Lam, G.W.; Schmiedel, S.; Schuz, J.; Hansen, A.B.; Horn, T. & Guldberg, P. (2011). Integrated genetic and epigenetic analysis of bladder cancer reveals an additive diagnostic value of FGFR3 mutations and hypermethylation events. *Int J Cancer*, Vol.129, No.1, pp. 78-87

Serrano, M.; Hannon, G.J. & Beach, D. (1993). A new regulatory motif in cell-cycle control causing specific inhibition of cyclin D/CDK4. *Nature*, Vol.366, No.6456, pp. 704-707

Serth, J.; Kuczyk, M.A.; Bokemeyer, C.; Hervatin, C.; Nafe, R.; Tan, H.K. & Jonas, U. (1995). p53 immunohistochemistry as an independent prognostic factor for superficial transitional cell carcinoma of the bladder. *Br J Cancer*, Vol.71, No.1, pp. 201-205

Sgambato, A.; Migaldi, M.; Faraglia, B.; Garagnani, L.; Romano, G.; De Gaetani, C.; Ferrari, P.; Capelli, G.; Trentini, G.P. & Cittadini, A. (1999). Loss of P27Kip1 expression correlates with tumor grade and with reduced disease-free survival in primary superficial bladder cancers. *Cancer Res*, Vol.59, No.13, pp. 3245-3250

Shariat, S.F.; Monoski, M.A.; Andrews, B.; Wheeler, T.M.; Lerner, S.P. & Slawin, K.M. (2003). Association of plasma urokinase-type plasminogen activator and its receptor with clinical outcome in patients undergoing radical cystectomy for transitional cell carcinoma of the bladder. *Urology*, Vol.61, No.5, pp. 1053-1058

Shariat, S.F.; Tokunaga, H.; Zhou, J.; Kim, J.; Ayala, G.E.; Benedict, W.F. & Lerner, S.P. (2004). p53, p21, pRB, and p16 expression predict clinical outcome in cystectomy with bladder cancer. *J Clin Oncol*, Vol.22, No.6, pp. 1014-1024

Shariat, S.F.; Ashfaq, R.; Sagalowsky, A.I. & Lotan, Y. (2006). Correlation of cyclin D1 and E1 expression with bladder cancer presence, invasion, progression, and metastasis. *Hum Pathol*, Vol.37, No.12, pp. 1568-1576

Shariat, S.F.; Ashfaq, R.; Karakiewicz, P.I.; Saeedi, O.; Sagalowsky, A.I. & Lotan, Y. (2007a). Survivin expression is associated with bladder cancer presence, stage, progression, and mortality. *Cancer*, Vol.109, No.6, pp. 1106-1113

Shariat, S.F.; Ashfaq, R.; Sagalowsky, A.I. & Lotan, Y. (2007b). Association of cyclin D1 and E1 expression with disease progression and biomarkers in patients with nonmuscle-invasive urothelial cell carcinoma of the bladder. *Urol Oncol*, Vol.25, No.6, pp. 468-475

Shariat, S.F.; Ashfaq, R.; Sagalowsky, A.I. & Lotan, Y. (2007c). Predictive value of cell cycle biomarkers in nonmuscle invasive bladder transitional cell carcinoma. *J Urol*, Vol.177, No.2, pp. 481-487;

Shariat, S.F.; Zlotta, A.R.; Ashfaq, R.; Sagalowsky, A.I. & Lotan, Y. (2007d). Cooperative effect of cell-cycle regulators expression on bladder cancer development and biologic aggressiveness. *Mod Pathol*, Vol.20, No.4, pp. 445-459

Shariat, S.F.; Bolenz, C.; Godoy, G.; Fradet, Y.; Ashfaq, R.; Karakiewicz, P.I.; Isbarn, H.; Jeldres, C.; Rigaud, J.; Sagalowsky, A.I. & Lotan, Y. (2009a). Predictive value of combined immunohistochemical markers in patients with pT1 urothelial carcinoma at radical cystectomy. *J Urol*, Vol.182, No.1, pp. 78-84;

Shariat, S.F.; Lotan, Y.; Karakiewicz, P.I.; Ashfaq, R.; Isbarn, H.; Fradet, Y.; Bastian, P.J.; Nielsen, M.E.; Capitanio, U.; Jeldres, C.; Montorsi, F.; Muller, S.C.; Karam, J.A.; Heukamp, L.C.; Netto, G.; Lerner, S.P.; Sagalowsky, A.I. & Cote, R.J. (2009b). p53 predictive value for pT1-2 N0 disease at radical cystectomy. *J Urol*, Vol.182, No.3, pp. 907-913

Shiff, C.; Naples, J.M.; Isharwal, S.; Bosompem, K.M. & Veltri, R.W. (2010). Non-invasive methods to detect schistosome-based bladder cancer: is the association sufficient for epidemiological use? *Trans R Soc Trop Med Hyg, Vol.104, No.1, pp. 3-5*

Shimazui, T.; Schalken, J.A.; Giroldi, L.A.; Jansen, C.F.; Akaza, H.; Koiso, K.; Debruyne, F.M. & Bringuier, P.P. (1996). Prognostic value of cadherin-associated molecules (alpha-, beta-, and gamma-catenins and p120cas) in bladder tumors. *Cancer Res*, Vol.56, No.18, pp. 4154-4158

Shinohara, A.; Sakano, S.; Hinoda, Y.; Nishijima, J.; Kawai, Y.; Misumi, T.; Nagao, K.; Hara, T. & Matsuyama, H. (2009). Association of TP53 and MDM2 polymorphisms with survival in bladder cancer patients treated with chemoradiotherapy. *Cancer Sci, Vol.100, No.12, pp. 2376-2382*

Sidransky, D.; Von Eschenbach, A.; Tsai, Y.C.; Jones, P.; Summerhayes, I.; Marshall, F.; Paul, M.; Green, P.; Hamilton, S.R.; Frost, P. & et al. (1991). Identification of p53 gene mutations in bladder cancers and urine samples. *Science*, Vol.252, No.5006, pp. 706-709

Sier, C.F.; Casetta, G.; Verheijen, J.H.; Tizzani, A.; Agape, V.; Kos, J.; Blasi, F. & Hanemaaijer, R. (2000). Enhanced urinary gelatinase activities (matrix metalloproteinases 2 and 9) are associated with early-stage bladder carcinoma: a comparison with clinically used tumor markers. *Clin Cancer Res*, Vol.6, No.6, pp. 2333-2340

Simon, R.; Burger, H.; Semjonow, A.; Hertle, L.; Terpe, H.J. & Bocker, W. (2000). Patterns of chromosomal imbalances in muscle invasive bladder cancer. *Int J Oncol*, Vol.17, No.5, pp. 1025-1029

Simon, R.; Struckmann, K.; Schraml, P.; Wagner, U.; Forster, T.; Moch, H.; Fijan, A.; Bruderer, J.; Wilber, K.; Mihatsch, M.J.; Gasser, T. & Sauter, G. (2002). Amplification pattern of 12q13-q15 genes (MDM2, CDK4, GLI) in urinary bladder cancer. *Oncogene*, Vol.21, No.16, pp. 2476-2483

Simoneau, M.; LaRue, H.; Aboulkassim, T.O.; Meyer, F.; Moore, L. & Fradet, Y. (2000). Chromosome 9 deletions and recurrence of superficial bladder cancer: identification of four regions of prognostic interest. *Oncogene*, Vol.19, No.54, pp. 6317-6323

Slaton, J.W.; Millikan, R.; Inoue, K.; Karashima, T.; Czerniak, B.; Shen, Y.; Yang, Y.; Benedict, W.F. & Dinney, C.P. (2004). Correlation of metastasis related gene expression and relapse-free survival in patients with locally advanced bladder cancer treated with cystectomy and chemotherapy. *J Urol*, Vol.171, No.2 Pt 1, pp. 570-574

Stadler, W.M. (2009). Randomized trial of p53 targeted adjuvant therapy for patients (pts) with organ- confined node-negative urothelial bladder cancer (UBC). *J Clin Oncol*, Vol.27, No.15s, abstract 5017

Stein, J.P.; Ginsberg, D.A.; Grossfeld, G.D.; Chatterjee, S.J.; Esrig, D.; Dickinson, M.G.; Groshen, S.; Taylor, C.R.; Jones, P.A.; Skinner, D.G. & Cote, R.J. (1998). Effect of p21WAF1/CIP1 expression on tumor progression in bladder cancer. *J Natl Cancer Inst*, Vol.90, No.14, pp. 1072-1079

Strope, S.A. & Montie, J.E. (2008). The causal role of cigarette smoking in bladder cancer initiation and progression, and the role of urologists in smoking cessation. *J Urol*, Vol.180, No.1, pp. 31-37;

Sun, C.H.; Chang, Y.H. & Pan, C.C. (2011). Activation of the PI3K/Akt/mTOR pathway correlates with tumour progression and reduced survival in patients with urothelial carcinoma of the urinary bladder. *Histopathology*, Vol.58, No.7, pp. 1054-1063

Svatek, R.S.; Herman, M.P.; Lotan, Y.; Casella, R.; Hsieh, J.T.; Sagalowsky, A.I. & Shariat, S.F. (2006). Soluble Fas--a promising novel urinary marker for the detection of recurrent superficial bladder cancer. *Cancer*, Vol.106, No.8, pp. 1701-1707

Swana, H.S.; Grossman, D.; Anthony, J.N.; Weiss, R.M. & Altieri, D.C. (1999). Tumor content of the antiapoptosis molecule survivin and recurrence of bladder cancer. *N Engl J Med*, Vol.341, No.6, pp. 452-453

Sylvester, R.J.; van der Meijden, A.P.; Oosterlinck, W.; Witjes, J.A.; Bouffioux, C.; Denis, L.; Newling, D.W. & Kurth, K. (2006). Predicting recurrence and progression in individual patients with stage Ta T1 bladder cancer using EORTC risk tables: a combined analysis of 2596 patients from seven EORTC trials. *Eur Urol*, Vol.49, No.3, pp. 466-465; discussion 475-467

Szarvas, T.; Jager, T.; Totsch, M.; vom Dorp, F.; Kempkensteffen, C.; Kovalszky, I.; Romics, I.; Ergun, S. & Rubben, H. (2008). Angiogenic switch of angiopietins-Tie2 system and its prognostic value in bladder cancer. *Clin Cancer Res*, Vol.14, No.24, pp. 8253-8262

Takahashi, R.; Hashimoto, T.; Xu, H.J.; Hu, S.X.; Matsui, T.; Miki, T.; Bigo-Marshall, H.; Aaronson, S.A. & Benedict, W.F. (1991). The retinoblastoma gene functions as a growth and tumor suppressor in human bladder carcinoma cells. *Proc Natl Acad Sci U S A*, Vol.88, No.12, pp. 5257-5261

Teng, D.H.; Hu, R.; Lin, H.; Davis, T.; Iliev, D.; Frye, C.; Swedlund, B.; Hansen, K.L.; Vinson, V.L.; Gumpper, K.L.; Ellis, L.; El-Naggar, A.; Frazier, M.; Jasser, S.; Langford, L.A.; Lee, J.; Mills, G.B.; Pershouse, M.A.; Pollack, R.E.; Tornos, C.; Troncoso, P.; Yung, W.K.; Fujii, G.; Berson, A.; Steck, P.A. & et al. (1997). MMAC1/PTEN mutations in primary tumor specimens and tumor cell lines. *Cancer Res*, Vol.57, No.23, pp. 5221-5225

Theodoropoulos, V.E.; Lazaris, A.; Sofras, F.; Gerzelis, I.; Tsoukala, V.; Ghikonti, I.; Manikas, K. & Kastriotis, I. (2004). Hypoxia-inducible factor 1 alpha expression correlates with angiogenesis and unfavorable prognosis in bladder cancer. *Eur Urol*, Vol.46, No.2, pp. 200-208

Theodoropoulos, V.E.; Lazaris, A.C.; Kastriotis, I.; Spiliadi, C.; Theodoropoulos, G.E.; Tsoukala, V.; Patsouris, E. & Sofras, F. (2005). Evaluation of hypoxia-inducible factor 1alpha overexpression as a predictor of tumour recurrence and progression in superficial urothelial bladder carcinoma. *BJU Int*, Vol.95, No.3, pp. 425-431

Thogersen, V.B.; Sorensen, B.S.; Poulsen, S.S.; Orntoft, T.F.; Wolf, H. & Nexo, E. (2001). A subclass of HER1 ligands are prognostic markers for survival in bladder cancer patients. *Cancer Res*, Vol.61, No.16, pp. 6227-6233

Tsuruta, H.; Kishimoto, H.; Sasaki, T.; Horie, Y.; Natsui, M.; Shibata, Y.; Hamada, K.; Yajima, N.; Kawahara, K.; Sasaki, M.; Tsuchiya, N.; Enomoto, K.; Mak, T.W.; Nakano, T.; Habuchi, T. & Suzuki, A. (2006). Hyperplasia and carcinomas in Pten-deficient mice and reduced PTEN protein in human bladder cancer patients. *Cancer Res*, Vol.66, No.17, pp. 8389-8396

Turkeri, L.N.; Erton, M.L.; Cevik, I. & Akdas, A. (1998). Impact of the expression of epidermal growth factor, transforming growth factor alpha, and epidermal growth factor receptor on the prognosis of superficial bladder cancer. *Urology*, Vol.51, No.4, pp. 645-649

Tut, V.M.; Braithwaite, K.L.; Angus, B.; Neal, D.E.; Lunec, J. & Mellon, J.K. (2001). Cyclin D1 expression in transitional cell carcinoma of the bladder: correlation with p53, waf1, pRb and Ki67. *Br J Cancer*, Vol.84, No.2, pp. 270-275

van Oers, J.M.; Wild, P.J.; Burger, M.; Denzinger, S.; Stoehr, R.; Rosskopf, E.; Hofstaedter, F.; Steyerberg, E.W.; Klinkhammer-Schalke, M.; Zwarthoff, E.C.; van der Kwast, T.H. & Hartmann, A. (2007). FGFR3 mutations and a normal CK20 staining pattern define low-grade noninvasive urothelial bladder tumours. *Eur Urol*, Vol.52, No.3, pp. 760-768

van Oers, J.M.; Zwarthoff, E.C.; Rehman, I.; Azzouzi, A.R.; Cussenot, O.; Meuth, M.; Hamdy, F.C. & Catto, J.W. (2009). FGFR3 mutations indicate better survival in invasive upper urinary tract and bladder tumours. *Eur Urol*, Vol.55, No.3, pp. 650-657

van Rhijn, B.W.; Lurkin, I.; Radvanyi, F.; Kirkels, W.J.; van der Kwast, T.H. & Zwarthoff, E.C. (2001). The fibroblast growth factor receptor 3 (FGFR3) mutation is a strong indicator of superficial bladder cancer with low recurrence rate. *Cancer Res*, Vol.61, No.4, pp. 1265-1268

van Rhijn, B.W.; van der Kwast, T.H.; Vis, A.N.; Kirkels, W.J.; Boeve, E.R.; Jobsis, A.C. & Zwarthoff, E.C. (2004). FGFR3 and P53 characterize alternative genetic pathways in the pathogenesis of urothelial cell carcinoma. *Cancer Res*, Vol.64, No.6, pp. 1911-1914

van Rhijn, B.W.; Burger, M.; Lotan, Y.; Solsona, E.; Stief, C.G.; Sylvester, R.J.; Witjes, J.A. & Zlotta, A.R. (2009). Recurrence and Progression of Disease in Non-Muscle-Invasive Bladder Cancer: From Epidemiology to Treatment Strategy. *Eur Urol, Vol.56, No.3, pp. 430-442*

van Rhijn, B.W.; Zuiverloon, T.C.; Vis, A.N.; Radvanyi, F.; van Leenders, G.J.; Ooms, B.C.; Kirkels, W.J.; Lockwood, G.A.; Boeve, E.R.; Jobsis, A.C.; Zwarthoff, E.C. & van der

Kwast, T.H. (2010). Molecular grade (FGFR3/MIB-1) and EORTC risk scores are predictive in primary non-muscle-invasive bladder cancer. *Eur Urol*, Vol.58, No.3, pp. 433-441

Vasala, K.; Paakko, P. & Turpeenniemi-Hujanen, T. (2003). Matrix metalloproteinase-2 immunoreactive protein as a prognostic marker in bladder cancer. *Urology*, Vol.62, No.5, pp. 952-957

Wada, T.; Louhelainen, J.; Hemminki, K.; Adolfsson, J.; Wijkstrom, H.; Norming, U.; Borgstrom, E.; Hansson, J.; Sandstedt, B. & Steineck, G. (2000). Bladder cancer: allelic deletions at and around the retinoblastoma tumor suppressor gene in relation to stage and grade. *Clin Cancer Res*, Vol.6, No.2, pp. 610-615

Waldman, T.; Lengauer, C.; Kinzler, K.W. & Vogelstein, B. (1996). Uncoupling of S phase and mitosis induced by anticancer agents in cells lacking p21. *Nature*, Vol.381, No.6584, pp. 713-716

Wallard, M.J.; Pennington, C.J.; Veerakumarasivam, A.; Burtt, G.; Mills, I.G.; Warren, A.; Leung, H.Y.; Murphy, G.; Edwards, D.R.; Neal, D.E. & Kelly, J.D. (2006). Comprehensive profiling and localisation of the matrix metalloproteinases in urothelial carcinoma. *Br J Cancer*, Vol.94, No.4, pp. 569-577

Wang, P.; Nishitani, M.A.; Tanimoto, S.; Kishimoto, T.; Fukumori, T.; Takahashi, M. & Kanayama, H.O. (2007). Bladder cancer cell invasion is enhanced by cross-talk with fibroblasts through hepatocyte growth factor. *Urology*, Vol.69, No.4, pp. 780-784

Weikert, S.; Christoph, F.; Schrader, M.; Krause, H.; Miller, K. & Muller, M. (2005a). Quantitative analysis of survivin mRNA expression in urine and tumor tissue of bladder cancer patients and its potential relevance for disease detection and prognosis. *Int J Cancer*, Vol.116, No.1, pp. 100-104

Weikert, S.; Krause, H.; Wolff, I.; Christoph, F.; Schrader, M.; Emrich, T.; Miller, K. & Muller, M. (2005b). Quantitative evaluation of telomerase subunits in urine as biomarkers for noninvasive detection of bladder cancer. *Int J Cancer*, Vol.117, No.2, pp. 274-280

Weiss, C.; von Romer, F.; Capalbo, G.; Ott, O.J.; Wittlinger, M.; Krause, S.F.; Sauer, R.; Rodel, C. & Rodel, F. (2009). Survivin expression as a predictive marker for local control in patients with high-risk T1 bladder cancer treated with transurethral resection and radiochemotherapy. *Int J Radiat Oncol Biol Phys*, Vol.74, No.5, pp. 1455-1460

Williams, S.G. & Stein, J.P. (2004). Molecular pathways in bladder cancer. *Urol Res*, Vol.32, No.6, pp. 373-385

Williams, S.V.; Sibley, K.D.; Davies, A.M.; Nishiyama, H.; Hornigold, N.; Coulter, J.; Kennedy, W.J.; Skilleter, A.; Habuchi, T. & Knowles, M.A. (2002). Molecular genetic analysis of chromosome 9 candidate tumor-suppressor loci in bladder cancer cell lines. *Genes Chromosomes Cancer*, Vol.34, No.1, pp. 86-96

Williamson, M.P.; Elder, P.A.; Shaw, M.E.; Devlin, J. & Knowles, M.A. (1995). p16 (CDKN2) is a major deletion target at 9p21 in bladder cancer. *Hum Mol Genet*, Vol.4, No.9, pp. 1569-1577

Wolf, H.K.; Stober, C.; Hohenfellner, R. & Leissner, J. (2001). Prognostic value of p53, p21/WAF1, Bcl-2, Bax, Bak and Ki-67 immunoreactivity in pT1 G3 urothelial bladder carcinomas. *Tumour Biol*, Vol.22, No.5, pp. 328-336

Wu, X.; Bayle, J.H.; Olson, D. & Levine, A.J. (1993). The p53-mdm-2 autoregulatory feedback loop. *Genes Dev*, Vol.7, No.7A, pp. 1126-1132

Wu, X.; Obata, T.; Khan, Q.; Highshaw, R.A.; De Vere White, R. & Sweeney, C. (2004). The phosphatidylinositol-3 kinase pathway regulates bladder cancer cell invasion. *BJU Int*, Vol.93, No.1, pp. 143-150

Wu, X. (2005). Urothelial tumorigenesis: a tale of divergent pathways. *Nat Rev Cancer*, Vol.5, No.9, pp. 713-725

Wu, X.; Ye, Y.; Kiemeney, L.A.; Sulem, P.; Rafnar, T.; Matullo, G.; Seminara, D.; Yoshida, T.; Saeki, N.; Andrew, A.S.; Dinney, C.P.; Czerniak, B.; Zhang, Z.F.; Kiltie, A.E.; Bishop, D.T.; Vineis, P.; Porru, S.; Buntinx, F.; Kellen, E.; Zeegers, M.P.; Kumar, R.; Rudnai, P.; Gurzau, E.; Koppova, K.; Mayordomo, J.I.; Sanchez, M.; Saez, B.; Lindblom, A.; de Verdier, P.; Steineck, G.; Mills, G.B.; Schned, A.; Guarrera, S.; Polidoro, S.; Chang, S.C.; Lin, J.; Chang, D.W.; Hale, K.S.; Majewski, T.; Grossman, H.B.; Thorlacius, S.; Thorsteinsdottir, U.; Aben, K.K.; Witjes, J.A.; Stefansson, K.; Amos, C.I.; Karagas, M.R. & Gu, J. (2009). Genetic variation in the prostate stem cell antigen gene PSCA confers susceptibility to urinary bladder cancer. *Nat Genet*, Vol.41, No.9, pp. 991-995

Xia, G.; Kumar, S.R.; Hawes, D.; Cai, J.; Hassanieh, L.; Groshen, S.; Zhu, S.; Masood, R.; Quinn, D.I.; Broek, D.; Stein, J.P. & Gill, P.S. (2006). Expression and significance of vascular endothelial growth factor receptor 2 in bladder cancer. *J Urol*, Vol.175, No.4, pp. 1245-1252

Xu, H.J.; Cairns, P.; Hu, S.X.; Knowles, M.A. & Benedict, W.F. (1993). Loss of RB protein expression in primary bladder cancer correlates with loss of heterozygosity at the RB locus and tumor progression. *Int J Cancer*, Vol.53, No.5, pp. 781-784

Yamana, K.; Bilim, V.; Hara, N.; Kasahara, T.; Itoi, T.; Maruyama, R.; Nishiyama, T.; Takahashi, K. & Tomita, Y. (2005). Prognostic impact of FAS/CD95/APO-1 in urothelial cancers: decreased expression of Fas is associated with disease progression. *Br J Cancer*, Vol.93, No.5, pp. 544-551

Part 2

Epidemiology, Biomarkers and Prognostic Factors

2

Biomarkers of Bladder Cancer in Urine: Evaluation of Diagnostic and Prognostic Significance of Current and Potential Markers

Daben Dawam
Medway NHS Foundation Trust
Medway Maritime Hospital
Associate Teaching Hospital, University of London,
United Kingdom

1. Introduction

The diagnosis of bladder cancer is generally made by cystoscopy and biopsy. Moreover, bladder cancer has a very high frequency of recurrence and therefore requires follow-up cystoscopy, along with urine cytology, as periodic surveillance to identify recurrence early. Cystoscopy is invasive and apt with complications like urine infection which sometimes lead to septicaemia with serious consequencies. Patient experience is most times not pleasant. Therefore, there needs to be a better way of surveillance for bladder cancer which is non-invasive and more acceptable to the patient experience. Consequently, urine biomarkers might be used to either supplement or supplant these tests.

Urinary bladder carcinoma, the fourth most common cancer in men and ninth most common in women results in significant morbidity and mortality.

Bladder cancer (urothelial carcinoma) typically presents as a tumour confined to the superficial mucosa of the bladder. The most common symptom of early bladder cancer is haematuria; however, urinary tract symptoms (i.e., urinary frequency, urgency and dysuria) may also occur. Most urologists follow the American Urological Association (AUA) guidelines for haematuria which recommend cystoscopic evaluation of all adults greater than 40 years old with microscopic haematuria and for those less than 40 years old with risk factors for developing bladder cancer. Confirmatory diagnosis of bladder cancer must by made by cystoscopic examination and biopsy which is considered to be the "gold standard."

At initial diagnosis, about 70 percent of patients have cancers confined to the epithelium or sub-epithelial connective tissue. Non-muscle invasive disease is usually treated with transurethral resection with or without intravesical therapy, depending on depth of invasion and tumour grade. However, there is a 75 percent incidence of recurrence in these patients with 10-15 percent progressing to muscle invasion over a five year period. Current follow-up protocols include flexible cystoscopy and urine cytology every three months for one to three years, every six months for an additional two to three years, and then annually, assuming no recurrence.

While urine cytology is a specific test (from 90 percent–100 percent), its sensitivity is lower, ranging from 50 percent–60 percent overall and is considered even lower for low-grade tumours. Therefore, there has been interest in identifying tumour markers in voided urine that would provide a more sensitive and objective test for tumour recurrence.

2. Background

Bladder cancer is very common, ranking second only to prostate cancer for cancers of the urinary tract. Approximately 54 000 new cases of bladder cancer are diagnosed and ~12 000 people die from this disease every year in the United States alone. Most patients are diagnosed with superficial tumours, which can be completely resected. However, two-thirds of these patients will experience recurrence within 5 years, and almost 90% will have a recurrence by 15 years. Early diagnosis leads to better clinical outcomes, underscoring the importance of finding new ways for screening the general population. Currently, potential bladder tumour markers can be used in various clinical scenarios, including (14):

- Serial testing for earlier detection of recurrence;
- Complementary testing to urine cytology to improve the detection rate;
- Providing a less expensive and more objective alternative to the urine cytology test; and
- Directing the cytoscopic evaluation of patient follow-up.

The gold standard for the detection of urothelial neoplasia is cytologic examination of urothelial cells from voided urine, urinary bladder washings, and urinary tract brushing specimens in combination with cystoscopic examination [12,13]. Because cystoscopy is an invasive procedure and urinary cytology suffers from low sensitivity and specificity, particularly for lower grade tumours, it is desirable to identify novel biomarkers for this cancer. Biochemical testing of urine is a non-invasive and less expensive procedure for diagnosing and monitoring this disease. Because none of the markers mentioned above has sufficient sensitivity and specificity, the quest for identifying additional bladder cancer biomarkers continues.

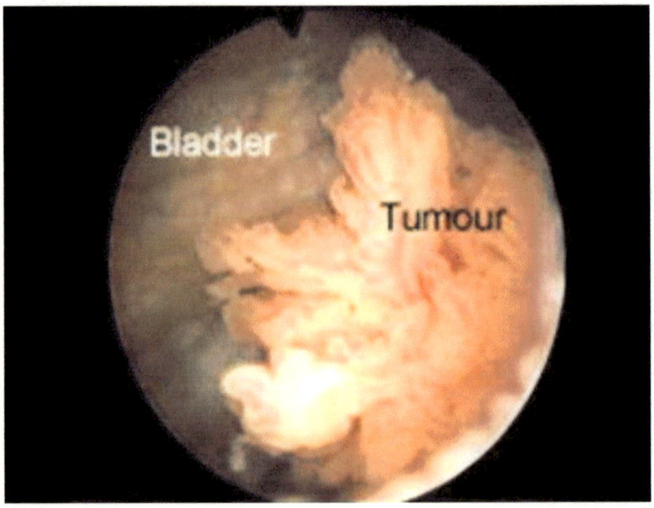

Fig. 1. Cystoscopic appearance of bladder tumour

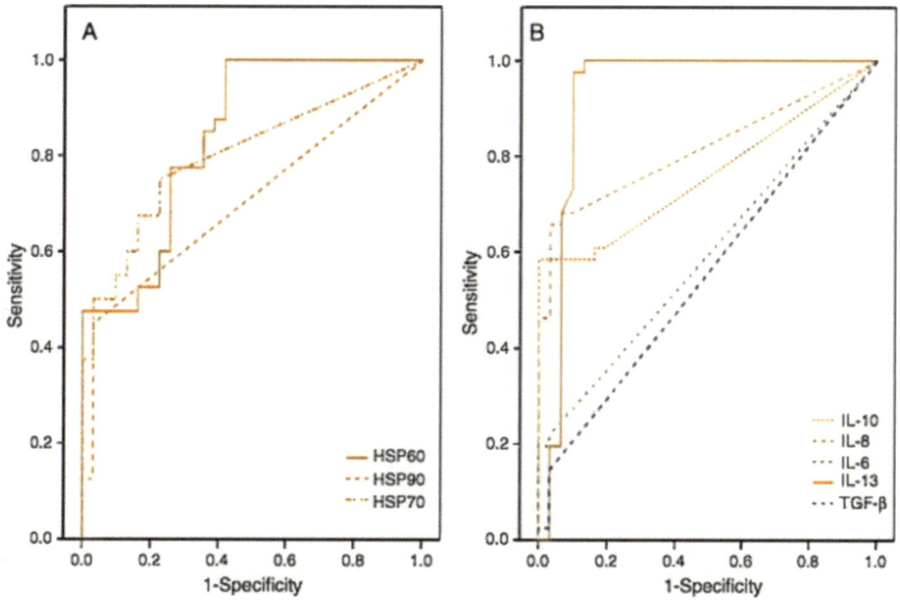

Fig. 2. Relationship between sensitivity and specificity

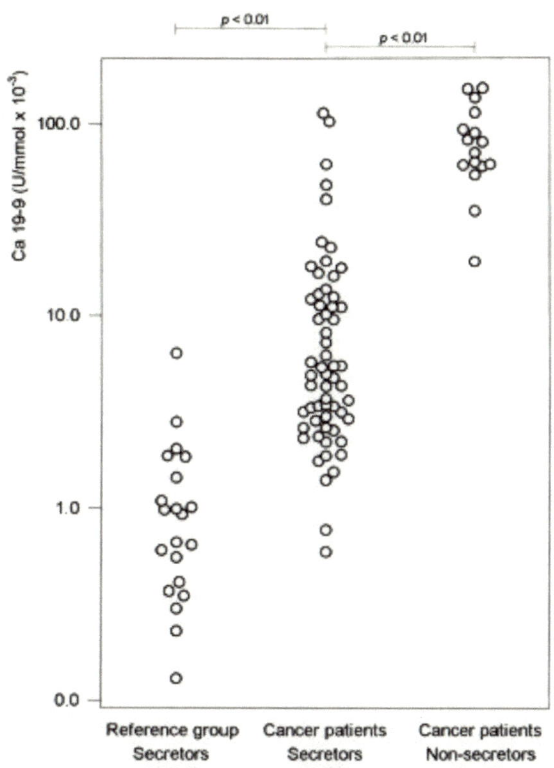

Fig. 3. Ca 19-9 levels in urine (Adapted from ClinChem.org)

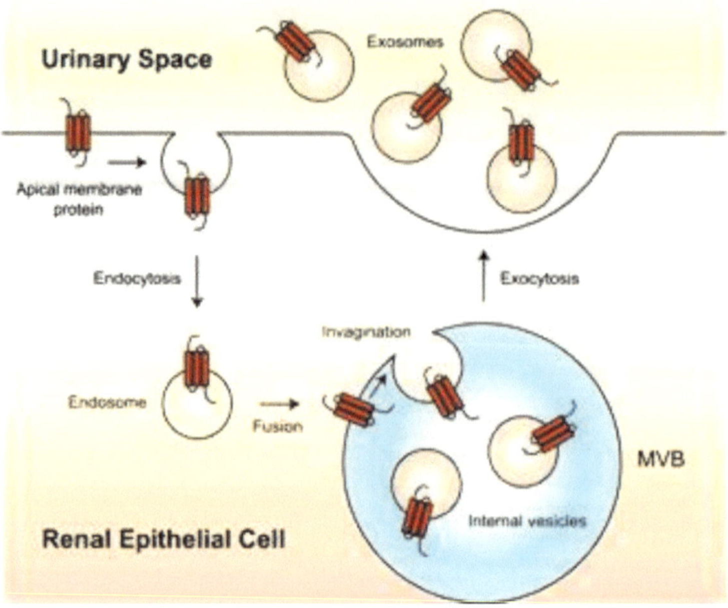

Fig. 4. Mechanism of cancer marker production and appearance in urine (Adapted from flipper.diff.org)

Kageyama et al. propose proteomic analysis of urine as a new way to identify bladder cancer biomarkers. Previously, Celis et al. utilised two-dimensional gel electrophoresis and developed a comprehensive database for bladder cancer profiles of both transitional and squamous cell carcinomas.

Biochemical testing of urine should be able to diagnose early bladder carcinoma because candidate informative molecules could be excreted into the urine during cancer development. Proteomic profiling of urine has been suggested as a diagnostic test for bladder carcinoma [11]. In addition, many other biochemical molecules or genetic markers have been discovered that could be used to diagnose bladder carcinoma with fair sensitivity and specificity. Such molecules (or methods) include, but are not limited to, the following (the approximate diagnostic sensitivities and specificities are in parentheses): BTA stat (68%; 66%); BTA-TRAK (71%; 62%); NMP22 (64%; 71%); telomerase (74%; 89%); HA-HAase (91%; 86%); Immunocyt (68%; 79%); F/FDP (68%; 86%); multicolor fluorescence in situ hybridization assays (84%; 90%); cytokeratins (76%; 84%); metalloproteinases (60%; 80%); and p53 mutation (32%; 100%). The most common noninvasive test, however, is voided urine cytology (VUC), which has a sensitivity of ~50%and a specificity of 97% [12]. This test has higher sensitivity for higher grade tumors.

Through their studies, Kageyama et al. were able to identify a potential tumour marker, calreticulin, which is found in the urine of patients with bladder carcinoma. The authors used a differential display method of bladder cancer vs healthy urothelial tissue and mass spectrometry to identify proteins that are increased in cancer tissue. In addition to calreticulin, an endoplasmic reticulum chaperone, they found nine other candidate proteins that could constitute new biomarkers for bladder carcinoma. The authors confirmed their data with quantitative Western blot analysis, immunoprecipitation, and immunohistochemistry. Their reported sensitivity and specificity were 73% and 86%, respectively, similar to the values reported for other biochemical bladder markers (see above). However, the diagnostic accuracy of their test was vulnerable to urinary tract infections.

The main question surrounding bladder cancer and urinary biomarkers is how these molecules can be used in clinical practice. Clearly, these tests are not useful for population screening because of their low sensitivity and specificity. In addition, none of the available tests is sufficiently accurate to replace cystoscopy in the investigation of a patient with a possible bladder tumour. VUC has relatively low sensitivity, especially for low-grade tumours, but it is currently the most specific test for bladder carcinoma. Consequently, when VUC is positive, it indicates a high-risk tumour that requires definitive treatment. VUC is currently used for monitoring of patients with known high-risk disease, and positive cytology with negative cystoscopy may indicate malignancy of the prostate or upper urinary tract.

Current guidelines suggest that low-risk patients should be surveyed once a year with cystoscopy and high-risk patients at 3-month intervals. Currently, cystoscopy is always combined with VUC. Because, as mentioned earlier, new urinary bladder tests such as BTA or NMP22 could detect lower-grade disease recurrence with higher sensitivity than VUC, it could be worthwhile to consider including one or more of these tests in the routine follow-up of patients with bladder carcinoma. However, large prospective studies will be necessary to test the clinical utility of these assays against cytology. Such trials could show the value of these new tests in reducing the frequency of cystoscopy and in contributing to the earlier and more sensitive detection of disease recurrence, leading to earlier therapeutic interventions and, fortunately, to improved clinical outcomes.

In conclusion, bladder cancer biomarkers have proliferated more than any other class of cancer markers over the last 10 years. We now have at hand a multitude of molecules that can be measured with automated, inexpensive, quantitative assays in urine. These markers may aid in the monitoring of patients with bladder carcinoma and have the potential to reduce the number of follow-up cystoscopy, thus reducing healthcare costs and patient discomfort and, at the same time, detecting relapsing disease more effectively than VUC. It is time to test these new possibilities with prospective clinical trials.

3. Evaluation of individual markers

Urine-based marker tests are being developed to fill some of the remaining needs. These newer tests are more accurate in detecting low-grade bladder cancer, so they are especially useful in monitoring for recurrence, may significantly improve and simplify workup, diagnosis, and follow-up, and hopefully allow for detection of disease at an earlier stage, thus improving the chances of curative therapy.

The urine marker assays discussed here have shown enhanced sensitivity in detecting bladder cancers. However, each still requires further validation and testing in clinical trials to determine how best to apply these tools for in individual patients. In recent years several of the newer tests are being used by urologists as another weapon in the arsenal. Although immunological markers are superior to standard urine cytology, at the present time urine bound tests are not specific enough to completely replace cystoscopy as a definite diagnostic tool.

In order to understand what these tests are about it's helpful to have an understanding of *Sensitivity vs. Specificity:*

A diagnostic test is one that predicts the presence of a disease. An ideal diagnostic test would always give the right answer, with a positive result in everyone with the disease and a negative result in everyone else - and would be quick, safe, simple, painless, reliable, and inexpensive, as well. Since no current diagnostic test is ideal, we need to evaluate each of them for their clinical usefulness. In practice, for any diagnostic test there is a trade-off between sensitivity and specificity. In cancer diagnosis, the need for this trade-off is rooted in the fact that cancer arises from our own tissues. It is not completely "foreign" to our systems like a virus or bacterium is.
It's important to remember that there are four possible results when a diagnostic test is run:
True positive - when the test is **positive** and the patient **does have** the disease
False positive - when the test is **positive** but the patient **does not have** the disease
True negative - when the test is **negative** and the patient **does not have** the disease
False negative - when the test is **negative** but the patient **does have** the disease
Here's another way of looking at this (often referred to as a "truth table"):

Test Result	The disease being tested for is present	The disease being tested for is not present
"Positive"	True positive	False positive
"Negative"	False negative	True negative

Calculating the disease sensitivity and specificity are ways of evaluating diagnostic tests, using the four possible results.
Sensitivity - is the ability of a test to correctly identify a positive specimen, and it tells you how good the test is at identifying the disease. Statistically, it's the proportion of patients with the disease who have a positive result, that is, the number of "true positives" out of all the situations where the disease is present.
For example, 100 patients with cancer are tested using a test that detects tumours. There are 80 positive results and 20 negative results. This means the test has a sensitivity of 80% - it correctly identified 80 of the 100 cancers - and it gave 20 false negative results.
Specificity - is the ability of a test to correctly identify a negative specimen, and it tells you how good the test is at identifying when the disease is absent. The statistical way of looking at this is the proportion of patients without the disease who have a negative test, that is, the number of "true negatives" out of all the situations where the disease is not present.
For example, 100 normal, healthy individuals are tested using a test that detects tumours. There are 80 positives and 20 negatives. This means the test has a specificity of 20% - it correctly identified 20 of the 100 negative specimens - and it gave 80 false positive results.
Both sensitivity and specificity are very important, and they can both be influenced by various factors, such as the characteristics of the population tested or the value used as a cut-off for the test (above which the test is positive and below which it is negative). A test with low sensitivity and many false negative results will fail to detect the tumour in a large portion of the patients being tested, while a test with low specificity with many false positive results may lead to unnecessary invasive or expensive procedures and cause undue alarm.
Many, but not all, patients report they would rather be "scared for nothing" than miss a tumour, and are therefore most interested in tests with high sensitivity.1

4. BTA stat test and the BTA TRAK assay

The original Bard BTA Test, which continues to be referred to in the literature from time to time, was a latex agglutination test detecting bladder tumour-associated antigen and is no longer distributed in the US. It is important to note that it has been replaced by two newer tests based on significantly improved technology with much better sensitivity and specificity.

Both of the new tests detect a human complement factor H-related protein (hCFHrp) which has been shown to be produced by several human bladder cancer cell lines, and by human bladder cancers, but not by other epithelial cell lines (Kinders, Clin Cancer Res 4:2511, 1998). It is thought that factor H acts to protect the tumor cell from the body's natural immune system (Corey, J Biol Chem 275:12917, 2000). Both the BTA stat and BTA TRAK tests can provide valuable but slightly different information for the bladder cancer patient and her doctor.

The BTA stat Test is a qualitative (positive or negative) test provided in a disposable format similar to a home pregnancy test. It uses five drops of urine and can be read in five minutes by the appearance of a coloured line in the patient window, while a coloured line appears in a "check" window to indicate the test is working properly. This test is cleared in the US for use by clinical laboratories, the physician or his staff right in the office, or even by the bladder cancer patient at home (with a physician's prescription). To date, it is the only tumour marker in the United States with this status. Besides being highly sensitive, fast, and easy to use, with a unique availability to be run by the physician and/or the patient, this test is significantly less costly than other diagnostic tests or cytology.

The BTA TRAK Assay is a quantitative immunoassay test and provides a numerical result of the hCFHrp level. Like the NMP22 test, urine must be sent to a reference laboratory where the test is performed by professional technologists. In addition to knowledge of the specific level, an advantage of the BTA TRAK test is the ability to monitor the rise or fall of hCFHrp.

Numerous clinical studies have been conducted with the new BTA tests. Most reports state findings in terms of "sensitivity" and "specificity." Briefly, sensitivity is the ability of the test to correctly identify a positive specimen, and specificity is the ability of the test to correctly identify a negative specimen.

4.1 BTA stat test studies

In the most recent study (June 2000) and the largest of its kind to date, Raitanen reported the overall sensitivity of BTA stat as 82%, and cytology as 30% . In another study, Pode reported 100% BTA stat sensitivity in tumors of stage T2 or higher, grade III, and all tumors greater than 2cm (Pode, J Urol 161:443, 1999). Specificity of the BTA stat Test has been reported as 72-95% (Sarosdy, Urology 50:349, 1997) and 98% in healthy individuals (Raitanen, Scand J Urol Nephrol 33:234, 1999).

4.2 BTA TRAK assay studies

In one study, the overall sensitivity of the BTA TRAK Assay was reported as 72% with a specificity of 75-97% (Ellis, Urology 50:882, 1997). Heicappell again reported an overall sensitivity of 72%, with 97% specificity in healthy individuals. He also reported that BTA

TRAK levels reflect tumour stage and grade, with levels in superficial bladder cancer at high risk of tumour progression significantly higher compared to low and intermediate grade superficial cancers (Heicappell, Eur Urol 35:81, 1999).

4.3 Comparison studies

In a study conducted at the Mayo Clinic, several urine tumour markers were evaluated, including urine cytology, BTA stat, NMP22, fibrin/fibrinogen degradation products (FDP), telomerase, chemiluminescent hemoglobin and hemoglobin dipstick. The telomerase test presented the highest combination of sensitivity and specificity for screening. However, other researchers have had difficulty reproducing the telomerase results of this study, possibly due to the technical difficulties of running the test. It's also important to note that telomerase is a "Research Use Only" test, and has not received FDA clearance for marketing in the US. In the same study, the BTA stat Test was shown to have the best overall sensitivity (74%), and the best sensitivity for T1-T3 and primary tumour detection (Ramakumar, J Urol 161:388, 1999).
Another comparison study (Giannopoulos, Urology 55:871, 2000) showed that the BTA stat Test was more sensitive than cytology in all stages and grades except G3, while NMP22 was more sensitive than cytology only in stage Ta and Grade 1 and 2. The BTA stat Test also had higher sensitivity than NMP22 in all stages and grades.
It is also important to note that in both of the BTA tests, and with NMP22 as well, results can be compromised if there is a urinary tract infection, inflammation, or kidney stones present, if there has been recent trauma to the bladder, or if the specimen is collected by catheter. The paper by Sharma, for example, shows the dramatic increase in specificity when these conditions are excluded from testing (Sharma, J Urol 162:53, 1999). As with any test, for the results to be most useful they should be interpreted in light of all the medical and clinical information available.

5. NMP22 'Bladder check'

In a study comparing cystoscopy, cytology, and Bladder Check; the NMP22/Bladderchek test had a considerably higher detection rate than cytology (67% vs. 20%). Cystoscopy detected 86% of bladder cancers.
More cost effective than cytology, the Bladder check test could also be a good adjunct to cystoscopy. The test costs in the range of $20 to $25, which Medicare reimburses for both bladder cancer monitoring and detection. It is a waived test under the Clinical Laboratory Improvement Amendments (CLIA).
While the test showed a high negative predictive value, it produced a false-positive result in 19 of the 194 patients without bladder cancer. Dr. Tomera advised that such patients need to be watched closely. Earlier data by Mark Soloway, MD, has shown that bladder cancer will be found in 70% of these individuals during the following 3 to 6 months (J Urol 1996; 156:363-7).
NMP22's core technology is based on the level of nuclear matrix proteins (NMPs) that are detected in body fluids. These levels are correlated to the presence of early-stage cancerous abnormalities, which have been validated in multiple clinical studies. The technology was discovered at the Massachusetts Institute of Technology and licensed to Matritech.

6. FISH

Florescence in situ hybridization (FISH) is an assay which uses a mixture of fluorescent labeled probes to assess urinary cells for chromosomal abnormalities associated with malignancy.
In a study at the Mayo clinic, researchers found that urine cytology detected cancerous cells in only 57 percent of the patients with bladder cancer while the FISH test picked up more than 95 percent of the high grade cancers, which are the most dangerous and important group of bladder cancers because they have a high probability of progressing to potentially incurable muscle-invasive bladder cancer. Cancers the test missed were low-grade tumours, which are less dangerous and have only a 3 to 5 percent chance of progressing to a higher stage tumour over five years. The FISH test also detected recurrence of the cancer three to six months earlier than by the cytology. This earlier detection capability should allow treatment to be initiated earlier and possibly give the patient a greater chance for survival, he said.
Fluorescence-in-situ-hybridization (FISH) for multiple centromeric probes has previously been shown to be a very sensitive test for diagnosing UC, however the test was limited by the requirement of multiple cytospins to evaluate 4 or more probe sets. Recently a new commercial test (VYSIS) for evaluating urinary cytology became available in which 4 probes are simultaneously evaluated on a per cell basis on a single cytospin. We performed a pilot study to test the efficacy of the new FISH test compared to standard urine cytology. This study showed that the multi-colour FISH probe test was more sensitive than cytology, easily performed and yielded a high number of cells with numerical chromosomal aberrations.

7. DiagnoCure's ImmunoCyt™ bladder cancer monitoring test

ImmunoCyt™ is a 510(k) cleared, by the FDA, qualitative direct immuno-cytofluorescence assay, intended for use in conjunction with cytology to increase the overall sensitivity for the detection of tumor cells exfoliated in the urine of patients previously diagnosed with bladder cancer.
ImmunoCyt™ contains a cocktail of three monoclonal antibodies labeled with fluorescent markers. The cocktail of antibodies have been shown to react with a mucin glycoprotein as well as to be specific to a glycoform of CEA. The test detects cellular markers specific for bladder cancer in exfoliated cells isolated from urine sample. This non-invasive test, when coupled with urine cytology proves to be more sensitive than urine cytology alone or other currently available tumour markers.
The current standard method for non-invasive detection of bladder cancer is urinary cytology, which consists of identifying the presence of cancer cells in urine. Urinary cytology has high specificity but poor sensitivity, typically no greater than 30% to 45%. This sensitivity varies according to the stage and grade of the tumor.
ImmunoCytT™is carried out in parallel with cytology to improve cytology's sensitivity at detecting tumour cells in the urine of patients, especially those with low stage, low grade tumors. The concomitant use of classical cytology and ImmunoCytTM can substantially improve the detection of bladder cancer. As shown in the ImmunoCytTM performance analysis (cumulative data from eleven publications and presentations from 3,203 cases), a sensitivity of 88% has been obtained when both cytology and ImmunoCyt™ were used together.

A multi-centre study in the United States, published in the Journal of Urology, concluded: ImmunoCyt™ enhances the sensitivity of cytology, which is a specific but not a sensitive method for detecting bladder cancer. The ability of this immuno-cytochemical test to detect low grade, superficial, small tumours makes it the most suitable available marker to test for monitoring strategies in patients with low risk bladder cancer. Performance of urine test in patients monitored for recurrence of bladder cancer: a multi-centre study in the United States.

8. FDP-Fibrin/Fibrinogen Degradation Products

FDP has shown high sensitivity even for low-grade and non-invasive tumours, and its diagnostic ability could be superior to NMP22 according to a recent study

The FDP test detects the presence of fibrin and fibrinogen degradation products in urine. It is a simple test that can be performed in the office, and results are available in about 10 minutes. Fibrin and fibrinogen degradation products are protein fragments generated by the action of the fibrinolytic system on fibrin and fibrinogen. Plasma proteins leak from blood vessels in tumours into the surrounding tissue. Clotting factors rapidly convert the fibrinogen in the plasma into an extravascular fibrin clot, which is degraded by plasmin and activated by urokinase. The FDP test can detect these degradation products and is positive in two thirds of patients with bladder cancer. The FDP assay is more accurate than urine cytology and has high specificity (negative in 96% of healthy subjects). The FDP test was found to be superior to the BTA test in at least one study*.

Telomerase is another substance currently being assessed for its potential usefulness in diagnosing transitional cell cancer (TCC) and in monitoring for recurrence. It will soon be made available to doctors and patients. Telomerase is a ribonucleoprotein enzyme responsible for production of telomeres, which are DNA sequences that occupy the ends of chromosomes and protect their integrity during DNA replication and may be involved in the immortalization of a cancer cell [3]

9. Comparison of screening methods in the detection of bladder cancer

In a study done in '99, researchers prospectively evaluated and compared the sensitivity and specificity of urine cytology, BTA stat, NMP22, fibrin/fibrinogen degradation products (FDP), telomerase, chemiluminescent hemoglobin and hemoglobin dipstick to detect bladder cancer ; within each tumour grade and stage telomerase had the strongest association with bladder cancer among all tests (69% overall concordance). Telomerase was positive in 91% of the patients (10 of 11) with carcinoma in situ. The combination of sensitivity and specificity (70 and 99%, respectively) was the highest for bladder cancer screening in these patients. Telomerase outperformed cytology, BTA stat, NMP22, FDP, chemiluminescent hemoglobin and hemoglobin dipstick in the prediction of bladder cancer. [4]

Telomerase - According to a study published in JAMA (2005; 294:2052-6) Italian researchers reported the assay showed 90% sensitivity and 88% specificity. Specificity increased to 94% for those aged 75 years or younger. The same predictive capacity of activity levels was observed for patients with low-grade tumours or with negative cytology results. In particular, sensitivity was 93%, 87%, and 89% for tumour grades 1, 2, and 3, respectively.

Although the test is proven to identify low-grade tumours, it is not recommended for use in routine screening programs because of the low incidence of bladder cancer and should be aimed at high-risk subgroups, noted the authors, from Morgagni-Pierantoni Hospital, Forli. Theoretically, urine telomerase appears more promising than do non-invasive tests for bladder cancer to date. The main advantages of the test, are that it is non-invasive, can be performed under local anaesthetic, and is significantly less expensive, at $20, than the approximately $100 for cystoscopy or $50 for urinary cytology. It could be a good marker for high-risk screening groups. Furthermore, it shows a high sensitivity for the diagnosis of low-grade tumours that can escape detection during cytological examination. Results are usually available in 2 to 3 days.

10. Hyaluronidase and hyaluronic acid

Hyaluronidase seems to be directly involved in tumour growth and progression, and recent reports have shown this marker has high accuracy in detecting bladder cancer and evaluating its grade, Hyaluronidase and hyaluronic acid are associated with induction of angiogenesis. It has been shown that Hyaluronic acid (HA), the urinary HAase levels of intermediate (G2) to high- grade (G3) bladder cancer patients are five- to seven-fold elevated as compared to those of normal individuals and patients with other genitourinary conditions or low-grade (G1) bladder cancer. The increase in urinary HAase levels is due to the secretion of a tumour-derived HAase which is elevated eight-fold in G2/G3 tumour tissues. The HAase in bladder tumour tissues is secreted by tumour epithelial cells and is associated with the invasive/ metastatic potential of the tumour cells.[5]
Researchers from Brazil investigated the usefulness of HA for the detection of residual tumours that may remain after incomplete TUR. [10] The authors concluded that HA- in addition to being one of the best markers for the initial evaluation of bladder carcinoma- can be used to determine the presence of a residual tumour. This is associated with poor prognosis. Furthermore, haematuria does not seem to influence the content of urinary HA. Other tumor markers such as FISH (Fluorescence in Situ Hybridization) and NMP22 might be affected by instrumentation and therefore could not be evaluated this early.

11. Low values of urinary HA after TUR indicate a favourable prognosis and could probably avoid the second procedure

The researchers suggest that after more experience and follow-up using this assay in the clinical setting, it might be possible to predict not only the cases with residual tumour, but also those who require early radical surgery or those in whom this can be delayed.
In addition to being a good marker in the initial evaluation of bladder carcinoma thanks to its excellent sensitivity (83.1%) and specificity (90.1%), HA potential uses include follow-up, prognostic evaluation, preventing unnecessary interventions and/or to indicate cases where early radical intervention is necessary.10

12. BLCA-4

Robert H. Getzenberg and colleagues at the University of Pittsburgh, USA have identified several components of the nuclear matrix, one of which is called BLCA-4, that differentiate human bladder tumour cells from normal bladder cells. Normal samples from unaffected individuals did not react with the antibody, and importantly, BLCA-4 appears to be present throughout the bladder (i.e., in both normal and tumour areas) in bladder cancer patients. This "field effect" permitted development of a urine immunoassay for BLCA-4 that detects the presence of tumour anywhere in the bladder, regardless of stage or grade. The BLCA-4-urine immunoassay has a specificity of 100% and a sensitivity of 95%. According to Dr. Getzenberg, the assay is currently being tested by the Pittsburgh researchers in a clinical trial of individuals at high risk for bladder cancer. [6]

Using a prospectively determined cut-off, 67 of the 75 samples from patients with bladder cancer were positive for BLCA-4, resulting in an assay sensitivity of 89%. Also, 62 of the 65 samples from individuals without bladder cancer were negative for BLCA-4, resulting in an assay specificity of 95%. The authors concluded that the high sensitivity and specificity of the sandwich BLCA-4 immunoassay may allow for earlier detection and treatment of disease, thus greatly improving patient care. [7]

BLCA-4, appears to be associated with a "field effect" of the disease, and in clinical trials is able to separate individuals with bladder cancer from those without the disease with high sensitivity and specificity. BLCA-4 is a bladder cancer marker that is highly specific and occurs early in the development of the disease. It appears to be a transcription factor that may play a role in the regulation of the gene expression in bladder cancer. BLCA-4 is a marker with significant clinical utility that may have an active role in the disease.

13. Other proposed markers

DD 23 monoclonal antibody recognizes a 185 kDa antigen expressed by bladder cancer cells and has been proposed as an adjunct to cytology for the detection of bladder cancer. Urine fibronectin and chorionic gonadotropin (protein and mRNA transcript) may also be markers for transitional cell carcinoma of the bladder .

14. Role of urine markers in early detection of bladder cancer

Almost all cases of bladder cancer are found during the work-up of patients who present with haematuria (71), but most cases of haematuria are not caused by bladder cancer. Urologic disease is detected in 10% of subjects who present with haematuria, and bladder cancer is detected in fewer than half of these subjects (72,73,74). The work-up of patients with haematuria is costly and often requires cytology, cystoscopy, intravenous urography or computed tomography (75). Thus, tumor markers could be useful in identifying the patients in this high-risk group, which requires more intensive clinical work-up for bladder cancer. Zippe et al reported on the value of the urine NMP22 test in the evaluation of 330 patients with haematuria (76). The NMP22 test when used with a cut-off value of 10.0 u/ml detected all 18 cases of bladder cancer with 45 false positive cases (sensitivity, 100%; specificity, 85%). In this study, 267 unnecessary cystoscopy could have been avoided if cystoscopy had been directed by the NMP22 test. In a clinical trial submitted to the Food and Drug Administration (as Pre-Market Approval Data), the NMP22 test was elevated in 69.6% of 56 bladder cancer that were detected in the high risk group. In this report, the specificity was 67.7% (77). The NMP22 test has been cleared by the FDA for use as an aid to diagnose bladder cancer in individuals with risk factors or who have symptoms of bladder cancer. It is highly likely that other urine markers (e.g. BTA, UroVysion and Immunocyt) may also have value for cancer detection in subjects who present with haematuria. The high false positive rate is the major criticism of the urine-based tests when they are used to assess patients who present with haematuria or are used in patient surveillance. The low false negative rate of these tests is their strength, leading to a high negative predictive value that effectively rules out disease in a significant proportion of patients, thereby eliminating unnecessary clinical work-ups for bladder cancer.

15. Role of tissue markers for prognosis

Considerable research effort continues to be directed towards the identification of markers that predict the aggressive potential of superficial bladder tumors. Such information could lead to more effective surveillance protocols and permit more aggressive treatment of those patients with tumors most likely to progress to invasive or metastatic disease. Stein et al have performed an exhaustive review of a variety of biological markers reported to have prognostic value. More recently, p53 and other cell cycle control genes, chorionic gonadotropin beta gene transcripts, various cell matrix and adhesion proteins and differentially expressed NACB.

16. Role of urine markers for patient surveillance

Many reports have established the value of urine tumor marker tests in the early detection of recurrent bladder tumors, but as yet these urine tests cannot replace routine cystoscopy and cytology in the management of bladder cancer patients. Instead, they may be used as complementary adjuncts that direct more effective utilization of clinical procedures, thus reducing the cost of patient surveillance. Patients with superficial lesions of low grade (Ta, Grade 1 and II) are at lower risk for recurrence than patients with Ta Grade III and T1 tumors, and these lower-risk patients may need less intensive follow-up .

The urine markers used in patient surveillance have on occasion been criticized for their low sensitivity in detecting disease, but in most studies they have significantly improved the detection of bladder cancer when used in conjunction with cytology and cystoscopy. Voided urine cytology has its own limitations in detecting carcinoma in situ (cis) and low-grade bladder tumors. It appears that urine markers can assist in the early detection of recurrence in patients with carcinoma in situ and low-grade superficial tumors.

17. Conclusion

The availability of many new markers for bladder cancer raises the possibility of improving the rate of cancer detection by combined use of selected markers, measured either simultaneously or sequentially. The objective of such panel testing should be to improve both the sensitivity and the specificity for bladder cancer detection. Prospective clinical trials are undoubtedly necessary to prove their clinical value, before such panels could be implemented in routine patient care. It should also be noted that the stability of these tumour marker antigens must be better defined in order to minimize false negative test results. Improved definition of the disease conditions which can produce false positive test results for urine based markers could lead to more effective use of these tests for cancer detection. It seems a long way before these markers replace invasive testing, but at least it can help define those group of patients who need cystoscopic surveillance while sparing the majority of patients who do not need the procedure. This will bring enormous cost saving to the increasing health care cost we face in the presence of dwinding health care budget allocations from other competing needs.

18. References

[1] Bailey MJ. Urinary markers in bladder cancer. BJUI 2003;91:772-773.
[2] Eissa S, Kassim S, El-Ahmady O. Detection of bladder tumours: role of cytology, morphology-based assays, biochemical and molecular markers. Curr Opin Obstet Gynecol 2003;15:395-403.
[3] Fritsche HA. Bladder cancer and urine tumor marker tests. Diamandis EP Fritsche HA Lilja H Chan DW Schwartz MK eds. Tumor markers: physiology, pathobiology, technology and clinical applications 2002:281-286 AACC Press Washington.
[4] Kageyama S, Isono T, Iwaki H, Wakabayashi Y, Okada Y, Kontani K, et al. Identification by proteomic analysis of calreticulin as a marker for bladder cancer and evaluation of the diagnostic accuracy of its detection in urine. Clin Chem 2004;50:857-866.
[5] Celis A, Rasmussen HH, Celis P, Basse B, Lauridsen JB, Ratz G, et al. Short-term culturing of low-grade superficial bladder transitional cell carcinomas leads to changes in the expression levels of several proteins involved in key cellular activities. Electrophoresis 1999;20:355-361.
[6] Bravaccini S, Sanchini MA, Granato AM, Gunelli R, Nanni O, Amadori D, Calistri D, Silvestrini R. Urine telomerase activity for the detection of bladder cancer in females. J Urol. 2007 Jul;178(1):57-61.
[7] Sanchini MA, Gunelli R, Nanni O, Bravaccini S, Fabbri C, Sermasi A, Bercovich E, Ravaioli A, Amadori D, Calistri D. Relevance of urine telomerase in the diagnosis of bladder cancer. JAMA. 2005 Oct 26;294(16):2052-6.
[8] Sanchini MA, Bravaccini S, Medri Urine telomerase: an important marker in the diagnosis of bladder cancer.
[9] Roberta Gunelli, ; Oriana Nanni, ; Sara Bravaccini, ; Carla Fabbri, Alice Sermasi, Eduard Bercovich, Alberto Ravaioli,; Dino Amadori,; Daniele Calistri. JAMA. 2005;294:2052-2056.
[10] Van Le TS, Myers J, Konety BR, Barder T, Getzenberg RH. Functional characterization of the bladder cancer marker, BLCA-4. J.Clin Cancer Res. 2004 ;15;10(4):1384-1391.
[11] Messing EM, Teot L, Korman H, Underhill E, Barker E, Stork B, Qian J, Bostwick DG. J Urol. 2005;174:1238-41.
[12] Oeda T, Manabe D. Nippon Hinyokika Gakkai Zasshi [The usefulness of urinary FDP in the diagnosis of bladder cancer: comparison with NMP22, BTA and cytology]. 2001;92(1):1-5.
[13] Tilki D, Burger M, Dalbagni G, Grossman HB, Hakenberg OW, Palou J, Reich O, Rouprêt M, Shariat SF, Zlotta AR. Urine Markers for Detection and Surveillance of Non-Muscle- Invasive Bladder Cancer. Eur Urol. 2011 Jun 12.
[14] Khadjavi A, Barbero G, Destefanis P, Mandili G, Giribaldi G, Mannu F, Pantaleo A, Ceruti C, Bosio A, Rolle L, Turrini F, Fontana D. Evidence of abnormal tyrosine phosphorylated proteins in the urine of patients with bladder cancer: the road toward a new diagnostic tool? J Urol. 2011 May;185(5):1922-1929.
[15] Sagnak L, Ersoy H, Gucuk O, Ozok U, Topaloglu H. Diagnostic Value of a Urine-Based Tumor Marker for Screening Lower Urinary Tract in Low-Risk Patients with Asymptomatic Microscopic Haematuria. Urol Int. 2011 Jun 3.

[16] Yamada Y, Enokida H, Kojima S, Kawakami K, Chiyomaru T, Tatarano S, Yoshino H, Kawahara K, Nishiyama K, Seki N, Nakagawa M. MiR-96 and miR-183 detection in urine serve as potential tumor markers of urothelial carcinoma: correlation with stage and grade, and comparison with urinary cytology. Cancer Sci. 2011 Mar;102(3):522-529.

[17] Kehinde EO, Al-Mulla F, Kapila K, Anim JT. Comparison of the sensitivity and specificity of urine cytology, urinary nuclear matrix protein-22 and multi-target fluorescence in situ hybridization assay in the detection of bladder cancer. Scand J Urol Nephrol. 2011 Mar;45(2):113-121.

[18] Roobol MJ, Bangma CH, el Bouazzaoui S, Franken-Raab CG, Zwarthoff EC. Urol Oncol. 2010 Nov-Dec;28(6):686-90. Feasibility study of screening for bladder cancer with urinary molecular markers (the BLU-P project).

[19] Costa VL, Henrique R, Danielsen SA, Duarte-Pereira S, Eknaes M, Skotheim RI, Rodrigues A, Magalhães JS, Oliveira J, Lothe RA, Teixeira MR, Jerónimo C, Lind GE. Three epigenetic biomarkers, GDF15, TMEFF2, and VIM, accurately predict bladder cancer from DNA-based analyses of urine samples. Clin Cancer Res. 2010 Dec 1;16(23):5842-51.

[20] Margel D, Pesvner-Fischer M, Baniel J, Yossepowitch O, Cohen IR. Stress proteins and cytokines are urinary biomarkers for diagnosis and staging of bladder cancer. Eur Urol. 2011 Jan;59(1):113-119.

[21] Szarvas T, Singer BB, Becker M, Vom Dorp F, Jäger T, Szendroi A, Riesz P, Romics I, Rübben H, Ergün S. Urinary matrix metalloproteinase-7 level is associated with the presence of metastasis in bladder cancer. BJU Int. 2011 Apr;107(7):1069-73.

[22] Lotan Y, Shariat SF, Schmitz-Dräger BJ, Sanchez-Carbayo M, Jankevicius F, Racioppi M, Minner SJ, Stöhr B, Bassi PF, Grossman HB. Considerations on implementing diagnostic markers into clinical decision making in bladder cancer. Urol Oncol. 2010 Jul-Aug;28(4):441-8.

[23] Yutkin V, Nisman B, Pode D. Can urinary biomarkers replace cystoscopic examination in bladder cancer surveillance? Expert Rev Anticancer Ther. 2010 Jun;10(6):787-90.

[24] Lai Y, Ye J, Chen J, Zhang L, Wasi L, He Z, Zhou L, Li H, Yan Q, Gui Y, Cai Z, Wang X, Guan Z. UPK3A: a promising novel urinary marker for the detection of bladder cancer. Urology. 2010 Aug;76(2):514.6-11.

[25] Horstmann M, Bontrup H, Hennenlotter J, Taeger D, Weber A, Pesch B, Feil G, Patschan O, Johnen G, Stenzl A, Brüning T. Clinical experience with survivin as a biomarker for urothelial bladder cancer.World J Urol. 2010 Jun;28(3):399-404.

[26] Tsui KH, Tang P, Lin CY, Chang PL, Chang CH, Yung BY. Bikunin loss in urine as useful marker for bladder carcinoma. J Urol. 2010 Jan;183(1):339-44.

[27] Mengual L, Burset M, Ars E, Lozano JJ, Villavicencio H, Ribal MJ, Alcaraz A. DNA microarray expression profiling of bladder cancer allows identification of non-invasive diagnostic markers. J Urol. 2009 Aug;182(2):741-748.

[28] Lotan Y, Elias K, Svatek RS, Bagrodia A, Nuss G, Moran B, Sagalowsky AI. Bladder cancer screening in a high risk asymptomatic population using a point of care urine based protein tumour marker. J Urol. 2009 Jul;182(1):52-7; discussion 58.

[29] Svatek RS, Karam J, Karakiewicz PI, Gallina A, Casella R, Roehrborn CG, Shariat SF. Role of urinary cathepsin B and L in the detection of bladder urothelial cell carcinoma. J Urol. 2008 Feb;179(2):478-84; discussion 484.

[30] Cai T, Mazzoli S, Meacci F, Tinacci G, Nesi G, Zini E, Bartoletti R. Interleukin-6/10 ratio as a prognostic marker of recurrence in patients with intermediate risk urothelial bladder carcinoma. J Urol. 2007 Nov;178(5):1906-11;discussion 1911-2.

[31] Yossepowitch O, Herr HW, Donat SM. Use of urinary biomarkers for bladder cancer surveillance: patient perspectives. J Urol. 2007 Apr;177(4):1277-82; discussion 1282.

[32] Shariat SF, Marberger MJ, Lotan Y, Sanchez-Carbayo M, Zippe C, Lüdecke G, Boman H, Sawczuk I, Friedrich MG, Casella R, Mian C, Eissa S, Akaza H, Serretta V, Huland H, Hedelin H, Raina R, Miyanaga N, Sagalowsky AI, Roehrborn CG, Karakiewicz PI. Variability in the performance of nuclear matrix protein 22 for the detection of bladder cancer. J Urol. 2006 Sep;176(3):919-26; discussion 926.

[33] Margel D, Pesvner-Fischer M, Baniel J, Yossepowitch O, Cohen IR. Stress proteins and cytokines are urinary biomarkers for diagnosis and staging of bladder cancer. Eur Urol. 2011 Jan;59(1):113-9.

[34] Renard I, Joniau S, van Cleynenbreugel B, Collette C, Naômé C, Vlassenbroeck I, Nicolas H, de Leval J, Straub J, Van Criekinge W, Hamida W, Hellel M, Thomas A, de Leval L, Bierau K, Waltregny D. Identification and validation of the methylated TWIST1 and NID2 genes through real-time methylation-specific polymerase chain reaction assays for the noninvasive detection of primary bladder cancer in urine samples. Eur Urol. 2010 Jul;58(1):96-104.

[35] Tilki D, Singer BB, Shariat SF, Behrend A, Fernando M, Irmak S, Buchner A, Hooper AT, Stief CG, Reich O, Ergün S. CEACAM1: a novel urinary marker for bladder cancer detection. Eur Urol. 2010 Apr;57(4):648-654.

[36] van Rhijn BW. Considerations on the use of urine markers for bladder cancer. Eur Urol. 2008 May;53(5):880-881.

[37] Vrooman OP, Witjes JA. Urinary markers in bladder cancer. Eur Urol. 2008 May;53(5):909-916.

[38] Fernandez-Gomez J, Rodríguez-Martínez JJ, Barmadah SE, García Rodríguez J, Allende DM, Jalon A, Gonzalez R, Alvarez-Múgica M. Urinary CYFRA 21.1 is not a useful marker for the detection of recurrences in the follow-up of superficial bladder cancer. Eur Urol. 2007 May;51(5):1267-74.

[39] Golshani R, Hautmann SH, Estrella V, Cohen BL, Kyle CC, Manoharan M, Jorda M, Soloway MS, Lokeshwar VB. HAS1 expression in bladder cancer and its relation to urinary HA test. Int J Cancer. 2007 Apr 15;120(8):1712-20.

[40] Grossman HB, Blute ML, Dinney CP, Jones JS, Liou LS, Reuter VE, Soloway MS. The use of urine-based biomarkers in bladder cancer. Urology. 2006 Mar;67(3 Suppl 1):62-4.

[41] Simon MA, Lokeshwar VB, Soloway MS. Current bladder cancer tests: unnecessary or beneficial? Crit Rev Oncol Hematol. 2003 Aug;47(2):91-107.

3

Epigenetic Biomarkers in Bladder Cancer

Daniela Zimbardi, Mariana Bisarro dos Reis,
Érika da Costa Prando and Cláudia Aparecida Rainho
*Department of Genetics, Institute of Biosciences, Sao Paulo State University – UNESP,
Botucatu – SP,
Brazil*

1. Introduction

1.1 Epigenetics and cancer: An overview

Genetic and epigenetic alterations are hallmarks of human cancer. In the last few decades, it has been well established that epigenetic changes are important events in human cancer development and progression in addition to genetic alterations (such as chromosomal rearrangements, aneuploidies and point mutations). Epigenetics refers to the study of changes in gene expression that are determined by mechanisms other than changes in the DNA sequence. Epigenetic phenomena include X-chromosome inactivation, genomic imprinting, cellular differentiation and the maintenance of cell identity. These events are mediated by several molecular mechanisms, including DNA methylation, post-translational histone modifications and various RNA-mediated processes. Many studies in the field of epigenetics have focused on the effects of histone modifications and DNA methylation in the transcription process because these mechanisms are often linked and interdependent (Ballestar, 2011). A variety of methods are currently being applied to detect epigenetic changes, and the past two decades have shown an exponential increase in novel approaches aimed at elucidating the molecular basis of epigenetic inheritance.

DNA methylation is the most well studied epigenetic modification in human diseases (Fernandez et al., 2011). It involves the addition of a methyl group to the 5 carbon of a cytosine that is immediately followed by one guanine; i.e., DNA methylation typically occurs in a CpG dinucleotide context. CpG dinucleotides are generally underrepresented in the genome due to the increased mutation frequencies of the methylcytosines that are spontaneously converted to thymines. However, within the regions that are known as CpG islands, these dinucleotides are found at higher frequencies than is expected. It is believed that the human genome is comprised of approximately 38,000 CpG islands, and a large proportion of them (~37%) are located in the 5′ gene regulatory regions (promoters). The aberrant content of DNA methylation (global genome hypomethylation) and patterns of cytosine methylation, especially hypermethylation in promoter-associated CpG islands, are known to be associated with cancer. Gene-specific promoter hypermethylation causes the breakdown of normal cell physiology by silencing tumor suppressor genes, while DNA hypomethylation can reactivate oncogenes and repetitive sequences of the genome and lead to chromosomal instability (Sawan et al., 2008).

Histones (H2A, H2B, H3 and H4) are the main protein components of chromatin that package and order DNA into structural units that are called nucleosomes. The histone code consists of post-translational covalent changes of specific amino acid residues that are located at histone tails (NH_2 terminal regions). These modifications include methylation, acetylation, phosphorylation, poly-ADP ribosylation, ubiquitinylation, sumoylation, carbonylation and glycosylation (Kouzarides, 2007). The histone code and DNA methylation interact to promote the regulation of specific gene activity and mediate chromatin accessibility and compaction by changing the local chromatin structure, as has been reported to occur during the silencing of tumor suppressor genes. In cancer cells, the hypermethylation of CpG islands in the promoter regions of tumor suppressor genes was associated with a specific profile of histone markers such as the loss of acetylation of histones H3 and H4, loss of H3K4 trimethylation, and gains of methylation in lysine residues of histone H3 (such as H3K9 and H3K27) (Portela & Esteller, 2010).

The most recently discovered epigenetic modification is mediated by a small class of RNAs that are also known as microRNAs (miRNAs). These molecules promote the silencing of target genes by associating with the 3′ untranslated region of messenger RNA (mRNA), which culminates in endonucleolytic cleavage, mRNA degradation by deadenylation or the inhibition of mRNA translation (Valeri et al., 2009). It is estimated that at least 30% of all human genes are regulated by miRNAs. Similar to the protein-coding genes, the down-regulation of miRNAs in cancer cells has been correlated with the presence of DNA hypermethylation in the regulatory regions. In addition, these molecules (named epi-miRNAs) were recently found to regulate epigenetic enzymes, such as DNA methyltransferases and histone deacetylases. Thus, it is possible that epi-miRNAs could indirectly affect the expression of cancer-related genes (Fabbri & Callin, 2010).

In summary, epigenetics is one of the most promising fields in biomedical research. Novel strategies for risk assessment, early detection and new therapeutic targets may be revealed by epigenetic studies (Boumber & Issa, 2011). This chapter will summarize the common epigenetic aberrations that are detected in bladder cancer, their translational implications and possible epigenetic therapies.

2. Translational implications of epigenetic changes in bladder cancer

Bladder cancer is the fifth most commonly diagnosed non-cutaneous solid tumor and the second most common in the urological tract. Although many tumors that originate in this organ are superficial, with low risks of metastasis, bladder cancer has a high recurrence risk; the 4-year recurrence rate for patients with superficial tumors is 50%. Currently, the diagnosis of bladder cancer is based on histological, pathological and morphological parameters and provides only a generalized outcome for patients (Tanaka & Sonpadvde, 2011). The gold standard for detecting bladder cancer is cystoscopic examination, but this analysis is costly, causes discomfort to the patient (invasive method) and has variable sensitivity, providing only a generalized outcome to patients. In addition, the sensitivity of the cytological analysis is questionable, especially in cases of low-grade carcinoma (Kim & Kim, 2009). With the advent of targeted therapy, molecular biomarkers are becoming increasingly important in both clinical research and practice. These markers are being identified with the purpose of reducing the need for invasive follow-up examinations and also to anticipate the prognosis of individual patients. Furthermore, the early diagnosis of bladder cancer by non-invasive methods could allow for more effective treatment and optimize the success of surgical therapy.

The DNA methylation of CpG islands that are mapped to promoter regions of specific genes, such as tumor suppressor genes, has been extensively reported in many cancer types. In bladder cancer, this epigenetic event has been related to tumor development, staging, recurrence, progression and clinical outcome. More specifically, DNA methylation has been strongly associated with higher stages, high rates of tumor progression and high mortality in patients with this cancer. As was demonstrated by Wolff et al. (2010), the analysis of epigenetic backgrounds can allow for the differentiation between noninvasive and invasive tumors by the identification of the different epigenetic characteristics that are present, such as the extensive DNA hypomethylation that is observed in noninvasive tumors compared to the high rates of DNA hypermethylation in invasive urothelial cancer. This may explain why ~15% of tumors will progress to invasive disease and have poor prognosis, while others will remain with low rates of generate metastasis.

Currently, some histone modifications and the aberrant expression of miRNAs have been linked to tumorigenesis and have also been identified to be reliable and strong biomarkers for bladder cancer. MicroRNAs are specifically interesting because they are very stable in body fluids due to their small sizes and thus are resistant to degradation by nucleases, which are present in large quantities in urine (Tilki et al., 2011).

2.1 Candidate epigenetic biomarkers in the diagnosis of bladder cancer

Because DNA methylation is chemically and biologically stable and can be detected early in the carcinogenesis process, this epigenetic change has been considered to be a valuable potential diagnostic marker that is feasible to assess in clinical routine analysis through the investigation of exfoliated cells in the urine or blood of patients with bladder cancer and appears to be more sensitive than conventional cytology. A number of genes have been identified as being hypermethylated in the urine or tissue samples of cancer patients compared to healthy tissues, indicating that the down-regulation of these genes has some clinical relevance to the origin and development of the disease (Table 1).

One example is the *RUNX3* (runt-related transcription factor 3) gene, which has been mapped to 1p36 and is thought to be a tumor suppressor gene that is frequently deleted or transcriptionally silenced in patients with cancer. In a study that analyzed 124 tumor tissue samples, 73% were found to have a methylation-positive pattern compared to the methylation-free pattern that was exhibited by the normal bladder mucosa. Moreover, the methylation of this gene was found to confer a significant increase (100-fold) in the risk of tumor development (Kim et al., 2005), suggesting that it may have potential as a potent bladder cancer detection marker.

Our group also contributed to the literature surrounding epigenetic markers in bladder cancer. We discovered high rates of DNA methylation in exfoliated urinary cells, in which the *RARB* gene had a sensitivity of 95% and specificity of 71% for detecting the presence of cancer (Negraes et al., 2008). These results are concordant with the increased methylation frequencies that have been previously described (Chan et al., 2002; Hoque et al., 2006) and suggest that this gene could be considered as a diagnostic biomarker. It encodes a member of the thyroid-steroid hormone receptor superfamily of nuclear transcriptional regulators that binds retinoic acid (the biologically active form of vitamin A) and also mediates cellular signaling during embryonic morphogenesis and cell growth and differentiation. It is thought that this protein limits the growth of many cell types by regulating gene expression (Soprano et al., 2004).

In the study conducted by Renard et al. (2010), it was demonstrated that 2 genes (*TWIST1* and *NID2*) were frequently methylated in urine samples collected from bladder cancer patients, including those with early-stage and low-grade diseases, with a specificity of 93% and sensitivity of 90%, which was an improvement from the cytological method of detection (48%).

Besides the identification of DNA hypermethylation at a single *locus*, some authors have demonstrated that several genes may be analyzed together to generate a profile of hypermethylated genes. These profiles may be able to allow for a more sensitive and reliable marker for the detection of bladder cancer (Table 1). Based on this, Chan et al. (2002) discovered that the sensitivity of the methylation analysis (90.9%) of four genes (*DAPK1, RARB, CDH1* and *CDKN2A*) was higher than that of urine cytology (45.5%) for cancer detection and was more striking in low-grade cases (100% versus 11.1%).

Similarly, Urakami et al. (2006) found that the identification of the increased methylation of six Wnt-antagonist genes (*SFRP1, SFRP2, SFRP4, SFRP5, WIF1* and *DKK3*) could predict bladder tumors with a sensitivity of 77.2% and specificity of 66.7%. These genes are known to inhibit Wnt signaling by binding to specific molecules that act in this pathway. The DNA methylation and consequent functional loss of these genes may result in the activation of the Wnt signaling pathway and promote the dysregulation of cell proliferation and differentiation. The authors also discovered that two of these genes (*SFRP2* and *DKK3*) were able to act as independent predictors of bladder tumors ($P < 0.05$ and $P < 0.01$, respectively).

Friedrich et al. (2004) also suggested that the presence of a combination of DNA methylation at the 5′ regions of three apoptosis-associated genes (*DAPK1, BCL2* and *TERT*) in urine sediment could be diagnostic of bladder cancer with a sensitivity of 78%, suggesting that this combined methylation analysis was a highly sensitive method for the noninvasive detection of bladder cancer.

In addition, Hoque et al. (2006) proposed a two-stage predictor for the classification of bladder cancer that was based on an investigation of a panel composed of nine genes (*APC, ARF, CDH1, GSTP1, MGMT, CDKN2A, RARB, RASSF1A* and *TIMP3*) in urine sediment. In the first stage, patients who presented with DNA methylation in the promoters of at least one of four specific genes (*CDKN2A, ARF, MGMT* and *GSTP1*) were classified as having cancer (100% specificity). Moreover, patients with no methylation in these genes were subjected to a second stage of investigation with a logistic prediction of risk scores based on the promoter methylation of the five remaining genes (sensitivity of 82% and specificity of 96%).

Three of these genes had previously been investigated by Dulaimi et al. (2004), who demonstrated the feasibility of obtaining reproducible highly sensitive (87%) and 100% positive identifications of hypermethylation in a panel composed of the *APC, RASSF1A* and *CDKN2A* tumor suppressor genes in urine in cases of early-stage disease. In addition to *RASSF1A* (a tumor suppressor gene that is frequently inactivated in several cancer types), the other two genes chosen were involved in the *p53/p14*^{ARF} tumor suppressor gene pathway (*CDKN2A* gene) (Sherr & McCormick, 2002) and the Wnt signaling pathway (*APC* gene) (Taipale & Beachy, 2001). The evaluation of this panel yielded superior results compared to those of cytology in the detection of bladder cancer. Yates et al. (2006) also investigated the *APC, RASSF1A* and *CDH1* genes in urine. This panel generated a lower sensitivity (69%) and specificity (60%) than the former; however, the diagnostic accuracy was 86%.

Many of the genes that have been chosen to be investigated in combined analyses to generate panels have frequently been suggested to be individually methylated in bladder cancer, such as *RASSF1A*. The DNA methylation of this gene had previously been reported to be able to detect bladder cancer in urine samples with 100% sensitivity by Chan et al. (2003). The authors advocated that the detection of gene methylation using multiple markers could increase both the sensitivity and specificity of cancer detection, and the addition of *RASSF1A* to this panel could improve the diagnostic accuracy even further.

Yu et al. (2007) discovered that the methylation of a panel composed by 11 genes (*SALL3, CFTR, ABCC6, HPSE, RASSF1A, MT1A, ALX4, CDH13, RPRM, APBA1* and *BRCA1*) in urine sediments showed positive correlations with diagnosis in 121 out of 132 bladder cancer cases with a sensitivity of 91.7% and accuracy of 87%. Remarkably, this approach was able to detect more than 75% of tumors at stage 0a and 88% of stage I tumors, indicating the value of this panel in the early diagnosis of bladder cancer.

Likewise, a three-gene (*GDF15, TMEFF2* and *VIM*) panel was able to detect bladder cancer in urine samples with a sensitivity of 94% and specificity of 100% (Costa et al., 2010), exceeding the detection rates that are normally obtained using conventional cytopathology and cytology. This panel of genes was selected based on stringent criteria after a screening test that employed a genome-wide approach and was distinctive because it was able to detect bladder cancer by noninvasive methods even when patients with kidney or prostate cancer were used as controls. These three genes are biologically relevant to carcinogenesis because *TMEFF2* (mapped at 2q32.3) and *VIM* (mapped at 10p13) were previously found to be silenced by promoter methylation in esophageal, colorectal (Shirahata et al., 2009; Tsunoda et al., 2009) and bladder cancer (Hellwinkel et al., 2008). *GDF15* (mapped to 19p13.11) is a member of the transforming growth factor (TGF)-β superfamily and may act as a tumor suppressor gene in early-stage cancers (Eling et al., 2006).

Another biomarker of interest for the detection of urothelial cancer, according to Ellinger et al. (2008), is cell-free serum DNA methylation. The authors detected that the diagnostic accuracy of this marker increased when hypermethylation at multiple gene sites was assessed simultaneously, particularly at the *GSTP1, RARRES1* or *APC* genes (80% sensitivity and 93% specificity).

The list of aberrant epigenetically regulated genes continues to grow. Is important to note that the same genes have been investigated by different groups, and the methylation rates found may vary from one report to another. Results may reflect the distinct methodologies employed, the numbers and types of samples (urine, surgical tissue and/or serum) as well as disease classifications. Nevertheless, the reports above highlight the high potential of DNA methylation markers for the effective early detection of bladder cancer using noninvasive urine tests.

The measurement of global cytosine methylation rates (%5-mC) concomitantly with the DNA methylation of specific genes could be a useful biomarker to assess a patient's susceptibility to bladder cancer. In a large case-control study conducted by Moore et al. (2008), the DNA hypomethylation of leukocytes was strongly associated with an increased bladder cancer risk, and this association was independent of smoking and other assessed risk factors.

Recently, evidence has emerged that circulating miRNAs are present in human body fluids (as urine) in concentrations that are subject to variation during cancer pathogenesis or development (Iguchi et al., 2010), as was reported by Dudziec et al. (2011). The authors discovered that the combined low expression levels of miR-152, -328 and -1224-3p allowed for accurate diagnosis with 81% sensitivity and 75% specificity. These miRNAs were found to be epigenetically regulated by DNA methylation at CpG islands and the shores (regions of less dense CpG dinucleotides) that surrounded them following a genome-wide screening. In addition, Hanke et al. (2010) found that the ratio of miR-126:miR-152 enabled the detection of bladder cancer from urine samples with a specificity of 82% and a sensitivity of 72%; thus, they may be used as a tumor markers for this disease.

In addition, Yamada et al. (2011) identified one microRNA (miR-96) that may be a useful diagnostic marker with high sensitivity and specificity (71.0% and 89.2%, respectively) when assessed in combination with urinary cytology (80% diagnostic accuracy). This molecule, which has been mapped to 7q32, is a putative onco-miRNA that has been demonstrated to be able to down-regulate tumor suppressor genes. It was found to be up-regulated in a previous study conducted by the same group (Ichimi et al., 2009), in which the microRNA expression signatures that are specific to bladder cancer were determined, and a subset of 7 microRNAs (miR-145, miR-30a-3p, miR-133a, miR-133b, miR-195, miR-125b and miR-199a*) that are significantly down-regulated in bladder cancer were validated. These microRNAs were sufficiently sensitive (>70%) and specific (>75%) to distinguish bladder cancer from normal epithelium.

As mentioned above, not only the DNA methylation but also the expression profile of the miRNA molecules have been closely associated with the diagnosis of bladder cancer.

Epigenetic biomarker	Samples	Sensitivity/ specificity/ OR	Supporting literature
DNA methylation			
RASSF1A	Urine	Sensitivity: 100%	Chan et al., 2003
RUNX3	Tissue	OR 107.55 (95% CI, 6.33-1827.39)	Kim et al., 2005
RARB	Bladder washing (exfoliated cells)	OR/Sensitivity/specificity: 48.89/95%/71%	Negraes et al., 2008
TWIST1 and *NID2*	Urine	Sensitivity/specificity: 90%/93%	Renard et a., 2010
DAPK1, RARB, CDH1 and *CDKN2A*	Urine	Sensitivity/specificity: 90.9%/76.4%	Chan et al., 2002
APC, RASSF1A and *CDKN2A*	Urine	Sensitivity/specificity: 87%/100%	Dulaimi et al., 2004
DAPK1, BCL2 and *TERT*	Urine	Sensitivity: 78%	Friedrich et al., 2004
APC, ARF, CDH1, GSTP1, MGMT, CDKN2A, RARB, RASSF1A and *TIMP3*	Urine	1st stage sensitivity: 100% 2nd stage Sensitivity/specificity: 82%/96%	Hoque et al., 2006
SFRP1, SFRP2, SFRP4, SFRP5, WIF1, DKK3	Tissue	Sensitivity/specificity: 77.2%/66.7%	Urakami et al., 2006
APC, RASSF1A and	Urine	Sensitivity/specificity:	Yates et al., 2006

Epigenetic biomarker	Samples	Sensitivity/ specificity/ OR	Supporting literature
CDH1		69%/60%	
SALL3, CFTR, ABCC6, HPSE, RASSF1A, MT1A, ALX4, CDH13, RPRM, APBA1 and *BRCA1*	Urine	Sensitivity/especificity: 91.7%/87%	Yu et al., 2007
GSTP1, RARRES1, APC	Cell-free serum DNA	Sensitivity/specificity: 80%/93%	Ellinger et al., 2008
GDF15, TMEFF2 and *VIM*	Urine	Sensitivity/specificity: 94%/100%	Costa et al., 2010
%5-mC of leukocytes	Blood cells	OR 1.38 (95% CI:1.05–1.08, p=0.02)	Moore et al., 2008
miRNAs			
miR-145, miR-30a-3p, miR-133a, miR-133b, miR-195, miR-125b and miR-199a*	Tissue	Sensitivity/specificity: >70%/>75%	Ichimi et al., 2009
RNA ratio of miR-126:miR-152	Urine	Sensitivity/specificity: 72%/82%	Hanke et al., 2010
miR-152, -328 and -1224	Urine	Sensitivity/specificity: 81%/75%	Dudziec et al., 2011
miR-96	Urine	Sensitivity/specificity: 71%/89.2%	Yamada et al., 2011

Table 1. Epigenetic diagnostic markers in bladder cancer. The genes were described as official symbols according recommendations of Guidelines for Human Gene Nomenclature. More information about specific genes can be achieved at http://www.genenames.org/guidelines.html.

2.2 Candidate epigenetic biomarkers in the prognosis of bladder cancer

The knowledge of prognostic factors is of great importance for the determination of therapeutic strategies and to enable the application of different modalities of therapy in cancer treatment. In cases of bladder cancer, patients are monitored for recurrence or progression by periodic cystoscopy and urine cytological analysis, the frequencies of which vary depending on the risk factors that are associated with the disease. Thus, the discovery of more sensitive and non-invasive tumor markers that can help to predict tumor recurrence, progression and metastasis are required, and epigenetic alterations may be promising new potential prognostic markers for bladder cancer.

Bladder tumors may be superficial, with low risks of metastasis, but may have high recurrence risks (McConkey et al., 2010). Several genes that are related to the progression and prognosis of bladder cancer have been identified in bladder washes, urine and tumor tissues using various molecular and epigenetic approaches (Mitra et al., 2006) and are considered to be potential markers (Table 2).

Maruyama et al. (2001) determined the methylation statuses of 10 genes in 98 fresh bladder tumor tissues and found that multiple genes are methylated during the process of bladder cancer development. Their results also indicated that the frequent methylation of four genes (*CDH1, CDH13, RASSF1A* and *APC*) together with high MIs (median methylation index) were correlated with poor prognosis (tumors showed high grade, nonpapillary growth patterns, muscle invasions, advanced tumor stages and aneuploidies). In addition, the methylation of *CDH1, FHIT* and high MIs were associated with reduced patient survival rates.

In a study performed by Catto et al. (2005) that employed a large cohort of urothelial carcinomas, CpG hypermethylation at *DAPK* was associated with higher progression rates (log-rank P = .014) in all of the transitional-cell carcinoma (TCC) samples that were investigated compared to unmethylated samples at this *locus*.

In another study, Christoph et al. (2006) selected related genes as targets of p53 in the apoptotic cycle to perform a quantitative analysis of 110 tumor samples. The authors found that *APAF1* methylation levels were correlated with tumor stages and grades. In addition, the methylation levels of the *APAF1* and *IGFBP3* genes enabled tumors with higher recurrence risks to be distinguished from low-risk tumors in non-muscle-invasive and muscle-invasive tumors. The epigenetic inactivation of pro-apoptotic genes may be important events that are related to the progression and increased aggressiveness of tumors that are hypermethylated in these *loci*.

In addition, the hypermethylation of the promoter region of the *TIMP3* gene detected in urine sediments was found to be associated with an increased risk of death (Hoque et al., 2008). Other genes also have been found to undergo aberrant promoter methylation and were associated with poor prognosis in bladder cancer, including the hypermethylation of the *RUNX3* promoter, which was correlated with the development of invasive tumors, tumor progression and cancer specific-survival in patients with TCC (Kim et al., 2008). The methylation of this gene was also shown to be related to an increased risk of developing bladder cancer (Kim et al., 2005), suggesting that this gene not only suppresses the aggressiveness of tumors but also inhibits the tumor development.

Beyond to the tumor size and grade parameters, response to treatment is also an important prognostic factor because multidrug resistance to chemotherapy is a major obstacle in the treatment of cancer patients. Tada et al. (2000) showed that the overexpression of the *ABCB1* gene may be a prognostic factor indicating recurrence in bladder cancer, and the hypomethylation of the promoter of this gene may be necessary for the development of increased *ABCB1* mRNA levels and multidrug resistance.

Global DNA hypomethylation is also a common phenomenon that has been reported in bladder cancer (Seifert et al., 2007). The loss of DNA methylation in repetitive sequences may account for a majority of the global hypomethylation that characterizes a large percentage of human cancers. Neuhausen et al. (2006) found that the hypomethylation of LINE-1 retrotransposons was present in 90% of the urothelial carcinoma specimens that were studied, and the absence of this epigenetic change was indicative of a better clinical prognosis. In a high-throughput DNA methylation analysis, a distinct hypomethylation pattern was found in non-invasive (Ta-T1) urothelial tumors compared to both normal urothelium and invasive tumors (Wolff et al., 2010). These researchers found a substantial number of probes to be hypomethylated in non-invasive tumors only, suggesting that lower levels of DNA methylation may be related to a less malignant phenotype.

A particularly interesting example of epigenetic regulation is genomic imprinting, in which one copy of a gene is silenced in a manner determined by its parental origin. Thus, imprinted genes show parental-specific monoallelic expression. The loss of allele-specific expression pattern is termed as loss of imprinting (LOI), an event described in several types of pediatric and adult cancers (Monk, 2010). LOI has already been identified as an

Clinical - histolopathological parameters	Epigenetic biomarker	Supporting literature
Grade	**DNA methylation** *CDKN2A, BCL2, TERT, EDNRB, CDH1, RASSF1A, APC, CDH13*	Maruyama et al., 2001; Domínguez et al., 2002; Friedrich et al., 2004
Stage	**DNA methylation** *TIMP3, CDKN2A, RASSF1A, BCL2, OPCML, CDH1, APC, CDH13* **Histone modification** H4K20me1	Maruyama et al., 2001; Domínguez et al., 2002; Friedrich et al., 2004; Hoque et al., 2008; Schneider et al. 2011; Duarte-Pereira et al., 2011
Recurrence	**DNA methylation** *DAPK1, H19, TIMP3*	Ariel *et al.*, 2000; Tada et al., 2002; Friedrich et al., 2005
Survival	**DNA methylation** *TIMP3, OPCML, RUNX3, FHIT, CDH1* **Histone modification** H4K20me3	Maruyama et al., 2001; Kim et al., 2008; Hoque et al., 2008; Schneider et al. 2011; Duarte-Pereira et al., 2011
Metastasis	**DNA methylation** *TIMP3* **miRNA expression** miR-452, miR-452*	Hoque et al., 2008; Veerla et al., 2009
Muscle invasion	**DNA methylation** *CDKN2A, CDH1, RASSF1A, APC, CDH13* **miRNA expression** miR-222, miR-125b	Maruyama et al., 2001; Domínguez et al., 2002; Veerla et al., 2009
Tumor progression	**DNA methylation** *RASSF1A, CDH1, TNFRSF25, EDNRB, APC, DAPK1, H19* **Histone modification** H3K4me1, H4K20me1, H4K20me2, H4K20me3 **miRNA expression** Set of miR-21, miR-510, miR-492, miR-20a, miR-198 and set of miR-455-5p, miR-143, miR-145, miR-125b, miR-503	Catto et al., 2005; Yates et al., 2007; Dyrskjøt et al., 2009; Schneider et al. 2011

Table 2. Epigenetic prognostic markers in bladder cancer. The genes were described as official symbols according recommendations of Guidelines for Human Gene Nomenclature. More information about specific genes can be achieved at http://www.genenames.org/guidelines.html.

epimarker of cancer development. The *IGF2* and *H19* imprinted genes have been well documented in the literature. Some studies showed that the *H19* gene is involved in the development of bladder cancer (Ariel et al., 1995; Elkin et al., 1995) and is associated with high recurrence risks for this tumor type (Ariel et al., 2000). Furthermore, insulin-like growth factor-II (IGF-II) loss of imprinting (LOI) in a series of paired tumoral and normal adjacent bladder tissues and E-cadherin (*CDH1*) immunolocalization suggested a possible mechanism underlying E-cadherin relocalization to the cytoplasm, that is, the presence of aberrant levels of IGF-II due in some cases to *IGF2* LOI (Gallagher et al., 2008). Furthermore, the finding of LOI in the tumoral adjacent normal samples holds promise of *IGF2* LOI as a predictor of tumor development.

Others epigenetic mechanisms in cancer patients remain less comprehensively understood. One of these epigenetic changes involves the histone modifications, which include changes in their levels and distribution at gene promoters, gene coding regions, repetitive DNA sequences and other genomic elements (Kurdistani, 2011). In a recent study, Schneider et al. (2011) found that global levels of H3K4me1, H4K20me1, H4K20me2 and H4K20me3 were decreased compared to normal urothelium. The distribution of these histone modifications were associated with the risk of metastasis in muscle-invasive compared to non-muscle-invasive bladder cancers. The authors also showed that H4K20me1 levels were increased in patients with non-muscle-invasive bladder cancer with advanced pT stages and less differentiated bladder cancer, and H4K20me3 levels were significantly correlated with mortality after radical cystectomy in patients with muscle-invasive cancer.

Recently, several groups have questioned whether the miRNA expression profiles or even single miRNAs could act as useful biomarkers not only for cancer diagnosis but also for prognosis and treatment optimization (Lu et al., 2005; Calin & Croce, 2006). Dyrskjøt et al. (2009) identified the aberrant expression of several miRNAs in 106 samples from patients with different stages of bladder cancer and associated their profiles with disease progression. Among the miRNAs that were differentially expressed in normal bladder tissue compared to that of bladder cancer, two subsets [(miR-21, miR-510, miR-492, miR-20a, miR-198) and (miR-455-5p, miR-143, miR-145, miR-125b, miR-503)] were up- and down-regulated by two-fold, respectively. In another large-scale study that evaluated miRNA expression, high expression levels of miR-222 and miR-125b were observed in muscle-invasive tumors, and miR-452 and miR-452* were shown to be over-expressed in node-positive tumors (Veerla et al., 2009).

Moreover, aberrant DNA methylation has been implicated in the deregulation of several miRNAs in different types of cancer (Lujambio et al., 2007). Wiklund et al. (2011) studied this relationship and found that the miR-200 family and miR-205 are concurrently silenced and that DNA hypermethylation would be associated with the silencing of these microRNAs in invasive bladder tumors. They also found that the loss of miR-200c expression was associated with disease progression of muscle-invasive cancers and with poor prognosis.

3. The promise of epigenetic therapy

The knowledge of epigenetic alterations that are associated with human cancers and their potential reversibility has prompted the development of drugs that target epigenetic enzymes. Either natural or synthetic modulators can be utilized to restore normal epigenetic and gene expression patterns; for example, by restoring the expression of the frequently silenced *RUNX3* gene, which is considered to be good target for this new therapeutic modality since the loss of its function in cancer cells due to genetic mutations is a rare event (Kim et al., 2005). The epigenetic therapy can be used alone or in combination with other therapeutic modalities, such as chemotherapy, immunotherapy or radiotherapy. This approach will eventually lead to targeted therapies that are suited for specific molecular defects, thereby significantly decreasing the morbidity associated with bladder cancer in addition to other cancers (Balmain, 2002; Kim & Kim, 2009; Mund & Lyko, 2010).

Two principal classes of epigenetic drugs have been demonstrated to be clinically relevant: DNA methyltransferase (DNMT) inhibitors and histone deacetylase (HDAC) inhibitors (Esteller, 2005) (Table 3). Novel epigenetic compounds that are of potential interest as clinical therapeutic drugs include the histone acetyltransferase inhibitors, such as anacardic acid, curcumin and peptide CoA conjugates. In addition, histone methyltransferase inhibitors and HDACis that are specific for SIRT1 (class III HDAC), such as nicotinamide and splitomycin, are now under intense analysis (Ballestar & Esteller, 2008; Greiner et al., 2005).

3.1 DNMTs inhibitors

Genes that are silenced by DNA hypermethylation may be reactivated by small molecules that are called DNMT inhibitors. These agents may be structural analogues of the nucleoside deoxycytidine or non-nucleoside analogues. The analogues, after being phosphorylated by kinases that convert the nucleosides into nucleotides, can be incorporated into DNA and subsequently inhibit DNMT activity by forming a covalent bond with the cysteine residue in the active DNMT site. However, it has also been shown that such incorporation may lead to instabilities in DNA structure and even DNA damage (Bouchard & Momparler, 1983; Goffin & Eisenhauer, 2002).

Two prominent examples are the cytosine analogs 5-azacytidine (azacytidine, Vidaza) and 2′-deoxy-5-azacytidine (decitabine, Dacogen), which are potent inhibitors of DNMTs (Table 3) and have been approved by the FDA (Food and Drug Administration) for the treatment of myelodysplastic syndrome, a pre-leukemic bone marrow disorder (Lübbert, 2000). Various additional molecules has been found to possess better stability and less toxicity and are currently being investigated as DNMT inhibitors in preclinical experiments, such as dihydro-5-azacytidine, arabinofuranosyl-5-azacytosine (fazarabine) and zebularine (Cheng et al., 2003).

Azacytidine and decitabine have been widely used in cell culture systems to reverse DNA hypermethylation and restore silenced gene expression. However, results from *in vivo* studies are not satisfactory, especially with solid tumors in which limited efficacy has been encountered. In general, both agents are unstable in aqueous solutions, have short half-lives and need to be freshly prepared before administration. In addition, both drugs have relatively poor bioavailabilities and high cytotoxic effects with potential risks, such as myelotoxicity, mutagenesis, and tumorigenesis, which have limited their clinical applications (Jackson-Grusby et al., 2007).

Despite this discouraging data, the orally administered zebularine shows some promise. It was shown to suppress the growth of TCC in bladder xenografts in nude mice and was less toxic than other nucleoside analogues. In addition, when zebularine was given at a lower dose after an initial dose of decitabine, a profound demethylation of the *CDKN2A* gene promoter was observed. These results provide a rationale for the strategy of combining an

initial administration of a parenteral DNMT inhibitor with a subsequent low dose of oral zebularine (Cheng et al., 2004; Zhang et al., 2006).
Another group of compounds are called non-nucleoside analogues. These small molecules inhibit DNA methylation by binding directly to the catalytic site of the DNMT enzyme without being incorporated into the DNA. The local anesthetic procaine and its derivative procainamide, which is an approved antiarrhythmic drug, have exhibited demethylating activities. For example, Lin et al. (2001) reported that procainamide was able to restore *GSTP1* gene expression by reversing the hypermethylation of the promoter CpG islands of androgen-sensitive human prostate adenocarcinoma (LNCaP) cells *in vitro* and *in vivo*. Because these agents do not incorporate into DNA, it is expected that they may have less genotoxicity than nucleoside DNMT inhibitors. In addition, (-)-epigallocatechin-3-gallate (EGCG), the main polyphenol compound in green tea, also acts as DNMT inhibitor . Cancer cells treated with micromolar concentrations of EGCG showed reduced DNA methylation and the increased transcription of tumor suppressor genes. However, it is still unknown whether EGCG has a direct inhibitory effect on DNMTs (Fang et al., 2003; Villar-Garea et al., 2003).

3.2 HDAC inhibitors

A variety of structurally distinct groups of compounds have been identified as histone deacetylase inhibitors (HDACi) (Table 3). These compounds inhibit histone deacetylase activity by binding to the catalytic site of the enzyme and chelating zinc ions because they share similar structures with the substrates (Finnin et al., 1999). Similar to their effects on gene expression and differentiation, HDACi have also been shown to be efficient inducers of apoptosis in several cellular systems. The precise mechanism of this effect is under investigation, and it has been suggested that they may affect cellular oxidative stress and DNA damage induction. They have shown impressive activities in preclinical studies as well as selectivity for neoplastic cells. Many HDACi are being tested in clinical trials for various malignancies (Bolden et al., 2006; Xu et al., 2007).
The class of the HDAC inhibitors is divided into four groups: hydroxamic acids, cyclic tetrapeptides, short-chain fatty acids and benzamides. The hydroxamate compounds are more potent and have higher inhibitory effects. Trichostatin A from *Streptomyces hygroscopicus* is active at nanomolar concentrations, while the synthetic compounds, such as suberoylanilide hydroxamic acid (SAHA), can function in low micromolar or nanomolar ranges. Cyclic tetrapeptides are very potent compounds and can inhibit histone deacetylase at nanomolar concentrations. Short-chain fatty acid compounds usually require millimolar concentrations to inhibit histone deacetylase activities *in vivo*; therefore, their clinical applicability could be limited. The fourth class is the benzamides, such as MS-275 and CI-994, which are effective at micromolar concentrations (Rosato et al., 2003; Zhang et al., 2006).
The clinical potentials of histone deacetylase inhibitors have been suggested by several promising *in vivo* studies. For example, SAHA was FDA approved in Oct. 2006 for the treatment of cutaneous T cell lymphoma (CTCL), and it is under a phase I clinical trial for use in patients with TCC (Mann et al., 2007). Preliminary reports have indicated that 2 out of 6 patients with metastatic TCC disease have had objective tumor regression and tumor-related symptom relief (Kelly et al., 2003). The induction of *CDKN1A* messenger RNA and

Group	Drug	Clinical status
DNMT inhibitor		
Nucleoside analogues	5-Azacyticine	Approved 2004 for MDS
	2´-Deoxy-5-azacytidine	Approved 2006 for MDS
	Zebularine	Preclinical
Non-nucleoside analogues	Hydralazine	Phase I > II for cervical Ca
	MG98	Phase I > II for advanced metastatic tumors
	Procaine	Preclinical
	RNAi	Preclinical
	Epigallocatichin-3-gallate	Preclinical
	Psammaplin A	Preclinical
HDAC inhibitor		
Hydroxamic acids	Suberoylanilide hydroxamic acid (SAHA)	Approved 2006 for CTCL
	Panobinostat	Phase I > II > III for breast Ca, gliomas, prostate Ca, NSCLC, CTCL, leukemia
	Belinostat	Phase I > II for ovarian Ca, CTCL, lymphoma, multiple myeloma, leukemia
	Trichostatin A	Preclinical
Cyclic tetrapeptides	Depsipeptide, Romidepsin	Approved 2009 for CTCL
Short-chain fatty acids	Valproic acid	Phase I > II > III for melanoma, myelodysplastic syndrome, leukemia, chronic lymphocytic leukemia, cervical Ca, breast Ca
	AN-9	Phase I > II for malignant melanoma, leukemia, lymphoma, NSCLC
Benzamides	Entinostat	Phase I > II for breast Ca, acute lymphoblastic leukemia, Hodgkin's lymphoma, MDS, renal Ca, colorectal Ca, lung Ca
	Mocetinostat	Phase I > II for breast Ca, NSCLC, prostate Ca, stomach Ca, non-Hodgkin's lymphoma, Hodgkin's lymphoma, AML, CLL, lymphoma
	N-Acetyldinaline	Phase I > II > III for multiple myeloma, lung Ca, pancreatic Ca

Table 3. List of the main DNMT and HDAC inhibitors and their current clinical trial status. MDS: myelodysplastic syndrome, CTCL: cutaneous T cell lymphoma, NSCLC: non small cell lung cancer, AML: acute myeloid leukemia, CLL: Chronic lymphocytic leukemia, Ca: cancer. Clinical status source: clinicaltrials.gov.

protein levels in T24 cells following SAHA exposure mediated by increased acetyl H3 and H4 levels in the respective promoter region may contribute to its tumor inhibitory effect

(Richon et al., 2000). Other researchers have reported similar inhibitory effects on bladder tumor growth using trichostatin A and pyroxamide on T24 cells. Additionally, trichostatin A is able to suppress 70% of tumor growth with no detectable toxicity in EJ and UM-UC-3 xenograft models (Canes et al., 2005).

3.3 Combination therapy

The emerging concept of gene silencing involves the interaction of multiple factors that may act in a sequential manner. It is also known that a single agent may not be able to eradicate a tumor mass that is derived from a very heterogeneous population of cells. Moreover, the adverse toxic effects that are caused by single-agent treatments, especially at high doses, call for a rationalized therapeutic approach with low-dosage drug combinations. Accumulating evidence has shown that the combination of histone deacetylase inhibitors and DNMT inhibitors is very effective (and synergistic) in inducing apoptosis, differentiation and/or cell growth arrest in various human cancer cell lines (Gottlicher et al., 2001; Mei et al., 2004; Stirzaker et al., 2004).

In urologic cancers, Cameron et al. (1999) showed that the combination of decitabine and trichostatin A stimulated a synergistic reactivation of several tumor suppressor genes. Dunn et al. (2005) reported that the combination of DNMT inhibitors and histone deacetylase inhibitors was able to reactivate the sensitivities of LNCaP cells to interferon treatment by the re-expression of JAK1 kinase, which is a key mediator of both interferon-gamma and interferon-alpha/beta receptor-elicited effects. Another strategy is to combine either histone deacetylase inhibitors or DNMT inhibitors with conventional therapies, as was demonstrated by Zhang et al. (2007), who indicated that the combination of FK228 (a HDAC inhibitor) and docetaxel (chemotherapeutic drug) caused a synergistic growth inhibition in androgen-independent prostate cancer cell lines. Moreover, single treatments with SAHA or MS-275 show enhanced radiation-induced cytotoxicity in DU-145 cells both *in vitro* and *in vivo* (Chinnaiyan et al., 2005).

4. Future

There is a great deal of evidence that demonstrates the connections between epigenetic modification enzymes and cancer. Epigenetic alterations contribute to tumorigenesis by the activation of oncogenes or inactivation of tumor suppressor genes. The identification of molecules that can modulate epigenetic enzymes could lead to the prevention of oncogene transcription and activation of tumor repressors, and thus it is an important topic to research (Zheng, 2008).

A major impediment to the use of such drugs is that they are nonspecific and may reactivate genes non-discriminately. However, this does not seem to be a problem in the present case because DNA methylation inhibitors only act on dividing cells and leave normal, non-dividing cells unaffected. Also, it seems that the drugs preferentially activate genes that have become abnormally silenced in cancer. Further studies are required to establish an unambiguous proof of concept for epigenetic cancer therapies (Jones & Baylin, 2007; Liang et al., 2002; Mund & Lyko, 2010).

For future clinical applications, researchers should focus on several aspects, including the biomarkers that predict drug responses. Researchers should also focus on the screening of new, more effective and less toxic agents. The psammaplin, for example, a family of bromotyrosine derivatives that have been extracted from the marine sponge *Pseudoceratina purpurea,* appear to be a novel class of compounds with the ability to inhibit both DNMT and histone deacetylase activities (Pina et al., 2003).

In addition, exploring the silencing of specific genes by RNA interference for key epigenetic regulatory complexes could enhance therapeutic indices. For example, DNMT-specific siRNA (single-interfering RNA) is able to elicit the demethylation of several epigenetically silenced genes. Additionally, the treatment of cultured cells *in vivo* with demethylating agents, either alone or in combination with HDACi, has been shown to re-activate the expression of tumor-suppressor miRNAs, such as miR-124a and miR-127, causing the corresponding repression of their oncogenic targets. Although the successful delivery of siRNAs to solid tumors has yet to be achieved, designing small-molecule siRNAs to mimic tumor-suppressor miRNAs could be a potential method to selectively repress the expression of oncogenes (Leu et al., 2003; Saito et al., 2006).

In the next decade, with the availability of gene profiling databases of epigenetic modifiers, it is expected that epigenetic therapy will be translated from the bench to the clinical arena and become a real alternative to conventional cancer treatments (Rodríguez-Paredes & Esteller, 2011; Zhang et al., 2006).

In summary, the field of epigenetic biomarker studies is still new but shows promise in the clinical management of cancer. Valuable progress has been made on this end, and the combination of existing and newly discovered biomarkers will likely allow for more accurate diagnosis. Thus, patients will be able to benefit from this new era of personalized medicine, in which biomarkers will allow for direct treatments with more effective therapeutic agents.

5. References

Ariel, I.; Sughayer, M.; Fellig, Y.; Pizov, G.; Ayesh, S.; Podeh, D.; Libdeh, B.A.; Levy, C.; Birman, T.; Tykocinski, M.L.; de Groot, N. & Hochberg, A. (2000). The imprinted H19 gene is a marker of early recurrence in human bladder carcinoma. *Molecular Pathology,* Vol.53, No.6, pp. 320-323.

Ariel, I.; Lustig, O.; Schneider, T.; Pizov, G.; Sappir, M.; De-Groot, N. & Hochberg, A. (1995). The imprinted H19 gene as a tumor marker in bladder carcinoma. *Urology,* Vol.45, No.2, pp. 335-338.

Ballestar, E. (2011). An introduction to epigenetics. *Advances in Experimental Medicine and Biology,* Vol.711, pp. 1-11.

Ballestar, E. & Esteller, M. (2008). Epigenetic gene regulation in cancer. *Advances in Genetics,* Vol.61, pp.247-67.

Balmain, A. (2002). Cancer: new-age tumour suppressors. *Nature,* Vol.417, No.6886, pp.235–7.

Bolden, J.E.; Peart, M.J. & Johnstone, R.W. (2006). Anticancer activities of histone deacetylase inhibitors. *Nature Reviews Drug Discovery,* Vol.5, No.9, pp.5 769–784.

Bouchard, J. & Momparler, R.L. (1983). Incorporation of 5-Aza-2′-deoxycytidine-5′-triphosphate into DNA. Interactions with mammalian DNA polymerase alpha and DNA methylase. *Molecular Pharmacology.* Vol.24, No.1, pp.109–14.

Boumber, Y. & Issa, J.P. (2011) Epigenetics in cancer: what's the future? *Oncology (Williston Park)*, Vol.25, No.3, pp. 220-6.

Calin, G.A. & Croce, C.M. (2006). MicroRNA signatures in human cancers. *Nature Review Cancer*, Vol.6, No.11, pp. 857-866.

Cameron, E.E.; Bachman, K.E.; Myöhänen, S.; Herman, J.G. & Baylin, S.B. (1999). Synergy of demethylation and histone deacetylase inhibition in the re-expression of genes silenced in cancer. *Nature Genetics,* Vol.21, No.1, pp.103–7.

Canes, D.; Chiang, G.J.; Billmeyer, B.R.; Austin, C.A.; Kosakowski, M.; Rieger-Christ, K.M.; Libertino, J.A. & Summerhayes, I.C. (2005). Histone deacetylase inhibitors upregulate plakoglobin expression in bladder carcinoma cells and display antineoplastic activity in vitro and in vivo. *International Journal of Cancer*, Vol.113, No.5, pp.841– 8.

Catto, J.W.; Azzouzi, A.R.; Rehman, I.; Feeley, K.M.; Cross, S.S.; Amira, N.; Fromont, G.; Sibony, M.; Cussenot, O.; Meuth, M. & Hamdy, F.C. (2005). Promoter hypermethylation is associated with tumor location, stage, and subsequent progression in transitional cell carcinoma. *Journal of Clinical Oncology*, Vol.23, No.13, pp. 2903-2910

Chan, M.W.; Chan, L.W.; Tang, N.L.; Tong, J.H.; Lo, K.W.; Lee, T.L.; Cheung, H.Y.; Wong, W.S.; Chan, P.S.; Lai, F.M. and To, K.F. (2002). Hypermethylation of multiple genes in tumor tissues and voided urine in urinary bladder cancer patients. *Clinical Cancer Research*, Vol.8, No.2, pp.464-470.

Chan, M.W.; Chan, L.W.; Tang, N.L.; Lo, K.W.; Tong, J.H.; Chan, A.W.; Cheung, H.Y.; Wong, W.S.; Chan, P.S.; Lai, F.M. & To, K.F. (2003). Frequent hypermethylation of promoter region of RASSF1A in tumor tissues and voided urine of urinary bladder cancer patients. *International Journal of Cancer,* Vol.104, No.5, pp.611-6.

Cheng, J.C.; Matsen, C.B.; Gonzales, F.A.; Ye, W.; Greer, S.; Marquez, V.E.; Jones, P.A. & Selker, E.U. (2003). Inhibition of DNA methylation and reactivation of silenced genes by zebularine. *Journal of the National Cancer Institute,* Vol.95, No.5, pp.399–409.

Cheng, J.C.; Weisenberger, D.J.; Gonzales, F.A.; Liang, G.; Xu, G.L., Hu, Y.G., Marquez, V.E. & Jones, P.A. (2004). Continuous zebularine treatment effectively sustains demethylation in human bladder cancer cells. *Molecular and Cellular Biology,* Vol.24, No.3, pp.1270–8.

Chinnaiyan, P.; Vallabhaneni, G.; Armstrong, E.; Huang, S.M. & Harari, P.M. (2005). Modulation of radiation response by histone deacetylase inhibition. *International Journal of Radiation Oncology, Biology, Physics,* Vol.62, No.1, pp.223–9.

Christoph, F.; Weikert, S.; Kempkensteffen, C.; Krause, H.; Schostak, M.; Miller, K. & Schrader, M. (2006). Regularly methylated novel pro-apoptotic genes associated with recurrence in transitional cell carcinoma of the bladder. *International Journal of Cancer*, Vol.119, No.6, pp. 1396-1402.

Costa, V.L.; Henrique, R.; Danielsen, S.A.; Duarte-Pereira, S.; Eknaes, M.; Skotheim, R.I.; Rodrigues, A.; Magalhães, J.S.; Oliveira, J.; Lothe, R.A.; Teixeira, M.R.; Jerónimo, C. & Lind, G.E. (2010) Three epigenetic biomarkers, GDF15, TMEFF2, and VIM, accurately predict bladder cancer from DNA-based analyses of urine samples. *Clinical Cancer Res*earch, Vol.16, No.23, pp.5842-51.

Domínguez, G.; Carballido, J.; Silva, J.; Silva, J.M.; García, J.M.; Menéndez, J.; Provencio, M.; España, P. & Bonilla, F. (2002). p14ARF promoter hypermethylation in plasma DNA as an indicator of disease recurrence in bladder cancer patients. *Clinical Cancer Research*, Vol.8, No.4, pp. 980-985.

Duarte-Pereira, S.; Paiva, F.; Costa, V.L.; Ramalho-Carvalho, J.; Savva-Bordalo, J.; Rodrigues, A.; Ribeiro, F.R.; Silva, V.M.; Oliveira, J.; Henrique, R. & Jerónimo, C. (2011). Prognostic value of opioid binding protein/cell adhesion molecule-like promoter methylation in bladder carcinoma. *European Journal of Cancer,* Vol.47, No.7, pp. 1106-1114.

Dudziec, E.; Miah, S.; Choudhry, H.M.; Owen, H.C.; Blizard, S.; Glover, M.; Hamdy, F.C. & Catto, J.W. (2011). Hypermethylation of CpG islands and shores around specific microRNAs and mirtrons is associated with the phenotype and presence of bladder cancer. *Clinical Cancer Research,* Vol.17, No.6, pp.1287-96.

Dulaimi, E.; Uzzo, R.G.; Greenberg, R.E.; Al-Saleem, T.; Cairns, P. (2004). Detection of bladder cancer in urine by a tumor suppressor gene hypermethylation panel. *Clinical Cancer Research,* Vol.10, No.6, pp.1887-1893

Dunn, G.P.; Sheehan, K.C.; Old, L.J. & Schreiber, R.D. (2005). IFN unresponsiveness in LNCaP cells due to the lack of JAK1 gene expression. *Cancer Research,* Vol.65, No.8, pp.3447–53.

Dyrskjøt, L.; Ostenfeld, M.S.; Bramsen, J.B.; Silahtaroglu, A.N.; Lamy, P.; Ramanathan, R.; Fristrup, N.; Jensen, J.L.; Andersen, C.L.; Zieger, K.; Kauppinen, S.; Ulhøi, B.P.; Kjems, J.; Borre, M. & Orntoft, T.F. (2009). Genomic profiling of microRNAs in bladder cancer: miR-129 is associated with poor outcome and promotes cell death in vitro. *Cancer Research,* Vol.69, No.11, pp.4851-4860.

Eling, T.E.; Baek, S.J.; Shim, M. & Lee, C.H. (2006). NSAID activated gene (NAG-1), a modulator of tumorigenesis. *Journal of Biochemistry and Molecular Biology,* Vol.39, No.6, pp.649-55.

Elkin, M.; Shevelev, A.; Schulze, E.; Tykocinsky, M.; Cooper, M.; Ariel, I.; Pode, D.; Kopf, E.; de Groot, N. & Hochberg, A. (1995). The expression of the imprinted H19 and IGF-2 genes in human bladder carcinoma. *FEBS Letters,* Vol.374, No.1, pp. 57-61.

Ellinger, J.; El Kassem, N.; Heukamp, L.C.; Matthews, S.; Cubukluoz, F.; Kahl, P.; Perabo, F.G.; Müller, S.C.; von Ruecker, A. & Bastian, P.J. (2008). Hypermethylation of cell-free serum DNA indicates worse outcome in patients with bladder cancer. *The Journal of Urology,* Vol.179, No.1, pp.346-52.

Esteller, M. (2005). DNA methylation and cancer therapy: New developments and expectations. *Current Opinion in Oncology,* Vol.17, No.1, pp.55–60.

Fabbri, M. & Calin, G.A. (2010). Epigenetics and miRNAs in human cancer. *Advances in Genetics*. Vol.70, pp.87-99.

Fang, M.Z.; Wang, Y.; Ai, N.; Hou, Z.; Sun, Y.; Lu, H.; Welsh, W. & Yang, C.S. (2003). Tea polyphenol (-)-epigallocatechin-3-gallate inhibits DNA methyltransferase and reactivates methylation-silenced genes in cancer cell lines. *Cancer Research,*Vol.63, No.22, pp.7563–70.

Fernandez, A.F.; Assenov, Y.; Martin-Subero, J.I.; Balint, B.; Siebert, R.; Taniguchi, H.; Yamamoto, H.; Hidalgo, M.; Tan, A.C.; Galm, O.; Ferrer, I.; Sanchez-Cespedes, M.; Villanueva, A.; Carmona, J.; Sanchez-Mut, J.V.; Berdasco, M.; Moreno, V.; Capella, G.; Monk, D.; Ballestar, E.; Ropero, S.; Martinez, R.; Sanchez-Carbayo, M.; Prosper, F.; Agirre, X.; Fraga, M.F.; Graña, O.; Perez-Jurado, L.; Mora, J.; Puig, S.; Prat, J.; Badimon, L.; Puca, A.A.; Meltzer, S.J.; Lengauer, T.; Bridgewater, J.; Bock, C. & Esteller, M. (2011). A DNA methylation fingerprint of 1628 human samples. *Genome Research*, Epub ahead of print.

Finnin, M.S.; Donigian, J.R.; Cohen, A.; Richon, V.M.; Rifkind, R.A.; Marks, P.A.; Breslow, R. & Pavletich, N.P. (1999). Structures of a histone deacetylase homologue bound to the TSA and SAHA inhibitors. *Nature*, Vol.401, No.6749, pp.88–93.

Friedrich, M.G.; Weisenberger, D.J.; Cheng, J.C.; Chandrasoma, S.; Siegmund, K.D.; Gonzalgo, M.L.; Toma, M.I.; Huland, H.; Yoo, C.; Tsai, Y.C.; Nichols, P.W.; Bochner, B.H.; Jones, P.A. & Liang, G. (2004). Detection of methylated apoptosis-associated genes in urine sediments of bladder cancer patients. *Clinical Cancer Research*, Vol.10, No.22, pp.7457-65.

Friedrich, M.G.; Chandrasoma, S.; Siegmund, K.D.; Weisenberger, D.J.; Cheng, J.C.; Toma, M.I.; Huland, H.; Jones, P.A. & Liang, G. (2005). Prognostic relevance of methylation markers in patients with non-muscle invasive bladder carcinoma. *European Journal of Cancer*, Vol.41, No.17, pp. 2769-2778.

Gallagher, E.M.; O'Shea, D.M.; Fitzpatrick, P.; Harrison, M.; Gilmartin, B.; Watson, J.A.; Clarke, T.; Leonard, M.O.; McGoldrick, A.; Meehan, M.; Watson, C.; Furlong, F.; O'Kelly, P.; Fitzpatrick, J.M.; Dervan, P.A.; O'Grady, A.; Kay, E.W. & McCann, A. (2008). Recurrence of urothelial carcinoma of the bladder: a role for insulin-like growth factor-II loss of imprinting and cytoplasmic E-cadherin immunolocalization. *Clinical Cancer Research*, Vol.14, No.21, pp.6829-6838.

Goffin, J. & Eisenhauer, E. (2002). DNA methyltransferase inhibitors-state of the art. *Annals of Oncology*, Vol.13, No.11, pp.1699 –716.

Gottlicher, M.; Minucci, S.; Zhu, P.; Krämer, O.H.; Schimpf, A.; Giavara, S.; Sleeman, J.P.; Lo Coco, F.; Nervi, C.; Pelicci, P.G. & Heinzel, T. (2001). Valproic acid defines a novel class of HDAC inhibitors inducing differentiation of transformed cells. *The EMBO Jornal*, Vol.20, No.24, pp.6969 –78.

Greiner, D.; Bonaldi, T.; Eskeland, R.; Roemer, E. & Imhof, A. (2005). Identification of a specific inhibitor of the histone methyltransferase SU (VAR) 3–9. *Nature Chemichal Biology*, Vol.1, No.3, pp.143–45.

Hanke, M.; Hoefig, K.; Merz, H.; Feller, A.C.; Kausch, I.; Jocham, D.; Warnecke, J.M. & Sczakiel, G. (2010) A robust methodology to study urine microRNA as tumor marker: microRNA-126 and microRNA-182 are related to urinary bladder cancer. *Urologic Oncology*, Vol.28, No.6, pp.655-61.

Hellwinkel, O.J.; Kedia, M.; Isbarn, H.; Budäus, L. & Friedrich, M.G. (2008) Methylation of the TPEF- and PAX6-promoters is increased in early bladder cancer and in normal mucosa adjacent to pTa tumours. *BJU International*, Vol.101, No.6, pp.753-7.

Hoque, M.O.; Begum, S.; Topaloglu, O.; Chatterjee, A.; Rosenbaum, E.; Van Criekinge, W.; Westra, W.H.; Schoenberg, M.; Zahurak, M.; Goodman, S.N. & Sidransky, D. (2006).

Quantitation of promoter methylation of multiple genes in urine DNA and bladder cancer detection. Journal of the National Cancer Institute, Vol.98, No.14, pp.996-1004.

Hoque, M.O.; Begum, S.; Brait, M.; Jeronimo, C.; Zahurak, M.; Ostrow, K.L.; Rosenbaum, E.; Trock, B.; Westra, W.H.; Schoenberg, M.; Goodman, S.N. & Sidransky, D. (2008). Tissue inhibitor of metalloproteinases-3 promoter methylation is an independent prognostic factor for bladder cancer. *Journal of Urology*, Vol.179, No.2, pp.743-747.

Ichimi, T.; Enokida, H.; Okuno, Y.; Kunimoto, R.; Chiyomaru, T.; Kawamoto, K.; Kawahara, K.; Toki, K.; Kawakami, K.; Nishiyama, K.; Tsujimoto, G.; Nakagawa, M. & Seki, N. (2009). Identification of novel microRNA targets based on microRNA signatures in bladder cancer. *International Journal of Cancer*, Vol.125, No.2, pp.345-52.

Iguchi, H.; Kosaka, N. & Ochiya, T. (2010). Versatile applications of microRNA in anti-cancer drug discovery: from therapeutics to biomarkers. *Current Drug Discovery Technologies*, Vol.7, No.2, pp.95-105.

Jackson-Grusby, L.; Laird, P.W.; Magge, S.N.; Moeller, B.J. & Jaenisch, R. (1997). Mutagenicity of 5-aza-2'-deoxycytidine is mediated by the mammalian DNA methyltransferase. *Proceedings of the National Academy of Sciences of the United States of America*, Vol.94, No.9, pp.4681–5.

Jones, P.A. & Baylin, S.B. (2007). The epigenomics of cancer. *Cell*, Vol.128, No.4, pp.683-92.

Kelly, W.K.; Richon, V.M.; O'Connor, O.; Curley, T.; MacGregor-Curtelli, B.; Tong, W.; Klang, M.; Schwartz, L.; Richardson, S.; Rosa, E.; Drobnjak, M.; Cordon-Cordo, C.; Chiao, J.H.; Rifkind, R.; Marks, P.A. & Scher, H. (2003). Phase I clinical trial of histone deacetylase inhibitor: Suberoylanilide hydroxamic acid administered intravenously. *Clinical Cancer Research*, Vol.9, No.10 Pt 1, pp.3578–88.

Kim, W.J. & Kim, Y.J. Epigenetic biomarkers in urothelial bladder cancer. (2009). *Expert Review of Molecular Diagnostics*. Vol.9, No.3, pp.259-69.

Kim, Y.K. & Kim, W.J. (2009). Epigenetic markers as promising prognosticators for bladder cancer. *International Journal of Urology*, Vol.16, No.1, pp.17-22.

Kim, E.J.; Kim, Y.J.; Jeong, P.; Ha, Y.S.; Bae, S.C. & Kim, W.J. (2008). Methylation of the RUNX3 promoter as a potential prognostic marker for bladder tumor. *Journal of Urology*, Vol.180, No.3, pp. 1141-1145.

Kim, W.J.; Kim, E.J.; Jeong, P.; Quan, C.; Kim, J.; Li, Q.L.; Yang, J.O.; Ito, Y. & Bae, S.C. (2005). RUNX3 inactivation by point mutations and aberrant DNA methylation in bladder tumors. *Cancer Research*, Vol.65, No.20, pp.9347-54.

Kouzarides T. (2007). Chromatin modifications and their functions. *Cell*, Vol.128, No.4, pp. 693-705.

Kurdistani, S.K. (2011). Histone modifications in cancer biology and prognosis. *Progress in Drug Research*, Vol.67, pp.91-106.

Leu, Y.W.; Rahmatpanah, F.; Shi, H.; Wei, S.H.; Liu, J.C.; Yan, P.S. & Huang, T.H. (2003). Double RNA interference of DNMT3b and DNMT1 enhances DNA demethylation and gene reactivation. *Cancer Research*, Vol.63, No.19, pp.6110 –5.

Liang, G.; Gonzales, F.A.; Jones, P.A.; Orntoft, T.F. & Thykjaer, T. (2002). Analysis of gene induction in human fibroblasts and bladder cancer cells exposed to the methylation inhibitor 5-aza-20-deoxycytidine. *Cancer Research,* Vol.62, No.4, pp.961–966.

Lin, X.; Asgari, K.; Putzi, M.J.; Gage, W.R.; Yu, X.; Cornblatt, B.S.; Kumar, A.; Piantadosi, S.; DeWeese, T.L.; De Marzo, A.M. & Nelson, W.G. (2001). Reversal of GSTP1 CpG island hypermethylation and reactivation of pi-class glutathione S-transferase (GSTP1) expression in human prostate cancer cells by treatment with procainamide. *Cancer Research,* Vol.61, No.24, pp.8611– 6.

Lu, J.; Getz, G.; Miska, E.A.; Alvarez-Saavedra, E.; Lamb, J.; Peck, D.; Sweet-Cordero, A.; Ebert, B.L.; Mak, R.H.; Ferrando, A.A.; Downing, J.R.; Jacks, T.; Horvitz, H.R. & Golub, T.R. (2005). MicroRNA expression profiles classify human cancers. *Nature,* Vol.435, No.7043, pp. 834-8.

Lübbert, M. (2000). DNA methylation inhibitors in the treatment of leukemias, myelodysplastic syndromes and hemoglobinopathies: Clinical results and possible mechanisms of action. *Current Topics in Microbiology and Immunology,* Vol.249, pp.135- 64.

Lujambio, A.; Ropero, S.; Ballestar, E.; Fraga, M.F.; Cerrato, C.; Setien, F.; Casado, S.; Suarez-Gauthier, A.; Sanchez-Cespedes, M.; Git, A.; Spiteri, I.; Das, P.P.; Calds, C.; Miska, E. & Esteller, M. (2007). Genetic unmasking of an epigenetically silenced microRNA in Human cancer cells. *Cancer Resesrch,* Vol.67, No.4, pp.1424-1429.

Maruyama, R.; Toyooka, S.; Toyooka, K.O.; Harada, K.; Virmani, A.K.; Zöchbauer-Müller, S.; Farinas, A.J.; Vakar-Lopez, F.; Minna, J.D.; Sagalowsky, A.; Czerniak, B. & Gazdar, A.F. (2001). Aberrant promoter methylation profile of bladder cancer and its relationship to clinicopathological features. *Cancer Research,* Vol.61, No.24, pp. 8659-8663.

Mann, B.S.; Johnson, J.R.; Cohen, M.H.; Justice, R. & Pazdur, R. (2007). FDA approval summary: vorinostat for treatment of advanced primary cutaneous T-cell lymphoma. *Oncologist.* Vol.12, No.10, pp.1247-1252.

McConkey, D.J.; Lee, S.; Choi, W.; Tran, M.; Majewski, T.; Lee, S.; Siefker-Radtke, A.; Dinney, C. & Czerniak, B. (2010). Molecular genetics of bladder cancer: Emerging mechanisms of tumor initiation and progression. *Urologic Oncology,* Vol.28, No.4, pp. 429-440.

Mei, S.; Ho, A.D. & Mahlknecht, U. (2004). Role of histone deacetylase inhibitors in the treatment of cancer. *International Journal of Oncology,* Vol.25, No.6, pp.1509 –19.

Mitra, A.P.; Datar, R.H & Cote, R.J. (2006). Molecular pathways in invasive bladder cancer: new insights into mechanisms, progression, and target identification. *Journal of Clinical Oncology,* Vol.24, No.35, pp.5552-5564.

Monk D. (2010). Deciphering the cancer imprintome. *Briefings in Functional Genomics and Proteomics,* Vol.9, No.4, pp.329-339.

Moore, L.E.; Pfeiffer, R.M.; Poscablo, C.; Real, F.X.; Kogevinas, M.; Silverman, D.; García-Closas, R.; Chanock, S.; Tardón, A.; Serra, C.; Carrato, A.; Dosemeci, M.; García-Closas, M.; Esteller, M.; Fraga, M.; Rothman, N. & Malats, N. (2008). Genomic DNA hypomethylation as a biomarker for bladder cancer susceptibility in the Spanish

Bladder Cancer Study: a case-control study. *The Lancet Oncology,* Vol.9, No.4, pp.359-66.

Mund, C. & Lyko, F. (2010). Epigenetic cancer therapy: Proof of concept and remaining challenges. *Bioessays,* Vol.32, No.11, pp.949-57.

Negraes, P.D.; Favaro, F.P.; Camargo, J.L.; Oliveira, M.L.; Goldberg, J.; Rainho, C.A.; Salvadori, D.M. (2008). DNA methylation patterns in bladder cancer and washing cell sediments: a perspective for tumor recurrence detection. *BMC Cancer.* Vol.8, pp.238-250.

Neuhausen, A.; Florl, A.R.; Grimm, M.O. & Schulz, W.A. (2006). DNA methylation alterations in urothelial carcinoma. *Cancer Biology and Therapy,* Vol.5, No.8, pp. 993-1001.

Pina, I.C.; Gautschi, J.T.; Wang, G.Y.; Sanders, M.L.; Schmitz, F.J.; France, D.; Cornell-Kennon, S.; Sambucetti, L.C.; Remiszewski, S.W.; Perez, L.B.; Bair, K.W. & Crews, P. (2003). Psammaplins from the sponge Pseudoceratina purpurea: Inhibition of both histone deacetylase and DNA methyltransferase. *The Journal of Organic Chemistry,* Vol.68, No.10, pp.3866 –73.

Portela, A. & Esteller, M. (2010). Epigenetic modifications and human disease. *Nature Biotechnology,* Vol.28, No.10, pp. 1057-68.

Renard, I.; Joniau, S.; van Cleynenbreugel, B.; Collette, C.; Naômé, C.; Vlassenbroeck, I.; Nicolas, H.; de Leval, J.; Straub, J.; Van Criekinge, W.; Hamida, W.; Hellel, M.; Thomas, A.; de Leval, L.; Bierau, K. & Waltregny, D. (2010). Identification and validation of the methylated TWIST1 and NID2 genes through real-time methylation-specific polymerase chain reaction assays for the noninvasive detection of primary bladder cancer in urine samples. *European Urology,* Vol.58, No.1, pp.96-104.

Richon, V.M.; Sandhoff, T.W.; Rifkind, R.A. & Marks, P.A. (2000). Histone deacetylase inhibitor selectively induces p21WAF1 expression and gene-associated histone acetylation. *Proceedings of the National Academy of Sciences of the United States of America,* Vol.97, No.18, pp.10014–9.

Rodríguez-Paredes, M. & Esteller, M. (2011). Cancer epigenetics reaches mainstream oncology. *Nature Medicine.* Vol.17, No.3, pp.330-339.

Rosato, R.R.; Almenara, J.A. & Grant, S. (2003). The histone deacetylase inhibitor MS-275 promotes differentiation or apoptosis in human leukemia cells through a process regulated by generation of reactive oxygen species and induction of p21CIP1/WAF1. *Cancer Research,* Vol.63, No.13, pp.3637–45.

Saito, Y.; Liang, G.; Egger, G.; Friedman, J.M.; Chuang, J.C.; Coetzee, G.A. & Jones, P.A. (2006). Specific activation of microRNA-127 with downregulation of the proto-oncogene BCL6 by chromatin-modifying drugs in human cancer cells. *Cancer Cell,* Vol. 9, No.6, pp. 435–43.

Sawan, C.; Vaissière, T.; Murr, R. & Herceg, Z. (2008). Epigenetic drivers and genetic passengers on the road to cancer. *Mutation Research,* Vol.642, No.1-2, pp. 1-13.

Schneider, A.C.; Heukamp, L.C.; Rogenhofer, S.; Fechner, G.; Bastian, P.J.; von Ruecker, A.; Müller, S.C. & Ellinger, J. (2011). Global histone H4K20 trimethylation predicts cancer-specific survival in patients with muscle-invasive bladder cancer. *British Journal of Urology International*, doi:10.1111/j.1464-410X.2011.10203.x.

Seifert, H.H.; Schmiemann, V.; Mueller, M.; Kazimirek, M.; Onofre, F.; Neuhausen, A.; Florl, A.R.; Ackermann, R.; Boecking, A.; Schulz, W.A. & Grote, H.J. (2007). In situ detection of global DNA hypomethylation in exfoliative urine cytology of patients with suspected bladder cancer. *Experimental and Molecular Pathology*, Vol.82, No.3, pp. 292-297.

Sherr, C.J. & McCormick, F. (2002). The RB and p53 pathways in cancer. *Cancer Cell*, Vol.2, No.2, pp.103–12.

Shirahata, A.; Sakata, M.; Sakuraba, K.; Goto, T.; Mizukami, H.; Saito, M.; Ishibashi, K.; Kigawa, G.; Nemoto, H.; Sanada, Y. & Hibi, K. (2009). Vimentin methylation as a marker for advanced colorectal carcinoma. *Anticancer Research*, Vol.29, No.1, pp.279-81.

Soprano, D.R.; Qin, P. & Soprano, K.J. Retinoic acid receptors and cancers. (2004). *Annual Review of Nutrition*, Vol.24, pp.201-21.

Stirzaker, C.; Song, J.Z.; Davidson, B. & Clark, S.J. (2004). Transcriptional gene silencing promotes DNA hypermethylation through a sequential change in chromatin modifications in cancer cells. *Cancer Research*, Vol.64, No.11, pp.3871–7.

Tada, Y.; Wada, M.; Kuroiwa, K.; Kinugawa, N.; Harada, T.; Nagayama, J.; Nakagawa, M.; Naito, S. & Kuwano, M. (2000). MDR1 gene overexpression and altered degree of methylation at the promoter region in bladder cancer during chemotherapeutic treatment. *Clinical Cancer Research*, Vol.6, No.12, pp. 4618-4627.

Tada, Y.; Wada, M.; Taguchi, K.; Mochida, Y.; Kinugawa, N.; Tsuneyoshi, M.; Naito, S. & Kuwano, M. (2002). The association of death-associated protein kinase hypermethylation with early recurrence in superficial bladder cancers. *Cancer Research*, Vol.62, No.14, pp. 4048-4053.

Taipale, J. & Beachy, P.A. (2001). The Hedgehog and Wnt signalling pathways in cancer. *Nature*, Vol.411, No.6835, pp.349–54.

Tanaka, M.F. & Sonpavde, G. (2011). Diagnosis and management of urothelial carcinoma of then bladder. *Postgraduate Medicine*, Vol.123, No.3, pp. 43-55.

Tilki, D.; Burger, M.; Dalbagni, G.; Grossman, H.B.; Hakenberg, O.W.; Palou, J.; Reich, O.; Rouprêt, M.; Shariat, S.F. & Zlotta, A.R. (2011). Urine Markers for Detection and Surveillance of Non-Muscle-Invasive Bladder Cancer. *European Urology*, doi:10.1016/j.eururo.2011.05.053.

Tsunoda, S.; Smith, E.; De Young, N.J.; Wang, X.; Tian, Z.Q.; Liu, J.F.; Jamieson, G.G. & Drew, P.A. (2009). Methylation of CLDN6, FBN2, RBP1, RBP4, TFPI2, and TMEFF2 in esophageal squamous cell carcinoma. *Oncology Reports*, Vol.21, No.4, pp.1067-73.

Urakami, S.; Shiina, H.; Enokida, H.; Kawakami, T.; Kawamoto, K.; Hirata, H.; Tanaka, Y.; Kikuno, N.; Nakagawa, M.; Igawa, M. & Dahiya, R. (2006). Combination analysis of hypermethylated Wnt-antagonist family genes as a novel epigenetic biomarker panel for bladder cancer detection. *Clinical Cancer Research*, Vol. 12, No.7 Pt 1, pp.2109-16.

Valeri, N.; Vannini, I.; Fanini, F.; Calore, F.; Adair, B. & Fabbri, M. (2009). Epigenetics, miRNAs, and human cancer: a new chapter in human gene regulation. *Mammalian genome: official journal of the International Mammalian Genome Society*, Vol.20, No.9-10, pp. 573-80.

Veerla, S.; Lindgren, D.; Kvist, A.; Frigyesi, A.; Staaf, J.; Persson, H.; Liedberg, F.; Chebil, G.; Gudjonsson, S.; Borg, A.; Månsson, W.; Rovira, C. & Höglund, M. (2009). MiRNA expression in urothelial carcinomas: important roles of miR-10a, miR-222, miR-125b, miR-7 and miR-452 for tumor stage and metastasis, and frequent homozygous losses of miR-31. *International Journal of Cancer*, Vol.124, No.9, pp. 2236-2242.

Villar-Garea, A.; Fraga, M.F.; Espada, J. & Esteller, M. (2003). Procaine is a DNAdemethylating agent with growth-inhibitory effects in human cancer cells. *Cancer Research*, Vol.63, No.16, pp.4984 -9.

Wiklund, E.D.; Bramsen, J.B.; Hulf, T.; Dyrskjøt, L.; Ramanathan, R.; Hansen, T.B.; Villadsen, S.B.; Gao, S.; Ostenfeld, M.S.; Borre, M.; Peter, M.E.; Ørntoft, T.F.; Kjems, J. & Clark, S.J. (2011). Coordinated epigenetic repression of the miR-200 family and miR-205 in invasive bladder cancer. *International Journal of Cancer*, Vol.128, No.6, pp. 1327-1334.

Wolff, E.M.; Chihara, Y.; Pan, F.; Weisenberger, D.J.; Siegmund, K.D.; Sugano, K.; Kawashima, K.; Laird, P.W.; Jones, P.A. & Liang, G. (2010). Unique DNA methylation patterns distinguish noninvasive and invasive urothelial cancers and establish an epigenetic field defect in premalignant tissue. Cancer Research, Vol.70, No.20, pp.8169-78.

Xu, W.S.; Parmigiani, R.B. & Marks, P.A. (2007). Histone deacetylase inhibitors: molecular mechanisms of action, *Oncogene*, Vol.26, No.37, pp.5541–5552.

Yamada, Y.; Enokida, H.; Kojima, S.; Kawakami, K.; Chiyomaru, T.; Tatarano, S.; Yoshino, H.; Kawahara, K.; Nishiyama, K.; Seki, N. & Nakagawa, M. (2011). MiR-96 and miR-183 detection inurine serve as potential tumor markers of urothelial carcinoma: correlation with stage and grade, and comparison with urinary cytology. *Cancer Science*, Vol.102, No.3, pp.522-9.

Yates, D.R.; Rehman, I.; Meuth, M.; Cross, S.S.; Hamdy, F.C. & Catto, J.W. (2006) Methylational urinalysis: a prospective study of bladder cancer patients and age stratified benign controls. *Oncogene*, Vol.25, No.13, pp.1984-8.

Yates, D.R.; Rehman, I.; Abbod, M.F.; Meuth, M.; Cross, S.S.; Linkens, D.A.; Hamdy, F.C. & Catto, J.W. (2007). Promoter hypermethylation identifies progression risk in bladder cancer. *Clinical Cancer Research*, Vol.13, No.7, pp. 2046-53.

Yu, J.; Zhu, T.; Wang, Z.; Zhang, H.; Qian, Z.; Xu, H.; Gao, B.; Wang, W.; Gu, L.; Meng, J.; Wang, J.; Feng, X.; Li, Y.; Yao, X. & Zhu, J. (2007). A novel set of DNA methylation markers in urine sediments for sensitive/specific detection of bladder cancer. *Clinical Cancer Research*, Vol.13, No.24, pp.7296-304.

Zhang, Z.; Karam, J.; Frenkel, E.; Sagalowsky, A. & Hsieh, J.T. (2006). The application of epigenetic modifiers on the treatment of prostate and bladder cancer. *Urologic Oncology*, Vol.24, No.2, pp.152-60.

Zhang, Z.; Stanfield, J.; Frenkel, E.; Kabbani, W. & Hsieh, J.T. (2007). Enhanced therapeutic effect on androgen-independent prostate cancer by depsipeptide (FK228), a histone deacetylase inhibitor, in combination with docetaxel. Urology, Vol.70, No.2, pp.396-401.

Zheng, Y.G.; Wu, J.; Chen, Z. & Goodman, M. (2008). Chemical regulation of epigenetic modifications: opportunities for new cancer therapy. *Medicinal Research Reviews*, Vol.28, No.5, pp.645-87.

4

Angiogenesis, Lymphangiogenesis and Lymphovascular Invasion: Prognostic Impact for Bladder Cancer Patients

Julieta Afonso[1,2,3], Lúcio Lara Santos[4,5] and Adhemar Longatto-Filho[1,3,6]
[1]*Life and Health Sciences Research Institute - ICVS, University of Minho*
[2]*ICVS/3B's - PT Government Associate Laboratory*
[3]*Alto Ave Superior Institute of Health – ISAVE*
[4]*Portuguese Institute of Oncology – IPO*
[5]*University Fernando Pessoa – UFP*
[6]*Faculty of Medicine, São Paulo State University*
[1,2,3,4,5]*Portugal*
[6]*Brazil*

1. Introduction

Bladder cancer is the second most common tumor of the urogenital tract. Urothelial carcinoma is the most frequent histologic type, being unique among epithelial carcinomas in its divergent pathways of tumorigenesis. Surgery continues to have a predominant role in the management of urothelial bladder cancer (Kaufman et al., 2009). However, the debate about the best treatment approach for T1G3 and muscle invasive tumors continually challenges all urologic surgeons and oncologists. This debate involves several aspects. First, a significant number of T1G3 tumors recurs and progresses rapidly after transurethral resection and BCG treatment (Wiesner et al., 2005). Second, half of patients with invasive tumors have a dismal outcome despite an effective treatment by radical cystectomy (Sternberg et al., 2007). Third, the extension of lymphadenectomy remains an issue of controversy, although clinical evidence suggests that an extended lymph node dissection may not only provide prognostic information, but also a significant therapeutic benefit for both lymph node-positive and lymph node-negative patients undergoing radical cystectomy (May et al., 2011). In muscle invasive bladder cancer, the presence of tumor foci in lymph nodes is an early event in progression, and the lymphatic vessels within or in the proximity to the primary tumor serve as the primary conduits for tumor dissemination (Youssef et al., 2011). Fourth, although urothelial bladder cancer is a chemo-sensitive tumor (Kaufman et al., 2000; von der Maase et al., 2000), adjuvant systemic chemotherapy does not reveal benefits (Walz et al., 2008), and neoadjuvant chemotherapy is not yet accepted as the best approach in invasive bladder cancer (Clark, 2009). Therefore, in order to solve the aforementioned problems, it is crucial to improve the knowledge about tumor microenvironment, regulation of cancer metabolism and neovascularization.

Blood and lymphatic neovascularization are essential for tumor progression and metastasis, by promoting oxygenation and fluid drainage, and establishing potential routes of dissemination (Adams and Alitalo, 2007). Therefore, the inhibition of tumor-induced neovascularization represents a powerful option for target therapy, in order to restrain the most efficient pathway of cancer spread.

2. Angiogenesis and lymphangiogenesis: Molecular regulation of vasculature development

During embryogenesis, the formation of the blood vascular system initiates by vasculogenesis: haemangioblasts proliferate, migrate and differentiate into endothelial cells, which in turn will organize a primitive vascular plexus. In parallel, angiogenesis promotes the remodeling and expansion of the primary capillary network, originating a hierarchical structure of different sized vessels that will mature into functional capillaries, veins and arteries (Risau, 1997). The lymphatic vascular system develops latter, when a group of blood endothelial cells differentiates into a lymphatic endothelium that subsequently sprouts to form the primary lymph sacs. By lymphangiogenesis, the lymphatic endothelial cells from the lymph sacs will further sprout, originating the peripheral lymphatic system (Sabin, 1902, as cited by Oliver & Detmar, 2002).

During postnatal life, blood and lymphatic vascular systems are, normally, in a quiescent state. Physiological angiogenesis and/or lymphangiogenesis occur to maintain or restore the integrity of tissues, namely during wound healing and the ovarian cycle. Conversely, the neovascularization machinery may be activated in pathological processes such as cancer and inflammatory diseases (reviewed in Lohela et al., 2009).

Similarly to physiological neovascularization, tumor-induced angiogenesis and/or lymphangiogenesis occur to satisfy the metabolic demands of a new tissue — the malignant tissue. Therefore, the molecular factors involved in the formation of the vascular systems during embryogenesis are newly recruited by the growing tumor (Papetti & Herman, 2002).

2.1 From angiogenesis to lymphangiogenesis in the embryo

The proliferation, sprouting and migration of endothelial cells during vasculogenesis and angiogenesis is mainly guided by the vascular endothelial growth factor (VEGF) signaling through VEGF receptor-2 (VEGFR-2) (Risau, 1997).

VEGF (or VEGF-A), initially termed as vascular permeability factor (VPF) (Senger et al., 1983), is a specific mitogen and pro-survival factor for blood endothelial cells, also stimulating vascular permeability. It binds and activates two tyrosine kinase receptors primarily found on the blood endothelium: VEGFR-1 (or Flt-1, fms-like tyrosine kinase 1) and VEGFR-2 (or KDR/Flk-1, human kinase insert domain receptor/mouse foetal liver kinase 1) (reviewed in Carmeliet, 2005). Interaction of VEGF with VEGFR-1 negatively regulates vasculogenesis and angiogenesis during early embryogenesis (Fong et al., 1999). On the contrary, VEGFR-2 is the earliest marker for endothelial cell development: mouse embryos lacking VEGFR-2 die at embryonic day 8.5-9.5 due to no development of blood vessels as well as very low hematopoiesis (Shalaby et al., 1995). Regarding the ligand, even heterozygote mice for *Vegf* deficiency die at embryonic day 11-12: blood islands, endothelial cells and vessel-like tubes fail to develop (Carmeliet et al., 1996; Ferrara et al., 1996).

In humans, five weeks after fertilization, certain blood endothelial cells become responsive to lymphatic inducing-signals. The lymphatic vessel endothelial hyaluronan receptor-1 (LYVE-1), a CD44 homologous transmembrane protein, is the first marker of lymphatic endothelial commitment. Initially, it is evenly expressed by the blood endothelium of the cardinal vein, which causes the blood endothelium to acquire the ability to differentiate in lymphatic endothelium (Banerji et al., 1999). The polarized expression of the prospero related homeobox gene-1 (Prox-1) transcription factor in a subpopulation of blood endothelial cells determines the establishment of the lymphatic identity and initiates the formation of the lymphatic vascular system. In mice, Prox-1 expressing cells are first observed at embryonic day 10 in the jugular vein (Wigle & Oliver, 1999). *Prox1* deletion leads to a complete absence of the lymphatic vasculature (Wigle et al., 2002). The expression of the transcription factor Sox18 [SRY (sex determining region Y) box 18] acts as a molecular switch to induce differentiation of lymphatic endothelial cells: it activates Prox-1 transcription by binding to its proximal promoter. Sox18-null embryos show a complete blockade of lymphatic endothelial cell differentiation (François et al., 2008). Later, the sprouting, migration and survival of the newly formed lymphatic endothelial cells depends on the expression of VEGF-C by the mesenchymal cells surrounding the cardinal veins (Karkkainen et al., 2004) (Fig. 1).

VEGF-C, like VEGF, is a member of the VEGF family of growth factors and a mitogen for lymphatic endothelial cells. VEGF-D is also a pro-lymphangiogenic factor, although its deletion does not affect the development of the primitive lymphatic vessels (Baldwin et al. 2001). Conversely, in *Vegfc*$^{-/-}$ mice, Prox-1 positive cells appear in the cardinal veins, but fail to migrate and proliferate to form primary lymph sacs (Karkkainen et al., 2004). VEGF-C and VEGF-D interact with VEGFR-3 (of Flt-4, fms-like tyrosine kinase 4). Their affinity to VEGFR-3 is increased by proteolytic cleavage; the fully processed forms can also bind to VEGFR-2 (reviewed in Lohela et al., 2009).

VEGFR-3 is widely expressed at the early stages of embryonic blood vasculature, becoming virtually restricted to lymphatic endothelium in the later stages of embryonic development, (after the lymphatic commitment mediated by Prox-1 expression), and during adult life (Kaipainen et al., 1995). In mice, inhibition of VEGFR-3 expression at embryonic day 15 induces regression of the developing lymphatic vasculature by apoptosis of lymphatic endothelial cells (Makinen et al., 2001).

The subsequent development of the lymphatic vasculature involves the separation of the blood and lymphatic vascular systems, the maturation of lymphatic vessels and the formation of secondary lymphoid organs. The molecular regulation of these processes involves the coordinated expression of distinct genes from those involved in the early events of lymphangiogenesis (reviewed in Alitalo et al., 2005) (Fig. 1). Moreover, several other growth factors, namely cyclooxygenase-2 (COX-2) fibroblast growth factor-2 (FGF-2), hepatocyte growth factor (HGF), insulin-like growth factors (IGFs) and platelet-derived growth factor-B (PDGF-B) have been shown to induce lymphangiogenesis and/or angiogenesis in experimental models (reviewed in Cao, 2005). These are mainly protein tyrosine kinases, which play central roles in signal transduction networks and regulation of cell behavior. In the lymphatic endothelium, these tyrosine kinases are collectively involved in processes such as the maintenance of existing lymphatic vessels, growth and maturation of new vessels and modulation of their identity and function (Williams et al., 2010).

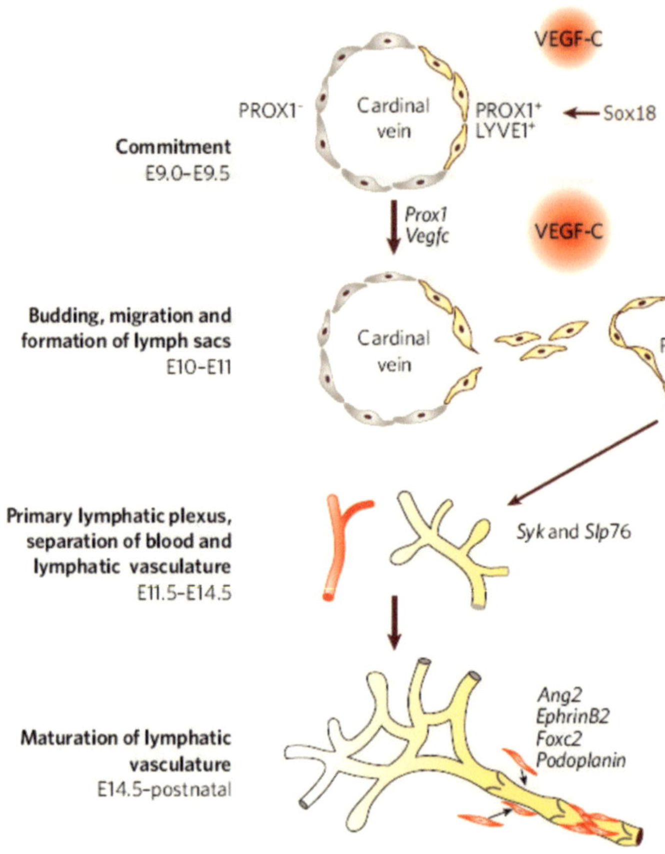

Fig. 1. Model for the development of mouse lymphatic vasculature (E- embryonic day; Syk- protein-tyrosine kinase SYK; Slp76- SH2 domain-containing leucocyte protein, 76-kDa; Ang2- angiopoietin 2; Foxc2- Forkhead Box C2) (adapted by permission from © 2005 Nature Publishing Group. Originally published in *Nature*. 438: 946-953)

2.2 Promotion of angiogenesis and lymphangiogenesis in the malignancy context

The major cause of cancer mortality is the metastatic spread of tumor cells that can occur via multiple routes, including blood and lymphatic vasculatures. For metastasis to occur, selected clones of malignant cells must be able to invade the newly formed vessels and disseminate. Induction of angiogenesis and/or lymphangiogenesis is, therefore, one of the first steps of the metastatic cascade (Alitalo & Carmeliet, 2002; Tobler & Detmar, 2006).

During the pre-vascular phase, the malignant tumor remains small (up to 1 or 2 mm^3); the preexistent surrounding blood vessels ensure the supply of oxygen and nutrients necessary for its survival. However, the expansion of the tumor mass is angiogenesis-dependent. As a compensatory response to hypoxia, proangiogenic factors such as VEGF are released by the malignant cells and infiltrating immune cells, namely monocytes. As a result, angiogenesis occurs and the tumor acquires its own blood supply. Neoplastic growth is thus promoted, as well as the potential for invasion and haematogenic metastasis (Kerbel, 2000).

Vegf is upregulated in hypoxia via the oxygen sensor hypoxia-inducible factor (HIF)-1α (Pugh & Ratcliffe, 2003). Another recently described VEGF activation mechanism is the induction of

the transcriptional coactivator peroxisoma proliferator-activated receptor-gamma coactivator-1α (PGC-1α) in response to the lack of nutrients and oxygen (Arany et al., 2008). Additionally, VEGF gene expression can be upregulated by oncogene signaling, several growth factors, inflammatory cytokines and hormones (reviewed in Ferrara, 2004). Tumor cells secrete VEGF mainly in a paracrine manner, although it can also act in an autocrine manner to promote a protective/survival effect to endothelial cells, among other cell types (Brusselmans et al., 2005).
The mechanisms underlying tumor lymphangiogenesis are not clearly defined. Inflammation seems to promote lymphatic neovascularization: inflammatory cells that infiltrate in the growing tumor produce lymphangiogenic growth factors. Another lymphangiogenesis trigger mechanism may be the high interstitial pressure generated inside the tumors due to the excessive production of interstitial fluid (reviewed in Cao, 2005). On the other hand, the extracellular matrix is of central importance for the generation of new lymphatic vessels as a response to the pathological stimulus. Integrins, a superfamily of cell adhesion molecules, are able to influence cell migration: integrin α9β1 is a target gene for Prox1, and its direct binding to VEGF-C and VEGF-D stimulates cell migration (reviewed in Wiig, 2010).
VEGF-C and VEGF-D, via signaling through VEGFR-3, appear to be essential for tumor-associated lymphangiogenesis, leading to lymphatic vessel invasion, lymph node involvement and distant metastasis (reviewed in Achen & Stacker, 2008). Moreover, VEGF interaction with VEGFR-2 may also promote lymphatic neovascularization, namely inside the regional draining lymph nodes, even before lymph node metastasis occurrence. This probably corresponds to a pathophysiologic strategy of "soil" preparation by the primary tumor to ensure the success of its future dissemination (Hirakawa et al., 2005). In fact, sentinel lymph node metastasis is the first step in the spreading of many cancer types.
Preexisting blood and lymphatic vessels in the vicinity of the malignant mass may contribute to tumor spread. However, *de novo* formed vessels by tumor-induced angiogenesis and lymphangiogenesis seem to be the preferential routes for dissemination (reviewed in Cao, 2005). This is a consequence of the ultra-structure of the tumor-associated blood and lymphatic vessels.

2.3 Ultra-structure of tumor-associated blood and lymphatic vessels

Blood vessels present in malignant tissues show remarkable differences with vessels present in normal tissues. Tumor blood vessels are highly disorganized: they are tortuous, excessively branched and dilated. The basement membrane and the muscular coverage are incomplete or absent. The endothelial cells, abnormal in shape, overlap and are projected into the lumen rather than organizing a pavement layer below the basement membrane. Blood vessel invasion is facilitated by this aberrant structure, but the extravasation rate is high, and blood flow is variable. As a result, interstitial tumor hypertension occurs, and delivery of therapeutic agents into tumors is compromised (Jain & Carmeliet, 2001; reviewed in Cao, 2005). The intratumoral edema is pernicious to malignant cells; therefore, homeostasis needs to be re-established. The formation of a tumoral lymphatic vasculature could potentially resolve this problem.
The key function of lymphatic vessels is to collect the excessive amount of interstitial fluid back to the blood circulation for immune surveillance in lymph nodes. Unlike normal blood capillaries, lymphatic capillaries have a discontinuous or fenestrated basement membrane and are not ensheathed by pericytes or smooth muscle cells; the endothelial cells are arranged in a slightly overlapping pattern and lack tight interendothelial junctions. Specialized anchoring

filaments of elastic fibers connect the endothelial cells to the extracellular matrix, which causes the vessels to dilate rather than to collapse when hydrostatic pressure rises (Alitalo et al., 2005; Tobler & Detmar, 2006). This structure facilitates the collection of interstitial fluid and is ideal for malignant cells' entry into the lymphatic flow.

A highly debated question is whether there are functional lymphatic vessels inside tumors (reviewed in Alitalo & Carmeliet, 2002; reviewed in Detmar & Hirakawa, 2002). On one hand, the elevated interstitial pressure generated by the proliferation of the malignant cells and by the high extravasion rate compromises the infiltration of new lymphatic vessels in the tumor stroma. Although intratumoral lymphangiogenesis may occur, the newly formed vessels are compressed and nonfunctional (Jain & Fenton, 2002). To compensate the lack of an intratumoral draining mechanism, the peritumoral lymphatic vessels enlarge due to an excess of pro-lymphangiogenic factors in that area. Therefore, in this model, the peritumoral lymphatic vessels passively collect interstitial fluid and, eventually, malignant cells (Carmeliet & Jain, 2000) (Fig. 2, A). However, some studies have demonstrated a relationship between the existence of functional intratumoral lymphatics, with cycling lymphatic endothelial cells and tumor emboli, and lymph node involvement (reviewed in Da et al., 2008). Additionally, peritumoral lymphangiogenesis occurs, and the new vessels actively contribute to metastatic spread (Padera et al., 2002) (Fig. 2, B). Probably, there are some organ-specific determinants that influence the occurrence of peritumoral and/or intratumoral lymphangiogenesis, as well as the function of the newly formed vessels.

2.4 Lymphovascular invasion and metastasis

Tumor metastasis involves a coordinated series of complex events that include promotion of angiogenesis and lymphangiogenesis, detachment of malignant cells from the primary tumor, microinvasion of the surrounding stroma, blood and/or lymphatic vessel invasion, survival of the malignant cells in the blood and/or lymphatic flow, and extravasion and growth in secondary sites. Because the large lymphatic vessels reenter the blood vascular system, malignant cells spread via the lymphatic system to the regional lymph nodes and, from this point, to distant organs (Alitalo & Carmeliet, 2002; Tobler & Detmar, 2006) (Fig. 3). Follow-up data have shown that 80% of the tumors, mainly those of epithelial origin, disseminate through the lymphatic vasculature; the remaining 20% use the blood circulation to colonize secondary organs (reviewed in Saharinen et al., 2004; reviewed in Wilting et al., 2005).

The blood vessels are not the best route for the success of malignant dissemination. Although their disorganized structure may contribute to the intravasion of malignant cells or emboli, in the bloodstream these cells experience serum toxicity, high shear stresses and mechanical deformation. Consequently, the viability of the tumor cells is seriously compromised (reviewed in Swartz, 2001). Conversely, the success rate of lymphogenous spread is high. As previously referred, the structure and function of the lymphatic capillaries facilitates intravasion of tumor cells or emboli. On the other hand, the composition of the lymph is similar to interstitial fluid, which provides an optimal medium for the survival of malignant cells. In collecting lymphatic vessels, muscle fibers assure lymph propulsion, that flows slowly, and valves prevent its backflow. Lymph nodes are areas of flow stagnation that represent ideal "incubators" for malignant cells' growth. Some cells exit the lymph node through the efferent channels or high endothelial venules. Other cells may remain mechanically entrapped for long periods of time, originating

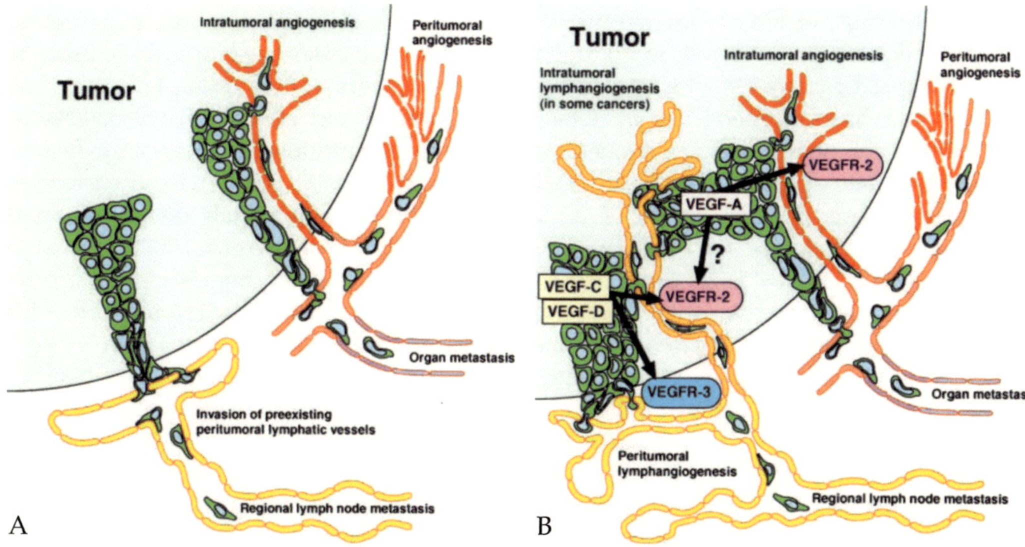

Fig. 2. (A) Traditional model of tumor metastasis via lymphatic and blood vessels. (B) Active lymphangiogenesis model of tumor metastasis (reprinted by permission from © 2002 Rockefeller University Press. Originally published in *J. Exp. Med.* 196: 713-718)

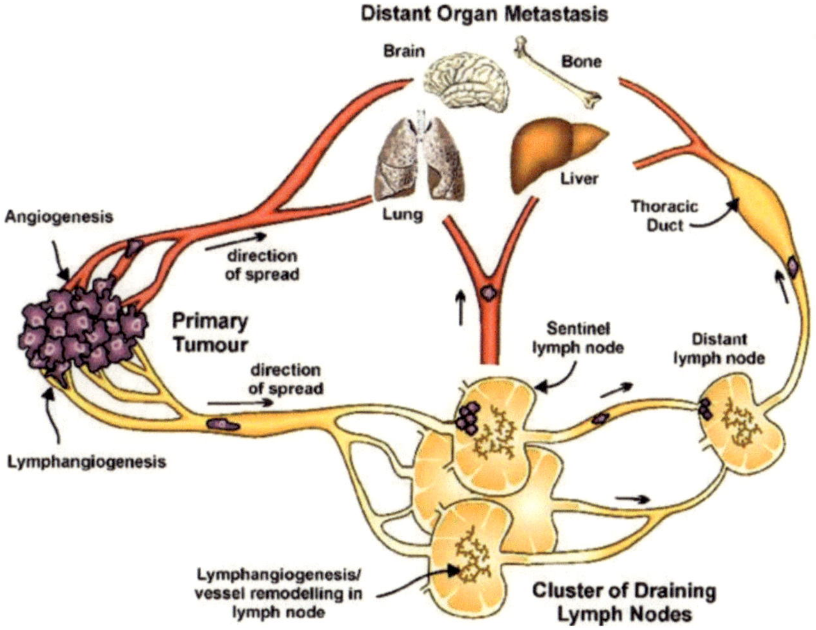

Fig. 3. Pathways of dissemination of malignant cells (reprinted by permission from © 2008 John Wiley & Sons, Inc. Originally published in *Ann. N. Y. Acad. Sci.* 1131: 225-234)

micrometastases (Swartz, 2001; Van Trapen & Pepper, 2002). Martens and colleagues described the expression of a gene signature of scavenger and lectin-like receptors in the lymph node sinus, which are known mediators of tumour cell adhesion and, therefore, can contribute to selective metastasis in an organ-specific context (Martens et al., 2006). Probably, tumor-cell-specific characteristics, microenvironmental factors and crosstalk between tumor and host cells have a pivotal role in determining survival and growth of micrometastasis. Moreover, lymph node lymphangiogenesis may provide an additional mechanism to facilitate further metastatic spread throughout the lymphatic system (Ji, 2009). The occurrence of lymphangiogenesis prior to arrival of tumor cells indicates that signals derived from the primary tumor are transported to the draining lymph nodes (Hirakawa et al., 2005).
Different tumors metastasize preferentially to different organs, suggesting that tumor spread is a guided process. It has been reported that malignant cells may use chemokine receptor ligand interactions to guide the colonization of target organs (reviewed in Saharinen et al., 2004; reviewed in Achen & Stacker, 2008). Chemokines are a family of chemoattractant cytokines that bind to G protein-coupled receptors expressed on target cells, namely malignant cells (Laurence, 2006). For instance, breast cancer cells, that normally choose regional lymph nodes, bone marrow, lung and liver as their first sites of destination, overexpress CCR7 (chemokine, CC motif, receptor 7) and CXCR4 (chemokine, CXC motif, receptor 4). Their ligands, SLC/CCL2 (secondary lymphoid chemokine / CC-type chemokine ligand 21) and SDF-1 CXCL12/ (stromal cell-derived factor 1 / chemokine, CXC motif, ligand 12) are expressed at high levels by isolated lymphatic endothelial cells and lymphatic endothelium from vessels present in the preferred sites of metastasis (Muller et al., 2001). This guides chemoattraction and migration of tumor cells, and characterizes lymphatic vessel invasion as an active event.

3. Angiogenesis, lymphangiogenesis and lymphovascular invasion in urothelial bladder cancer

The metastatic profile of urothelial bladder carcinoma implies, as in most malignant tumors, the dissemination of tumor cells through the lymphatic vasculature, and the colonization of regional lymph nodes is an early event in progression. Smith & Whitmore reported the involvement of the internal iliac and obturator groups of lymph nodes in about 74% of patients who underwent radical cystectomy; the external iliac nodes were involved in 65% of the patients, and the common iliac nodes were involved in 20% of the cases (Smith & Whitmore, 1981). As already referred, controversy exists regarding the optimal extent of lymphadenectomy and the number of lymph nodes to be retrieved at radical cystectomy. An extended pelvic lymph node dissection (encompassing the external iliac vessels, the obturator fossa, the lateral and medial aspects of the internal iliac vessels, and at least the distal half of the common iliac vessels together with its bifurcation) has been suggested as potentially curative in patients with metastasis or micrometastasis to a few nodes (Karl et al., 2009; Abol-Enein et al., 2011). Wright and colleagues observed that an increased number of lymph nodes removed at the time of radical cystectomy associates with improved survival in patients with lymph node-positive bladder cancer (Wright et al., 2008). The recommendation from the Bladder Cancer Collaboration Group is that ten to fourteen lymph nodes should be removed at the time of radical cystectomy (Herr et al., 2004). The concept of lymph node density (the number of positive lymph nodes divided by the total number of lymph nodes) was introduced by Stein and colleagues and helps to select lymph node-positive patients after radical cystectomy for adjuvant treatment (Stein et al., 2003). However, the lymph node density threshold is a debatable question (Gilbert, 2008). In large series, the median number of total lymph nodes removed was nine, with high lymph node density (25%), which can lead to misleading N0 staging (Wright et al., 2008). Therefore, in this subgroup of patients (lymph nodes removed ≤ 9 and N0), another prognostic factor is needed to better select patients for adjuvant treatment. Moreover, according to Malmström, extending the boundaries of surgery will not drastically improve survival. The focus should be on exploring biomarkers that predict extravesical dissemination and improving on the systemic treatment concept (Malmström, 2011). In this line of investigation, angiogenesis, lymphangiogenesis and lymphovascular invasion occurrence have been implicated in bladder cancer progression, invasion and metastasis, and represent potential targets for guided therapy.

Several studies reported a significant association between VEGF overexpression — both in tumor tissue (Crew et al., 1997; O'Brien et al., 1995) and urine (Crew et al., 1999; Jeon et al., 2001) —, high blood vessel density (Goddard et al., 2003; Santos et al., 2003) and the occurrence of recurrence and progression in patients with non-muscle invasive bladder cancer. In this group of patients, it has been observed that angiotensin II type 1 receptor (AT1R) expression associates with high blood vessel density and is related to early intravesical recurrence (Shirotake et al., 2011). AT1R supports tumor-associated macrophage infiltration, which results in enhanced tissue VEGF protein levels (Egami et al., 2009). These results suggest that AT1R is involved in bladder tumor angiogenesis and may become a new molecular target and a prognostic factor for urothelial bladder cancer patients

In the subset of invasive urothelial bladder cancer, most studies also reported the association between angiogenesis occurrence and unfavorable prognosis. High blood vessel density was identified as an independent prognostic factor by several authors (Bochner et al., 1995; Chaudhary et al., 1999; Dickinson et al., 1994; Jaeger et al., 1995). Moreover, overexpression of VEGF associates with high blood vessel density (Sato et al., 1998; Yang et al., 2004). Analysis of serum levels of VEGF has demonstrated its optimal sensitivity and specificity for predicting metastatic disease (Bernardini et al., 2001). Inoue and colleagues reported the importance of measuring blood vessel density and VEGF immunoexpression in identifying patients with invasive tumors who are at high risk of recurrence and development of metastasis after radical cystectomy and neoadjuvant systemic chemotherapy. The author highlighted the role of VEGF as a cell survival factor, not only by protecting the malignant cells in situations of hypoxia, but also during the occurrence of chemotherapy-induced apoptosis (Inoue et al., 2000).

Beyond VEGF signaling, other angiogenesis-related molecules have been implicated in bladder cancer recurrence, progression and metastasis, namely several proangiogenic factors — matrix metalloproteinases, fibroblast growth factors, platelet derived-growth factors, cyclooxygenases, integrins, angiopoietins, Notch signaling — and several antiangiogenic factors — thrombospondin-1, angiostatin-endostatin, platelet factor-4 (Chikazawa et al., 2008; Durkan et al., 2001; Grossfeld et al., 1997; Patel et al., 2006; reviewed in Pinto et al., 2010; Shariat et al., 2010).

The relevance of lymphangiogenesis in bladder cancer setting has gained recent attention. A few articles suggest that lymphangiogenesis occurrence, detected using specific lymphatic markers, is associated with poor prognosis (Fernández et al., 2008; Ma et al., 2010; Miyata et al., 2006; Zhou et al., 2011; Zu et al., 2006). VEGF-C, VEGF-D and VEGFR-3 are overexpressed in bladder cancer and promote tumor-induced lymphangiogenesis. This correlates with tumor upstaging and lymph node involvement, and results in a worse prognosis (Afonso et al., 2009; Miyata et al., 2006; Suzuki et al., 2005; Herrmann et al., 2007; Zhou et al., 2011; Zu et al., 2006). Interestingly, VEGF-C overexpression also associates with angiogenic events, probably by interaction of the fully processed form with VEGFR-2 (Afonso et al., 2009; Miyata et al., 2006). On the other hand, tumor associated macrophages play an important role in promoting lymphangiogenesis by producing VEGF-C and VEGF-D, mainly in peritumoral areas (Schoppmann et al., 2002). The blockade of VEGF-C/D with a soluble VEGF receptor-3 markedly inhibited lymphangiogenesis and lymphatic metastasis in an orthotopic urinary bladder cancer model. In addition, the depletion of tumor associated macrophages exerted similar effects (Yang et al. 2011).

Lymphovascular invasion has been identified as an independent prognostic factor for bladder cancer patients in several studies (Cho et al., 2009; Leissner et al., 2003; Lotan et al., 2005; Quek et al., 2005). In patients with newly diagnosed T1 urothelial bladder cancer, lymphovascular invasion in transurethral resection of bladder tumor specimens predicts disease progression and metastasis (Cho et al., 2009). Lotan and colleagues observed that blood and lymphatic vessel invasion (accessed by Haematoxylin-eosin stain) is an independent predictor of recurrence and low overall survival in patients who undergo radical cystectomy for invasive urothelial bladder cancer and are lymph node negative. They emphasized that these patients represent a high risk group that may benefit from neoadjuvant or adjuvant treatments. However, in this study, the mean number of lymph nodes removed per patient at the time of radical cystectomy was 20,1±10,2 (Lotan et al., 2005).

The prognostic impact of lymphovascular invasion in patients with lymph node-negative urothelial bladder cancer treated by radical cystectomy has been recently validated in large multicentre trials (Bolenz et al., 2010; Shariat et al, 2010). May and colleagues emphasized that, besides the importance of performing extended lymphadenectomies, the information resulting from an assessment of lymphovascular invasion is critical for stratification of risk groups and identification of patients who might benefit from adjuvant treatments (May, 2011). Algaba underlined that, in this field, it would be necessary to reach a consensus on strict diagnostic criteria as soon as possible, to be able to incorporate this prognostic factor in clinical practice (Algaba, 2006). Leissner and colleagues endorsed that blood and lymphatic vessel invasion should be commented on separately in the pathology report (Leissner et al., 2003).

Afonso and colleagues reported the prognostic contribution of molecular markers of blood vessels (like CD31) (Fig. 4, A) and lymphatic vessels (like D2-40) (Fig. 4, B) to accurately assess the occurrence of blood and/or lymphatic vessel invasion. The use of endothelial markers is encouraged because immunohistochemistry antibodies are significantly more sensitive in detecting invasive events than the standard Haematoxylin-eosin staining method and, additionally, facilitate the discrimination between blood and lymphatic vessel invasion. This is particularly important in identifying isolated malignant cells invading lymphatic vessels, because their viability is more probable in the lymphatic flow than in the blood circulation. Conversely, emboli of malignant cells are better suited to survive in the bloodstream, and are more easily identified, even by the traditional Haematoxylin-eosin staining method. This advocates the use of lymphatic markers for purposes of counting invaded lymphatic vessels. In this study, blood vessel invasion by malignant emboli assessed by CD31 staining (Fig. 5, A), and lymphatic vessel invasion by isolated malignant cells assessed by D2-40 staining (Fig. 5, B) significantly affected patients' prognosis; blood vessel invasion remained as an independent prognostic factor (Afonso et al., 2009). When included in a model of bladder cancer aggressiveness, these parameters contributed to a clear separation between low and high aggressiveness groups (Afonso et al., 2011).

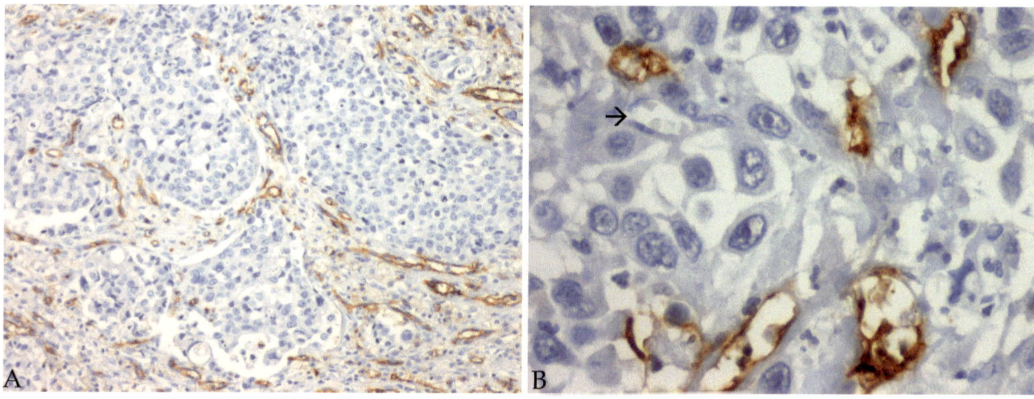

Fig. 4. Intratumoral blood vessels highlighted by CD31 (A), and intratumoral lymphatic vessels highlighted by D2-40 (B), in invasive urothelial bladder carcinoma. Evidence of internal negative control in A (D2-40 negative blood vessel →) (original magnification x100) (reprinted by permission from © 2009 John Wiley & Sons, Inc. Originally published in *Histopathol.* 55: 514-524)

Both peritumoral and intratumoral lymphatic vessels seem to be functional for urothelial cells' dissemination. Some articles reported the existence of intratumoral lymphatic vessels in bladder tumors, and their possible participation in metastatic events. No intratumoral edema has been observed, which is consistent with the occurrence of efficient lymphatic neovascularization (Afonso et al., 2009; Fernández et al., 2008; Ma et al., 2010; Miyata et al. 2006). Lymphatic vessel invasion occurrence correlates with high lymphatic vessel density values, mainly in the intratumoral areas. Although most of the invaded lymphatic vessels were distorted and collapsed, single malignant cells were significantly observed in the well-preserved intratumoral lymphatic vessels (Fig. 5, B). Moreover, the absence of intratumoral edema is a surrogate marker of an efficient lymphatic flow (Afonso et al., 2009).

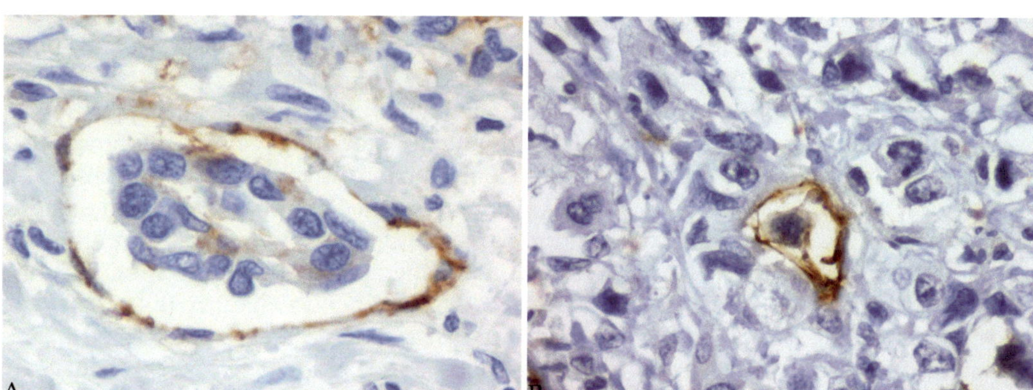

Fig. 5. Intratumoral blood vessel highlighted by CD31 invaded by a small malignant embolus (A), and intratumoral lymphatic vessel highlighted by D2-40 invaded by an isolated malignant cell (B), in invasive urothelial bladder carcinoma (original magnification x100) (reprinted by permission from © 2009 John Wiley & Sons, Inc. Originally published in *Histopathol.* 55: 514-524)

4. Angiogenesis and Lymphangiogenesis as therapeutic targets in urothelial bladder cancer

Our current understanding of the importance of tumor-induced angiogenesis and lymphangiogenesis for the occurrence of haematogenous and lymphogenous metastasis suggests that, by blocking the activity of key molecules involved in these processes, it should be possible to suppress the onset of metastasis following diagnosis of cancer and its subsequent therapy. Moreover, prophylactic suppression of metastasis would be useful for patients who are at risk of recurrence (Thiele & Sleeman, 2006). Therefore, clinical trials evaluating novel agents and combinations including chemotherapeutic drugs, as well as targeted inhibitors, are desperately needed (Iyer et al., 2010).

Two types of neovascularization inhibitors have been described. The direct inhibitors refer to compounds that function directly on endothelial cells by blocking a common pathway of vessel growth. Indirect inhibitors are molecules that neutralize the functions of angiogenic and lymphangiogenic growth factors; due to their mode of action, these are preferred over the direct inhibitors (Cao, 2005; Folkman, 2003). The main strategies that have been tested focus on modulating the signaling of VEGF family of growth factors and receptors, and are based on the use of monoclonal antibodies or soluble versions of receptors to neutralize the ligand-receptor interaction, and the inhibition of the kinase activity of the receptors (Achen et al., 2006; Thiele & Sleeman, 2006).

In 2004, the U.S. Food and Drug Administration (FDA) has approved bevacizumab (Avastin®), a humanized monoclonal antibody that binds to VEGF-A, as the first drug developed solely for antiangiogenesis anticancer use in humans. Antiangiogenic drugs are presently approved in a wide number of tumor types, namely in breast, colorectal, lung, liver, glioblastoma and kidney cancer. Other compounds are currently in preclinical development, with many of them now entering the clinic and/or achieving approval (reviewed in Boere et al., 2010; reviewed in Cook & Figg, 2010; reviewed in Pinto et al., 2010).

In anticancer therapy, an angiogenesis inhibitor may prevent the growth of new blood vessels. This should decrease the delivery of oxygen and nutrients - the "starving therapy" - which are indispensable elements for the support of uncontrolled cell division and tumor expansion. Angiogenesis inhibitors are predicted to be cytostatic, stabilizing tumors and perhaps preventing metastasis, rather than being curative (Zhi-chao & Jie, 2008). Therefore, there is the need to administrate this type of therapy for long periods of time. As a consequence, problems with bleeding, blood clotting, heart function and depletion of the immune system are common (Cohen et al., 2007). Nevertheless, inhibition of circulating VEGF reduces vascular permeability and thus tumoral interstitial pressure, permitting easier penetration of the tumor by conventional chemotherapeutic targets (Ferrara, 2005).

A second concern of anti-angiogenesis therapy is the approach to objectify the response to anti-angiogenic drugs. Chan and colleagues found that targeted contrast enhanced micro-ultrasound imaging enables investigators to detect and monitor vascular changes in orthotopic bladder tumors. Therefore, this technique may be useful for direct, noninvasive and in vivo evaluation of angiogenesis inhibitors (Chan et al., 2011). Lassau and colleagues demonstrated that dynamic ultrasound can be used to quantify dynamic changes in tumor vascularity as early as three days after the administration of the anti-angiogenic drug. These changes may be potential surrogate measures of the effectiveness of antiangiogenic therapy, namely by predicting progression-free survival and overall survival (Lassau et al., 2011).

Regarding antilymphangiogenic strategies, numerous compounds that could be used to block lymphangiogenesis already exist, although there is some delay in the translation to the clinic. These act mainly by targeting lymphangiogenic protein tyrosine kinases (Williams et al., 2010) (Table 1) or other indirect regulators of lymphangiogenic events. For instance, rapamycin (sirolimus), a classical immunosuppressant drug used to prevent rejection in organ transplantation, and a known inhibitor of the mTOR (mammalian target of rapamycin) signaling, has demonstrated potent antilymphangiogenic properties (Huber et al., 2007), and may suppress lymphatic metastasis (Kobayashi et al., 2007). mTOR is a member of the phosphoinositide-3-kinase-related kinase family, and is centrally involved in growth regulation, proliferation control and cancer cell metabolism (Rosner et al., 2008). Its inhibition impairs downstream signaling of VEGF-A as well as VEGF-C via mTOR to the ribosomal p70S6 kinase (a regulator of protein translation, and a major substrate of mTOR) in lymphatic endothelial cells (Huber et al., 2007). Other derivative compounds of rapamycin, like everolimus (RAD001) and temsirolimus (Torisel), have also demonstrated anti-tumor properties, namely by inhibiting tumor neovascularization (reviewed in Garcia & Danielpour, 2008). Recently, in patients with lymphangioleiomyomatosis (LAM, a progressive, cystic lung disease in women, which is associated with inappropriate activation of mTOR) sirolimus stabilized lung function, reduced serum VEGF-D levels, and was associated with a reduction in symptoms and improvement in the quality of life (McCormack et al., 2011).

Inhibition of lymphangiogenesis has been shown to block lymphatic metastasis by 50-70% in preclinical animal models, with good safety profiles, which suggests that anti-lymphangiogenic therapy could possibly be used safely in cancer patients, without disrupting normal lymphatic function (reviewed in Holopainen et al., 2011). Optimally, the gold-standard strategy would be the one that could inhibit both angiogenic and lymphangiogenic cascades, in order to compromise the success of haematogenous and lymphogenous dissemination. Some potential compounds are being investigated (reviewed in Boere et al., 2010; reviewed in Cook & Figg, 2010; reviewed in Pinto et al., 2010; reviewed in Stacker & Achen, 2008).

Urothelial bladder carcinoma has experienced very few therapeutic successes, regarding antineovascularization therapy, in the last years. Compounds like bevacizumab (Avastin®), aflibercept (VEGF-Trap, AVE0005), sunitinib malate (Sutent, SU11248), sorafenib (BAY 43-9006), vandetanib (Zactima, ZD6474) and pazopanib (Votrient, GW786034) are being tested in preclinical and clinical trials (reviewed in Pinto et al., 2010) (Table 2).

Bevacizumab, as has been already referred, is a monoclonal antibody that binds and neutralizes VEGF in the serum. Aflibercept is a soluble fusion protein of the human extracellular domains of VEGFR-1 and VEGFR-2, and the Fc portion of human immunoglobulin G. It binds, with a higher affinity than other monoclonal antibodies, to VEGF and additional VEGF-family members, namely VEGF-B and placental growth factor (PlGF). Sunitinib is an oral multi-targeted receptor tyrosine kinase inhibitor, with activity against VEGF receptors and PDGF receptors, among others. Sorafenib is a small, oral molecule that inhibits various targets along the EGFR/MAPK (epidermal growth factor receptor / mitogen-activated protein kinase) signal transduction pathway, and also through VEGFR and PDGFR families. Vandetanib is a tyrosine kinase inhibitor, antagonist of VEGFR and EGFR. Pazopanib is a multitargeted tyrosine kinase inhibitor against VEGF receptors, c-kit, and PDGF receptors (Cook & Figg, 2010).

Gene	Role in lymphatic vessels	Inhibitors available	Effect of pathway inhibition
VEGFR-2	Receptor for the VEGF family of ligands. Can also heterodimerize with VEGFR-3.	Yes	Secreted VEGFR-2 is a naturally occurring inhibitor of lymphatic vessel growth; however, Sorafenib† did not block VEGF-C/D induced tumor lymphangiogenesis.
VEGFR-3	Predominant receptor for VEGF-C and VEGF-D. Transduces survival, proliferation and migration signals.	Yes	Cediranib‡ blocks VEGFR-3 activity and inhibits lymphangiogenesis. Anti-VEGFR-3 antibody prevented tumor lymphangiogenesis with no effect on preexisting vessels.
Tie1	Not critical for lymphatic cell commitment during development, and no ligand has been shown.	None reported.	Tie1 knockout mouse has lymphatic vascular abnormalities that precede the blood vessel phenotype.
Tie2	Receptor for Ang-1 and Ang-2. Appears to control vessel maturation.	Yes	Tie2-/- mice are embryonic lethal due to vascular defects. Inhibition of Ang-2 leads to tumor blood vessel normalization.
EphB4	Expressed on lymphatic capillary vessels. Involved in vascular patterning. Binds to the ephrinB2 ligand.	Yes	Mice expressing a mutant form of ephrinB2 lacking the PDZ binding domain show major lymphatic defects in capillary vessels and collecting vessel valve formation.
FGFR3	The ligands FGF-1 and FGF-2 promote proliferation, migration, and survival of cultured lymphatic endothelial cells. FGFR3 is a direct transcriptional target of Prox1.	Yes	Knockdown of FGFR3 reduced lymphatic endothelial cells' proliferation.
IGF1R	Both of the IGF1R ligands, IGF-1 and IGF-2, significantly stimulated proliferation and migration of primary lymphatic endothelial cells.	Yes	None reported.
PDGFRβ	The ligand PDGF-BB stimulated MAP kinase activity and cell motility of isolated lymphatic endothelial cells.	Yes	None reported.

Gene	Role in lymphatic vessels	Inhibitors available	Effect of pathway inhibition
MET	The ligand for c-Met, hepatocyte growth factor, has lymphangiogenic effect, but it is unclear if c-Met is expressed on lymphatic endothelial cells.	Yes	May be indirect effect.

†Sorafenib inhibits B-Raf, PDGFRb, VEGFR-2 and c-Kit. ‡Cediranib inhibits VEGFR-1, -2, -3, PDGFRb and c-Kit.

Table 1. Protein tyrosine kinases involved in lymphatic biology, and available inhibitors (Tie- tyrosine kinase with immunoglobulin and EGF homology domain; EphB4- ephrin type-B receptor 4) (reprinted by permission from © 2010 BioMed Central Ltd. Originally published in *J. Ang. Res.* 2: 1-13)

Principal investigator / organization	Regimen	Patient population	Phase
Siefker-Radtke/MDACC	Methotrexate + vinblastine + doxorubicin+ cisplatin + bevacizumab	Neoadjuvant (muscle-invasive)	II
Kraft/MUSC	Gemcitabine + cisplatin + bevacizumab → cystectomy → paclitaxel + bevacizumab	Neoadjuvant/adjuvant (muscle-invasive)	II
Hahn/HOG	Gemcitabine + cisplatin + bevacizumab	First-line metastatic	II
Bajorin/MSKCC	Gemcitabine + carboplatin + bevacizumab	First-line metastatic (cisplatin-ineligible)	II
Rosenberg/CALGB	Gemcitabine + cisplatin ± bevacizumab	First-line metastatic	III
Garcia/Cleveland Clinic	Sunitinib	Neoadjuvant (muscle-invasive)	II
Sonpavde/HOG	Gemcitabine + cisplatin + sunitinib	Neoadjuvant (muscle-invasive)	II
Bellmunt	Sunitinib	First-line metastatic (cisplatin-ineligible)	II
Galsky/US Oncology	Gemcitabine + cisplatin + sunitinib	First-line metastatic	II
Hussain/University of Michigan	Sunitinib versus placebo	Maintenance after first-line chemotherapy	II
Gallagher/MSKCC	Sunitinib	Second-line metastatic	II
Milowsky/MSKCC	Gemcitabine + cisplatin + sorafenib	First-line metastatic	II
Kelly/Yale	Gemcitabine + carboplatin + sorafenib	First-line metastatic (cisplatin-ineligible)	II

Principal investigator / organization	Regimen	Patient population	Phase
Sternberg/EORTC	Gemcitabine + carboplatin ± sorafenib	First-line metastatic	II
Dreicer/ECOG	Sorafenib	Second-line metastatic	II
Choueiri/DFCI	Docetaxel ± vandetanib	Second-line metastatic	II
Vaishampayan/Mayo Clinic	Pazopanib	Second-line metastatic	II

MDACC = MD Anderson Cancer Center; MUSC = Medical University of South Carolina; HOG = Hoosier Oncology Group; MSKCC = Memorial Sloan-Kettering Cancer Center; CALGB = Cancer and Leukemia Group B; EORTC = European Organization for Research and Treatment of Cancer; ECOG = Eastern Cooperative Oncology Group; DFCI = Dana-Farber Cancer Institute

Table 2. Selected ongoing or recently completed trials exploring antiangiogenic therapies in urothelial bladder carcinoma (reprinted by permission from © 2010 Elsevier. Originally published in *Commun. Oncol.* 7: 500-504)

4.1 Preclinical studies

In the preclinical scenario, Videira and colleagues studied the effect of bevacizumab on autocrine VEGF stimulation in bladder cancer cell lines, and concluded that, at clinical bevacizumab concentrations, cancer cells compensate the VEGF blockade, by improving the expression of VEGF and related genes. This highlights the need to follow the patient's adaptation response to bevacizumab treatment (Videira et al., 2011). The antiangiogenic treatment of tumours may restore vascular communication and, thereby, normalize flow distribution in tumour vasculature. The use of antiangiogenic drugs leads to improved tumour oxygenation and chemotherapy drug delivery (Pries et al., 2010). However, these mechanisms may be also the cause of malignant dissemination, because tumours elicit evasive resistance. Caution is recommended, due to the divergent effects that VEGF inhibitors can induce on primary tumor growth and metastasis (Loges et al., 2009).

Yoon and colleagues, when exposing six human bladder cancer cell lines to an escalating dose of sunitinib alone or in combination with cisplatin/gemcitabine, demonstrated that sunitinib malate has a potent antitumor effect and may synergistically enhance the known antitumor effect of gemcitabine (Yoon et al, 2011).

The first study with vandetanib in bladder cancer cell lines demonstrated its potential to sensitize tumor cells to cisplatin. At vandetanib concentrations of ≤2microM, the combination with cisplatin was synergistic, especially when given sequentially after cisplatin , and additive with vandetanib followed by cisplatin (Flaig et al., 2009).

Li and colleagues studied the efficacy of pazopanib, both alone and in combination with docetaxel, in bladder cancer cell lines. They demonstrated that single-agent pazopanib has modest activity, but when given in combination with docetaxel, acted synergistically in docetaxel-resistant bladder cancer cells, with the potential of improved toxicity (Li et al., 2001).

Urothelial bladder carcinoma expresses mTOR signaling molecules, providing a rationale for clinical trials evaluating agents targeting this pathway (Tickoo et al., 2011). In fact, some studies using bladder cancer cell lines have demonstrated that sirolimus and related drugs inhibit the growth of cancer cells and decrease their viability (Fechner et al., 2009; Hansel et al., 2010; Pinto-Leite et al., 2009; Schedel et al., 2011). Similar results were obtained when treating bladder cancer animal models with sirolimus or everolimus (Chiong et al., 2011; Oliveira et al., 2011; Parada et al., 2011; Seager et al., 2009; Vasconcelos-Nóbrega et al., 2011).

4.2 Phase II studies

The results of a phase II trial of cisplatin, gemcitabine, and bevacizumab (CGB) as first-line therapy for metastatic urothelial carcinoma revealed that CGB may improve overall survival — with a median follow-up of 27.2 months, overall survival time was 19.1 months. However, the rate of side effects was high, namely neutropenia, thrombocytopenia, anemia, and deep vein thrombosis/pulmonary embolism (Hahn et al., 2011).

In a phase II trial of gemcitabine, carboplatin, and bevacizumab in patients with advanced/metastatic urothelial carcinoma, Balar and colleagues concluded that addition of bevacizumab does not improve the response rate. However, bevacizumab can be safely added to gemcitabine and carboplatin, because the rate of venous thromboembolisms is similar to the one observed with gemcitabine and carboplatin alone (Balar et al., 2011). Moreover, in a pooled analysis of cancer patients in randomized phase II and III studies, the addition of bevacizumab to chemotherapy did not statistically significantly increase the risk of venous thromboembolisms *versus* chemotherapy alone. Probably, the risk for venous thromboembolisms is driven predominantly by tumor and host factors (Hurwitz et al., 2011). This type of side effect is primarily prevented by using anticoagulants simultaneously with cytotoxic chemotherapy (Riess et al., 2010). However, anticoagulant use during bevacizumab therapy may increase the risk of serious hemorrhage, although it is generally well tolerated (Bartolomeo et al., 2010). This controversial issue is still under scrutiny and more data are needed to clarify the optimal regime to reduce venous thromboembolisms in bladder cancer patients, particularly in those who are being treated with antiangiogenic drugs.

Patients with recurrent or metastatic urothelial carcinoma who had received a prior platinum-containing regimen were entered in a phase II trial with aflibercept as a second-line therapy. Aflibercept was well tolerated, but it had limited single agent activity in platinum-pretreated bladder cancer patients (Twardowski et al., 2009).

In a phase II study of sunitinib in patients with metastatic urothelial cancer designed to assess the efficacy and tolerability of this drug in patients with advanced, previously treated urothelial cancer, anti-tumour responses were observed. However, sunitinib did not achieve the predetermined threshold of ≥20% activity defined by the Response Evaluation Criteria in Solid Tumors, and side effects such as embolic events were reported (Gallagher et al., 2010).

In a multicenter phase II trial with sunitinib as first-line treatment in patients with metastatic urothelial cancer ineligible for cisplatin, on intention-to-treat analysis revealed that 38% of the patients showed partial responses (PRs), and 50% presented with stable disease (SD), the majority more than 3 months. Clinical benefit (PR + SD) was 58%. Median time to progression was 4.8 months and median overall survival 8.1 months (Bellmunt et al., 2011).

In a multicentre phase II trial of sorafenib as second-line therapy in patients with metastatic urothelial carcinoma, there were no objective responses to therapy. The 4-month progression-free survival rate was 9.5%, and the overall survival was 6.8 months (Dreicer et al., 2009).

Choueiri and colleagues conducted a double-blind randomized trial in which patients with metastatic bladder cancer and as many as three previous chemotherapy regimens received intravenous docetaxel with or without vandetanib. The results demonstrated that the

addition of vandetanib to second-line docetaxel did not result in significant improvements in progression-free survival, overall survival or response rates (Choueiri et al., 2011).
The final results of a phase II study of everolimus in metastatic urothelial cell carcinoma have been presented at 2011 ASCO (American Society of Clinical Oncology) Annual Meeting. It was demonstrated that everolimus has clinical activity in patients with advanced urothelial bladder cancer. For the thirty-seven evaluable patients, the median progression-free survival was 3.3 months, and the median overall-survival was 10.5 months. Some side effects possibly related to everolimus were observed, namely anemia, infection, hyperglycemia, lymphopenia, hypophosphatemia and fatigue (Milowsky et al., 2011).
Dovitinib (TKI258) is an oral investigational drug that inhibits angiogenic factors, including FGFR and VEGFR. A multicenter, open-label phase II trial of dovitinib in advanced urothelial carcinoma patients with either mutated or wild-type FGFR3 is currently underway (Milowsky et al., 2011).

4.3 Phase III studies

A randomized double-blinded phase III study comparing gemcitabine, cisplatin, and bevacizumab to gemcitabine, cisplatin, and placebo in patients with advanced urothelial carcinoma is open to enrollment. The primary end point is to compare the overall survival of patients with advanced urothelial carcinoma treated with gemcitabine hydrochloride, cisplatin, and bevacizumab *versus* gemcitabine hydrochloride, cisplatin, and placebo. The secondary end points are to compare the progression-free survival, the objective response rate and the grade 3 and greater toxicities of these regimens in the patients (Cancer and Leukemia Group B, 2011).

5. Conclusion

Bladder cancer represents a significant health problem, and the costliest type of cancer to treat. Although the majority of cases present as non-muscle invasive disease, the recurrence and progression rates are high, which demands for long-term follow-up and repeated interventions. Moreover, patients with advanced tumors treated by neoadjuvant or adjuvant regiments frequently progress and may develop chemotherapy resistance. Therefore, biomarkers of tumour aggressiveness and response to therapy are urgently needed, since the classical formulae based on stage and grade classification are insufficient to characterize bladder cancer. In this sense, angiogenesis, lymphangiogenesis and lymphovascular invasion have been described as surrogate markers of bladder cancer progression, invasion and metastasis, and represent potential fields of intervention. On one hand, the combined analysis of these biological parameters in tumor samples with the classical clinicopathological parameters may improve the individual characterization of bladder cancer, in what concerns to its clinical and prognostic course, and should allow therapeutic adequacy. On the other hand, the knowledge and modulating of biological phenomena related with bladder cancer progression may represent a significant improvement in the development of new drugs and in the pathological response to therapy, which ultimately will lead to an increase in disease-free survival and overall survival rates.
Targeted therapy has caused dramatic changes in the treatment of other types of tumors. However, in bladder cancer setting, clinical trials with molecularly targeted agents have been few in number and largely unsuccessful. Regarding antiangiogenic and

antilymphangiogenic agents, these are still considered an investigational option for urothelial bladder cancer patients, and more results are needed to establish their roles in the treatment armamentarium. Research studies with anti-neovascularization drugs should not only provide effective agents to treat bladder cancer patients, but also predictive biomarkers for response to anti-neovascularization therapy, in order to implement the concept of personalized therapy.

6. Acknowledgements

We thank Nuno Sousa, from the Department of Medical Oncology of the Portuguese Institute of Oncology - IPO, for a critical review of the chapter.

7. References

Abol-Enein, H.; Tilki, D.; Mosbah, A. et al. (2011). Does the Extent of Lymphadenectomy in Radical Cystectomy for Bladder Cancer Influence Disease-Free Survival? A Prospective Single-Center Study. *European Urology*, (June 2011), [Epub ahead of print], ISSN 0302-2838.

Achen, M.G. & Stacker, S. (2008). Molecular Control of Lymphatic Metastasis. *Annals of the New York Academy of Sciences*, Vol.1131, pp. 225-234, ISSN 0077-8923.

Achen, M.G.; Mann, G.B. & Stacker, S.A. (2006). Targeting lymphangiogenesis to prevent tumor metastasis. *British Journal of Cancer*, Vol.94, No.10 (May 2006), pp.1355-1360.

Adams, R.H. & Alitalo, K. (2007). Molecular regulation of angiogenesis and lymphangiogenesis. *Nature Reviews Cancer*, Vol.8, No.6 (June 2007), pp. 464-478, ISSN 1474-175X.

Afonso, J.; Santos, L.L.; Amaro, T.; Lobo, F. & Longatto-Filho, A. (2009). The aggressiveness of urothelial carcinoma depends to a large extent on lymphovascular invasion - the prognostic contribution of related molecular markers. *Histopathology*, Vol.55, No.5 (November 2009), pp: 514-524, ISSN 1365-2559.

Afonso, J.; Longatto-Filho, A.; Baltazar, F. et al. (2011). CD147 overexpression allows an accurate discrimination of bladder cancer patients' prognosis, *European Journal of Surgical Oncology*, (July 2011), doi:10.1016/j.ejso.2011.06.006, ISSN 0748-7983.

Algaba, F. (2006). Lymphovascular invasion as a prognostic tool for advanced bladder cancer. *Current Opinion in Urology*, Vol.16, No.5 (September 2006), pp. 367-371, ISSN 1473-6586.

Alitalo, K. & Carmeliet, P. (2002). Molecular mechanisms of lymphangiogenesis in health and disease. *Cancer Cell*. Vol.1, No.3 (April 2002), pp. 219-227, ISSN 1535-6108.

Alitalo, K.; Tammela, T. & Petrova, T. (2005). Lymphangiogenesis in development and human disease. *Nature*, Vol.438, No.7070 (December 2005), pp. 946-953, ISSN 0028-0836.

Arany, Z.; Foo, S.Y.; Ma, Y. et al. (2008). HIF-independent regulation of VEGF and angiogenesis by the transcriptional coactivator PGC-1alpha. *Nature*, Vol.451, No.7181 (February 2008), pp. 1008-1012, ISSN 0028-0836.

Balar, A.V.; Milowsky, M.I.; Apolo, A.B. et al. (2011). Phase II trial of gemcitabine, carboplatin, and bevacizumab in chemotherapy-naive patients with advanced/metastatic urothelial carcinoma. *Proceedings of the 2011 Genitourinary Cancers Symposium*, Abstract No 248, Orlando, Florida, USA, February 17-19, 2011.

Baldwin, M.E.; Halford, M.M.; Roufail, S. et al. (2005). Vascular Endothelial Growth Factor D is dispensable for Development of the Lymphatic System. *Molecular and Cellular Biology*, Vol.25, No.6 (March 2005), pp. 2441-2449, ISSN 1098-5549.

Banerji, S.; Ni, J.; Wang, S.X. et al. (1999). LYVE-1, a new homologue of the CD44 glycoprotein, is a lymph-specific receptor for hyaluronan. *The Journal of Cell Biology*, Vol.144, No.4 (February 1999), pp. 789-801, ISSN 1540-8140.

Bartolomeo, J.; Norden, A.D.; Drappatz, J. et al. (2010). Safety of concurrent bevacizumab therapy and anticoagulation in high-grade glioma patients. *Proceedings of the 2010 ASCO Annual Meeting*, Abstract No 2043, Chicago, Illinois, USA, June 4-8, 2010.

Bellmunt, J.; González-Larriba, J.L.; Prior, C. et al. (2011). Phase II study of sunitinib as first-line treatment of urothelial cancer patients ineligible to receive cisplatin-based chemotherapy: baseline interleukin-8 and tumor contrast enhancement as potential predictive factors of activity. *Annals of Oncology*, (March 2011), [Epub ahead of print], ISSN 1569-8041.

Bernardini, S.; Fauconnet, S.; Chabannes, E. et al. (2001). Serum levels of vascular endothelial growth factor as a prognostic factor in bladder cancer. *The Journal of Urology*, Vol.166, No.4 (October 2001), pp. 1275-1279, ISSN 0022-5347.

Bochner, B.H.; Cote, R.J.; Weidner, N. et al. (1995). Angiogenesis in bladder cancer: relationship between microvessel density and tumor prognosis. *Journal of the National Cancer Institute*, Vol.87, No.21 (November 1995), pp. 1603-1612, ISSN 1460-2105.

Boere, I.A.; Hamberg, P. & Sleijfer, S. (2010). It takes two to tango: combinations of conventional cytotoxics with compounds targeting the vascular endothelial growth factor-vascular endothelial growth factor receptor pathway in patients with solid malignancies. *Cancer Science*, Vol.101, No.1 (January 2010), pp. 7-15, ISSN 1349-7006.

Bolenz, C.; Herrmann, E.; Bastian, P.J. et al. (2010). Lymphovascular invasion is an independent predictor of oncological outcomes in patients with lymph node-negative urothelial bladder cancer treated by radical cystectomy: a multicentre validation trial. *British Journal of Urology International*, Vol.106, No.4 (August 2010), pp. 493-499, ISSN 2042-2997.

Brusselmans, K.; Bono, F.; Collen, D. et al. (2005). A novel role for vascular endothelial growth factor as an autocrine survival factor for embryonic stem cells during hypoxia. *The Journal of Biological Chemistry*, Vol.280, No.5 (February 2005), pp. 3493-3499, ISSN 1083-351X.

Cancer and Leukemia Group B (2011). CALGB90601 A Randomized Double-Blinded Phase III Study Comparing Gemcitabine, Cisplatin, and Bevacizumab to Gemcitaine, Cisplatin, and Placebo in Patients with Advanced Transitional Cell Carcinoma, In: University of Colorado Hospital, 08.07.2010, Available from: http://www.uch.edu/ClinicalTrials/clinical-trials-detail/?id=117

Cao, Y. (2005). Emerging mechanisms of tumour lymphangiogenesis and lymphatic metastasis. *Nature Reviews Cancer*, Vol.5, No.9 (September 2005), pp. 735-743, ISSN 1474-175X.

Carmeliet, P. & Jain, R.K. (2000). Angiogenesis in cancer and other diseases. *Nature*, Vol.407, No.6801 (September 2000), pp. 249-257, ISSN 0028-0836.

Carmeliet, P. (2005). VEGF as a Key Mediator of Angiogenesis in Cancer. *Oncology*, Vol.69, No.3 (November 2005) pp. 4-10, ISSN 1423-0232.

Carmeliet, P.; Ferreira, V.; Breier, G. et al. (1996). Abnormal blood vessel development and lethality in embryos lacking a single VEGF allele. *Nature*, Vol.380, No.6573 (April 1996), pp. 435-439, ISSN 0028-0836.

Chan, E.S.; Patel, A.R.; Larchian, W.A. & Heston, W.D. (2011). In vivo targeted contrast enhanced micro-ultrasound to measure intratumor perfusion and vascular endothelial growth factor receptor 2 expression in a mouse orthotopic bladder cancer model. *The Journal of Urology*, Vol.185, No.6 (June 2011), pp. 2359-2365, ISSN 0022-5347.

Chaudhary, R.; Bromley, M.; Clarke, N.W. et al. (1999). Prognostic relevance of micro-vessel density in cancer of the urinary bladder. *Anticancer Research*, Vol.19, No.4C (July-August 1999), pp. 3479-3484, ISSN 1791-7530.

Chikazawa, M.; Inoue, K.; Fukata, S.; Karashima, T. & Shuin, T. (2008). Expression of angiogenesis-related genes regulates different steps in the process of tumor growth and metastasis in human urothelial cell carcinoma of the urinary bladder. *Pathobiology*, Vol.75, No.6 (December 2008), pp.335-345, ISSN 1423-0291.

Chiong, E.; Lee, I.L.; Dadbin, A. et al. Effects of mTOR inhibitor everolimus (RAD001) on bladder cancer cells. *Clinical Cancer Research*, Vol.17, No.9 (May 2011), pp. 2863-2873, ISSN 1557-3265.

Cho, K.S.; Seo, H.K.; Joung, J.Y. et al. (2009). Lymphovascular invasion in transurethral resection specimens as predictor of progression and metastasis in patients with newly diagnosed T1 bladder urothelial cancer. *The Journal of Urology*, Vol.182, No.6 (December 2009), pp.2625-2630, ISSN 0022-5347.

Choueiri, T.K.; Vaishampayan U.N.; Yu, E.Y. et al. (2011). A double-blind randomized trial of docetaxel plus vandetanib versus docetaxel plus placebo in platinum-pretreated advanced urothelial cancer. *Proceedings of the 2011 Genitourinary Cancers Symposium*, Abstract LBA239, Orlando, Florida, USA, February 17-19, 2011.

Clark, P.E. (2009). Neoadjuvant versus adjuvant chemotherapy for muscle-invasive bladder cancer. *Expert Review of Anticancer Therapy*, Vol.9, No.6 (June 2009), pp. 821-830, ISSN 1473-7140.

Cohen, M.H.; Gootenberg, J.; Keegan, P. & Pazdur, R. (2007). FDA drug approval summary: Bevacizumab plus FOLFOX4 as second-line treatment of colorectal cancer. *The Oncologist*, Vol.12, No.3 (March 2007), pp. 356-361, ISSN 1549-490X.

Cook, K.M. & Figg, W.D. (2010). Angiogenesis inhibitors: current strategies and future prospects. *CA: A Cancer Journal for Clinicians*, Vol.60, No.4 (July-August 2010), pp. 222-243, ISSN 1542-4863.

Crew, J.P.; O'Brien, T.; Bicknell, R. et al. (1999). Urinary vascular endothelial growth factor and its correlation with bladder cancer recurrence rates. *The Journal of Urology*, Vol.161, No.3 (March 1999), pp. 799-804, ISSN 0022-5347.

Crew, J.P.; O'Brien, T.; Bradburn, M. et al. (1997). Vascular endothelial growth factor is a predictor of relapse and stage progression in superficial bladder cancer. *Cancer Research*, Vol.57, No.23 (December 1997), pp. 5281-5285, ISSN 1538-7445.

Da, M.X.; Wu, Z. & Tian, H.W. (2008). Tumor lymphangiogenesis and lymphangiogenic growth factors. *Archives of Medical Research*, Vol.39, No.4 (May 2008), pp. 365-372, ISSN 0188-4409.

Detmar, M. & Hirakawa, S. (2002). The Formation of Lymphatic Vessels and Its Importance in the Setting of Malignancy. *The Journal of Experimental Medicine*, Vol.196, No.6 (September 2002), pp. 713-718, ISSN 1540-9538.

Dickinson, A.J.; Fox, S.B.; Persad, R.A. et al. (1994). Quantification of angiogenesis as an independent predictor of prognosis in invasive bladder carcinomas. *British Journal of Urology International*, Vol.74, No.6 (December 1994), pp. 762-766, ISSN 2042-2997.

Dreicer, R.; Li, H.; Stein, M. et al. (2009). Phase 2 trial of sorafenib in patients with advanced urothelial cancer: a trial of the Eastern Cooperative Oncology Group. *Cancer*, Vol.115, No.18 (September 2009), pp. 4090-4095, ISSN 1097-0142.

Durkan, G.C.; Nutt, J.E.; Rajjayabun, P.H. et al. (2001). Prognostic significance of matrix metalloproteinase-1 and tissue inhibitor of metalloproteinase-1 in voided urine samples from patients with transitional cell carcinoma of the bladder. *Clinical Cancer Research*, Vol.7, No.11 (November 2001), pp. 3450-3456, ISSN 1557-3265.

Egami, K.; Murohara, T.; Shimada, T. et al. (2003). Role of host angiotensin II type 1 receptor in tumor angiogenesis and growth. *The Journal of Clinical Investigation*, Vol.112, No.1 (July 2003), pp. 67-75, ISSN 0021-9738.

Fechner, G.; Classen, K.; Schmidt, D.; Hauser, S. & Müller, S.C. (2009). Rapamycin inhibits in vitro growth and release of angiogenetic factors in human bladder cancer. *Urology*, Vol.73, No.3 (March 2009), pp. 665-668 (discussion 668-669), ISSN 0090-4295.

Fernández, M.I.; Bolenz, C.; Trojan, L. et al. (2007). Prognostic Implications of Lymphangiogenesis in Muscle-Invasive Transitional Cell Carcinoma of the Bladder. *European Urology*, Vol.53, No.3 (March 2008), pp.571-578, ISSN 0302-2838.

Ferrara, N. (2004). Vascular endothelial growth factor: basic science and clinical progress. *Endocrine Reviews*, Vol.25, No.4 (August 2004), pp. 581-611, ISSN 1945-7189.

Ferrara, N. (2005). VEGF as a Therapeutic Target in Cancer. *Oncology*, Vol. 69, No.3 (November 2005), pp. 11-16, ISSN 1423-0232.

Ferrara, N.; Carver-Moore, K.; Chen, H. et al. (1996). Heterozygous embryonic lethality induced by targeted inactivation of the VEGF gene. *Nature*, Vol.380, No.6573 (April 1996), pp. 439-442, ISSN 0028-0836.

Flaig, T.W.; Su, L.J.; McCoach, C. et al. (2009). Dual epidermal growth factor receptor and vascular endothelial growth factor receptor inhibition with vandetanib sensitizes bladder cancer cells to cisplatin in a dose- and sequence-dependent manner. *British Journal of Urology International*, Vol.103, No.12 (June 2009), pp. 1729-1737, ISSN 2042-2997.

Folkman, J. (2003). Angiogenesis inhibitors: a new class of drugs. *Cancer Biology & Therapy*, Vol.2, No.4 Suppl 1 (July-August 2003), pp. S127-S133, ISSN 1555-8576.

Fong, G.H.; Zhang, L.; Bryce, D.M. & Peng, J. (1999). Increased hemangioblast commitment, not vascular disorganization, is the primary defect in flt-1 knock-out mice. *Development*, Vol.126, No.13 (July 1999), pp. 3015-3025, ISSN 1477-9129.

François, M.; Caprini, A.; Hosking, B. et al. (2008). Sox18 induces development of the lymphatic vasculature in mice. *Nature*, Vol.456, No.7222 (December 2008), pp. 643-647, ISSN 0028-0836.

Gallagher, D.J.; Milowsky, M.I.; Gerst, S.R. et al. (2010). Phase II study of sunitinib in patients with metastatic urothelial cancer. *Journal of Clinical Oncology*, Vol.28, No.8 (March 2010), pp. 1373-1379, ISSN 1527-7755.

Galsky, M.D. (2010). Integrating antiangiogenic therapy for advanced urothelial carcinoma: rationale for a phase II study of gemcitabine, cisplatin, and sunitinib. *Community Oncology*, Vol.7, No.11 (November 2010), pp. 500-504, ISSN 1548-5315.

Garcia, J.A. & Danielpour, D. (2008). Mammalian target of rapamycin inhibition as a therapeutic strategy in the management of urologic malignancies. *Molecular Cancer Therapeutics*, Vol.7, No.6 (June 2008), pp. 1347-1354, ISSN 1538-8514.

Gilbert, S.M. (2008). Separating surgical quality from causality-gaining perspective in the debate on lymph node count and extent of lymphadenectomy. *Cancer*, Vol.112, No. (June 2008), pp. 2331-2233, ISSN 1097-0142.

Goddard, J.C.; Sutton, C.D.; Furness, P.N.; O'Byrne, K.J. & Kockelbergh, R.C. (2003). Microvessel Density at Presentation Predicts Subsequent Muscle Invasion in Superficial Bladder Cancer. *Clinical Cancer Research*, Vol.9, No.7 (July 2003), pp. 2583-2586, ISSN 1557-3265.

Grossfeld, G.D.; Ginsberg, D.A.; Stein, J.P. et al. (1997). Thrombospondin-1 expression in bladder cancer: association with p53 alterations, tumor angiogenesis, and tumor progression. *Journal of the National Cancer Institute*, Vol.89, No.3 (February 1997), pp. 219-227, ISSN 1460-2105.

Hahn, N.M.; Stadler, W.M.; Zon, R.T. et al. (2011). Phase II trial of cisplatin, gemcitabine, and bevacizumab as first-line therapy for metastatic urothelial carcinoma: Hoosier Oncology Group GU 04-75. *Journal of Clinical Oncology*, Vol.29, No.12 (April 2011), pp. 1525-1530, ISSN 1527-7755.

Hansel, D.E.; Platt, E.; Orloff, M. et al. (2010). Mammalian target of rapamycin (mTOR) regulates cellular proliferation and tumor growth in urothelial carcinoma. *American Journal of Pathology*, Vol.176, No.6 (June 2010), pp. 3062-3072, ISSN 0002-9440.

Herr, H.; Lee, C.; Chang, S.; Lerner, S. & Bladder Cancer Collaborative Group (2004). Standardization of radical cystectomy and pelvic lymph node dissection for bladder cancer: a Collaborative Group report. *The Journal of Urology*, Vol.171, No.5 (May 2004), pp. 1823-1828, ISSN 0022-5347.

Herrmann, E.; Eltze, E.; Bierer, S. et al. (2007). VEGF-C, VEGF-D and Flt-4 in transitional bladder cancer: relationships to clinicopathological parameters and long-term survival. *Anticancer Research*, Vol.27, No.5A (September-October 2007), pp. 3127-3133, ISSN 1791-7530.

Hirakawa, S.; Kodama, S.; Kunstfeld, R. et al. (2005). VEGF-A induces tumor and sentinel lymph node lymphangiogenesis and promotes lymphatic metastasis. *The Journal of Experimental Medicine*, Vol.201, No.7 (April 2005), pp. 1089-1099, ISSN 1540-9538.

Holopainen, T.; Bry, M.; Alitalo, K. & Saaristo, A. (2011). Perspectives on lymphangiogenesis and angiogenesis in cancer. *Journal of Surgical Oncology*, Vol.103, No.6 (May 2011), pp. 484-488, ISSN 1096-9098.

Huber, S.; Bruns, C.J.; Schmid, G. et al. (2007). Inhibition of the mammalian target of rapamycin impedes lymphangiogenesis. *Kidney International*, Vol.71, No.8 (April 2007), pp. 771-777, ISSN 0085-2538.

Hurwitz, H.I.; Saltz, L.B.; Van Cutsem, E. et al. (2011). Venous thromboembolic events with chemotherapy plus bevacizumab: a pooled analysis of patients in randomized phase II and III studies. *Journal of Clinical Oncology*, Vol.29, No.13 (May 2011), pp. 1757-1764, ISSN 1527-7755.

Inoue, K.; Slaton, J.W.; Karashima, T. et al. (2000). The prognostic value of angiogenesis factor expression for predicting recurrence and metastasis of bladder cancer after neoadjuvant chemotherapy and radical cystectomy. *Clinical Cancer Research*, Vol.6, No.12 (December 2000), pp. 4866-4873, ISSN 1557-3265.

Iyer, G.; Milowsky, M.I. & Bajorin, D.F. (2010). Novel strategies for treating relapsed/ refractory urothelial carcinoma. *Expert Review of Anticancer Therapy*, Vol.10, No.12 (December 2010), pp. 1917-1932, ISSN 1473-7140.

Jaeger, T.M.; Weidner, N. & Chew, K. (1995). Tumor angiogenesis correlates with lymph node metastases in invasive bladder cancer. *The Journal of Urology*, Vol.154, No.1 (July 1995), pp. 69-71, ISSN 0022-5347.

Jain, R.K. & Carmeliet, P.F. (2001). Vessels of death or life. *Scientific American*, Vol. 285, No.6 (December 2001), pp. 38-45, ISSN 0036-8733.

Jain, R.K. & Fenton, B.T. (2002). Intratumoral lymphatic vessels: a case of mistaken identity or malfunction? *Journal of the National Cancer Institute*, Vol.94, No.6 (March 2002), pp. 417-421, ISSN 1460-2105.

Jeon, S.H.; Lee, S.J. & Chang, S.G. (2001). Clinical significance of urinary vascular endothelial growth factor in patients with superficial bladder tumors. *Oncology Reports*, Vol.8, No.6 (November-December 2001), pp. 1265-1267, ISSN 1791-2431.

Ji, R.C. (2009). Lymph node lymphangiogenesis: a new concept for modulating tumor metastasis and inflammatory process. *Histology and Histopathology*, Vol.24, No.3 (March 2009), pp. 377-384, ISSN 1699-5848.

Kaipainen, A.; Korhonen, J.; Mustonen, T. et al. (1995). Expression of the fms-like tyrosine kinase 4 gene becomes restricted to lymphatic endothelium during development. *Proceedings of the National Academy of Sciences USA*, Vol.92, No.8 (April 1995), pp. 3566-3570, ISSN 0027-8424.

Karkkainen, M.J.; Haiko, P.; Sainio, K. et al. (2004). Vascular endothelial growth factor C is required for sprouting of the first lymphatic vessels from embryonic veins. *Nature Immunology*, Vol.5, No.1 (January 2004), pp.74-80, ISSN 1529-2908.

Karl, A.; Carroll, P.R.; Gschwend, J.E. et al. (2009). The impact of lymphadenectomy and lymph node metastasis on the outcomes of radical cystectomy for bladder cancer. *European Urology*, Vol.55, No.4 (April 2009), pp. 826-35, ISSN 0302-2838.

Kaufman, D.; Raghavan, D.; Carducci, M. et al. (2000). Phase II trial of gemcitabine plus cisplatin in patients with metastatic urothelial cancer. *Journal of Clinical Oncology*, Vol.18, No.9 (May 2000), pp. 1921-1927, ISSN 1527-7755.

Kaufman, D.S.; Shipley, W.U. & Feldman, A.S. (2009). Bladder Cancer. *The Lancet*, Vol.374, No 9685, (July 2009), pp. 239-49, ISSN 0140-6736.

Kerbel, R.S. (2000). Tumor angiogenesis: past, present and the near future. *Carcinogenesis*, Vol.21, No.3 (March 2000), pp. 505-515, ISSN 1460-2180.

Kobayashi, S.; Kishimoto, T.; Kamata, S. et al. (2007). Rapamycin, a specific inhibitor of the mammalian target of rapamycin, suppresses lymphangiogenesis and lymphatic metastasis. *Cancer Science*, Vol.98, No.5 (May 2007), pp. 726-733, ISSN 1349-7006.

Lassau, N.; Koscielny, S.; Chami, L. et al. (2011). Advanced hepatocellular carcinoma: early evaluation of response to bevacizumab therapy at dynamic contrast-enhanced US with quantification - preliminary results. *Radiology*, Vol.258, No.1 (January 2011), pp. 291-300, ISSN 1527-1315.

Laurence A.D. (2006). Location, movement and survival: the role of chemokines in haematopoiesis and malignancy. *British Journal of Haematology*, Vol. 132, No.3 (February 2006), pp. 255-267, ISSN 0007-1048.

Leissner, J.; Koeppen, C. & Wolf, H.K. (2003). Prognostic significance of vascular and perineural invasion in urothelial bladder cancer treated with radical cystectomy. *The Journal of Urology*, Vol.169, No.3 (March 2003), pp. 955-960, ISSN 0022-5347.

Li, Y.; Yang, X.; Su, L.J. & Flaig, T.W. (2011). Pazopanib synergizes with docetaxel in the treatment of bladder cancer cells. *Urology*, Vol.78, No.1 (July 2011), pp. 233.e7-233.e13, ISSN 0090-4295.

Loges, S.; Mazzone, M.; Hohensinner, P. & Carmeliet, P. (2009). Silencing or fueling metastasis with VEGF inhibitors: antiangiogenesis revisited. *Cancer Cell*, Vol.15, No.3 (March 2009), pp. 167-70, ISSN 1535-6108.

Lohela, M.; Bry, M.; Tammela, T. & Alitalo, K. (2009). VEGFs and receptors involved in angiogenesis versus lymphangiogenesis. *Current Opinion in Cell Biology*, Vol.21, No.2, (February 2009), pp. 154-165, ISSN 0955-0674.

Lotan, Y.; Gupta, A.; Shariat, S.F. et al. (2005). Lymphovascular invasion is independently associated with overall survival, cause-specific survival, and local and distant recurrence in patients with negative lymph nodes at radical cystectomy. *Journal of Clinical Oncology*, Vol.23, No.27 (September 2005), pp. 6533-6539, ISSN 1527-7755.

Ma, Y.; Hou, Y.; Liu, B. et al. (2010). Intratumoral lymphatics and lymphatic vessel invasion detected by D2-40 are essential for lymph node metastasis in bladder transitional cell carcinoma. *Anatomical Record (Hoboken)*, Vol.293, No.11 (November 2010), pp. 1847-1854, ISSN 1932-8494.

Mäkinen, T.; Jussila, L.; Veikkola, T. et al. (2001). Inhibition of lymphangiogenesis with resulting lymphedema in transgenic mice expressing soluble VEGF receptor-3. *Nature Medicine*, Vol.7, No.2 (February 2001), pp.199-205, ISSN 1078-8956.

Malmström, P.U. (2011). Bladder tumours: time for a paradigm shift? *British Journal of Urology International*, Vol.107, No.10 (May 2011), pp.1543-1545, ISSN 2042-2997.

Martens, J-H.; Kzhyshkowska, J.; Falkowski-Hansen, M. et al. (2006). Differential expression of a gene signature for sacavanger/lectin receptors by endothelial cells and macrophages in human lymph node sinuses, the primary sites of regional metastasis. *The Journal of Pathology*, Vol.208, No.4 (March 2006), pp. 574-589, ISSN 1096-9896

May, M.; Herrmann, E.; Bolenz, C. et al. (2011). Association Between the Number of Dissected Lymph Nodes During Pelvic Lymphadenectomy and Cancer-Specific Survival in Patients with Lymph Node-Negative Urothelial Carcinoma of the Bladder Undergoing Radical Cystectomy. *Annals of Surgical Oncology*, Vol.18, No.7 (July 2011), pp. 2018-2025, ISSN 1534-4681.

McCormack, F.X.; Inoue, Y.; Moss, J. et al. (2011). Efficacy and safety of sirolimus in lymphangioleiomyomatosis. *The New England Journal of Medicine*, Vol.364, No.17 (April 2011), pp. 1595-1606, ISSN 1533-4406.

Milowsky, M.I.; Carlson, L.; Shi, M.M. et al. (2011). A multicenter, open-label phase II trial of dovitinib (TKI258) in advanced urothelial carcinoma patients with either mutated or wild-type FGFR3. *Proceedings of the 2011 Genitourinary Cancers Symposium*, Abstract TPS186, Orlando, Florida, USA, February 17-19, 2011.

Milowsky, M.I.; Regazzi, A.M.; Garcia-Grossman, I.R. et al. (2011). Final results of a phase II study of everolimus (RAD001) in metastatic transitional cell carcinoma (TCC) of the urothelium. *Proceedings of the 2011 Genitourinary Cancers Symposium,* Abstract 4606, Orlando, Florida, USA, February 17-19, 2011.

Miyata, Y.; Kanda, S.; Ohba, K. et al. (2006). Lymphangiogenesis and Angiogenesis in Bladder Cancer: Prognostic implications and Regulation by Vascular Endothelial Growth Factors-A, -C and -D. *Clinical Cancer Research,* Vol.12, No.3Pt1 (February 2006), pp. 800-806, ISSN 1557-3265.

Muller, A.; Homey, B.; Soto, H. et al. (2001). Involvement of chemokine receptors in breast cancer metastasis. *Nature,* Vol.410, No.6824 (March 2001), pp. 50-56, ISSN 0028-0836.

O'Brien, T.; Cranston, D.; Fuggle, S.; Bicknell, R. & Harris, A.L. (1995). Different Angiogenic Pathways Characterize Superficial and Invasive Bladder Cancer. *Cancer Research,* Vol.55, No.3 (February 1995), pp. 510-513, ISSN 1538-7445.

Oliveira, P.A.; Arantes-Rodrigues, R.; Sousa-Diniz, C. et al. (2009). The effects of sirolimus on urothelial lesions chemically induced in ICR mice by BBN. *Anticancer Research.* Vol.29, No.8 (August 2009), pp. 3221-3226, ISSN 1791-7530.

Oliver, G. & Detmar, M. (2002). The rediscovery of the lymphatic system: old and new insights into the development and biological function of the lymphatic vasculature. *Genes & Development,* Vol.16, No.7 (April 2002), pp. 773-783, ISSN 1549-5477.

Padera, T.P.; Kadambi, A. & di Tomaso, E. (2002). Lymphatic metastasis in the absence of functional intratumor lymphatics. *Science,* Vol.296, No.5574 (June 2002), pp. 1883-1886, ISSN 1095-9203.

Papetti, M. & Herman, I.M. (2002). Mechanisms of normal and tumor-derived angiogenesis. *American Journal of Physiology – Cell Physiology,* Vol. 282, No.5 (May 2002), pp. 947-970, ISSN 1522-1563.

Parada, B.; Reis, F.; Figueiredo, A. et al. (2011). Inhibition of bladder tumour growth by sirolimus in an experimental carcinogenesis model. *British Journal of Urology International,* Vol.107, No.1 (January 2011), pp. 135-143, ISSN 2042-2997.

Patel, N.S.; Dobbie, M.S.; Rochester, M. et al. (2006). Up-regulation of endothelial delta-like 4 expression correlates with vessel maturation in bladder cancer. *Clinical Cancer Research,* Vol.12, No.16 (August 2006), pp. 4836-4844, ISSN 1557-3265.

Pinto, A.; Redondo, A.; Zamora, P.; Castelo, B. & Espinosa, E. (2010). Angiogenesis as a therapeutic target in urothelial carcinoma. *Anticancer Drugs,* Vol.21, No.10 (November 2010), pp. 890-896, ISSN 1473-5741.

Pinto-Leite, R.; Botelho, P.; Ribeiro, E.; Oliveira, P.A. & Santos, L. (2009). Effect of sirolimus on urinary bladder cancer T24 cell line. *Journal of Experimental & Clinical Cancer Research,* Vol.28, No.3 (January 2009), ISSN 1557-3265.

Pries, A.R.; Höpfner, M.; le Noble, F.; Dewhirst, M.W. & Secomb, T.W. (2010). The shunt problem: control of functional shunting in normal and tumour vasculature. *Nature Reviews Cancer,* Vol.10, No.8 (August 2010), pp. 587-593, ISSN 1474-175X.

Pugh, C.W. & Ratcliffe, P.J. (2003). Regulation of angiogenesis by hypoxia: role of the HIF system. *Nature Medicine,* Vol.9, No.6 (June 2003), pp. 677-684, ISSN 1078-8956.

Quek, M.L.; Stein, J.P.; Nichols, P.W. et al. (2005). Prognostic significance of lymphovascular invasion of bladder cancer treated with radical cistectomy. *The Journal of Urology,* Vol.174. No.1 (July 2005), pp. 103-106, ISSN 0022-5347.

Riess, H.; Pelzer, U.; Opitz, B. et al. (2010). A prospective, randomized trial of simultaneous pancreatic cancer treatment with enoxaparin and chemotherapy: Final results of the CONKO-004 trial. *Proceedings of the 2010 ASCO Annual Meeting*, Abstract No 4033, Chicago, Illinois, USA, June 4-8, 2010.

Risau W. (1997). Mechanisms of angiogenesis. *Nature*, Vol.386, No.6626 (April 1997), pp. 671-674, ISSN 0028-0836.

Rosner, M.; Hanneder, M.; Siegel, N. et al. (2008). The mTOR pathway and its role in human genetic diseases. *Mutation Research*, Vol.659, No.3 (September-October 2008), pp. 284-292, ISSN 1383-5742.

Saharinen, P.; Tammela, T.; Karkkainen, M. & Alitalo, K. (2004). Lymphatic vasculature: development, molecular regulation and role in tumor metastasis and inflammation. *TRENDS in Immunology*, Vol.25, No.7 (July 2004), pp. 387-395, ISSN 1471-4906.

Santos, L.; Costa, C.; Pereira, S. et al. (2003). Neovascularization is a prognostic factor for early recurrence in T1/G2 urothelial bladder tumours. *Annals of Oncology*. Vol.14, No.9 (September 2003), pp. 1419-1424, ISSN 1569-8041.

Sato, K.; Sasaki, R.; Ogura, Y. et al. (1998). Expression of vascular endothelial growth factor gene and its receptor (flt-1) gene in urinary bladder cancer. *The Tohoku Journal of Experimental Medicine*, Vol.185, No.3 (July 1998), pp. 173-184, ISSN 1349-3329.

Schedel, F.; Pries, R.; Thode, B. et al. (2011). mTOR inhibitors show promising in vitro activity in bladder cancer and head and neck squamous cell carcinoma. *Oncology Reports*, Vol.25, No.3 (March 2011), pp. 763-768, ISSN 1791-2431.

Schoppmann, S.F.; Birner, P.; Stockl, J. et al. (2002). Tumor-associated macrophages express lymphatic endothelial growth factors and are related to peritumoral lymphangiogenesis. *The American Journal of Pathology*, Vol.161, No.3 (September 2002), pp. 947-956, ISSN 0002-9440.

Seager, C.M.; Puzio-Kuter, A.M.; Patel, T. et al. (2009). Intravesical delivery of rapamycin suppresses tumorigenesis in a mouse model of progressive bladder cancer. *Cancer Prevention Research (Philadelphia, Pa.)*, Vol. 2, No.12 (December 2009), pp.1008-1014, ISSN 1940-6215.

Senger, D.R.; Galli, S.J.; Dvorak, A.M. et al. (1983). Tumor cells secrete a vascular permeability factor that promotes accumulation of ascites fluid. *Science*, Vol. 219, No. 4587 (February 1983), pp. 983-985, ISSN 1095-9203.

Shalaby, F.; Rossant, J.; Yamaguchi, T.P. et al. (1995). Failure of blood-island formation and vasculogenesis in Flk-1-deficient mice. *Nature*, Vol. 376, No. 6535 (July 1995), pp. 62-66, ISSN 0028-0836.

Shariat, S.F.; Svatek, R.S.; Tilki, D. et al. (2010). International validation of the prognostic value of lymphovascular invasion in patients treated with radical cystectomy. *British Journal of Urology International*, Vol.105, No.10 (May 2010), pp. 1402-1412, ISSN 2042-2997.

Shariat, S.F.; Youssef, R.F.; Gupta, A. et al. (2010). Association of angiogenesis related markers with bladder cancer outcomes and other molecular markers. *The Journal of Urology*, Vol.183, No.5 (May 2010), pp. 1744-1750, ISSN 0022-5347.

Shirotake, S.; Miyajima, A.; Kosaka, T. et al. (2011). Angiotensin II type 1 receptor expression and microvessel density in human bladder cancer. *Urology*, Vol.77, No.4 (April 2011), pp. 1009.e19-25, ISSN 0090-4295.

Si, Z.C. & Liu, J. (2008). What "helps" tumors evade vascular targeting treatment? *Chinese Medical Journal (English)*, Vol.121, No.9 (May 2008), pp.844-849, ISSN 0366-6999.

Smith, J.A. & Whitmore, W.F.Jr. (1981). Regional lymph node metastasis from bladder cancer. *The Journal of Urology*. Vol.126, No.5 (November 1981), pp. 591-593, ISSN 0022-5347.

Stacker, S.A. & Achen, M.G. (2008). From anti-angiogenesis to anti-lymphangiogenesis: emerging trends in cancer therapy. *Lymphatic Research and Biology*, Vol.6, No.3-4, pp. 165-172, ISSN 1557-8585.

Stein, J.P.; Cai, J.; Groshen, S. & Skinner, D.G. (2003). Risk factors for patients with pelvic lymph node metastasis following radical cystectomy with en bloc pelvic lymphadenectomy: concept of lymph node density. *The Journal of Urology*, Vol.170, No.1 (July 2003), pp. 35-41, ISSN 0022-5347.

Sternberg, C.N.; Donat, S.M.; Bellmunt, J. et al. (2007). Chemotherapy for bladder cancer: treatment guidelines for neoadjuvant chemotherapy, bladder preservation, adjuvant chemotherapy, and metastatic cancer. *Urology*, Vol.69, No.1 (January 2007), pp. 62-79, ISSN 0090-4295.

Suzuki, K.; Morita, T. & Tokue, A. (2005). Vascular endothelial growth factor-C (VEGF-C) expression predicts lymph node metastasis of transitional cell carcinoma of the bladder. *International Journal of Urology*, Vol.12, No.2 (February 2005), pp. 152-158, ISSN 1442-2042.

Swartz, M.A. (2001). The physiology of the lymphatic system. *Advanced Drug Delivery Reviews*, Vol.50, No1-2 (August 2001), pp. 3-20, ISSN 0169-409X.

Thiele, W. & Sleeman, J.P. (2006). Tumor-induced lymphangiogenesis: a target for cancer therapy? *Journal of Biotechnology*, Vol.124, No.1 (June 2006), pp. 224-241, ISSN 0168-1656.

Tickoo, S.K.; Milowsky, M.I.; Dhar, N. et al. (2011). Hypoxia-inducible factor and mammalian target of rapamycin pathway markers in urothelial carcinoma of the bladder: possible therapeutic implications. *British Journal of Urology International*, Vol.107, No.5 (March 2011), pp. 844-849, ISSN 2042-2997.

Tobler, N.E. & Detmar, M. (2006). Tumor and lymph node lymphangiogenesis - impact on cancer metastatis. *Journal of Leukocyte Biology*, Vol.80, No.4 (October 2006), pp. 691-696, ISSN 0741-5400.

Twardowski, P.; Stadler, W.M.; Frankel, P. et al. (2010). Phase II study of Aflibercept (VEGF-Trap) in patients with recurrent or metastatic urothelial cancer, a California Cancer Consortium Trial. *Urology*, Vol.76, No.4 (October 2010), pp.923-926, ISSN 0090-4295.

Van Trappen, P.O. & Pepper, M.S. (2002). Lymphatic dissemination of tumour cells and the formation of micrometastases. *Lancet Oncology*, Vol.3, No.1 (January 2002), pp. 44-52. ISSN 1470-2045.

Vasconcelos-Nóbrega, C.; Colaço, A.; Santos, L. et al. Experimental study of the anticancer effect of gemcitabine combined with sirolimus on chemically induced urothelial lesions. *Anticancer Research*, Vol.31, No.5 (May 2011), pp. 1637-1642, ISSN 1791-7530.

Videira, P.A.; Piteira, A.R.; Cabral, M.G. et al. (2011). Effects of bevacizumab on autocrine VEGF stimulation in bladder cancer cell lines. *Urologia Internationalis*, Vol.86, No.1 (February 2011), pp. 95-101, ISSN 1423-0399.

von der Maase, H.; Hansen, S.W.; Roberts, J.T. et al. (2000). Gemcitabine and cisplatin versus methotrexate, vinblastine, doxorubicin and cisplatin in advanced or metastatic bladder cancer: results of a large, randomized, multinational, multicenter, phase III study. *Journal of Clinical Oncology*, Vol.18, No.17 (September 2000), pp. 3068-3077, ISSN 1527-7755.

Walz. J.; Shariat, S.F.; Suardi, N. et al. (2008). Adjuvant chemotherapy for bladder cancer does not alter cancer-specific survival after cystectomy in a matched case control study. *British Journal of Urology International*, Vol.101, No.11 (June 2008), pp. 1356-1361, ISSN 2042-2997.

Wiesner, C.; Pfitzenmaier, J.; Faldum, A. et al. (2005). Lymph node metastases in non-muscle invasive bladder cancer are correlated with the number of transurethral ressections and tumor upstaging at radical cystectomy. *British Journal of Urology International*, Vol.95, No. 3 (February 2005), pp. 301-305, ISSN 2042-2997.

Wigle, J.T. & Oliver, G. (1999). Prox1 function is required for the development of the murine lymphatic system. *Cell*, Vol.98, No.6 (September 1999), pp. 769-778, ISSN 0092-8674.

Wigle, J.T.; Harvey, N.; Detmar, M. et al. (2002). An essential role for Prox1 in the induction of the lymphatic endothelial cell phenotype. *The EMBO Journal*, Vol.21, No.7 (April 2002),pp. 1505-1513, ISSN 1460-2075.

Wiig, H.; Keskin, D. & Kalluri, R. (2010). Interaction between the extracellular matrix and lymphatics: consequences for lymphangiogenesis and lymphatic function. *Matrix Biology*, Vol.29, No.8 (August 2010), pp. 645-656, ISSN 0945-053X.

Williams, S.P.; Karnezis, T.; Achen, M.G. & Stacker SA. (2010). Targeting lymphatic vessel functions through tyrosine kinases. *Journal of Angiogenesis Research*, Vol.2 (August 2010), pp. 1-13, ISSN 2045-824X.

Wilting, J.; Hawighorst, T.; Hecht, M.; Christ, B. & Papoutsi, M. (2005). Development of lymphatic vessels: tumour lymphangiogenesis and lymphatic invasion. *Current Medicinal Chemistry*, Vol.12, No.26, pp. 3043-3053, ISSN 0929-8673.

Wright, J.L.; Lin, D.W. & Porter, M.P. (2008). The association between extent of lymphadenectomy and survival among patients with lymph node metastases undergoing radical cystectomy. *Cancer*, Vol.112, No.11 (June 2008), pp. 2401-2408, ISSN 1097-0142.

Yang, C.C.; Chu, K.C. & Yeh, W.M. (2004). The expression of vascular endothelial growth factor in transitional cell carcinoma of urinary bladder is correlated with cancer progression. *Urologic Oncology*, Vol.22, No.1 (January-February 2004), pp. 1-6, ISSN 1078-1439.

Yang, H.; Kim, C.; Kim, M.J. et al. (2011). Soluble vascular endothelial growth factor receptor-3 suppresses lymphangiogenesis and lymphatic metastasis in bladder cancer. *Molecular Cancer*, Vol.10 (April 2011), pp.36, ISSN 1476-4598.

Yoon, C.Y.; Lee, J.S.; Kim, B.S. et al. (2011). Sunitinib malate synergistically potentiates anti-tumor effect of gemcitabine in human bladder cancer cells. *Korean Journal of Urology*, Vol.52, No.1 (January 2011), pp. 55-63, ISSN 2005-6745.

Youssef, R.F. & Lotan, Y. (2011). Predictors of outcome of non-muscle-invasive and muscle-invasive bladder cancer. *Scientific World Journal*, Vol.11 (February 2011), pp. 369-381, ISSN 1537-744X.

Zhou, M.; He, L.; Zu, X. et al. (2011). Lymphatic vessel density as a predictor of lymph node metastasis and its relationship with prognosis in urothelial carcinoma of the bladder. *British Journal of Urology International*, Vol.107, No.12 (June 2011), 1930-1935, ISSN 2042-2997.

Zu, X.; Tang, Z.; Li, Y. et al. (2006). Vascular endothelial growth factor-C expression in bladder transitional cell cancer and its relationship to lymph node metastasis. *British Journal of Urology International*, Vol.98, No.5 (November 2006), pp. 1090-1093, ISSN 2042-2997.

5

Angiogenesis and Lymphangiogenesis in Bladder Cancer

Yasuyoshi Miyata, Hideki Sakai and Shigeru Kanda
Nagasaki University Graduate School of Biomedical Sciences
Japan

1. Introduction

In cancer patients, the majority of deaths occur as a consequence of metastatic diseases. In addition, metastasis is a marker for poor prognosis and low quality of life in many malignancies. Several groups have investigated the mechanism of tumor metastasis. Metastatic lesions are formed through a multi-step complex process and then spread either locally at the site of the primary tumor, or into distant organs through the blood or lymphatic vessels.

Another important feature of cancers is the chaotic behavior of tumor growth and cancer cell cycle progression. To maintain such activities, abundant supply of oxygen and nutrients are necessary. Angiogenesis refers to the formation of new blood vessels and development of new branching vessels from the existing tumor tissue vasculature and this pathological process is important to secure adequate blood supply including oxygen and nutrients to the rapidly dividing malignant cells. In fact, there is a good correlation between tumor growth/cancer cell proliferation and the extent of angiogenesis in almost of all cancers.

While there is abundant information on the mechanisms that are involved in the initiation, regulation and maintenance of angiogenesis in cancer tissue, little is known about the mechanisms involved in the formation of new lymphatic vessels (lymphangiogenesis) in cancers. Furthermore, the current knowledge about cancer dissemination through the lymphatics lacks details about the mode of transport of cancer cells within the lymphatic vessels and the mechanisms involved in their exit and seeding into the distant organs.

In this paper, we review the clinical and pathological significance of angiogenesis and lymphangiogenesis in bladder cancer. In addition, the mechanisms that regulate the formation of new vessels in bladder cancer are discussed. Specifically, we focus on the factors that co-regulate these two different vessels and their potential use as predictive marker of outcome in patients with bladder cancer. In addition, we also discuss the limitation of quantification of these vessels in human tissues.

2. Angiogenesis and lymphangiogenesis

2.1 Angiogenesis in cancer tissues

Angiogenesis is defined as the formation of new blood vessels from pre-existing vasculature, and it is an integrated process of tumor growth, maintenance, and progression in solid tumors (Folkmann, 1992). Angiogenesis is a multistep processes involving changes in the extracellular matrix, cell proliferation, cell migration, and tube formation. Blood vessel density (BVD), a surrogate marker for angiogenesis, correlates with the malignant potential and poor prognosis of patients with various types of cancers. In addition, anti-angiogenic therapy that targets the tumor vascular supply and pathways of cancer cell dissemination was first introduced in 1971 (Folkman, 1971). Since then, numerous investigators have focused on the mechanisms of angiogenesis, including molecular mechanisms. At present, there is a general agreement that the regulation of tumor angiogenesis depends on a complex mechanism that dynamically balances angiogenic and anti-angiogenic factors. In this regard, these factors are secreted by both tumor cells and stromal cells in complicated systems. To complicate the issue, the mechanisms and pathological roles of these factors vary according to the type of cancer, its malignant potential, and systemic condition.

2.2 Lymphangiogenesis in cancer tissues

In addition to angiogenesis, many investigators have examined the process of lymphangiogenesis, i.e., the formation of new lymphatic vessels, due to its importance in lymph node metastasis and distant metastasis. Lymph node metastasis occurs in various types of malignancies and its presence is considered a strong predictor of recurrence and poor survival of patients with bladder cancer. However, the clinical role and prognostic value of lymphangiogenesis in cancer patients remain unclear, largely due to the lack of specific endothelial markers for lymphatic vessels as well as the lack of proper imaging procedures for lymphatic vessels in human tissues (Pepper, 2001). In recent years, various specific antibodies for lymphatic endothelial cells have been developed and used to investigate the clinical and pathological significance of lymphangiogenesis in cancer patients. Similar to angiogenesis, evidence suggests that lymphangiogenesis is also regulated by complex mechanisms that include a variety of factors. While various common mechanisms regulate the processes of angiogenesis and lymphangiogenesis, other mechanisms vary according to these processes. For example, in contrast to angiogenesis, no intrinsic anti-lymphangiogenic molecules have yet been isolated.

Thus, to discuss the pathological roles, predictive values, and potential therapeutic targets of angiogenesis and lymphangiogenesis, it is important to understand the various complex mechanisms and cooperative functions involved in these two processes.

2.3 Angiogenesis and lymphangiogenesis in bladder cancer

BVD is often used in the analysis of human cancer tissues as a surrogate and semi-quantitative marker of angiogenesis. Previous studies suggested that BVD provides significant information on prognosis and survival in patients with bladder cancer (Streeter & Harris, 2002; Goddard, 2003). However, other investigators were less supportive for the prognostic value of BVD, especially in patients with non-muscle-invasive bladder cancer (NMIBC) (Korkolopoulou, et al., 2001; Ioachim, et al., 2006; Miyata, et al., 2006). Table 1 provides a summary of the currently held opposing views on BVD.

Such discrepancy could be attributed to differences in methodology, such as methods used for counting, size of the field of view, definition of microvessel, and antibodies used in different assays. For example, measurement at periphery or growth from of the tumor (Stavropoulos et al., 2004) or at highest vascularity "hot spots" (Korkolopoulou et al., 2001). Furthermore, the diameter of the microvessel was no mentioned in some studies; though other provided descriptive terms (the lumen diameter was smaller than approximately eight red blood cells) (Stavropoulos, 2004). More detailed problems are described in the following section.

Patients	Findings	Reference
109 NMIBC	Predictor of muscle invasion in G3 patients, though not an independent factor.	Starvropoulos
66 NMIBC	Independent predictor of recurrence-free survival, particularly in T1G2 tumors	Santos
35 NMIBC + 80 MIBC	Independent predictor for overall survival in MIBC. No significant role in NMIBC	Korkolopoulou
87 NMIBC + MIBC	Independent predictor of lymph node metastasis.	Susuki
104 NMIBC + 22 MIBC	Not significant for recurrence-free, metastasis-free, or cause-specific survival.	Miyata

NMIBC: non-muscle-invasive bladder cancer, MIBC: muscle-invasive bladder cancer

Table 1. Predictive value of blood vessel density (BVD) for progression and survival.

In addition to semi-quantitative measures of BVD, vascular invasion by tumor cells (blood vessel invasion, BVI) has also been identified as a prognostic factor in bladder cancer (Harada et al., 2005). Furthermore, vascular area and various parameters related to the shape, relapse, and/or complexity of the vessels have been suggested as important for more detailed discussion on the relationship between angiogenesis and pathological role, prognosis, and survival. In this regard, several investigators paid special attention to the morphological variability in the vascular pattern (Korkolopoulou et al., 2001; Sharma et al., 2005), and one study reported that the vascular area was an independent predictor of overall survival in patients with T1 disease whereas BVD was not (Korkolopoulou et al., 2001).

In contrast to angiogenesis, there is little or no information on the clinical and pathological significance and predictive value of lymphangiogenesis in patients with bladder cancer. Several studies reported that higher LVD correlates significantly with malignant behavior, cancer cell progression, and prognosis (Fernández et al., 2008; Miyata et al., 2006). In addition, one report indicated that the pathological role of lymphangiogenesis was depended on the location of lymphatic vessels, such as intra-tumoral and peri-tumoral area. In other words, intra-tumoral LVD correlated with histological differentiation, and peri-tumoral LVD correlated with lymph node metastasis (Fernández, et al., 2008). Similar to BVI, of lymphatic vessel invasion (LVI) by tumor cells was also identified as a prognostic factor in bladder cancer (Algaba, 2006). In general, however, information on lymphangiogenesis in human bladder cancer is to a large extent scarce, compared to that on angiogenesis.

2.4 Regulation of angiogenesis and/or lymphangiogenesis

Members of the vascular endothelial growth factor (VEGF) family are the most important molecules involved in the processes of angiogenesis and lymphangiogenesis. This family consists of 7 members, including VEGF-A, -B, -C, -D, and -E, svVEGF, and placental growth factor. In addition, three types of receptors have so far been identified: VEGFR-1, -2, and -3 (Takahashi et al., 2005). The angiopoietin (Ang) family also encompasses several pro-angiogenic factors. This family consists of Ang-1 and -2 and Tie2 tyrosine kinase receptors, and the system is influenced by VEGF family. In addition, several factors, for example, fibroblast growth factor (FGF)-2, hepatocyte growth factor (HGF), and insulin-like growth factor (IGF), are also reported to be involved in the regulation of both angiogenesis and lymphangiogenesis.

Angiostatin and endostatin, which are both produced by proteolytic cleavage of plasminogen and collagen XVIII, respectively, are well characterized anti-angiogenic factors. (O'Reilly, et al., 1994, 1997). In addition, thrombospondins (TSPs) also inhibits angiogenesis (Lawler, 2000). Another report indicated that down-regulation of TSP-1 secretion in bladder cancer tissues was a key event in the change from an anti-angiogenic to an angiogenic phenotype during carcinogenesis (Campbell, et al., 1998). On the other hand, there are conflicting results on the relationship between TSP-1 expression and BVD in human bladder cancer. Specifically, TSP-1 staining correlated negatively with BVD (Grossdfeld et al., 1997), whereas other investigators reported that TSP-1 expression correlated positively with BVD (Ioachim et al., 2006).

We review here in detail two representative pro-angiogenic factors; VEGF family and Ang family. Their selection was based on the finding that they are potential therapeutic targets in various cancers. Actually, targeted therapies based on these factors have been tested already in patients with bladder cancer. Unfortunately, however, anti-angiogenic factor-targeted therapy is still in its infancy and there is little possibility to use such drugs for treatment of bladder cancer in the near future.

2.5 VEGF family

Among the VEGF family members, VEGF-A is a major regulator of angiogenesis. On the other hand, both VEGF-C and VEGF-D have been found to play major roles in lymphangiogenesis. Furthermore, VEGFR-2 and VEGFR-3 are reported to be the major mediators of angiogenic response in blood endothelial cells and lymphangiogenic response in lymphatic endothelial cells, respectively. In other words, VEGF-A signaling through VEGFR-2 is the major pathway that activates angiogenesis by stimulating cell proliferation, survival, and migration of endothelial cells (Shibuya & Claesson-Welsh, 2006). Furthermore, the VEGF-C/D-VEGFR-3 signaling pathway is important for the growth of lymphatic endothelial cells (Skobe et al. 2001; Stacker et al., 2001; Lin, et al., 2005). In support of this notion, blocking the VEGF-C/D-VEGFR-3 signaling pathway was reported to inhibit tumor lymphangiogenesis and lymph node metastasis in several xenograft and transgenic tumor models (He et al., 2002; Lin et al., 2005; Roberts et al., 2006).

In contrast to the above studies, several groups reported that VEGF-A could stimulate lymphangiogenesis *in vivo* (Nagy et al., 2002; Cursiefen et al., 2004). In addition, in an animal model of chemically-induced skin cancer, VEGF-A induced lymphangiogenesis and promoted lymphatic metastasis (Hirakawa et al., 2005). Conversely, VEGF-C and VEGF-D were reported to play important roles in angiogenesis under various physiological and pathological conditions (Cao 1998, Jussila & Alitalo, 2002).

VEGFR-1 has a high affinity for VEGF-A, VEGF-B, and PIGF. However, its tyrosine kinase activity is comparatively weak (Autiero, et al., 2003; Shibutya & Claesson-Welsh, 2006). VEGFR-1 is expressed in endothelial cells. In addition, it is also expressed in monocytes/macrophages, hemopoietic cells, and pericytes. Its tyrosine kinase activity is required for stimulation of hemopoietic cell migration towards VEGFs and PIGFs (Barleon, et al., 1996; Clauss, et al. 1996). Based on these results, VEGF-B, PIGF, and VEGFR-1 are thought to play minimal roles in angiogenesis. In fact, they do not activate angiogenesis during development. However, they have been reported to exhibit angiogenic activity under a variety of pathological conditions (Fisher et al., 2008). For examples, in animal experiments, PIGF was associated with angiogenesis in various pathological conditions including ischemia, inflammation, and tumor growth (Carmeliet, et al., 2001; Luttun, et al., 2002).

The role of VEGFR-2 in lymphangiogenesis is still controversial. VEHGR-2 is expressed at low levels in lymph vessels, and VEGF-VEGFR-2 signaling can induce lymphatic vessel formation (Hong et al., 2004). On the other hand, evidence suggests that lymphangiogenesis induced by such system involves the recruitment of immune cells producing VEGF-C and -D (Crusiefen, et al., 2004).

The following schematic diagram illustrates the relationship between VEGFs and VEGFRs and angiogenesis and lymphangiogenesis:

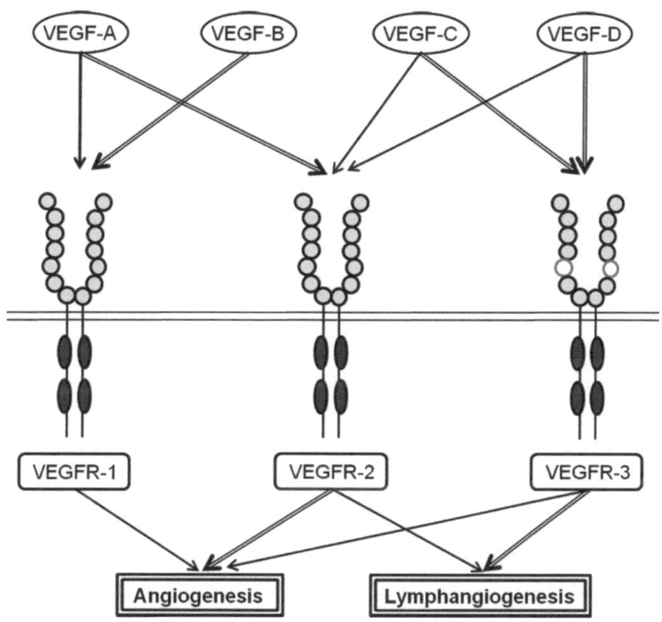

2.6 VEGF family in bladder cancer

Angiogenesis in bladder cancer involves the VEGF-A signaling through the receptor VEGFR-2. The interaction between VEGF-A and VEGFR-2 plays a crucial role in tumor growth, progression, and prognosis via regulation of angiogenesis in patients with bladder cancer.

VEGF-C and -D are highly expressed in cancer cells than in normal urothelial cells (O'Breien, et al., 1995; Zu et al., 2006; Miyata, et al.). Several investigators have reported that the expression of VEGF-C in bladder cancer is closely associated with tumor progression including lymph node metastasis (Suzuki, et al., 2005; Zu, et al., 2006). In addition, the expression of VEGF-C was a significant predictor of poor cause-specific survival in 87 patients. However, multivariate analysis in the same study showed that VEGF-C was not an independent factor and its expression did not correlate with various clinicopathological features (Suzuki, et al, 2005). On the other hand, the same analysis showed that the expression of VEGF-C in bladder cancer was a significant and independent predictor of pelvic lymph node metastasis. Thus, these reports have demonstrated that VEGF-C plays important role in the malignant aggressiveness and its overexpression is associated with poor prognosis of patients with bladder cancer. On the other hand, controversy exists regarding the prognostic value of VEGF-C expression in bladder cancer (Mylona, et al., 2006).

The fact that VEGF-C binds to and stimulates phosphorylation of tyrosine kinase receptor VEGFR-3 is well-known. In addition to VEGFR-3, VEGF-C also binds and activates VEGFR-2, but not VEGFR-1 (Roberts, et al., 2006). Because VEGFR-2 is the major pathway of angiogenesis, it is possible that VEGF-C also correlates with angiogenesis in bladder cancer. One study of 45 patients with bladder cancer reported that VEGF-C expression did not correlate with microvessel density (Zu, et al., 2006). On the other hand, we found that VEGF-C expression correlated positively with both MVD and LVD in 126 patients with bladder cancer. Another group reported that VEGF-C expression correlated with intra-tumoral BVD, but not with overall BVD. They also showed that VEGF-C expression correlated significantly with both intra-tumoral and peri-tumoral LVD (Afonso, et al., 2009). The reasons for these discrepancies are probably related to differences in antibodies used to measure MVD and also differences in sample size.

VEGF-D expression is also reported to be significantly associated with pathological features and prognosis of patients with bladder cancer (Miyata et al, 2006; Herrmann, et al., 2007). In addition, several studies demonstrated that VEGF-D expression also correlated with tumor growth, metastasis, and survival of patients with bladder cancer (Miyata, et al., 2006; Herrmann, et al, 2007). However, in comparison with VEGF-C, information regarding pathological significance and predictive value of VEGF-D in patients with bladder cancer is very limited.

Similarly, there is a little information on VEGF-B expression in bladder cancer. To our knowledge, there is only one study on VEGF-B m-RNA expression in bladder cancer tissues (Fauconett, et al., 2009). These authors used Northern blot analysis and reported the lack of VEGF-B mRNA expression in 37 bladder cancer specimens.

2.7 Ang family in cancers including bladder cancer

Angiopoietin (Ang)-1 and -2 have angiogenic function acting on Tie2 tyrosine kinase receptors (Maisonpierre, et al., 1997; Papapetropoulos, et al., 1999). Ang-1 is known as stabilizing factor because it helps to maintain and stabilize mature vessels by promoting interactions between endothelial cells and neighboring cells including pericytes and smooth muscle cells (Maisonpierre, et al., 1997; Papapetropoulos, et al., 1999, 2000). In contrast, Ang-2 is known as an antagonist to Ang-1 because it is expressed at sites of vascular remodeling and acts to destabilize vessels (Maisonpierre, et al., 1997). Interestingly, Ang-2 is reported to potentiate angiogenesis in the presence of VEGF, but causes regression of this process in the absence of VEGF (Maisonpierre, et al., 1997; Holash, et al., 1999). Thus, the angiopoietin-Tie2 system, comprising Ang-1, Ang-2, Tie2, and VEGF, seems to be regulated by complex mechanisms.

In bladder cancer, there are conflicting results on the clinical and pathological significance of angiopoietin-Tie2 system. One study demonstrated a significant correlation between Ang-2 protein expression and high stage, high grade tumors, and poor prognosis, whereas Ang-1 protein expression did not show the same trend (Oka, et al., 2005). It also showed that Ang-2 expression was an independent predictor of overall survival in patients with bladder cancer. On the other hand, Ang-2 mRNA expression in early stage superficial carcinomas and low grade tumors was reported to be significantly higher than in advanced stage muscle invasive carcinomas and high grade tumors (Quentin, et al., 2004). In comparison, the same study also reported that Ang-1 mRNA was expressed at significantly low levels in low grade and early stage tumors compared to high grade or advanced stage tumors. Other studies on Ang-1 and Ang-2 demonstrated the presence of significantly higher serum levels of Ang-1 in patients with bladder cancer relative to the control; and conversely, Ang-2 and Tie2 levels were significantly lower. (Szarvas, et al., 2009). The same study also showed that high Tie2 serum level was an independent prognostic factor for metastasis in multivariate analysis model that included tumor grade and stage.

2.8 Limitation of quantification of angiogenesis and lymphangiogenesis

BVD is often used as a quantitative marker of angiogenesis. The method used for quantification was first described after antibodies to factor VIII-related antigen became commercially availability; these antibodies were used to immunohistochemically stain blood vessels. Since then, various immunohistochemical pan-endothelial markers, such as CD31, CD34, von-Willebrand factor, have been used to stain and study blood vessels. CD31, also known as PECAM-1 (Platelet Endothelial Cell Adhesion Molecule-1), is a 130 KDa integral membrane protein, and is expressed constitutively on the surface of adult and embryonic endothelial cells. The CD34 protein is a member of a family of single-pass transmembrane proteins expressed on blood vessel endothelial cells (Nielsen & McNagny, 2008). However, these markers cannot distinguish between small and large blood vessels (Hassan, et al., 2002). On the other hand, CD105, also known as endoglin, is a disulphide-linked, proliferation-associated, hypoxia-inducible homodynamic cell membrane glycoprotein, and is known to be over-expressed in proliferating endothelial cells and is strongly up-regulated in endothelial cells of neoplastic tissues compared with normal cells (Fonasanti, et al., 2002; Minhajat, et al., 2006). Based on these properties, many recent studies have recommended the use of CD105 for evaluation of angiogenesis in tumor tissues because it reflects the dynamic status of tumor-related angiogenesis compared to other pan-endothelial markers (Sharma, et al., 2005). In fact, so far, CD105 antibody was demonstrated to have a greater specificity for tumor vasculature than other pan-endothelial markers, such as CD31, CD34, and Factor VIII in a clinical study of colorectal cancer (Saadi, et al., 2004).

In bladder cancer tissues, several antibodies have been used to evaluate angiogenesis. These include factor VIII (Lianes, et al., 1998; Shirotake, et al., 2011), CD31 (Korkolopoulos, et al., 2001; Afonso, et al., 2009), and CD34 (Shirotake, et al., 2011; Stavropoulos, et al., 2004; Ioachim, et al., 2006); whereas CD105 has rarely been used in bladder cancer tissues.

It is suggested that CD31, CD34, and CD105 are more useful because they efficiently recognize small-caliber vessels that are associated with angiogenesis in bladder cancer than factor VIII (Santos, et al., 2003). However, this study did not discuss the difference between these markers. Thus, to date, there is no ideal antibody to truly reflect the clinical and pathological significance of angiogenesis in bladder cancer. To this effect, some investigators have doubted the pathological significance and predictive value of BVD in patients with bladder cancer (Table 2).

Similar to angiogenesis, there is no ideal antibody that reflects the significance of lymphangiogenesis. In general, three different antibodies such as anti-lymphatic vessel endothelial hyaluronan receptor (LYVE)-1 (Yang, et al., 2011), anti-VEGFR-3 (Zhou et al., 2011) and anti-D2-40 (Miyata, et al., 2006; Afonso, et al., 2009,) have been used to detect lymphatic vessels. However, detailed information on the differences and characteristics of each of these factors is not available. Further studies are necessary to discuss the methods of quantification and evaluation of lymphangiogenesis in bladder cancer tissues.

	n	Antibody	Progression	Survival	Reference	year
NMIBC	35	CD31	No	No	Korkolopoulou	2001
NMIBC	66	CD31+CD34+FVIII	Yes*	-	Santos	2003
NMIBC	109	CD34	Yes**	-	Stavropoulos	2004
MIBC	109	FVIII	No	No	Linanes	1998
MIBC	80	CD31	Yes	No	Korkolpoulou	2001
Both	113	CD31+CD34	No	Yes	Bochener	1995
Both	148	CD34	No	No	Ioachim	2006
Both	42	CD31+FVIII	-	-	Gehani	2011

NMIBC, non-muscle invasive bladder cancer; MIBC, muscle invasive bladder cancer;
FVIII, factor VIII. * In T1/grade 2 patients. ** In grade 3 patients.

Table 2. Prognostic significance of blood vessel density (BVD)

3. Conclusion

Angiogenesis and lymphangiogensis play important roles for tumor growth and progression in bladder cancer. VEGF family and Ang family are well known to be associated with these phenomenon in bladder cancer. However, other factors and molecules are also speculated to regulate them by complex mechanism. So, detailed mechanism of their regulations is still fully understood. In addition, further studies are necessary to discuss the methods of quantification and evaluation of angiogenesis and lymphangiogenesis in bladder cancer tissues.

4. Acknowledgement

We are grateful to Mr. Takumi Shimogama, Mr. Yoshikazu Tsuji, Mrs. Miki Yoshimoto, and Mrs. Miho M. Kuninaka, for their outstanding support. This manuscript was supported in no funding.

5. References

Afonso, J.; Santos, L.L.; Amaro, T. et al. (2009). The aggressiveness of urothelial carcinoma depends to a large extent on lymphvascular invasion – the prognostic contribution of related molecular markers. Histopathology, Vol.55, No.5, (July), pp. 514-524.

Algaba, F. (2006). Lymphovascular invasion as aprognotic tool for advanced bladder cancer. Curr Opin Urol, Vol.16, No.5 (September), pp. 367-371.

Autiero, M.; Waltenberger, J.; Communi, D. et al. (2003). Role of PIGF in the intra- and intermolecular cross talk between the VEGF receptors Flt1 and Flk1. Nat Med, Vol.9, No.7, (July), pp. 936-943.

Barleon, B.; Sozzani, S.; Zhou, D. et al. (1996). Migration of human monocytes in response to vascular endothelial growth factor (VEGF) is mediated via the VEGF receptor flt-1. Blood, Vol.87, No.8, (April), pp. 3336-3343.

Campbell, SC.; Volpert, O.V.; Ivanovich, M. et al. (1998). Molecular mediators of angiogenesis in bladder cancer. Cancer Res, Vol.58, No.6 (March), pp. 1298-1304.

Cao, Y.; Linden, P.; Famebo, J. et al. (1998). Vascular endothealil growth factor C induceds angiogenesis in vivo. Proc Natl Acd Sci USA, Vol.95, No24. (November), pp. 14389-14394.

Carmeliet, P.; Moons, L.; Luttun, A. et al. (2001). Synergism between vascular endothelial growth factor and placental growth factor contributes to angiognenesis and plasma extravasation in pathological conditions. Nat Med, Vol.7, No.5, (May), pp. 575-583.

Clauss, M.; Weich, H.; Breier, G. et al. (1996). The vascular endothelial growth factor receptor Flt-1 mediates biological activities. Implications for a functional role of placenta growth factor in monocyte activation and chemotaxis. J Biol Chem, Vol.271, No.30, (July), pp.17629-17634.

Cursiefen, C.; Chen, L.; Borges, L.P. (2004). VEGF-A stimulates lymphangiogensis and hemangiogenesis in inflammatory neovasculalization via macrophage recruitment. J Clin Invest, Vol.113, No.7, (April), pp.1040-1050.

Fauconnet, S.; Bernardini, S.; Lascombe, I. et al. (2009). Expression analysis of VEGF-A and VEGF-B: relationship with clinicopathological parameters in bladder cancer. Oncol Rep, Vol.21, No.6, (June), pp. 1495-1504.

Fernández, M.I.; Bolenz, C.; Smith, N.; et al. (2008). Prognostic implications of lymphangiogenesis in muscle-invasive transitional cell carcinoma of the bladder. Eur Urol, Vol.53, No.3, (March), pp. 571-578.

Fischer, C.; Mazzone, M.; Jonckx, B. et al. (2008). Flt1 and its ligands VEGFB and PIGF: during targets for anti-agniogenic therapy? Nat Rev Cancer, Vol.8, No.12, (December), pp. 942-956.

Folkman, J. (1971). Tumor angiogenesis: Thrapeutic implications. N Engl J Med, Vol.285, No.21, (November), pp. 285: 1182-1186.

Folkman, J. (1992). The role of angiogenesis in tumor growth. Semin Cancer Biol Vol.3, No.2, (April), pp. 65-71.

Fonsatti, E.; Altomonte, M.; Nicotra, M.R. et al. (2003). Endoglin (CD105): a powerful therapeutic target on tumor-associated angiognenenic blood vessels. Oncogene, Vol.22, No.42, (May), pp. 6557-6563.

Goddard, J.C.; Sutton, C.D.; Furness, P.N.; et al. (2003). Microvessel density at presentation predicts subsequent muscle invasion in superficial bladder cancer. Clin Cancer Res 2003, Vol.9, No.7, (July), pp. 2583-2586.

Grossfeld, G.D.; Ginsberg, D.A.; Stein, J.P. et al. (1997). Thrombospondin-1 expression in bladder cancer: association with p53 alternations, tumor angiogenesis, and tumor progression. J Natl Cancer Inst, Vol.89, No.3, (February), pp. 219-227.

Harada, K.; Sakai, I, Hara, I.; et al. (2005). Prognostic significance of vascular invasion in patients with bladder cancer who underwent radical cystectomy. J Urol. Vol.12, No.3, (March), pp.250-255.

Hasan, J.; Byers, R. & Jayson, GC. (2002). Intra-tumoural microvessel density in human solid tumours. Br J Cancer, Vol.86, No. 1566 - 1577.

He, Y.; Kozaki, K.; Karpanen, T. et al. (2002). Suppression of tumor lymphangiogensis and lymph node metastasis by blocking vascular endothelial growth factor 3 signaling. J Natl Cancer Inst, Vol.94, No.11, (June), pp. 819-825.

Herrmann, E.; Eltze, E.; Bierer, S. et al. (2007). VEGF-C, VEGF-D, and Flt-4 in transitional bladder cancer: relationships to clinicopathological parameters and long-term survival. Anticancer Res, Vol.27, No.5A, (September-October), pp. 3127-3133.

Hirakawa, S.; Kodama, S.; Kunstfeld, R. et al. (2005). VEGF-A induces tumor and sentinel lymph node lymphangiogensis and promotes lymphatic metastasis. J Exp Med, Vol.201, No.7, (April), pp. 1089-1099.

Hong, Y.K.; Lange-Asschenfeldt, B.; Velasco, P. et al. VEGF-A promotes tissue repair-associated lymphatic vessel formation via VEGFR-2 and the alpha1beta1 and alpha2beta1 integrins. FASEB J, Vol.18, No.10, (July), pp. 1111-1113.

Holash, J.; Maisonpierre, P.C.; Olsson, L.E. et al. (1999). Vessel cooption, regression, and growth in tumors mediated by angiogenesis and VEGF. Science, Vol.284, No.5422 : pp. 1994-1998.

Jussila, L. & Alitalo, K. (2002). Vascular growth factors and lymphangiogensis. Physiol Rev, Vol.82, No.3, (July), pp. 673-700.

Ioachim, E.; Michael M.C.; Salmas, M.; et al. (2006) Thrombospondin-1 expression in urothelial carcinoma: prognostic significance and association with p53 alterations, tumour angiogenesis and extracellular matrix components. BMC Cancer Vol. 29, No.6, (May), p140.

Korkolopoulou, P.; Konstantinidou, A.E.; Kavantzas, N.; et al. (2001). Morphometric microvascular characteristics predict prognosis in superficial and invasive bladder cancer. Virchow Arch (2001) Vol.438, No. 6, (June): 603-611.

Lawler, J. (2000). The functions of thromboospondin-1 and -2. Curr Opin Cell Biol, Vol.12, No.5, (October), pp. 634-640.

Lianes, P.; Chartytonowicz, E.; Cordon-Cardo, C. et al. (1998). Biomarker study of primary nonmetastatic versus metastatic invasive bladder cancer. Clin Cancer Res, Vol.4, No.5, (May), pp. 1267-1271.

Lin, J.; Lalani, A.S.; Harding, T.C., et al. (2005). Inhibition of lymphogenous metastasis using adeno-associated virus-mediated gene transfer of a soluble VEGFR-3 decoy receptor. Cancer Res, Vol.65, No.15, (August), pp. 6901-6909.

Luttun, A.; Tjwa, M,; Moons, L. et al. (2002). Revascularization of ischemic tissues by PIGF treatment, and inhibition of tumor angiogenesis, arthritis, and atherosclerosis by anti-Flt1. Nat Med, Vol.8, No.8, (August), pp. 831-840.

Maisonpierre, P.C.; Suri, C.; Jones, P.F. et al. (1997). Angiopoietin-2, a natural antagonists for Tie 2 that discupts in vivo angiogeensis. Science, Vol.227, No.5322, (July), pp. 55-60.

Miyata, Y.; Kanda, S.; Ohba, K.; et al. (2006). Lymphangiogenesis and angiogenesis in bladder cancer: prognostic implications and regulation by vascular endothelial growth factors-A, -C, and -D. Clin Cancer Res Vol.12, No.3 pt 1, (February), pp. 300-306.

Mylona, E.; Magkou, C.; Gorantonakis, G. et al. (2006). Evaluation of the vascular endothelial growth factor (VEGF)-C role in urothelial carcinomas of the bladder. Anticancer Res, Vol.26, No.5A, (Deptember-October), pp. 3567-3571.

Nagy, J.A.; Vasile, E.; Feng, D. et al. (2002). Vascular permeability factor/vascular endothelial growth factor induces lymphangiogenesis as well as angiogenesis. J Exp Med, Vol.196, No.11, (December), pp. 1497-1506.

Nielsen, J.S. & McNagny, K.M. (2008). Novel functions of the CD34 family. J of Cell Science, Vol.121, Vol.Pt 22, (November), pp. 3682-3692

O'Brien, T.; Cranston, D.; Fuggle, S. et al. (1995). Different angiogenic pathways characterize superficial and invasive bladder cancer. Cancer Res, Vol.55, No3, (February), pp. 510-513.

Oka, N.; Yamamoto, Y.; Takahashi, M. et al. (2005). Expression of angiopoietin-1 and -2, and its clinical significance in human bladder cancer. BJU Int, Vol.95, No.4, (March), pp. 660-773.

O'Reilly, M.S.; Holmgren, L.; Shing, Y. et al. (1994). Angiostatin: a novel angiogenesis inhibitor that medicates the suppression of metastases by a Lewis lung carcinoma. Cell, Vol.79, No.2, (October), pp. 315-328.

O'Reilly, M.S.; Boehm, T.; Shing, Y.; et al. (1997). Endostatin: an endogenous inhibitor of angiogenesis and tumor growth. Cell 1997, Vol.88, No.2 (January), pp277-285.

Papapetropoulos, A.; Garcia-Cardena, G.; Dengler, T.J. et al. (1999), Direct actions of angiopoietin-1 on human endothelium: evidence for network stabilization, cell survival, and interaction with other angiogenic growth factors. Lab Invest, Vol.79, No.2, (February), pp. 213-223.

Papapetropoulos, A.; Fulton, D.; Mahboubi, K. et al. (2000). Angiopoietin-1 inhibits endothelial cell apoptosis via the Akt/survival pathway. J Biol Chem, Vol.275, No.13, (March), pp. 9102-9105.

Pepper, M.S. (2001). Lymphangiogenesis and tumor metastasis: myth or reality? Clin Cancer Res, Vol.7, No.3, (March): pp.462-468.

Roberts, N.; Kloos, B.; Cassella, M. et al. (2006). Inhibition of VEGFR-3 activation with the antagonistic antibody more potentially suppresses lymph node and distant metastases than inactivation of VEGFR-2. Cancer Res, Vol.66, No.5, (March), pp. 2650-2657.

Quentin, T.; Schlott, T.; Korabiowska, M. et al. (2004). Alternation of the vascular endothelial growth factor and angiopoientin-1 and -2 pathways in transitional cell carcinoma of the urinary bladder asscoaited with tumor progression. Anticancer Res, Vol.24, No.5A, (September-October), pp. 2745-2756.

Santos, L.; Costa, C.; Pereira, S. et al. (2003). Neovascularisation is a prognostic factor of early recurrence in T1/G2 urothelial bladder cancer. Ann Oncol, Vol.14, No.9, (September): pp.1419-1424.

Sharma, S.; Sharma, M.C. & Sarkar, C. (2005). Morphology of angiogenesis in human cancer: a conceptual overview, histoprognostic perspective and significance of neoangiogenesis. Histopathology, Vol.46, No.5, pp. 481-489.

Shibuya, M. & Claesson-Welsh L. (2006). Sinal transduction by VEGF receptors in regulation of angiogenesis and lymphangiogensis. Exp Cell Res, Vol.312, No.5, (March), pp. 549-560.

Shirotake, S.; Miyajima, A.; Kosaka, T. et al. (2011). Angiotensin II type 1 receptor expression and microvessel density in human bladder cancer. Urology, Vol.77, No.4, (April), 1009.e19pe25.

Skobe, M.; Hawighorst, T.; Jackson, D.G., et al. (2001). Induction of tumor lymphangiogensis by VEGF-C promotes breast cancer metastasis. Nat Med, Vol.7, No.2, (February), pp. 192-198.

Stacker SA, Caesar C, Baldwin ME, et al. (2001). VEGF-D promotes the metastatic spread of tumor cells via the lymphatics. Nat Med, Vol.7, No.2, (February), pp. 186-191.

Stavropoulos, N.E.; Bouropoulos, C.; Ioachim, I.E.; et al. (2004). Prognostic significance of angiogenesis in superficial bladder cancer. Int Urol Nephrol Vol.36, No.2, : pp. 163-167.

Streeter, E.H. & Harris, A.L. (2002). Angiogenesis in bladder cancer - prognostic marker and target for further therapy. Surg Oncol Vol.11, No.1-2 (March): pp. 85-100.

Szarvas, T.; Jäger, T.; Droste, F. et al. (2009). Serum levels of angiogenic factors and their prognostic releavance in bladder cancer. Pathol Oncol Res, Vol.15, No.2, (June), pp. 193-201.

Takahashi, H. & Shibuya, M. (2005). The vascular endothelial growth factor (VEGF)/VEGF receptor system and its role under physiological and pathological conditions. Clin Sci (Lond), Vol.109, No. 3, pp. 227-241.

Yang, H.; Kim, C.; Kim, M-J. et al. (2011). Soluble vascular endothelial growth factor receptor-3 suppresses lymphangiogensis and lymphatic metastasis in bladder cancer. Mol Cancer, Vol.10, No.10, (April), pp. 36-48.

Zhou, M.; He, L.; Zu, X. et al. Lymphatic vessel density as a predictor of lymph node metastasis and its relationship with prognosis in urothelial carcinoma of the bladder. BJU Int, in press.

Zu, X.; Tang, Z.; Li, Y. et al. (2006). Vascular endothelial growth factor-C expression in bladder transitional cell cancer and its relationship to lymph node metastasis. BJU Int, Vol.98, No.5, (November), pp. 1090-1093.

6

UHRF1 is a Potential Molecular Marker for Diagnosis and Prognosis of Bladder Cancer

Motoko Unoki
Division of Epigenomics, Department of Molecular Genetics, Medical Institute of Molecular Genetics, Kyushu University, Japan

1. Introduction

Bladder cancer is the second most common cancer of the urinary system. An estimated 386,300 new cases and 150,200 deaths from bladder cancer occurred in 2008 worldwide (**Jemal et al., 2011**). The highest rates of bladder cancer incidence are found in industrially developed countries, particularly in North America and Western Europe (**Parkin et al., 2005**). Bladder cancer is more common in males. The cancer is the 7th most common cancer in males worldwide and 4th most common cancer in males in industrially developed countries, while the cancer is not ranked in the top 10 most common cancers in females even in industrially developed countries (**Jemal et al., 2011**). In industrially developed countries, approximately 90% of the cancers are transitional cell carcinomas (TCCs), while the remaining 10% are squamous cell carcinomas and adenocarcinomas (**Stein et al., 2001**).
There are several potential biomarkers for diagnosis and prognosis for bladder cancer, including Nuclear matrix protein-22 (NMP-22), human complement factor H related protein, telomerase, fibrin degradation product, and hyaluronic acid (**Dey, 2004**). Among these, only two biomarkers, NMP-22 and human complement factor H related protein, are in clinical use in Japan. Although these two markers are in clinical use, sensitivity and specificity of these markers are not perfect (**van Rhijn et al., 2005**); NMP-22 staining shows false positivity reactions in patients with hematuria, and the BTA (bladder tumour antigen) stat/BTA TRAK assay, which detects human complement factor H related protein, shows false positivity reactions in patients with urinary tract inflammation, recent genitourinary tumours and in cases of bladder stone (**Dey, 2004**). Cytology is still the most accurate diagnosis method, although sensitivity is not enough high (**van Rhijn et al., 2005**). Thus, discovery of a novel biomarker, which is sensitive and specific for bladder cancer, is an urgent subject.

2. UHRF1 is a potential molecular marker for diagnosis and prognosis of bladder cancer

UHRF1 (ubiquitin-like with PHD and ring finger domains 1), also known as ICBP90 (Inverted CCAAT box-binding protein of 90 kDa), was identified as a protein, whose expression is only detectable in proliferating cells, not in quiescent cells (**Hopfner et al., 2000; Unoki et al., 2004**). UHRF1 plays a central role in transferring DNA methylation status from mother cells to daughter cells. Its SET and RING finger-associated (SRA) domain recognizes hemi-methylated DNA that appears in newly synthesized daughter DNA strands during duplication of DNA strands through the S phase (**Arita et al., 2008; Avvakumov et al., 2008; Hashimoto et al., 2008**). UHRF1 recruits DNA methyltransferase 1 (DNMT1) to the site with proliferating cell nuclear antigen (PCNA) and methylates the newly synthesized strands (**Achour et al., 2008; Sharif et al., 2007**). UHRF1 also recognizes tri/di-methylated H3K9, and recruits the H3K9 methyltransferase G9a, the histone deacetylase 1 (HDAC1), and the histone acetylase Tip60 (**Achour et al., 2009; Hashimoto et al., 2009; Karagianni et al., 2008; Kim et al., 2009; Unoki et al., 2004**), indicating that UHRF1 links DNA methylation and histone modification status (Fig. 1).

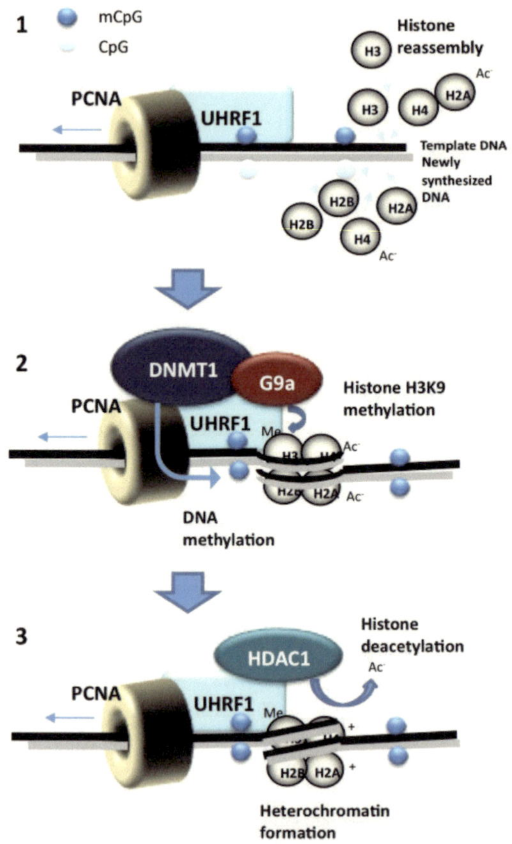

Fig. 1. Proposed mechanism of heterochromatin formation through UHRF1 at DNA replication fork or DNA repair site. 1) UHRF1 binds to PCNA and the SRA domain of UHRF1 recognizes hemi-methylated CpG on newly synthesized DNA. Then histones are reassembled. 2) UHRF1 recruits DNMT1 to methylate both DNA strands to transfer methylation status. UHRF1 also recruits G9a to methylate histone H3K9. Methylated histone H3K9 interacts with the Tudor-PHD domain of UHRF1. 3) UHRF1 recruits HDAC1 to the site and deacetylates histones. Then, histones become charged positively and bind to negatively charged DNA tightly, causing heterochromatin formation. This figure is cited from our article (**Unoki et al., 2009a**).

UHRF1 promotes G1/S transition (**Arima et al., 2004; Jeanblanc et al., 2005**) and is a direct target of E2F transcription factor 1 (E2F1) (**Abbady et al., 2005; Mousli et al., 2003; Unoki et al., 2004**). The tumour suppressor p53, which is deficient in 50% of all human cancers (**Hussain & Harris, 2000**), indirectly down-regulates UHRF1 through up-regulation of p21/WAF1 and subsequent deactivation of E2F1 (**Arima et al., 2004**) (Fig. 2).

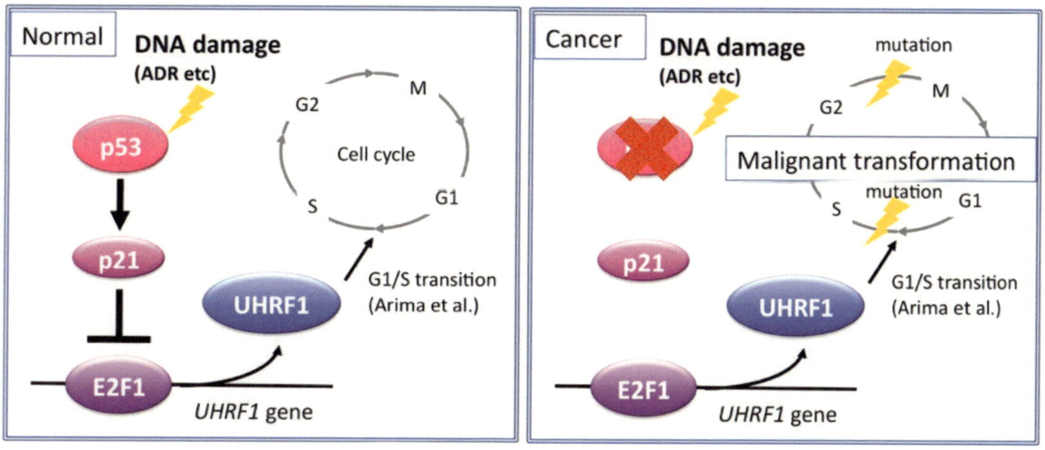

Fig. 2. Proposed p53-UHRF1 pathway model.

Expression of UHRF1 is up-regulated in various cancers, including breast cancer (Fig. 3), lung cancer (Fig. 4), prostate cancer, astrocytoma, pancreatic cancer, cervical cancer, and poorly differentiated thyroid carcinoma (**Crnogorac-Jurcevic et al., 2005; Jenkins et al., 2005; Lorenzato et al., 2005; Mousli et al., 2003; Oba-Shinjo et al., 2005; Pita et al., 2009; Unoki et al., 2010; Unoki et al., 2004**). Overexpression of UHRF1 in these cancers could be partially due to the inactivation of p53, although there could be several pathways, which regulate expression of UHRF1. Knock down of UHRF1 expression in cancer cells suppressed cell growth, indicating that UHRF1 is essential for progression of cancers and thus could be an anticancer drug target (**Tien et al., 2011; Unoki, 2011; Unoki et al., 2009a; Unoki et al., 2004; Yan et al., 2011**). Moreover, knockdown or inactivation of UHRF1 is reported to enhance sensitivity against current chemotherapies and radiation therapy *in vitro* (**Alhosin et al., 2010; Jenkins et al., 2005; Jin et al., 2010; Li, X. et al., 2011; Li, X. L. et al., 2009; Muto et al., 2002**). Therefore, UHRF1 is also an attractive target of cancer combination therapies (**Bronner et al., 2007; Unoki, 2011; Unoki et al., 2009a**).

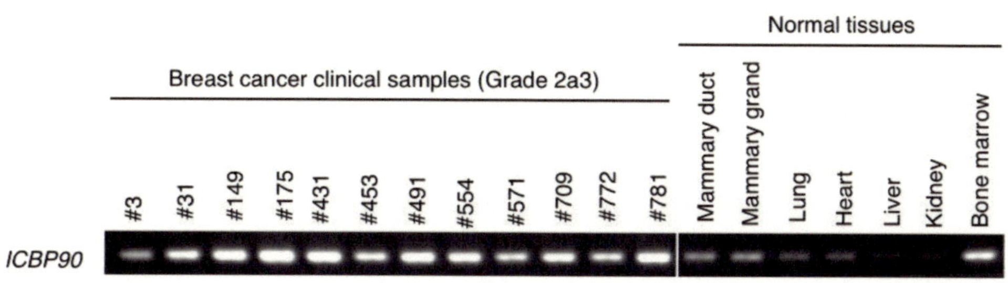

Fig. 3. Expression of *UHRF1* in breast cancer clinical samples detected by semi-quantitative RT-PCR. This figure is cited from our article (**Unoki et al., 2004**).

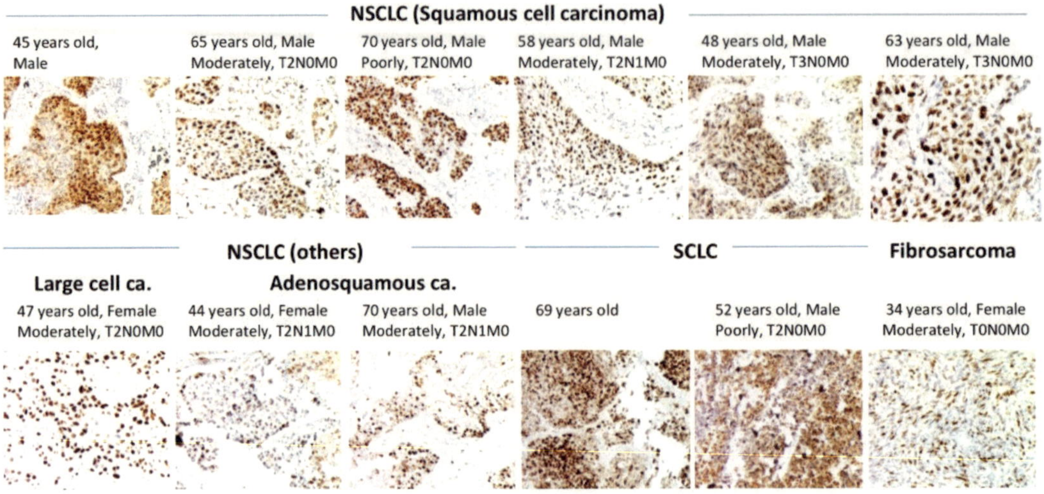

Fig. 4. Expression of UHRF1 in lung cancer clinical samples detected by immunohistochemistry. Representative data of UHRF1 staining in small cell lung carcinoma (SCLC), fibrosarcoma, and non-adenocarcinoma (ADC) histological types of non-small-cell lung carcinoma including squamous cell carcinoma (SCC), large cell carcinoma, and adenosquamous carcinoma (x 200). This figure is cited from our article (**Unoki et al., 2010**).

2.1 UHRF1 is overexpressed in bladder cancer

Considering these features of UHRF1, we thought that UHRF1 could be also important for bladder carcinogenesis, and examined expression of UHRF1 in bladder cancer specimens obtained from 124 UK cases (Table 1) and 36 Japanese cases (**Unoki et al., 2009b**). As a result, we found that UHRF1 was significantly overexpressed in bladder cancers at the mRNA and protein level (Fig. 5 and Fig. 6).

Because overexpression of UHRF1 in the cancer was detected both in UK cases and also in Japanese cases, the overexpression of UHRF1 could be common worldwide. Recently, another group showed that UHRF1 is also overexpressed in superficial, non-muscle-invasive bladder cancer of Chinese cases (**Yang et al., 2011**). Their result supports our observation. We also examined correlation between expression of UHRF1, p53, and *p21/WAF1*, and observed accumulation of stabilized p53 protein, which is probably mutated, in cancer tissues at grade II-III. However, we did not observe any accumulation of p53 in cancer tissues at grade I, although overexpression of UHRF1 was observed in this grade (Fig. 7). There was no relationship between expression levels of *UHRF1* and *p21* mRNA. Therefore, UHRF1 seems to be superior to p53 as a potential diagnostic marker of bladder cancer. This result is concordant with the fact that p53 is mutated only in 10-30 % of bladder cancer cases (**Berggren et al., 2001**; **Lorenzo Romero et al., 2004**).

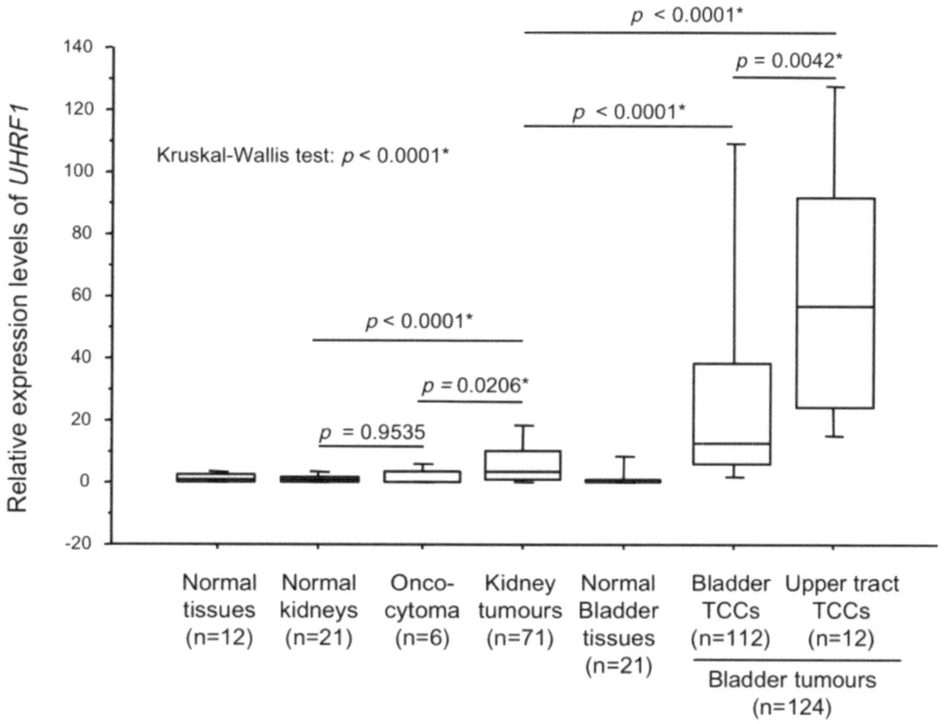

Fig. 5. Expression levels of *UHRF1* mRNA in urinary system tumours and normal tissues detected by TaqMan qRT-PCR. Expression of *UHRF1* in 12 different normal tissues, 21 normal kidneys, 6 oncocytomas, 71 kidney tumours, 21 normal bladders, and 124 bladder tumours, including 112 bladder located transitional cell carcinomas (TCCs) and 12 TCCs occurred in upper tract, were compared. Expression of *UHRF1* differed among the seven groups ($p<0.0001$, Kruskal-Wallis' test). Expression of *UHRF1* in the kidney cancers was higher than that in the normal kidneys and also in the oncocytomas significantly ($p<0.0001$, and $p=0.0206$, respectively, Mann-Whiteney's U-test), but expression levels of *UHRF1* in the bladder cancers were much higher than those in the kidney cancers ($p<0.0001$, Mann-Whiteney's U-test). Among the bladder cancers, expression of *UHRF1* was significantly high in upper tract TCCs (n=12) compared with the bladder-origin bladder tumours (n=112) (Mann-Whiteney's U-test; $p=0.0042$). *β2-microgloblin* was used for normalization. Asterisk indicates statistically significant *p*-values. This figure is cited from our article (**Unoki et al., 2009b**).

Characteristics	[a]n (%)	Characteristics	n (%)
Total numbers of patients	124	Sex	
Anatomic site		Male	75 (72%)
Bladder	112 (90%)	Female	29 (28%)
Upper tract	12 (10%)	Numbers of tumours	
Type		<4	53 (85%)
TCC	122 (>99%)	>4	9 (15%)
Others	1 (<1%)	Tumour size	
Invasiveness		<5	38 (66%)
Superficial	71 (63%)	>5	20 (34%)
Invasive	41 (37%)	Growth pattern	
T-category		[c]CIS	1 (2%)
Ta	40 (35%)	Papillary	32 (52%)
T1	32 (28%)	Solid	19 (31%)
T2	24 (21%)	Solid/Papillary	9 (15%)
T3	14 (12%)	Recurrence	
T4	4 (4%)	No	19 (29%)
WHO grading		Yes	46 (71%)
Grade 1	9 (8%)	5-years survival	
Grade 2	59 (51%)	Alive	46 (49%)
Grade 3	47 (41%)	Dead	48 (51%)
Risk after [b]TURBT		Smoking	
Low	7 (13%)	Non-smoker	22 (35%)
Intermediate	26 (46%)	Smoker	40 (65%)
High	23 (41%)		

[a]Total numbers of the patients are not always 124, because not all patients have all the clinical information; [b]TURBT, transurethral resection of the bladder tumour; [c]CIS, carcinoma *in situ*.

Table 1. Base line characteristics of bladder cancer patients used for our analyses (Unoki et al., 2009b).

We also examined expression of UHRF1 in kidney cancer, another urinary system tumour, together with the bladder cancer by immunohistochemistry. Although overexpression of *UHRF1* is significant at mRNA level (Fig. 5), expression of UHRF1 in kidney cancer was not detected at protein level (Fig. 8A). Therefore, immunohistochemical staining of UHRF1 in the cancer seems not to be useful. However, overexpression of *UHRF1* at the mRNA level was associated with several characteristics of kidney cancer patients including 5-year survival rates, pathological staging and histological grade (Fig. 8B-D). Thus, detection of

UHRF1 mRNA overexpression in surgical specimen might be useful as a prognosis tool in kidney cancer.

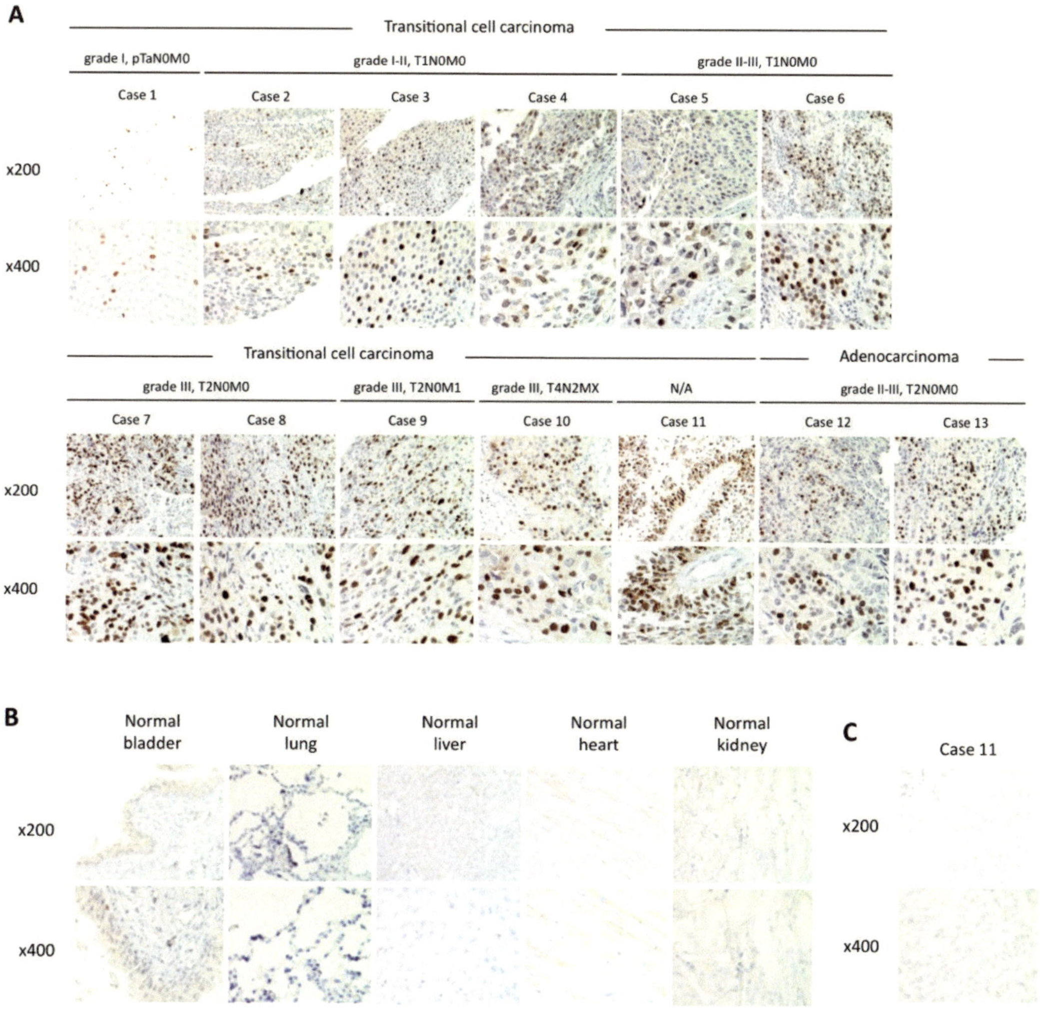

Fig. 6. Immunohistochemical staining of UHRF1 in 13 bladder tumour cases. A. Expression of UHRF1 in 11 transitional cell carcinomas and two adenocarcinomas with the different stage and grade. High expression of UHRF1 was detected only in nucleus of cancer cells, not in stromal cells. B. Expression of UHRF1 in normal tissues including bladder, lung, liver, heart, and kidney. No expression was observed in these normal tissues. Original magnifications, x 200 (top), and x 400 (bottom). C. Representative images of normal IgG staining as a negative control (Case 11 used for Fig. 6A). Original magnifications, x 200 (top), and x 400 (bottom). This figure is cited from our article **(Unoki et al., 2009b)**.

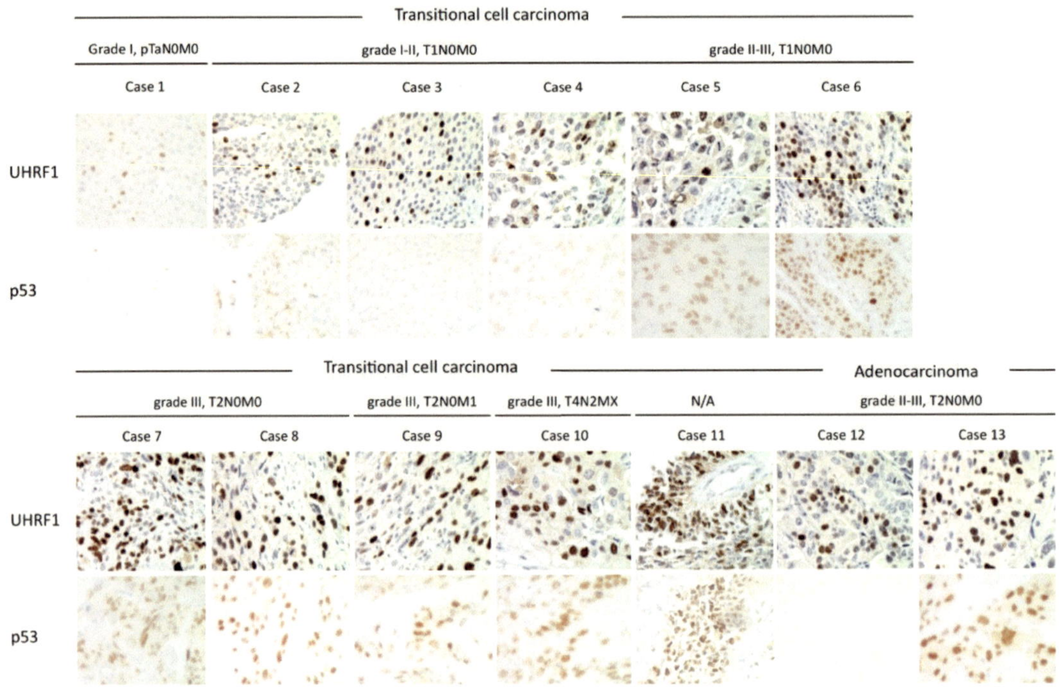

Fig. 7. Expression of p53 and UHRF1 in bladder cancers detected by immunohistochemistry. This figure is cited from our article (**Unoki et al., 2009b**).

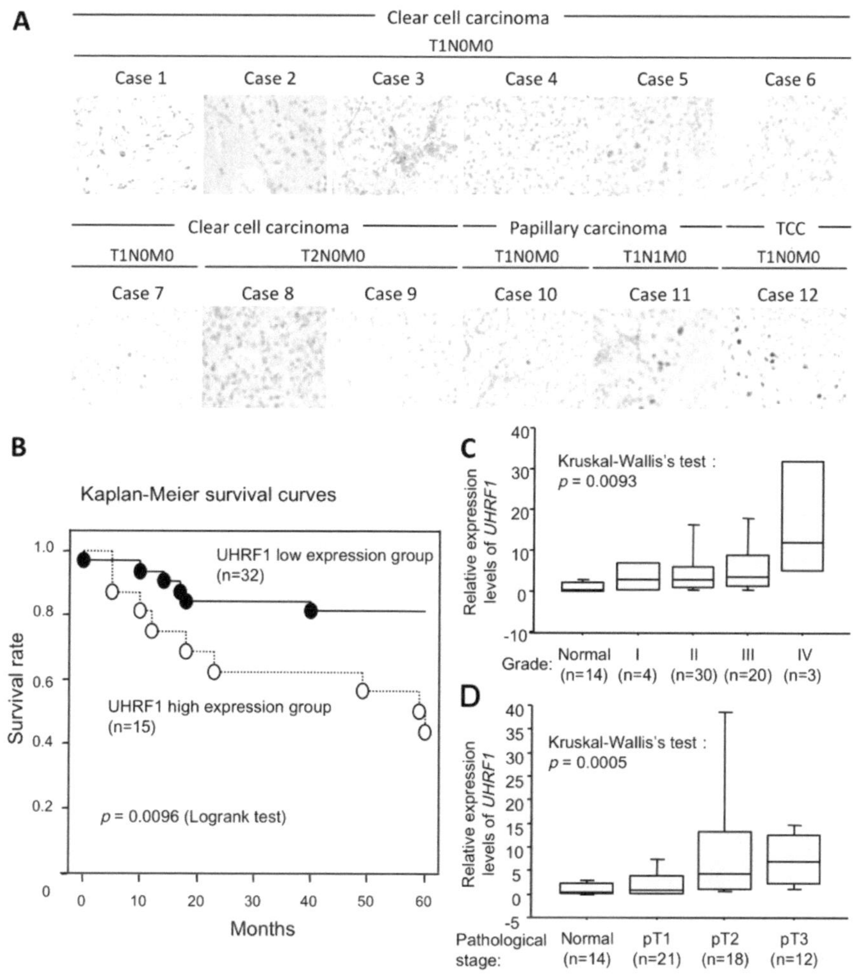

Fig. 8. Expression of UHRF1 in kidney cancer. A. UHRF1 expression in kidney cancers examined by immunohistochemistry. Magnification level is x400. B. Expression levels of *UHRF1* correlate with 5-years' survival rate of kidney tumours detected by TaqMan qRT-PCR. Patients were categorized into two groups by expression levels of *UHRF1*. The *UHRF1* high expression group is a group, which expresses *UHRF1* eight or more (≥8) and the low expression group is a group, which expresses *UHRF1* less than eight fold (<8) compared with average of *UHRF1* expression level in normal kidney from 21 individuals as 1.0. In the result of Kaplan-Meier survival analysis, the *UHRF1* high expression group showed significantly poor survival rate compared with the *UHRF1* low expression group (p=0.0096: Logrank test). *β2-microgloblin* was used for normalization. C. Expression levels of *UHRF1* correlated with histological grade of kidney tumours detected by TaqMan qRT-PCR. Patients were categorized into four groups by histological grade (I to IV). High expression of *UHRF1* correlated with advanced grade (p=0.0093: Kruskal-Wallis's test). *β2-microgloblin* was used for normalization. D. Expression levels of *UHRF1* correlated with pathological staging and histological grade of renal cancers detected by TaqMan qRT-PCR. Patients were categorized into three groups with pathological stages, pT1 to pT3. High expression of

UHRF1 correlated with advanced stage (p=0.0005: Kruskal-Wallis's test). *β2-microgloblin* was used for normalization. This figure is cited from our article (Unoki et al., 2009b).

2.2 Expression level of *UHRF1* correlates with malignancy of bladder cancer

We examined correlations between *UHRF1* expression in bladder cancer and various clinical features of the patients (Table 1). Among these features, the expression of *UHRF1* correlated with the T-category and the WHO histological grading significantly (Fig. 9A and 9B). Expression level of *UHRF1* in superficial bladder cancers (T-category: Ta and T1) and invasive bladder cancers (T-category classification: T2, T3 and T4) was both significantly higher than that in normal bladders. This result is concordant with data from the another group (**Yang et al., 2011**). In addition, expression of *UHRF1* in invasive bladder cancers was higher than that in superficial cancers, when we compared the three groups, normal bladders, invasive bladder cancers (pTa, pT1), and superficial bladder cancers (pT2-4), by Kruskal-Wallis's test (Fig. 9A). In addition, expression level of *UHRF1* in cancers with grade-II and -III was up-regulated compared with that in normal bladders (Fig. 9B). Therefore, up-regulation level of *UHRF1* reflects progression level of bladder cancer.

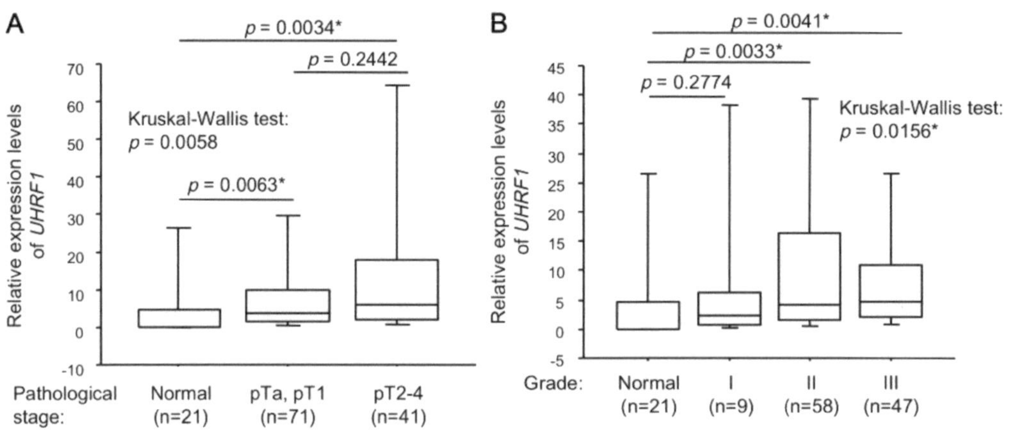

Fig. 9. Expression of *UHRF1* correlated with the stage, and grade. A. Expression of *UHRF1* in 21 normal bladders, 71 superficial bladder tumours (T-category is pTa and pT1), and 41 invasive bladder tumours (T-category is pT2, pT3, and pT4) detected by TaqMan qRT-PCR. Expression levels of *UHRF1* in superficial bladder tumours and in invasive tumours were significantly higher compared with those in normal bladders by Mann-Whiteney's U-test (p=0.0063 and p=0.0034, respectively). Although its expression in superficial tumours and invasive tumours did not differ (p=0.2442, Mann-Whiteney's U-test), it differed among the three different groups (p=0.0058, Kruskal-Wallis' test). *β2-microgloblin* was used for normalization. B. Expression of *UHRF1* differed among four groups with the different grade (p=0.0156, Kruskal-Wallis' test) detected by TaqMan qRT-PCR. Expression of *UHRF1* in grade II, and III tumour was higher than that in the normal bladders (p=0.0033 and p=0.0041). *β2-microgloblin* was used for normalization.

In our result, expression of *UHRF1* was not associated with difference of gender, numbers of tumour, tumour size, growth pattern (papillary or solid), incidence of recurrence, survival status after five years from surgery, and smoking history (Fig. 10), although the another group showed an association between UHRF1 expression levels and tumour recurrence in superficial bladder cancer of Chinese cases (**Yang et al., 2011**). Therefore, UHRF1 could be a molecular marker for predicting the recurrence of superficial bladder cancers in some ethnic groups.

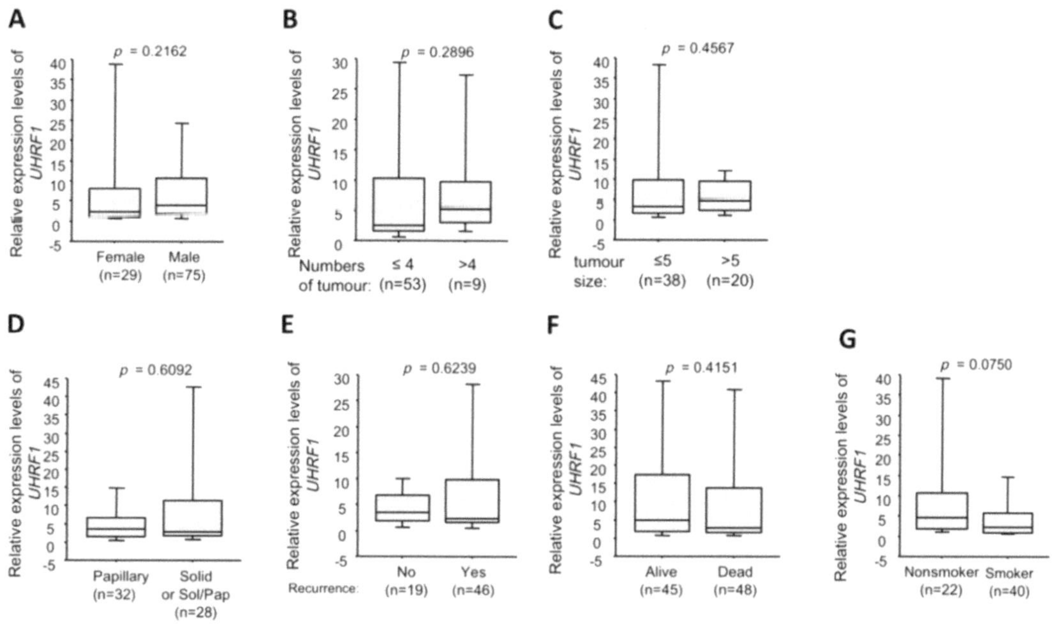

Fig. 10. Expression of *UHRF1* detected by TaqMan qRT-PCR and many characteristics of patients were compared by Mann-Whiteney's U-test. A. Expression levels of *UHRF1* in female patients (n=29) and male patients (n=75). Gender was not associated with expression levels of *UHRF1* (p=0.2162). B. Expression levels of *UHRF1* in patients with tumours four and less (n=53) and more than four (n=9) were not different (p=0.2896). C. Expression levels of *UHRF1* in patients with ≤ 5cm tumours (n=38) and with >5 cm tumours (n=20) were not different (p=0.4567). D. Expression levels of *UHRF1* in patients with papillary type tumours (n=32) and with solid or solid/papillary tumours (n=28) were not different (p=0.4567). E. Expression levels of *UHRF1* in patients who did not have a recurrence (n=19) and have a recurrence (n=46) were not different (p=0.6239). F. Expression levels of *UHRF1* in patients who survived 5 years after surgery (n=45) and died within 5 years (n=48) were not different (p=0.4151). G. Expression levels of *UHRF1* in non-smoker patients (n=22) and smoker patients including 4 ex-smokers (n=40) was not different (p=0.0750). *β2-microgloblin* was used for normalization.

2.3 Expression *UHRF1* can be used for predicting recurrence risk after TURBT

Over 75% bladder cancer patients have one or more superficial bladder cancers, and two thirds of them will develop recurrent disease (**Lutzeyer et al., 1982**), with 10–20% progressing to an invasive phenotype (**Torti & Lum, 1984**). The outcome of patients with invasive tumours remains still poor, with distant metastasis occurring in over 50% within 2 years and an average 5-year survival of only 50% (**Raghavan et al., 1990**). Currently, superficial bladder cancers are resected by a procedure called TURBT (TransUrethral

Resection of Bladder Tumour), and patients are treated differently based on estimated recurrence risk after TURBT. Thus, diagnosis of bladder cancer at non-advanced stage and also precise estimation of the risk after the TURBT, are very important for prognosis of patients. Currently, the risk after the surgery is estimated by a scoring system and risk tables developed by European Organization for Research and Treatment of Cancer (EORTC). The EORTC scoring system was developed based on the six most significant clinical and pathological factors, which are tumour stage, tumour grade, numbers of tumour, tumour size, prior recurrence rate, and presence of carcinoma *in situ* (CIS). Bladder cancer patients with pTaG1 tumours (50% of all patients) are at very low risk, and those with CIS or with pT1G3 tumours are at the highest risk (15% of all patients). Intermediate risk patients are those with pTa/pT1 G1/G2 disease who develop multiple recurrent cancers (35% of all patients). Our TaqMan qRT-PCR result showed that high expression of *UHRF1* was associated with high risk after TURBT (Fig. 11), probably because reflecting the association between high expression of *UHRF1* and stage, and/or grade (Fig. 9A and 9B). Based on these results, detection of *UHRF1* in tissue samples after TURBT will be a prognostic marker of future recurrence and may help to determine the risk together with the current prognostic factors.

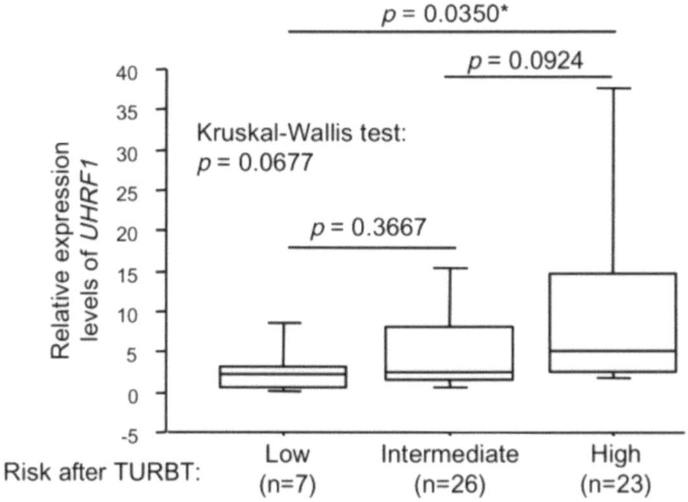

Fig. 11. Expression of *UHRF1* correlated with the recurrence risk after TURBT. Significant high expression of *UHRF1* in the high risk group after TURBT (n=23) was observed compared with that in the low risk group (n=7) by Mann-Whiteney's U-test (p=0.0350). Asterisk indicates statistically significant p-values. *β2-microgloblin* was used for normalization. This figure is cited from our article (Unoki et al., 2009b).

2.4 UHRF1 is a possible marker of bladder cancers and upper tract TCCs

Because *UHRF1* was significantly overexpressed in bladder cancers and upper tract TCCs (Fig. 5), UHRF1 might be a useful diagnostic marker especially for upper tract TCCs. Upper tract TCCs are often very malignant when it is diagnosed, partially because it is relatively difficult to find at an early stage. If the cancer is found at an early stage, the prognosis of patients is improved. The development of a sensitive urine based detection marker is still being sought. Examination of voided urine or bladder barbotage for exfoliated cancer cells is useful for diagnosis of urothelial tumours anywhere in the urinary tract, from the calyx, through the ureters, into bladder and urethra. However, cytological interpretation can be problematic; low cellular yields, atypia, degenerative changes, urinary tract infections, stones and intravesical instillations hamper a correct diagnosis. Because the current two biomarker tests in clinical use, NMP-22 detection and BTA stat/BTA TRAK assay, can be hampered by existence of bleeding, inflammation, recent genitourinary tumours, and bladder stone (**Dey, 2004**), these markers have not improved the traditional cytology-based bladder cancer diagnosis largely. Thus, cytology is still the mainstay for diagnosing bladder cancer. Because the expression of *UHRF1* in peripheral blood mononuclear cells (PBMCs) was under detection limit of qRT-PCR (Fig. 12), the presence of these cells in urine would not impede the diagnosis. Additionally, expression of UHRF1 was not detected in adjacent normal bladder tissues by immunohistochemistry (Fig. 6A and 6B). Thus, contamination of these stromal cells also would not disturb the diagnosis, either. Therefore, an immunohistochemistry or Enzyme-Linked ImmunoSorbent Assay (ELISA)-based UHRF1 detection in urine sediment can be a sensitive and cancer-specific diagnostic method, and may greatly improve the current diagnosis based on cytology.

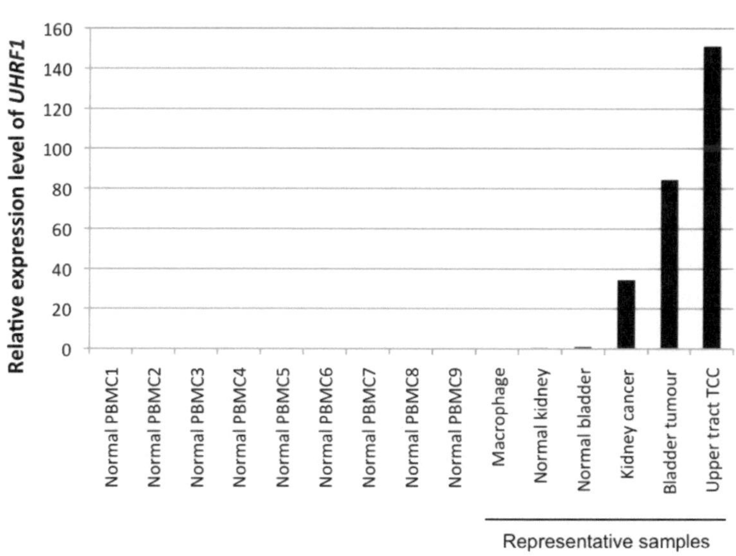

	Fold
Normal PBMC1	0.06
Normal PBMC2	0.00
Normal PBMC3	0.00
Normal PBMC4	0.01
Normal PBMC5	0.01
Normal PBMC6	0.01
Normal PBMC7	0.01
Normal PBMC8	0.01
Normal PBMC9	0.00
Macrophage	0.00
Normal kidney	0.53
Normal bladder	1.00
Kidney cancer	34.30
Bladder tumour	84.45
Upper tract TCC	151.17

Fig. 12. Relative expression levels of *UHRF1* in peripheral blood mononuclear cells (PBMCs) were examined by TaqMan qRT-PCR. Almost no expression of *UHRF1* was detected in PBMCs.

3. Conclusion

Although UHRF1 expression in muscle invasive cancer was greater than in non-invasive (pTa) or superficially invasive (pT1) cancers, UHRF1 could still be detected by immunohistochemistry in the early stage bladder cancers. In addition, overexpression of *UHRF1* was associated with increased risk of progression after TURBT. Therefore, our result indicates that detection of UHRF1 may be a useful marker for early stage bladder cancers, and also for estimation of risk after TURBT, although it should be tested in larger series to determine if it can improve current strategies for diagnosis and prognosis of bladder cancer.

4. Acknowledgement

I thank Professor Yusuke Nakamura for his continuous support of my research, Dr. Ryuji Hamamoto, Professor John D. Kelly, Professor David E. Neal, and Professor Sir Bruce A. J. Ponder for providing us UK bladder cancer specimens and for helpful discussion, Professor Tomoaki Fujioka for providing us Japanese bladder cancer specimens, and Drs. Ryo Takata, Hitoshi Zembutsu, and Yoichiro Kato for very useful advice and discussion.

5. References

Abbady, A. Q.; Bronner, C.; Bathami, K.; Muller, C. D.; Jeanblanc, M.; Mathieu, E.; Klein, J. P.; Candolfi, E. & Mousli, M. (2005). TCR pathway involves ICBP90 gene down-regulation via E2F binding sites. *Biochem Pharmacol,* Vol.70, No.4, (Aug 2005), pp.570-579, ISSN 0006-2952

Achour, M.; Jacq, X.; Ronde, P.; Alhosin, M.; Charlot, C.; Chataigneau, T.; Jeanblanc, M.; Macaluso, M.; Giordano, A.; Hughes, A. D.; Schini-Kerth, V. B. & Bronner, C. (2008). The interaction of the SRA domain of ICBP90 with a novel domain of DNMT1 is involved in the regulation of VEGF gene expression. *Oncogene,* Vol.27, No.15, (Apr 2008), pp.2187-2197, ISSN 1476-5594

Achour, M.; Fuhrmann, G.; Alhosin, M.; Ronde, P.; Chataigneau, T.; Mousli, M.; Schini-Kerth, V. B. & Bronner, C. (2009). UHRF1 recruits the histone acetyltransferase Tip60 and controls its expression and activity. *Biochem Biophys Res Commun,* Vol.390, No.3, (Oct 2009), pp.523-528, ISSN 1090-2104

Alhosin, M.; Abusnina, A.; Achour, M.; Sharif, T.; Muller, C.; Peluso, J.; Chataigneau, T.; Lugnier, C.; Schini-Kerth, V. B.; Bronner, C. & Fuhrmann, G. (2010). Induction of apoptosis by thymoquinone in lymphoblastic leukemia Jurkat cells is mediated by a p73-dependent pathway which targets the epigenetic integrator UHRF1. *Biochem Pharmacol,* Vol.79, No.9, (May 2010), pp.1251-1260, ISSN 1873-2968

Arima, Y.; Hirota, T.; Bronner, C.; Mousli, M.; Fujiwara, T.; Niwa, S.; Ishikawa, H. & Saya, H. (2004). Down-regulation of nuclear protein ICBP90 by p53/p21Cip1/WAF1-dependent DNA-damage checkpoint signals contributes to cell cycle arrest at G1/S transition. *Genes Cells,* Vol.9, No.2, (Feb 2004), pp.131-142, ISSN 1356-9597

Arita, K.; Ariyoshi, M.; Tochio, H.; Nakamura, Y. & Shirakawa, M. (2008). Recognition of hemi-methylated DNA by the SRA protein UHRF1 by a base-flipping mechanism. *Nature,* Vol.455, No.7214, (Oct 2008), pp.818-821, ISSN 1476-4687

Avvakumov, G. V.; Walker, J. R.; Xue, S.; Li, Y.; Duan, S.; Bronner, C.; Arrowsmith, C. H. & Dhe-Paganon, S. (2008). Structural basis for recognition of hemi-methylated DNA by the SRA domain of human UHRF1. *Nature,* Vol.455, No.7214, (Oct 2008), pp.822-825, ISSN 1476-4687

Berggren, P.; Steineck, G.; Adolfsson, J.; Hansson, J.; Jansson, O.; Larsson, P.; Sandstedt, B.; Wijkstrom, H. & Hemminki, K. (2001). p53 mutations in urinary bladder cancer. *Br J Cancer,* Vol.84, No.11, (Jun 2001), pp.1505-1511, ISSN 0007-0920

Bronner, C.; Achour, M.; Arima, Y.; Chataigneau, T.; Saya, H. & Schini-Kerth, V. B. (2007). The UHRF family: oncogenes that are drugable targets for cancer therapy in the near future? *Pharmacol Ther,* Vol.115, No.3, (Sep 2007), pp.419-434, ISSN 0163-7258

Crnogorac-Jurcevic, T.; Gangeswaran, R.; Bhakta, V.; Capurso, G.; Lattimore, S.; Akada, M.; Sunamura, M.; Prime, W.; Campbell, F.; Brentnall, T. A.; Costello, E.; Neoptolemos, J. & Lemoine, N. R. (2005). Proteomic analysis of chronic pancreatitis and pancreatic adenocarcinoma. *Gastroenterology,* Vol.129, No.5, (Nov 2005), pp.1454-1463, ISSN 0016-5085

Dey, P. (2004). Urinary markers of bladder carcinoma. *Clin Chim Acta,* Vol.340, No.1-2, (Feb 2004), pp.57-65, ISSN 0009-8981

Hashimoto, H.; Horton, J. R.; Zhang, X.; Bostick, M.; Jacobsen, S. E. & Cheng, X. (2008). The SRA domain of UHRF1 flips 5-methylcytosine out of the DNA helix. *Nature,* Vol.455, No.7214, (Oct 2008), pp.826-829, ISSN 1476-4687

Hashimoto, H.; Horton, J. R.; Zhang, X. & Cheng, X. (2009). UHRF1, a modular multi-domain protein, regulates replication-coupled crosstalk between DNA methylation and histone modifications. *Epigenetics,* Vol.4, No.1, (Jan 2009), pp.8-14, ISSN 1559-2308

Hopfner, R.; Mousli, M.; Jeltsch, J. M.; Voulgaris, A.; Lutz, Y.; Marin, C.; Bellocq, J. P.; Oudet, P. & Bronner, C. (2000). ICBP90, a novel human CCAAT binding protein, involved in the regulation of topoisomerase IIalpha expression. *Cancer Res,* Vol.60, No.1, (Jan 2000), pp.121-128, ISSN 0008-5472

Hussain, S. P. & Harris, C. C. (2000). Molecular epidemiology and carcinogenesis: endogenous and exogenous carcinogens. *Mutat Res,* Vol.462, No.2-3, (Apr 2000), pp.311-322, ISSN 0027-5107

Jeanblanc, M.; Mousli, M.; Hopfner, R.; Bathami, K.; Martinet, N.; Abbady, A. Q.; Siffert, J. C.; Mathieu, E.; Muller, C. D. & Bronner, C. (2005). The retinoblastoma gene and its product are targeted by ICBP90: a key mechanism in the G1/S transition during the cell cycle. *Oncogene,* Vol.24, No.49, (Nov 2005), pp.7337-7345, ISSN 0950-9232

Jemal, A.; Bray, F.; Center, M. M.; Ferlay, J.; Ward, E. & Forman, D. (2011). Global cancer statistics. *CA Cancer J Clin,* (Feb 2011), ISSN 1542-4863

Jenkins, Y.; Markovtsov, V.; Lang, W.; Sharma, P.; Pearsall, D.; Warner, J.; Franci, C.; Huang, B.; Huang, J.; Yam, G. C.; Vistan, J. P.; Pali, E.; Vialard, J.; Janicot, M.; Lorens, J. B.; Payan, D. G. & Hitoshi, Y. (2005). Critical role of the ubiquitin ligase activity of

UHRF1, a nuclear RING finger protein, in tumor cell growth. *Mol Biol Cell,* Vol.16, No.12, (Dec 2005), pp.5621-5629, ISSN 1059-1524

Jin, W.; Liu, Y.; Xu, S. G.; Yin, W. J.; Li, J. J.; Yang, J. M. & Shao, Z. M. (2010). UHRF1 inhibits MDR1 gene transcription and sensitizes breast cancer cells to anticancer drugs. *Breast Cancer Res Treat,* Vol.124, No.1, (Nov 2010), pp.39-48, ISSN 1573-7217

Karagianni, P.; Amazit, L.; Qin, J. & Wong, J. (2008). ICBP90, a novel methyl K9 H3 binding protein linking protein ubiquitination with heterochromatin formation. *Mol Cell Biol,* Vol.28, No.2, (Jan 2008), pp.705-717, ISSN 1098-5549

Kim, J. K.; Esteve, P. O.; Jacobsen, S. E. & Pradhan, S. (2009). UHRF1 binds G9a and participates in p21 transcriptional regulation in mammalian cells. *Nucleic Acids Res,* Vol.37, No.2, (Feb 2009), pp.493-505, ISSN 1362-4962

Li, X.; Meng, Q.; Rosen, E. M. & Fan, S. (2011). UHRF1 confers radioresistance to human breast cancer cells. *Int J Radiat Biol,* Vol.87, No.3, (Mar 2011), pp.263-273, ISSN 1362-3095

Li, X. L.; Meng, Q. H. & Fan, S. J. (2009). Adenovirus-mediated expression of UHRF1 reduces the radiosensitivity of cervical cancer HeLa cells to gamma-irradiation. *Acta Pharmacol Sin,* Vol.30, No.4, (Apr 2009), pp.458-466, ISSN 1745-7254

Lorenzato, M.; Caudroy, S.; Bronner, C.; Evrard, G.; Simon, M.; Durlach, A.; Birembaut, P. & Clavel, C. (2005). Cell cycle and/or proliferation markers: what is the best method to discriminate cervical high-grade lesions? *Hum Pathol,* Vol.36, No.10, (Oct 2005), pp.1101-1107, ISSN 0046-8177

Lorenzo Romero, J. G.; Salinas Sanchez, A. S.; Gimenez Bachs, J. M.; Sanchez Sanchez, F.; Escribano Martinez, J.; Hernandez Millan, I. R.; Segura Martin, M. & Virseda Rodriguez, J. A. (2004). p53 Gene mutations in superficial bladder cancer. *Urol Int,* Vol.73, No.3, (2004), pp.212-218, ISSN 0042-1138

Lutzeyer, W.; Rubben, H. & Dahm, H. (1982). Prognostic parameters in superficial bladder cancer: an analysis of 315 cases. *J Urol,* Vol.127, No.2, (Feb 1982), pp.250-252, ISSN 0022-5347

Mousli, M.; Hopfner, R.; Abbady, A. Q.; Monte, D.; Jeanblanc, M.; Oudet, P.; Louis, B. & Bronner, C. (2003). ICBP90 belongs to a new family of proteins with an expression that is deregulated in cancer cells. *Br J Cancer,* Vol.89, No.1, (Jul 2003), pp.120-127, ISSN 0007-0920

Muto, M.; Kanari, Y.; Kubo, E.; Takabe, T.; Kurihara, T.; Fujimori, A. & Tatsumi, K. (2002). Targeted disruption of Np95 gene renders murine embryonic stem cells hypersensitive to DNA damaging agents and DNA replication blocks. *J Biol Chem,* Vol.277, No.37, (Sep 2002), pp.34549-34555, ISSN 0021-9258

Oba-Shinjo, S. M.; Bengtson, M. H.; Winnischofer, S. M.; Colin, C.; Vedoy, C. G.; de Mendonca, Z.; Marie, S. K. & Sogayar, M. C. (2005). Identification of novel differentially expressed genes in human astrocytomas by cDNA representational difference analysis. *Brain Res Mol Brain Res,* Vol.140, No.1-2, (Oct 2005), pp.25-33, ISSN 0169-328X

Parkin, D. M.; Bray, F.; Ferlay, J. & Pisani, P. (2005). Global Cancer Statistics, 2002. *CA-Cancer J Clin,* Vol.55, No.2, (Mar-Apr 2005), pp.74-108, ISSN 0007-9235

Pita, J. M.; Banito, A.; Cavaco, B. M. & Leite, V. (2009). Gene expression profiling associated with the progression to poorly differentiated thyroid carcinomas. *Br J Cancer,* Vol.101, No.10, (Nov 2009), pp.1782-1791, ISSN 1532-1827

Raghavan, D.; Shipley, W. U.; Garnick, M. B.; Russell, P. J. & Richie, J. P. (1990). Biology and management of bladder cancer. *N Engl J Med,* Vol.322, No.16, (Apr 1990), pp.1129-1138, ISSN 0028-4793

Sharif, J.; Muto, M.; Takebayashi, S.; Suetake, I.; Iwamatsu, A.; Endo, T. A.; Shinga, J.; Mizutani-Koseki, Y.; Toyoda, T.; Okamura, K.; Tajima, S.; Mitsuya, K.; Okano, M. & Koseki, H. (2007). The SRA protein Np95 mediates epigenetic inheritance by recruiting Dnmt1 to methylated DNA. *Nature,* Vol.450, No.7171, (Dec 2007), pp.908-912, ISSN 1476-4687

Stein, J. P.; Lieskovsky, G.; Cote, R.; Groshen, S.; Feng, A. C.; Boyd, S.; Skinner, E.; Bochner, B.; Thangathurai, D.; Mikhail, M.; Raghavan, D. & Skinner, D. G. (2001). Radical cystectomy in the treatment of invasive bladder cancer: long-term results in 1,054 patients. *J Clin Oncol,* Vol.19, No.3, (Feb 2001), pp.666-675, ISSN 0732-183X

Tien, A. L.; Senbanerjee, S.; Kulkarni, A.; Mudbhary, R.; Goudreau, B.; Ganesan, S.; Sadler, K. C. & Ukomadu, C. (2011). UHRF1 depletion causes a G2/M arrest, activation of DNA damage response and apoptosis. *Biochem J,* Vol.435, No.1, (Apr 1 2011), pp.175-185, ISSN 1470-8728

Torti, F. M. & Lum, B. L. (1984). The biology and treatment of superficial bladder cancer. *J Clin Oncol,* Vol.2, No.5, (May 1984), pp.505-531, ISSN 0732-183X

Unoki, M.; Nishidate, T. & Nakamura, Y. (2004). ICBP90, an E2F-1 target, recruits HDAC1 and binds to methyl-CpG through its SRA domain. *Oncogene,* Vol.23, No.46, (Oct 2004), pp.7601-7610, ISSN 0950-9232

Unoki, M.; Brunet, J. & Mousli, M. (2009a). Drug discovery targeting epigenetic codes: The great potential of UHRF1, which links DNA methylation and histone modifications, as a drug target in cancers and toxoplasmosis *Biochem Pharmacol.,* Vol.78, No.10, (Nov 2009a), pp.1279-1288, ISSN 1873-2968

Unoki, M.; Kelly, J. D.; Neal, D. E.; Ponder, B. A. J.; Nakamura, Y. & Hamamoto, R. (2009b). UHRF1 is a novel molecular marker for diagnosis and the prognosis of bladder cancer. *Br J Cancer,* Vol.101, No.1, (Jul 2009b), pp.98-105, ISSN 1532-1827

Unoki, M.; Daigo, Y.; Koinuma, J.; Tsuchiya, E.; Hamamoto, R. & Nakamura, Y. (2010). UHRF1 is a novel diagnostic marker of lung cancer. *Br J Cancer,* Vol.103, No.2, (Jul 2010), pp.217-222, ISSN 1532-1827

Unoki, M. (2011). Current and potential anticancer drugs targeting members of the UHRF1 complex including epigenetic modifiers. *Recent Pat Anticancer Drug Discov,* Vol.6, No.1, (Jan 2011), pp.116-130, ISSN 1574-8928

van Rhijn, B. W.; van der Poel, H. G. & van der Kwast, T. H. (2005). Urine markers for bladder cancer surveillance: a systematic review. *Eur Urol,* Vol.47, No.6, (Jun 2005), pp.736-748, ISSN 0302-2838

Yan, F.; Tan, X. Y.; Geng, Y.; Ju, H. X.; Gao, Y. F. & Zhu, M. C. (2011). Inhibition Effect of siRNA-Downregulated UHRF1 on Breast Cancer Growth. *Cancer Biother Radiopharm,* Vol.26, No.2, (Apr 2011), pp.183-189, ISSN 1557-8852

Yang, G. L.; Zhang, L. H.; Bo, J. J.; Chen, H. G.; Cao, M.; Liu, D. M. & Huang, Y. R. (2011). UHRF1 is associated with tumor recurrence in non-muscle-invasive bladder cancer. *Med Oncol,* (May 25 2011), ISSN 1559-131X

7

Epidemiology and Polymorphisms Related to Bladder Cancer in Ecuadorian Individuals

César Paz-y-Miño and María José Muñoz
Instituto de Investigaciones Biomédicas, Facultad de Ciencias de la Salud, Universidad de las Américas
Quito
Ecuador

1. Introduction

Bladder cancer (BC) is the fourth most common cancer in men and the eighth most common in women being the responsible for annual deaths of 150,000 and is the seventh most prevalent type of cancer worldwide (Parkin, et al., 2005; Jemal, et al., 2009; Altayli, et al., 2009; Covolo, et al., 2008; Marmot, et al., 2007). In Ecuador the incidence rates of BC are 5.4% in males and 1.6% in females taking into account all cases of cancer diagnosed (Cueva & Yepez, 2009). In Argentina, it was reported as the fourth and the fourteenth most commonly diagnosed malignancy in men and women, respectively, with age-standardized incidence rate per 100,000 people around 15.1 (men) and 2.6 (women) in the period 1998 - 2002 (Pou, et al., 2011). The estimated downward trend in bladder cancer mortality over the last decades has been previously reported in countries of the European Union (Bosetti, et al., 2008) as well as South and North America (Bosetti, et al., 2005).

Susceptibility to BC is considered to depend on interaction between genetic factors and environmental chemical carcinogens. Bladder cancer involves a heterogeneous cell population, and numerous factors are likely to be involved in tumorigenesis (Hirao, et al., 2009). These factors result in uncontrolled growth of the cell population, decreased cell death, invasion and metastasis, and may influence the patient´s prognosis. Identification of the aggressive features of the cancer in patients with BC is very important for adequate management of this disease (Ha, et al., 2011).

Many studies have investigated the effects of gene polymorphism on the risk of cancer in humans (Paz-y-Miño, at al., 2010; Wacholder, et al., 2004; Marchini, et al., 2004). Single nucleotide polymorphisms (SNPs) are the most common type of gene polymorphism. Several millions of SNP variants have been identified. The risk of cancer associated with this type of polymorphism probably is not high, and the proportion of malignant tumors associated with a distinct polymorphism depends on the frequency of occurrence of this variant in the human population (Zaridze, 2008). Genetic polymorphisms that alter the activity of enzymes of biotransformation pathways have been reported to be associated with cancer development and progression (Franekova, et al., 2008).

In the other hand, molecular epidemiology of cancer studies, molecular markers of distribution of malignant tumors in the populations and their effects on individual are important to understand the risk of developing a disease. For an epidemiological study is very important not only the source of the biological material, but also the individual information, that could be the factors influencing the risk of developing cancer. Among these can mention lifestyle factors as smoking, alcohol consumption, nutrition/diet, physical activity, environmental factors as occupation and exposure to carcinogens at workplace, familial and individual medical history, and many other variables (Zaridze, 2008). Many epidemiological studies have been conducted to investigate the putative association between polymorphic genes for biometabolism, environmental carcinogens, and the development of urinary tract cancer (Souto Grando, et al., 2009).

The association between cigarette smoking and cancer of the urinary tract has been extensively investigated in epidemilogy (Zeegers, et al., 2000). Cigarette smoking is the main bladder cancer risk factor for both men (60%) and women (25%) (Paz-y-Miño, et al., 2010); approximately half of male urinary tract cancers and one third of female urinary tract cancers may be attributable to cigarette smoking (Hecht, 2003). Over 60 carcinogens have been identified in cigarette smoke. Among these are polycyclic aromatic hydrocarbons (PAHs) such as benzo[a]pyrene and aromatic amines, such as 2-naphtylamine and 4-aminobiphenyl, the organic benzene derivatives found in cigarettes and the reactive oxygen species (ROS) such molecular oxygen, hydrogen peroxide, and hydroxyl radicals (Ichimura, et al., 2004) increase the risk of developing this neoplasm by 25% (Paz-y-Miño, et al., 2010; Hecht, 2003; Luch, 2005). Molecular markers can be detected in tissues and biological liquids and characterize individual exposure to carcinogens, biological effect of the exposure, genetic susceptibility to the development of disease, and final result of carcinogenesis, i.e. tumor (Zaridze, 2008).

Many studies have indicated the relationship between different genetic polymorphisms and bladder cancer among the may appoint enzymes that perform a detoxifying function deactivate compounds and anions that are dangerous for the cell (Paz-y-Miño, et al., 2010). Cells are protected against metabolic ROS by several enzymatic and non-enzymatic defense systems, including superoxide dismutase (SOD), glutathione peroxidase (GPX) and reduced glutathione (Heistad, 2003). Three isoforms of SOD are present: Cu,Zn-SOD (SOD1 gene, cytosolic protein), Mn-SOD (SOD2 gene, mitochondrial protein) and EC-SOD (SOD3 gene, extracellular SOD) (Faraci & Didion, 2004). Manganese superoxide dismutase (MnSOD) has been the subject of particular interest as it is located in mitochondria and can be induced by several cytokines and by superoxide anion; it also appears to be involved in other processes, including tumor suppression and cellular differentiation (Charniot, et al., 2011).

In regards to GPX1, this is a major intracellular enzyme that catalyzes the degradation of peroxides by oxidizing glutathione with the formation of its conjugates, thereby preventing cellular injury (Deng, et al., 2008; Trošt, et al., 2010). Mutation in gene GPX1, which locates at chromosome 3p21, is one of the major factors regulating GPX1 activity. And among these, a genetic polymorphism at codon 198, resulting in either a proline (Pro) or leucine (Leu) at the corresponding position of the encoded peptide, have drawn increasing attention in the etiology of several cancers (Raaschou-Nielsen, et al., 2007; Ezzikouri, et al., 2010). In humans, the selenium-dependent activation of GPX 198Leu mutant enzyme is lower than for the GPX 198Pro wild-type enzyme (Hu, et al., 2010). And associations between low level of GPX1 activity in the circulation and increased risk of cancer were found in several cancer types including breast cancer (Arsova-Sarafinovska, et al., 2009; Hansen, et al., 2009); it is presumed that GPX1 Pro198Leu (C[T) polymorphism affecting GPX1 activity may be important for cancer development (Hu, et al., 2010).

The glutathione *S*-transferases (GSTs) are conjugation enzymes, which detoxify reactive chemical species, for example polycyclic aromatic hydrocarbons. Moreover these enzymes belong to a group of dimeric isozymes with various catalytic activities, which predominantly conjugate with electrophiles of glutathione conjugation and exert other noncatalytic functions. This isozyme is expressed in many tissues, including urinary bladder, and frequently overexpressed in carcinomas. The respiratory, urinary, and digestive tract epithelia express high levels of GSTP1 activity (Altayli, et al., 2009; Kopps, et al., 2008; Fishbain, et al., 2004)

There are five subclasses of the GST enzymes in humans: alpha, pi, mu, theta and zeta (Strange, et al., 2001). GSTM1, GSTT1, and GSTP1 are phase II enzymes (Rodriguez-Antona & Ingelman-Sundberg, 2006).

Altered substrate affinity has been shown in a polymorphism at exon 5 of the GSTP1 gene. Some studies have reported higher susceptibility to cancer in individuals carrying the variant GSTP1 allele, although contradictory results have also been obtained (Srivastava, et., 2005; Hu, et al., 1997).

A prevalent genetic polymorphism of the GSTP1 gene was reported differing only in a single A to G transition at nucleotide position 1578 corresponding to codon 105, resulting in an amino acid change from isoleucine to valine (Zimniak, et al., 1994; Harries, et al., 1997). The polymorphic forms were designated GSTP1a (Ile105, wild type) and b (Val105, mutant). Homozygosity for GSTP1 (Ile105Val) was found to be associated with a considerably higher risk for bladder cancer in patients in the United Kingdom (Harries, et al., 1997). In contrast, another study on Chinese benzidine workers diagnosed with bladder cancer indicated that GSTP1 Ile/Val and Val/Val polymorphism was a factor in disease occurrence (Ma, et al., 2003).

Association between oxidative stress and DNA damage has been well known and many studies have focused on the association between DNA damage and the development of certain diseases (Paz-y-Miño, et al., 2010; Padma, et al., 2011). DNA repair enzymes continuously monitor chromosomes to correct damaged nucleotide residues generated by exposure to cytotoxic compounds or carcinogens (Wood, et al., 2001). Recently, it has been hypothesized in many studies that polymorphisms in DNA repair genes reduce their capacity to repair DNA damage and thereby lead to enhanced cancer or other age-related disease susceptibility (Liu, et al., 2007; Povey, et al., 2007).

To date more than 100 DNA repair genes have been identified and their polymorphisms have been reported to be related with some diseases. Among them, polymorphisms of xeroderma pigmentosum complementation group D (XPD) and X-ray complementing group I (XRCC1) have been studied extensively (Clarkson & Wood, 2005; Paz-y-Miño, et al., 2011).

The human XRCC1 (X-ray repair cross-complementing group 1) gene is involved in single strand breaks and base excision repair (BER), it is located on chromosome 19q13.2, encodes for a 633 amino acids protein that plays an important role in BER and single-strand breaks repair (SSBR), following exposure to endogenous ROS or alkylating agents (Padma, et al., 2011; Vidal, et al., 2003; Marsin, et al., 2003). The XRCC1 is a scaffold protein that interacts with other many components of BER as DNA polymerase β, APE1, hOGG1, poly-(ADP-ribose) polymerase and DNA ligase III in the NH_2-terminal, central, and COOH-terminal regions, respectively (Sterpone & Cozzi, 2010). In 1998 Shen et al., described three polymorphisms of XRCC1 gene, which resulted in non-conservative aminoacid changes at evolutionary conserved regions: C → T substitution in codon 194 of exon 6 (Arg to Trp);

G → A substitution in codon 280 of exon 9 (Arg to His) and G → A substitution in codon 399 of exon 10 (Arg to Gln). All these single nucleotide polymorphisms (SNPs) could alter the XRCC1 function and impair DNA repair efficiency or accuracy (Shen, et al., 1998).
Given the large number of polymorphic variants and due to the existence of substantial differences in bladder cancer incidence in different ethnic groups, it is very important determine the frequencies of polymorphisms of many genes in Ecuadorian population affected with bladder cancer. These analyses are of great interest since it allows determining the genetic constitution of the population.

2. Materials and methods

2.1 Biological samples and data collection

A total of 97 formalin-fixed, paraffin-embedded (FFPE) bladder cancer samples were obtained from males and females individuals affected with bladder cancer. These samples were collected from the Department of Urology of Carlos Andrade Marín Hospital in Quito and the Department of Pathology of the Solón Espinoza Ayala Oncologic Hospital of Ecuador (SOLCA). One hundred twenty peripheral blood samples from male and female individuals with a medical history without malignancy served as control. In both cases, all the individuals signed informed consent after receiving information about the study. The study protocol and consent forms were approved by the University Institutional Bioethics Committee.
The distribution of selected characteristics between cases and control groups is summarized in Table 1. As for gender, the group of healthy individuals consisted of 33% of women and 67% of men, while de group of affected individuals consisted of 43% of women and 57% of men. In regard to histological subtype, transitional cell carcinoma accounted for 89%, of total cancer cases; 1% cases consisted of adenocarcinoma, 6% presented urothelial papillary carcinoma and 4% of affected individuals presented squamous cell carcinoma.

Characteristic	Cases Number	Control Number	Odds Ratio
Gender			5.3, 95% CI 2.9-9.5, $p<0.001$
Women	42	37	
Men	55	83	
Age	71 (>68)	41 (>66)	0.6, 95% CI 0.334-1.020, $p<0.05$
	26 (<68)	76 (<66)	
Age ($X \pm SD$)	68 ± 5.5	66 ± 4.5	
Smoking status			23.95, 95% CI 1.28-4.07. $p<0.05$
Smoker	72	67	
Non-smoker	25	53	
Histotype	Male	Female	
Transitional cell carcinoma	47 (55%)	39 (45%)	
Adenocarcinoma	1 (100%)	0 (0%)	
Urothelial papillary carcinoma	4 (67%)	2 (33%)	
Squamus cell carcinoma	3 (75%)	1 (25%)	

$X \pm SD$ medium $\pm$ standard deviation
CI confidence interval

Table 1. Clinical-Pathological characteristic of bladder cancer and control individuals

Concerning cigarette consumption as a risk factor to develop bladder cancer, 74% and 56% of affected individuals and healthy individuals respectively used to smoke, whereas 26% of affected and 44% of controls never smoked.

2.2 Genotyping

The DNA of affected individuals was obtained using the Purelink Genomic DNA extraction kit (Invitrogen, Carlsbad, CA), while, DNA from peripheral venous blood samples was isolated by a "salting out" method (Sambrook, et al., 1989), stored in the nucleic acid data bank of the Biomedical Research Institute at the Universidad de las Américas. The mean concentration of the DNA samples was 80ng/mL measured in a Qubit® Fluorometer (Invitrogen, Carlsbad, CA). We proceeded to study single nucleotide polymorphisms (SNPs) in the GSTP1 (Ile105Val), GPX-1 (Pro198Leu), MnSOD (Ile58Thr) and XRCC1 (Arg399Gln) genes. Genotyping was performed through the polymerase chain reaction–restriction fragment length polymorphism technique (PCR-RFLP).

For GPX-1, MnSOD, GSTP-1 and XRCC1 genes amplification, a PCR final volume of 50µl was prepared, containing 4µl of DNA template, 34µl H_2O Milli-Q, 0,4µM of forward and reverse primers, (Table 2) 1.5mM MgCl 2,5µl 10 × buffer (200 mM Tris-HCl pH 8.4, 500 mM KCl), 0,2µm each deoxynucleotide triphosphate (dNTPs), and 2.5 U Taq DNA polymerase (Invitrogen). For a 191-bp fragment amplification and the analysis of the Pro198Leu polymorphism found in chromosome 3, we used the initial denaturation step lasted 10 min at 95ºC, then 35 cycles of 30 s at 56ºC, 30 s at 56ºC, 45 s at 72ºC and 3 min at 72ºC were needed. Digestion of PCR product was carried out during 2h at 37ºC with the ApaI (Promega, Madison, USA) restriction enzyme. The PCR-RFLP test revealed homozygous individuals (Pro/Pro), (Leu/Leu) or heterozygous (Pro/Leu) (Paz-y-Miño, et al., 2010; Ichimura, et al., 2004). For the amplification of the 145-bp fragment of the Ile58Thr found in chromosome 6, for the PCR reaction, samples were placed in a thermo cycler MJ Research PTC 200® (MJ-Research Inc., Watertown, MA) for the amplification. The initial denaturation step lasted 10 min at 95ºC, followed by 35 cycles of 30 s at 95ºC, 30 s at 55ºC, 1 min at 72ºC, and 10 min at 72ºC. For the 177-bp fragment amplification and the analysis of the Ile105Val polymorphism found in chromosome 11, codon 105, exon 5, once the PCR reaction was obtained, the samples were placed in the MultiGene Thermal Cycler TC9600-G for amplification (Labnet, Edison, NJ, USA). The initial denaturation lasted 5 min at 95ºC, followed by 35 cycles of 45 s at 94ºC, 30 s at 62ºC, 30 s at 72ºC, and 1 min at 72ºC. Digestion of the amplified fragment was performed during 2 h at 37ºC with 5 U of the Alw26I

Genes	Primers
GPX-1	Forward, 5'-AAGGTGTTCCTCCCTCGTAGGT-3'
	Reverse, 5'-CTACGCAGGTACAGCCGCCGCT-3'
MnSOD	Forward, 5'-ACTTCAGTGCAGGCTGAACAGC-3'
	Reverse, 5'-CTGGTCCCATTATCTAATAGCTT-3'
GSTP-1	Forward, 5'-ACCCCAGGGCTCTATGGGAA-3'
	Reverse, 5'-TGAGGGCACAAGAAGCCCCT-3'
XRCC1	Forward, 5'-CCCCAAGTACAGCCAGGTC-3'
	Reverse, 5'-TGCCCCGCTCCTCTCAGTAG-3'

Table 2. Sequences of the PCR primers

(Promega, Madison, WI, USA) restriction enzyme. Electrophoresis analysis revealed homozygous individuals (Ile/Ile), (Val/Val) or heterozygous (Ile/Val) (Paz-y-Miño, et al., 2011); whereas for a 242-bp fragment amplification and the analysis of the Arg399Gln polymorphism found in chromosome 19, codon 399, exon 10, the initial denaturation step lasted 5 min at 95ºC, then 35 cycles of 45 s at 94ºC, 1 min at 59ºC, 30 s at 72ºC and 3 min at 72ºC. Digestion of amplicon was performed during 2 hours at 37ºC with the MspI (Promega) restriction enzyme. The analysis revealed homozygote individuals (Arg/Arg), (Gln/Gln) or heterozygote individuals (Arg/Gln) (Wong, et al., 2008).
All the polymorphisms were genotyped using a PCR-RFLP assay. After amplification, PCR products were cleaved by 5U of the corresponding enzyme. After digestion, the fragments were separated by electrophoresis on a 3.0% agarose gel and visualized using ethidium bromide in a transilluminator under ultraviolet light.

2.3 Statistical analysis

All information obtained from the studied individuals was kept in a database and statistical analyses were performed using PASW Statistics 17 for Windows (SPSS, Chicago, IL). The allelic and genotypic frequencies of each single nucleotide polymorphism were calculated from the information provided by the genotypes; and the Hardy-Weinberg equilibrium was determined by using software available on the Internet (http://www.genes.org.uk/software/hardy-weinberg.shtml). Chi-square (X) analysis was performed to determine significant differences between the presence of Ile105Val, Pro198Leu, and Arg399Gln polymorphisms of the studied population. The risk of developing disease in the presence of the studied polymorphisms between affected and control groups was determined using the odds ratio test (OR). Data were analyzed using a 2x2 contingency table.
Table 3 shows the Hardy-Weinberg equilibrium and the genotypic and allelic frequency of the studied polymorphisms. For the GPX1 and MnSOD genes, the genotypic frequencies

Gene	Group	Genotype	Individual (%)	Genotypic Frequency	Allele Frequency
GPX-1	Affected (n = 97)	Pro/Pro	28 (29%)	0.29	0.39
		Pro/Leu	19 (19%)	0.19	
		Leu/Leu	50 (52%)	0.52	061
	Control (n = 120)	Pro/Pro	73 (61%)	0.61	0.79
		Pro/Leu	42 (35%)	0.35	
		Leu/Leu	5 (4%)	0.04	0.21
MnSOD	Affected (n = 97)	Ile/Ile	43 (44%)	0.44	0.68
		Ile/Thr	47 (49%)	0.48	
		Thr/Thr	7 (7%)	0.07	0.32
	Control (n = 120)	Ile/Ile	75 (62%)	0.63	0.82
		Ile/Thr	45 (38%)	0.37	
		Thr/Thr	0 (0%)	0.0	0.18

Table 3. Genotype Distribution and Allele Frequency of the pro198leu and ile58thr

observed in both groups were in Hardy-Weinberg equilibrium (GPX1 cases, X = 0.36, p<0.05; controls, X = 0, p<0.05 and MnSOD; cases, X = 0.02; p<0.05; controls, X = 0.05; p<0.05), confirming that the study samples were obtained from a population in equilibrium. Regarding the GSTP1 Ile105Val polymorphism, we observed that the frequency of the Val allele in control individuals was 0.28 (Table 4). Concerning to the XRCC1 Arg399Gln polymorphism, we observed that the frequency of the Gln allele in control individuals was (0.98) (Table 4). The frequencies of both alleles for the individuals affected with bladder cancer are not shown but according to information reported in other studies could be correlated with the results obtained from the Ecuadorian population.

Genes	Genotype	Genotypic frequency Control	Allele frequency Control
	Ile/Ile	0.54	0.72
GSTP1 Ile105Val	Ile/Val	0.36	
	Val/val	0.10	0.28
XRCC1 Arg399Gln	Arg/Arg	0.01	0.02
	Arg/Gln	0.01	
	Gln/Gln	0.98	0.98

Table 4. Genotypic distribution and allelic frequency of GSTP1 Ile105Val and XRCC1 Arg399Gln polymorphisms

3. Conclusion

Bladder cancer is an important cause of death worldwide, there are many known risk factors for this cancer including age, male sex, smoking habit, and exposure to carcinogens (Pou, et al., 2011). The results obtained from the analysis of four genes using PCR-RFLP technique to determine the presence of the polymorphisms pro198leu in the GPX-1 gene, ile58thr in the MnSOD gene, Ile105Val in the GSTP1 gene and Arg399Gln in the XRCC1 gene in Ecuadorian individuals affected with bladder cancer, although small, support other evidence that genetic polymorphisms of the detoxification enzymes can modify bladder cancer risk.

GSTP1 participates in the detoxification of polycyclic aromatic hydrocarbon in promoting the conjugation of carcinogenic electrophiles with glutathione, thus enhancing excretion in the urine. This gene has been reported to possess two variant alleles. A single base substitution at position 313 of exon 5, guanine for adenine, results in the presence of valine (Val), where originally isoleucine (Ile) was present (Cao, et al., 2005). The prevalence rates of these isoforms are entirely dependent on which ethnic group is being considered (Shimada, 2006). Some have suggested that GSTP1 genes have an increased risk for tobacco-related cancers, including bladder cancer (Souto Grando, et al., 2009). Regarding genetics, the GSTP1 gene encodes proteins that are believed to function in xenobiotic metabolism and play the role as regulator of apoptosis (Moyer, et al., 2008). We found an association between the polymorphism and bladder cancer (data not shown), these findings could be suggesting that the presence of the Val/Val variant could be associated with an increased risk of acquiring detoxification problems, whereas the combination of the Ile/Val and

Val/Val alleles could be associated with the risk of presenting a GSTP1 gene dysfunction. Those individuals presenting the GSTP1 Val/Val and GPX-1 Leu/Leu variables may have a higher risk of acquiring problems in the detoxification (Paz-y-Miño, et al., 2011; Cao, et al., 2005).

Altayli, et al., had reported that smokers with GSTP1 Val105Leu heterozygous genotype had a reduced risk of bladder cancer. Some other authors reported a statistically significant association between the Leu/Leu and Val/Leu genotypes and bladder cancer risk. There are other authors that reported no association between the Ile105Val polymorphism of the GSTP1 gene and laryngeal squamous cell cancer, gastric cancer, and colorectal cancer (Unal, et al., 2004; Cao, et al., 2005).

The GSTP1 Ile105Val polymorphisms appear to be associated with a modest increase in the risk of bladder cancer. Some studies conducted in Asiatic population shows higher risk of developing bladder cancer when GSTP1 Ile/Val and Val/Val versus genotype Ile/Ile were compared, whereas the Chinese population did not have a significant influence on the unadjusted summary odds ratio for GSTP1 Ile/Val and Val/Val compared with GSTP1 Ile/Ile (Ma, et al., 2003). In conclusion, the GSTP1 polymorphisms Ile/Val and Val/Val compared with Ile/Ile seem to be associated with a modest increase in the risk of bladder cancer (data not published).

Our results indicate that the Ile105 allele was associated with an increased risk of bladder cancer. In previous articles, several types of carcinoma have been studied, in which there appeared to be an approximately threefold increase in risk between those with the GSTP1 (Val/Val) allele and those with GSTP1 (Ile/Ile) variant for bladder carcinoma (Harries, et al., 1997).

Successful repair of damaged DNA relies on the coordinated action of many repair enzyme systems. Age dependent decline or imbalance of the activities of the DNA repair enzymes will result in the compromise of the overall capacity of repair for the damaged DNA molecules. Common polymorphisms in DNA repair enzymes have been hypothesized to result in reduced capability to repair DNA damage. XRCC1 is a DNA repair gene that is emerging as an essential element in the repair of both damaged bases and SSBs (Padma, et al., 2011). Additionally, XRCC1 is important in BER, the major repair pathway for nonbulky damaged bases, abasic sites, and DNA single-stranded breaks after treatment with ionizing radiation. Some reports in human populations suggested the 399Gln variant of XRCC1 was associated with greater DNA and chromosomal damage (Yoon, et al., 2011).

It has been suggested that changes in the XRCC1 protein, mainly in amino acid 399, increase the susceptibility for tumor development via genomic instability (Meza-Espinoza, et al., 2009). Nevertheless, another study did not find any effect of the Arg399Gln polymorphisms with regard to DNA damage (Pastorelli et al., 2002), even though it is not well known whether these polymorphisms produce a functional change in the protein. In any case, the risk of cancer depends on the involvement of several factors, and not only on the presence or combination of certain common genetic polymorphisms (Naccarati et al., 2007).

Earlier investigators reported that reduced DNA repair capacity resulting from genetic polymorphism was associated with increased risk for various cancers (Mittal, et al., 2008). In our study the Arg allele was found mainly in the population affected with bladder cancer. In our study, the results obtained show that the XRCC1 Arg399Gln polymorphism, the frequency of the Gln allele was higher in affected individuals when compared to the control group (data not show). Among the polymorphisms of the XRCC1 gene the Arg399Gln amino acid change alters the phenotype of XRCC1 protein and thereby result in deficient DNA repair. According to our data in case of codon 399 our study exhibited no risk for bladder cancer which was in accord with the Northern Italian population (Shen, et al., 2003). Kelsey et al., 2004 indicated a 40% reduction in risk for bladder cancer among patients with homozygous variant XRCC1 399 (AA) compared with those with wild-type allele carriers. However, Stern et al., 2001 observed contrasting results by showing low risk for AA genotype in bladder cancer patients (OR = 0.7), but with not significant p value. One of the most interesting findings was the obtained by Mittal, et al., 2008 in which XRCC1 codon 399 where AA genotype exhibited 5.27 folds increased recurrence risk (HR=5.27, p=0.04).

On the one hand, GPX1 is suggested to play an important role in moderating H_2O_2 under pathological conditions (Ardanaz, et al., 2010). Over-expression of GPX-1 is associated with a wide range of effects, including the prevention of apoptosis, the protection against toxicity and the reduction of DNA damage (Zhuo, et al., 2009). Given human epidemiological data indicating significant associations between polymorphisms in GPx-1 and the risk of several cancer types due to the important biological activities of the essential trace element selenium are mediated through the function of selenoenzymes (Ichimura, et al., 2004; Hu & Diamond, 2003; Mak, et al., 2006; Choi, et al., 2007; Peters, et al., 2008). In this article we show the relationship between the presence of the Pro198Leu variant of the GPX-1 gene and its association with the risk of developing bladder cancer.

Among the ninety-seven patients analyzed for the GPX1 gene, 28.87% harbored the P/P homozygous genotype, 19,58% were P/L heterozygous and 51.55% were L/L homozygous. Of the 120 controls analyzed for the GPX-1 gene, 60.83% were P/P homozygous, 35% were P/L heterozygous and 4.17% were L/L homozygous (Table 3). For the MnSOD gene in the affected population, 44.33% were I/I homozygous, 48.45% I/T heterozygous, and 7.22% T/T homozygous. For controls 62.5% I/I homozygous, 39.17% I/T heterozygous and 0% T/T homozygous. The allelic frequency of the (I/I) allele was 0.68 for the group of affected individuals and 0.32 for control group (Table 3). The frequencies of the GPX-1 and MnSOD null genotypes were, respectively 39 and 82% in the patients and 79 and 18% in the control group.

When comparing control subjects and those affected with bladder cancer, we found that the presence of the Pro198Leu polymorphism has a relationship with the risk of developing bladder cancer (OR = 3.8; 95% CI 2.1-6.8; $p<0.001$), therefore the presence of the allelic variant (L/L) decreases the unique redox characteristics of the glutathione peroxidase, which can reduce reactive oxygen species and thereby prevent damage of important biomolecules, including DNA, RNA, lipids, proteins, and membranes; reactive oxygen species–induced DNA damage is known to promote tumor progression (Peters, et al., 2008), thereby conferring risk of developing bladder cancer in the Ecuadorian population. Previous studies demonstrate that the carriers of the variant L/L have a four times greater risk of developing bladder cancer than the individuals with the P/P variant (Ichimura, et al., 2004; Hu & Diamond, 2003).

Table 5 shows the respective OR values of the GPX1 and MnSOD genotypes. We found an increased risk of bladder cancer associated with the genotypes for the GPX1 (P/L or L/L) OR = 3.8; 95% CI=2.1-6.8; $p<0.001$), while the MnSOD was not statistically significant (OR = 2.1; 95% CI=1.3-3.5; $p>0.05$). Possible modification of associations between genetic polymorphisms and bladder cancer risk was also achieved by stratifying cases based on old age (OR = 5.3; 95% CI 2.9-9.5; $p<0.001$), sex (OR = 0.6; 95% CI 0.33-1.02; $p<0.05$), and smoking history (OR = 2.3; 95% CI 1.28-4.07; $p<0.05$).

Pro198Leu	Pro/Pro	Pro/Leu	Leu/Leu	Chi-Square	Odds Ratio
Affected	29%	19%	52%	69.9, $p>$ 0.001	3.8, 95% CI 2.1-6.8, p<0.001
Control	61%	35%	4%		
Ile58Thr	**Ile/Ile**	**Ile/Thr**	**Thr/Thr**	**Chi-square**	**Odds Ratio**
Affected	44%	49%	7%	0.25, $p > 0.05$	2.1, 85% CI 1.3-3.5, p>0.05
Control	62%	38%	0%		

Table 5. Statistical Analysis

Several studies in different populations worldwide have reported, and an association between these variants with the risk of developing different types of cancer (Raaschou-Nielsen, et al., 2007; Ezzikouri, et al., 2010; Hu, et al., 2010; Arsova-Sarafinovska, et al., 2009; Hansen, et al., 2009). The incidence of these polymorphisms according to the population analyzed, for example: the allelic frequency of L/L in the Japanese population is 0.05, and in the Caucasian population it is 0.36 (Ichimura, et al., 2004; Hu & Diamond, 2003). Furthermore, it has been determined that variants in different populations increases 2.6 times of developing bladder cancer and 1.43 times of developing breast cancer (Ratnasinghe, et al., 2000).

About the age of individuals under study, it has been determined that the risk of acquire bladder cancer is increased in old aged individuals (OR = 0.6; 95% CI 0.334-1.020; p<0.05), and can be considered as a risk factor for developing this disease. Furthermore, it was determined that men are at five times more risk to develop this type of cancer than women (OR = 5.3; 95% CI 2.9-9.5; p<0.001).

Current scientific evidence considers tobacco as a carcinogenic in human, with a causal relationship also to urinary bladder cancer (Lagiou, et al., 2005), being one of the most important risk factors, responsible for almost one-third of bladder cancer deaths (Parkin, 2008). It has been determined that individuals who used to smoke are at two times more risk to develop bladder cancer than individuals that never smoke (OR = 2.3; 95% CI 1.28-4.07; p<0.05). These findings are supported because it has previously been reported that smoking results in lower GPX activity (Ravn-Haren, et al., 2006).

As a result of the ethnic differences, the distribution of the polymorphisms is affected; some studies have found that the risk of developing bladder cancer when a significant incidence of the L/L allelic variant exists, with the proportion of homozygous individuals for the L/L allele being low for the Asian population and high for the Caucasian population (Ichimura, et al., 2004; Hu & Diamond, 2003). These findings have been corroborated for the Ecuadorian population, due to the L/L genotype being present in a high proportion of individuals diagnosed with bladder cancer (n = 51; 51%).

Free radicals, which are produced naturally in the body, can cause oxidative damage of DNA, lipids, proteins and other cell constituents, contributing to the onset of cancer and other chronic diseases (Evans, et al., 2004). Several enzymes, including MnSOD, GSTP, are involved in the scavenging of free radicals and prevention of oxidative damage. MnSOD catalyzes the dismutation of superoxide radicals in mitochondria by converting anion superoxide into hydrogen peroxide and oxygen, being a primary source of defense against cellular oxidants, regulating mitochondrial transport. It plays a key role in protecting cells from oxidative stress, especially in people with a low intake of natural antioxidants (Vineis,

et al., 2007) because low levels of MnSOD gene activity may cause oxidative stress, leading to the development of cancer, diabetes, and neurodegenerative diseases like Parkinson´s and Alzheimer´s (Paz-y-Miño, et al., 2010). Although low expression of MnSOD has often been suggested for different types of cancer, it has been demonstrated that overexpression of this protein inhibited cancerous growth implying it as a tumor suppressor gene (Tamimi, et al., 2004). In addition, MnSOD may exert its effect as a tumor suppressor, by altering pathways involving in cellular apoptosis and proliferation (Canan, et al., 2011).
It has been reported that the frequency of the ile58thr variant of the MnSOD gene does not have a high significance (Hu & Diamond 2003). However there are other reports that have found an association between genetic polymorphisms in MnSOD and myeloid leukemia (Vineis, et al., 2007) indicating that oxidative stress can play a role in cancer. When we compare the values reported with the values obtained in the study we performed, we confirmed that the incidence of the T/T allele maintains a low level within the Ecuadorian population. We have shown statistically that there is no significant difference between the bladder cancer group and the control group (Paz-y-Miño, et al., 2010).
In the same way when we calculate the related risk of this two polymorphism (Pro/Leu and Ile/Thr), a negative relationship between the tendency to develop bladder cancer was found (OR = 2.1; 95% CI 1.2-3.6; $p>0.05$), concluding that the individuals who present the pro198leu variant have an increased risk of developing bladder cancer; contrary to what we found for ile58thr polymorphism and being different from that reported by other authors (Clemente, et al., 2007). It is well known that the ile58thr polymorphism of the MnSOD gene varies within different populations, with an incidence of 11% in Japanese populations and 30% in Chinese populations, compared to the Caucasian populations, which has a 62% of incidence (Hori, et al., 2000; Ambrosone, et al. 1999).
Some authors have reported that the expression level of the manganese superoxide dismutase enzyme, varies within tissues and shows an increment in individuals with brain, skin, lung tumors, breast, bladder cancer and myeloid leukemia (Vineis, et al., 2007; Ichimura, et al., 2004; Clemente, et al., 2007; Ambrosone, et al., 1999), for this reason the present study is important because it allows a characterization of the Ecuadorian population with bladder cancer. Various ethnic groups exhibit significant differences in the distribution of alleles throughout the population, which may influence the interpretation of epidemiological and association studies, these region-specific epidemiological studies provide important information on the frequency of polymorphic allelic variants in various ethnic groups (Souto Grando, et al., 2009).
The very different findings in other populations might be caused by some confounding factors such as ethnicity, selection of control groups and characterization of cases, sample sizes, and gene–gene and gene–environment interactions. In conclusion, these results shown an association with increased risk of bladder cancer in the population studied. In addition, the results suggest that the genotypes of the polymorphisms may be associated with increased risk of bladder cancer.

4. References

Ambrosone, CB., Freudenheim, JL., Thompson, PA., Bowman, E., Vena, JE., Marshal, JR., Graham, S., Laughlin, R., Nemoto, T., & Shields, PG. (1999). Manganeso superoxide dismutase (MnSOD) genetic polymorphisms, dietary antioxidants and risk of breast cancer. *Cancer Research*; Vol.59, No.3, pp.602–606, ISSN 1538-7445.

Ardanaz, N., Yang, X-P., Cifuentes, ME., Haurani, MJ., Jackson, KW., Liao, T-W., Carretero, OA., & Pagano, PJ. (2010). Lack of Glutathione Peroxidase 1 Accelerates Cardiac-Specific Hypertrophy and Dysfunction in Angiotensin II *Hypertension*, Vol. 55, No.1 pp.116-123, ISSN 0194911X.

Arsova-Sarafinovska, Z., Matevska, N., Eken, A., Petrovski, D., Banev, S., Dzikova, S., Georgiev, V., Sikole, A., Erdem, O., Sayal, A., Aydin, A., & Dimovski, AJ. (2009). Glutathione peroxidase 1 (GPX1) genetic polymorphism, erythrocyte GPX activity, and prostate cancer risk. *International Urology and Nephrology*, Vol.41, No.1, pp.63–70, ISSN 1573-2584.

Altayli, E., Gunes, S., Yilmaz, AF., Goktas, S., & Bek, Y. (2009). CYP1A2, CYP2D6, GSTM1, GSTP1, and GSTT1 gene polymorphisms in patients with bladder cancer in a Turkish population. *International Urology and Nephrology*, Vol.41, No.2, pp.259–266, ISSN: 1573-2584.

Bosetti, C., Malvezzi, M., Chatenoud, L., Negri, E., Levi, F., & La Vecchia, C. (2005). Trends in cancer mortality in the Americas, 1970–2000. *Annals of Oncology*, Vol.16, No.3, pp. 489–511, ISSN 1569-8041.

Bosetti, C., Bertuccio, P., Levi, F., Lucchini, F., Negri, E., & La Vecchia, C. (2008). Cancer mortality in the European Union, 1970–2003, with a joinpoint analysis. *Annals of Oncology*, Vol.19, No. 4, pp. 631–640, ISSN 1569-8041.

Canan Kucukgergin, C., Sanli, O., Tefik, T., Aydın, M., Ozcan, F., & Seckin, Ş. (2011). Increased risk of advanced prostate cancer associated with MnSOD Ala-9-Val gene polymorphism. *Molecular Biology Reports* (on-line). ISSN 1573-4978.

Cao. W., Cai, L., Rao, JY., Pantuck, A., Lu, ML., Dalbagni, G., Reuter, V., Scher, H., Cordon-Cardo, C., Figlin, RA., Belldegrun, A., & Zhang, EF. (2005). Tobacco smoking, GSTP1 polymorphism, and bladder carcinoma. *Cancer*, Vol.104, No.11, pp.2400–2408, ISSN 1097-0142.

Charniot, JC., Sutton, A., Bonnefont-Rousselot, D., Cosson, C., Khani-Bittar, R., Giral, P., Charnaux, N., & Albertini, JP. (2011). Manganese superoxide dismutase dimorphism relationship with severity and prognosis in cardiogenic shock due to dilated cardiomyopathy. *Free Radical Research;* Vol.45, No.4, pp.379-388, ISSN 1029-2470.

Choi, JY., Neuhouser, ML., Barnett, M., Hudson, M., Kristal, AR., Thornquist, M., King, IB., Goodman, GE., & Ambrosone, GB. (2007). Polymorphisms in Oxidative Stress–Related Genes Are Not Associated with Prostate Cancer Risk in Heavy Smokers. *Cancer Epidemiology Biomarkers & Prevention*, Vol.16, No.6, pp.1115-1120, ISSN 1538-7755.

Clarkson, SG., & Wood, RD. (2005). Polymorphisms in the human XPD (ERCC2) gene, DNA repair capacity and cancer susceptibility: an appraisal. *DNA Repair* Vol.4, No.10, pp.1068-74, ISSN 1568-7864.

Clemente, C., Elba, S., Buongiorno, G., Guerra, V., D'Attoma, B., Orlando, A., & Russo, F. (2007). Manganese superoxide dismutase activity and incidence of hepatocellular carcinoma in patients with Child-Pugh class. A liver cirrhosis: A 7-year follow-up study. *Liver International*, Vol.277, No.6, pp.791-797, ISSN 1478-3223.

Covolo, L., Placidi, D., Gelatti, U., Carta, A., Scotto Di Carlo, A., Lodetti, P., Piccichè, A., Orizio, G., Campagna, M., Arici, C., & Porru, S. (2008). Bladder cancer, GSTs, NAT1, NAT2, SULT1A1, XRCC1, XRCC·, XPD genetic polymorphisms and coffee consumption: a case-control study. *European Journal of Epidemiology,* Vol.23, No.5, pp.355–362, ISSN 1573-7284.

Cueva, P., & Yépez, J. (2009). *Cancer Epidemiology in Quito 2003-2005.* Quito, AH, Editorial: National Cancer Registry (NCR), SOLCA. ISBN 9942-9958. Quito-Ecuador.

Deng, FY., Liu, YZ., Li, LM., Jiang, C., Wu, S., Chen, Y., Jiang, H., Yang, F., Xiong, JX., Xiao, P., Xiao, SM., Tan, LJ., Sun, X., Zhu, XZ., Liu, MY., Lei, SF., Chen, XD., Xie, JY., Xiao, GG., Lian, SP., & Deng, HW. (2008). Proteomic analysis of circulating monocytes in Chinese premenopausal females with extremely discordant bone mineral density. *Proteomics* Vol.8, No.20, pp. 4259–4272, ISSN, 1615-9861.

Evans, MD., Dizdaroglu, M., & Cooke, MS. (2004). Oxidative DNA damage and disease: induction, repair and significance. *Mutation Research,* Vol.567, No. 1, pp.1–61, ISSN 0027-5107.

Ezzikouri, S., El-Feydi, AE., Afifi, R., Benazzouz, M., Hassar, M., Pineau, P., & Benjelloun, S. (2010). Polymorphisms in antioxidant defence genes and susceptibility to hepatocellular carcinoma in a Moroccan population. *Free Radical Research;* Vol.44, No.2, pp.208-216, ISSN 1029-2470.

Faraci, FM., & Didion, SP. (2004). Vascular protection: superoxide dismutase isoforms in the vessel wall. *Arteriosclerosis, Thrombosis, and Vascular Biology,* Vol,24, No.8, pp.1367-1373 ISSN 10795642.

Franekova, M., Halasova, E., Bukovska, E., Luptak, J., & Dobrota, D. (2008). Gene polymorphisms in bladder cancer. *Urologic Oncology,* Vol.26, No.1, pp.1–8, ISSN, 1078-1439.

Fishbain, DA., Fishbain, D., Lewis, J., Cutler, RB., Cole, B., Rosomoff, HL., & Rosomofff, RS. (2004). Genetic testing for enzymes of drug metabolism: does it have clinical utility for pain medicine at the present time? *Pain Medicine,* Vol.5, No.1, pp.81–93, ISSN, 1526-4637.

Ha, Y-S., Yan, C., Jeong, P., Kim, W., Yun, S-J., Kim, I., Moon, S-K., & Kim, W-J. (2011). *GSTM1* Tissue Genotype as a Recurrence Predictor in Nonmuscle Invasive Bladder Cancer. *Journal of Korean Medical Science,* Vol. 26, No.2, pp. 231-236, ISSN 1598-6357.

Hansen, RD., Krath, BN., Frederiksen, K., Tjønneland, A., Overvad, K., Roswall, N., Loft, S., Dragsted, LO., Vogel, U., & Raaschou-Nielsen, O. (2009). GPX1 Pro(198)Leu polymorphism, erythrocyte GPX activity, interaction with alcohol consumption and smoking, and risk of colorectal cancer. *Mutation Research,* Vol.664, No. 1-2, pp.13–19, ISSN 0027-5107.

Harries, LW., Stubbins, MJ., Forman, D., Howard, GC., & Wolf, CR. (1997). Identification of genetic polymorphisms at the glutathione S-transferase Pi locus and association with susceptibility to bladder, testicular and prostate cancer. *Carcinogenesis* Vol.18, No.4, pp.641–644, ISSN 1460-2180.

Hecht, EM. (2003). Tobacco carcinogens, their biomarkers and tobacco induced cancer. *Nature Reviews Cancer,* Vol.3, No.10, pp.733–744, ISSN 1474-175X.

Heistad, DD. (2003). Oxidative stress and vascular disease. *Arteriosclerosis, Thrombosis, and Vascular Biology,* Vol,26, No.4, pp.689 - 695, ISSN 10795642.

Hirao, Y., Kim, W., & Fujimoto, K. (2009). Environmental factors promoting bladder cancer. *Current Opinion in Urology,* Vol.19, No.5, pp. 494-499, ISSN 1473-6586.

Hori, H., Ohmori, O., Shinkai, T., Kojima, H., Okano, C., Suzuki, T., & Nakamura, J. (2000). Manganese superoxide dismutase gene polymorphism and achizophrenia: Relation to tardive dyskinesia. *Neuropsychopharmacology*, Vol.23, No.2, pp.170-177. ISSN 0893-133X.

Hu, X., Ji, X., Srivastava, SK., Xia, H., Awasthi, S., Nanduri, B., Awasthi, YC., Zimniak, P., & Singh, SV. (1997). Mechanism of differential catalytic efficiency of the two polymorphic forms of the human glutathione Stransferase P1-1 in the glutathione conjugation of carcinogenic diol epoxide of chrysene. *Archives of Biochemestry and Biophysics* Vol.345, No.1, pp.32–38, ISSN 0003-9861.

Hu, YJ., & Diamond, AM. (2003). Role of glutathione peroxidase 1 in breast cancer: Loss of heterozygosity and allelic differences in response to selenium. *Cancer Research* Vol.63, No.12, pp.3347–3351, ISSN 1538-7445.

Hu, J., Zhou, GH., Wang, N., & Wang, YJ. (2010). GPX1 Pro198Leu polymorphism and breast cancer risk: a meta-analysis. *Breast Cancer Research and Treatment*, Vol.124, No.2, pp. 425–431, ISSN 1573-7217.

Ichimura, Y., Habuchi, T., Tsuchiya, N., Wang, L., Oyama, C., Sato, K., Nishiyama, H., Owag, O., & Kato, T. (2004). Increased risk of bladder cancer associated with a glutathione peroxidase 1 codon 198 variant. *The Journal of Urology*, Vol. 172, No.2, pp.728-32, ISSN 0022-5347.

Jemal, A., Siegel, R., Ward, E., Hao, Y., Xu, J., & Thun, M. (2009). Cancer statistics, 2009. *CA A Cancer Journal for Clinicians*, Vol.59, No.4, pp. 225-249, ISSN 1542-4863.

Kelsey, KT., Park, S., Nelson, HH., & Karagas, MR. (2004). A population-based case-control study of the XRCC1 Arg399Gln polymorphism and susceptibility to bladder cancer. *Cancer Epidemiology Biomarkers & Prevention*, Vol.13, pp.1337-1341, ISSN 1538-7755

Kopps, S., Angeli-Greaves, M., Blaszkewicz, M., Prager, HM., Roemer, HC., Löhlein, D., Weistenhöfer, W., Bolt, HM., & Golga, K. (2008). *Glutathione S-Transferase P1 Ile105Val* Polymorphism in Occupationally Exposed Bladder Cancer Cases. *Journal of Toxicology and Environmental Health, Part A*, Vol.71, No.13-14, pp.898–901, ISSN 1087-2620.

Lagiou, P., Adami, HO., & Trichopoulos, D. (2005). Causality in cancer epidemiology. *European Jounal of Epidemiology*, Vol.20, No.7, pp.565–574, ISSN 1573-7284.

Liu, G., Zhou, W., Yeap, BY., Su, L., Wain, JC., Poneros, JM., Nishioka, NS., Lynch, TJ., & Christiani, DC. (2007). XRCC1 and XPD polymorphisms and esophageal adenocarcinoma risk. *Carcinogenesis*, Vol.28, No.6, pp.1254-8, ISSN 1460-2180.

Luch, A. (2005). Nature and nurture—lessons from chemical carcinogenesis. *Nature Reviews Cancer*, Vol.5, No.2, pp.113–125, ISSN 1474-175X.

Ma, Q., Lin, G., Qin, Y., Lu, D., Golka, K., Geller, F., Chen JG., & Shen JH. (2003). GSTP1 A1578G (Ile105Val) polymorphism in benzidine-exposed workers: An association with cytological grading of exfoliated urothelial cells. *Pharmacogenetics*, Vol.13, No.7, pp.409–415, ISSN 0960-314X.

Marchini, J., Cardon, L., Phillips, M., & Donnelly, P. (2004). The effects of human population structure on large genetic association studies *Nature Genetics*, Vol.36, No.5, pp.512-517, ISSN 1061-4036.

Mak, JC., Leung, HC., Ho, SP., Kow, FW., Cheung, AH., & Chang-Yeung, MM. (2006). Polymorphisms in manganese superoxide dismutase and catalase genes: Functional study in Hong Kong Chinesse asthma patients. *Clinical and Experimental Allergy*, Vol.36, No.4, pp.440-447, ISSN 1365-2222.

Marsin, S., Vidal, AE., Sossou, M., Ménissier-de Murcia, J., Le Page, F., Boiteux, S., De Murcia, G., & Radicella, JP. (2003). Role of XRCC1 in the coordination and stimulation of oxidative DNA damage repair initiated by the DNA glycosylase hOGG1," *The Journal of Biological Chemistry;* Vol.278, No.45, pp.44068–44074, ISSN 1083-351X.

Marmot, M., Atinmo, T., Byers, T., Chen, J., & Hirohata, T. (2007). *Food, nutrition, physical activity, and the prevention of cancer: a global perspective*, World Cancer Research Fund / American Institute for Cancer Research, ISBN, 13-9780972252225, AICR, Washington DC.

Meza-Espinoza, JP., Peralta-Leal, V., Gutierrez-Angulo, M., Macias-Gomez, N., Ayala-Madrigal, ML., Barros-Nuñez, P., Duran-Gonzalez, J., Leal-Ugarte, E. (2009). *XRCC1* polymorphisms and haplotypes in Mexican patients with acute lymphoblastic leukemia. *Genetics and Molecular Research;* Vol.8, No.4, pp.1451-1458, ISSN 1676-5680.

Mittal, RD., Singh, R., Manchanda, PK., Ahirwar, D., Gangwar, R., Kesarwani, P., Mandhani, A. (2008). XRCC1 codon 399 mutant allele. A risk factor for recurrence of urothelial bladder carcinoma in patients on BCG immunotherapy. *Cancer Biology & Therapy,* Vol.7, No.5, pp.647-652. ISSN 1555-8576.

Moyer, A., Salavaggione, O., Wu, T., Moon, I., Eckloff, B., Hildebrandt, MA., Schaid, DJ., Wieben, ED., & Weinshilboum, RM. (2008). Glutathione S-transferase P1: gene sequence variation and functional genomic studies. *Cancer Research;* Vol.68, No.18, pp.4791-4801, ISSN 1538-7445.

Naccarati, A., Pardini, B., Hemminki, K. & Vodicka, P. (2007). Sporadic colorectal cancer and individual susceptibility: a review of the association studies investigating the role of DNA repair genetic polymorphisms. *Mutation Research* Vol.635, No.2–3, pp.118–145, ISSN 0027-5107.

Padma, G., Mamata, M., Ravi Kumar, K., & Padma, T. (2011). Polymorphisms in two DNA repair genes (*XPD* and *XRCC1*) - association with age related cataracts. *Molecular Vision;* Vol.12, No.17, pp.127-133, ISSN 1090-0535.

Pastorelli, R., Cerri, A., Mezzetti, M., Consonni, E., & Airoldi, L. (2002). Effect of DNA repair gene polymorphisms on BPDE-DNA adducts in human lymphocytes. *International Journal of Cancer.* Vol.100, No.1, pp.9-1, 1097-0215.

Parkin, DM. (2008). The global burden of urinary bladder cancer. *Scandinavian Journal of Urology and Nephrology. Supplementum.* Vol.218, pp.12–20, ISSN 03008886.

Parkin, D., Bray, F., Ferlay, J., & Pisani, P. (2005). Global cancer statistics, 2002. *CA A Cancer Journal for Clinicians,* Vol.55, No.2, pp. 74-108, ISSN 1542-4863.

Paz-y-Miño, C., Muñoz, MJ., López-Cortés, A., Cabrera, A., Palacios, A., Castro, B., Paz-y-Miño, N., & Sánchez, ME. (2010). Frequency of Polymorphisms pro198leu in *GPX-1* Gene and ile58thr in *MnSOD* Gene in the Altitude Ecuadorian Population With Bladder Cancer. *Oncology Research,* Vol.18, No.8, pp.395–400, ISSN 0965-0407.

Paz-y-Miño, C., Muñoz, MJ., Maldonado, A., Valladares, C., Cumbal, N., Herrera, C., Robles, P., Sánchez, ME., & López-Cortés, A. (2011). Baseline determination in social, health, and genetic areas in communities affected by glyphosate aerial spraying on the northeastern Ecuadorian border. *Reviews on Environmental Health,* Vol.26, No.1, pp.45-51, ISSN 2191-0308.

Peters, U., Chatterjee, N., Hayes, RB., Schoen, RE., Wang, Y., Chanock, SJ., & Foster, CB. (2008). Variation in the Selenoenzyme Genes and Risk of Advanced Distal Colorectal Adenoma. *Cancer Epidemiology Biomarkers & Prevention*, Vol.17, No.5, pp.1144-1154, ISSN 1538-7755.

Pou, S., Osella, A., & Diaz, M. (2011). Bladder cancer mortality trends and patterns in Córdoba, Argentina (1986–2006). *Cancer Causes Control*; Vol.22, No.3, pp. 407–415, ISSN 1573-7225

Povey, JE., Darakhshan, F., Robertson, K., Bisset, Y., Mekky, M., Rees, J., Doherty, V., Kavanagh, G., Anderson, N., Campbell, H., Mackie, RM., & Melton, DW. (2007). DNA repair gene polymorphisms and genetic predisposition to cutaneous melanoma. *Carcinogenesis*, Vol.28, No.5, pp.1087-93, ISSN 1460-2180.

Raaschou-Nielsen, O., Sørensen, M., Hansen, RD., Frederiksen, K., Tjønneland, A., Overvad, K., & Vogel, U. (2007). GPX1 Pro198Leu polymorphism, interactions with smoking and alcohol consumption, and risk for lung cancer. *Cancer Letters*, Vol.247, No.2, pp. 293–300, ISSN 0304-3835.

Ratnasinghe, D., Tangrea, JA., Andersen, MR.,Barrett, MJ., Virtamo, J., Taylor, PR., & Albanes, D. (2000). Glutathione peroxidase codon 198 polymorphism variant increases lung cancer risk. *Cancer Research* Vol.60, No.22, pp.6381–6383, ISSN 1538-7445.

Ravn-Haren, G., Olsen, A., Tjønneland, A., Dragsted, LO., Nexø, BA., Wallin, H., Overvad, K., Raaschou-Nielsen, O., & Vogel, U. (2006). Associations between GPX1 Pro198Leu polymorphism, erythrocyte GPX activity, alcohol consumption and breast cancer risk in a prospective cohort study. *Carcinogenesis*, Vol.27, No.4, pp.820 – 825, ISSN 0143-3334.

Rodriguez-Antona, C., & Ingelman-Sundberg, M. (2006). Cytochrome P450 pharmacogenetics and cancer. *Oncogene*, Vol.25, No.11, pp.1679–1691, ISSN, 0950-9232.

Sambrook, J., Fritsch, E.F., & Maniatis, T. (1989). *Molecular Cloning: A Laboratory Manual*. Cold Spring Harbor Laboratory Press, ISBN, 0-87969-577-3, New York, USA.

Shen, M., Hung, RJ., Brennan, P., Malaveille, C., Donato, F., Placidi, D., Carta, A., Hautefeuille, A., Boffetta, P., & Porru, S. (2003). Polymorphisms of the DNA Repair Genes XRCC1, XRCC3, XPD, Interaction with Environmental Exposures, and Bladder Cancer Risk in a Case-Control Study in Northern Italy. *Cancer Epidemiology Biomarkers & Prevention*, Vol.12, pp.1234-1240, ISSN 1538-7755

Shen, MR., Jones IM., & Mohrenweiser, H. (1998). Nonconservative amino acid substitution variants exist at polymorphic frequency in DNA repair genes in healthy humans," *Cancer Research*; Vol.58, No.4, pp.604–608, ISSN 1538-7445.

Shimada, T. (2006). Xenobiotic-metabolizing enzymes involved in activation and detoxification of carcinogenic polycyclic aromatic hydrocarbons. *Drug Metabolism and Pharmacokinetics*. Vol.21, No.4, pp.257-276, ISSN 1880-0920.

Souto Grando, J., Kuasne, H., Losi-Guembarovski, R., Rodrigues, I., Mitsu-Matsuda, H., Fuganti, PE., Pereira, E., Libos, F., Paes de Menezez, R., de Freitas, MA., & de Syllos, IM. (2009). Association between polymorphisms in the biometabolism genes CYP1A1, GSTM1, GSTT1 and GSTP1 in bladder cancer. *Clinical and Experimental Medicine*, Vol.9, No.1, pp.21–28, ISSN 1591-9528.

Srivastava, DSL., Mishra, DK., Mandhani, A., Mittal, B., Kumar, A., & Mittal, RD. (2005). Association of genetic polymorphism of glutathione S-transferase M1, T1, P1 and susceptibility to bladder cancer. *European Urology*, Vol.48, No2, pp.339–344, ISSN 1569-9056.

Stern. MC., Umbach, DM., van Gils, CH., Lunn, RM., & Taylor, JA. (2001). DNA Repair Gene *XRCC1* Polymorphisms, Smoking, and Bladder Cancer Risk. *Cancer Epidemiology Biomarkers & Prevention*, Vol.10, pp.125-131, ISSN 1538-7755.

Sterpone, S., & Cozzi, R. (2010). Influence of XRCC1 Genetic Polymorphisms on Ionizing Radiation-Induced DNA Damage and Repair. *Journal of Nucleic Acids*, pp.1-6 ISSN 2090-0201.

Strange, RC., Spiteri, MA., Ramachandran, S., & Fryer, AA. (2001). Glutathione-S-transferase family of enzymes. *Mutation Research* Vol.482, No.1–2, pp.21–26, ISSN 0027-5107.

Tamimi, RM., Hankinson, SE., Spiegelman, D., Colditz, GA., & Hunter, DJ. (2004). Manganese superoxide dismutase polymorphism, plasma antioxidants, cigarette smoking, and risk of breast cancer. *Cancer Epidemiology, Biomarkers & Prevention*, Vol.13, No.6, pp.989-996. ISSN 1538-7755.

Trošt, Z., Trebše, R., Preželj, J., Komadina, R., Bitenc-Logar, D., & Marc, J. (2010). A microarray based identification of osteoporosis related genes in primary culture of human osteoblasts, *Bone*, Vol. 46, No.1, pp.72–80, ISSN 8756-3282.

Unal, M., Tamer, L., Ateş, NA., Akbas, Y., Pata, YS., Vayisoğlu, Y., Ercan, B., Görür, K., & Atik, U. (2004). Glutathione S-transferase M1, T1, and P1 gene polymorphism in laryngeal squamous cell carcinoma. *American Journal of Otolaryngology*, Vol.25, No.5, pp.317–322 ISSN 1532-818X

Vidal, AE., Boiteux, S., Hickson, ID., & Radicella, JP. (2003). XRCC1 coordinates the initial and late stages of DNA abasic site repair through protein-protein interactions," *The EMBO Journal*, Vol.20, No.22, pp. 6530–6539, ISSN 0261-4189.

Vineis, P., Veglia, F., Garte, S., Malaveille, C., Matullo, G., Dunning, A., Peluso, M., Airoldi, L., Overvad, K., Raaschou-Nielsen, O., Clavel-Chapelon, F., Linseisen, JP., Kaaks, R., Boeing, H., Trichopoulou, A., Palli, D., Crosignani, P., Tumino, R., Panico, S., Bueno-De-Mesquita, HB., Peeters, PH., Lund, E., Gonzalez, CA., Martinez, C., Dorronsoro, M., Barricarte, A., Navarro, C., Quiros, JR., Berglund, G., Jarvholm, B., Day, NE., Key, TJ., Saracci, R., Riboli, E., & Autrup, H. (2007). Genetic susceptibility according to three metabolic pathways in cancers of the lung and bladder and in myeloid leukemias in nonsmokers. *Annals of Oncology*, Vo.18, pp. 1230–1242. ISSN 1569-8041.

Wacholder, S., Chanock, S., Garcia_Closas, M., El Ghormli, L., & Rottiman, N. (2004). Assessing the Probability That a Positive Report is False: An Approach for Molecular Epidemiology Studies *Journal of the National Cancer Institute*, Vol.96, No.6, pp.434-442, ISSN 1460-2105.

Wong, RH., Chang, SY., Ho, SW., Huang, PL., Liu, YJ., Chen, YC., Yeh, YH., & Lee, HS. (2008). Polymorphisms in metabolic GSTP1 and DNA - repair XRCC1 genes with an increased risk of DNA damage in pesticide exposed fruit growers. *Mutation Research*, Vol.654, No. 2, pp.168 - 75, ISSN 1383-5718.

Wood, RD., Mitchell, M., Sgouros, J., & Lindahl, T. (2001). Human DNA repair genes. *Science*, Vol.291, No.5507, pp.1284-1289, ISSN 1095-9203.

Yoon, HH., Catalano, PJ., Murphy, KM., Skaar, TC., Philips, S., Powell, M., Montgomery, EA., Hafez, MJ., Offer, SM., Liu, G., Meltzer SJ., Wu, X., Forastiere, AA., Benson, AB., Kleinberg, LR., & Gibson, MK. (2011). Genetic variation in DNA-repair pathways and response to radiochemotherapy in esophageal adenocarcinoma: a retrospective cohort study of the Eastern Cooperative Oncology Group. *Bio Med Central Cancer,* Vol.17, No.11, pp.176. ISSN 1471-2407.

Zaridze, D. (2008). Molecular Epidemiology of Cancer. *Biochemistry (Moscow),* Vol. 73, No.5, pp. 532-542, ISSN 0006-2979.

Zeegers, MPA., Tan, FES., Dorant, E., & Van den Brandt, P. (2000). The impact of characteristics of cigarette smoking on urinary tract cancer risk. A meta-analysis of epidemiologic studies. *Cancer,* Vol.89, No.3, pp.630–639, ISSN 1097-0142.

Zimniak, P., Nanduri, B., Pikula, S., Bandorowicz-Pikula, J., Singhal, SS., Srivastava, SK., Awasthi, S., & Awasthi, YC. (1994). Naturally occurring human glutathione S-transferase GSTP1-1 isoforms with isoleucine and valine in position 104 differ in enzymic properties. *European Journal of Biochemistry,* Vol.224, No.3, pp.893–899, ISSN 1742-4658.

Part 3

Clinical Presentation and Diagnosis

8

Clinical Presentation

Samer Katmawi-Sabbagh
Kettering General Hospital NHS Trust
United Kingdom

1. Introduction

Bladder cancer can occur at any age. However, it is known to be a disease of the middle-aged or elderly patient. The incidence is variable in different countries and the risk factors includes male sex, increasing age, smoking, occupational exposure to carcinogens, chronic inflammation, drugs such as phenacitin and cyclophosphamide, and pelvic radiation. In this chapter, we will discuss the different symptoms and signs that the bladder cancer patient could present with, keeping in mind that non of these presenting features are unique for bladder cancer.

2. Haematuria

Haematuria is the presenting symptom in up to 80% of patients with bladder cancer(Cummings et al., 1992). It could be Visible (previously called gross or frank haematuria), or Non Visible (previously called Dipstick or Microscopic haematuria). It is usually intermittent rather than constant, therefore, if a second urine specimen is free of any haematuria after a previous positive sample, investigations are still warranted in a bladder cancer age range patient. It may be initial or terminal if the lesion is at the bladder neck or in the prostatic urethra. The history of smoking or occupational exposure to certain chemicals is relevant. The Renal Association and British Association of Urological Surgeons joint consensus statement uses the abbreviations VH and NVH to refer to visible and non visible haematuria respectively (Kelly et al., 2009). They also define significant haematuria as the one that is visible (VH), Symptomatic non visible (sNVH)ie: associated with lower urinary tract symptoms, and persistent asymptomatic (aNVH)ie: without association with any urinary tract symptoms. Persistence was defined as 2 out of 3 positive urine samples. Microscopic or non visible haematuria (NVH) is defined as more than 3 Red blood cells (RBCs) per high-powered field(HPF) on a spun specimen by the American Urological Association. However, Campbell-Walsh definition is more than 5 RBCs per HPF for spun urine and more than 2 RBCs per HPF for unspun urine. The degree of haematuria does not correlate with the stage or the grade of the bladder cancer but cancer pick up rate is different. Cancer diagnosis is about 20-25% for the VH and 5-10% for the NVH (Khadra et al.,2000; Edwards et al.,2006). Majority of cancers discovered when investigating haematuria are bladder ones and the rarity relate to the upper urinary tract. Haematuria is an alarming presentation especially when asymptomatic. It requires extensive examination and investigations to rule out underlying pathologies and in particular bladder or upper urinary tract cancers. The role of purposely designed one-stop haematuria clinic has been developed

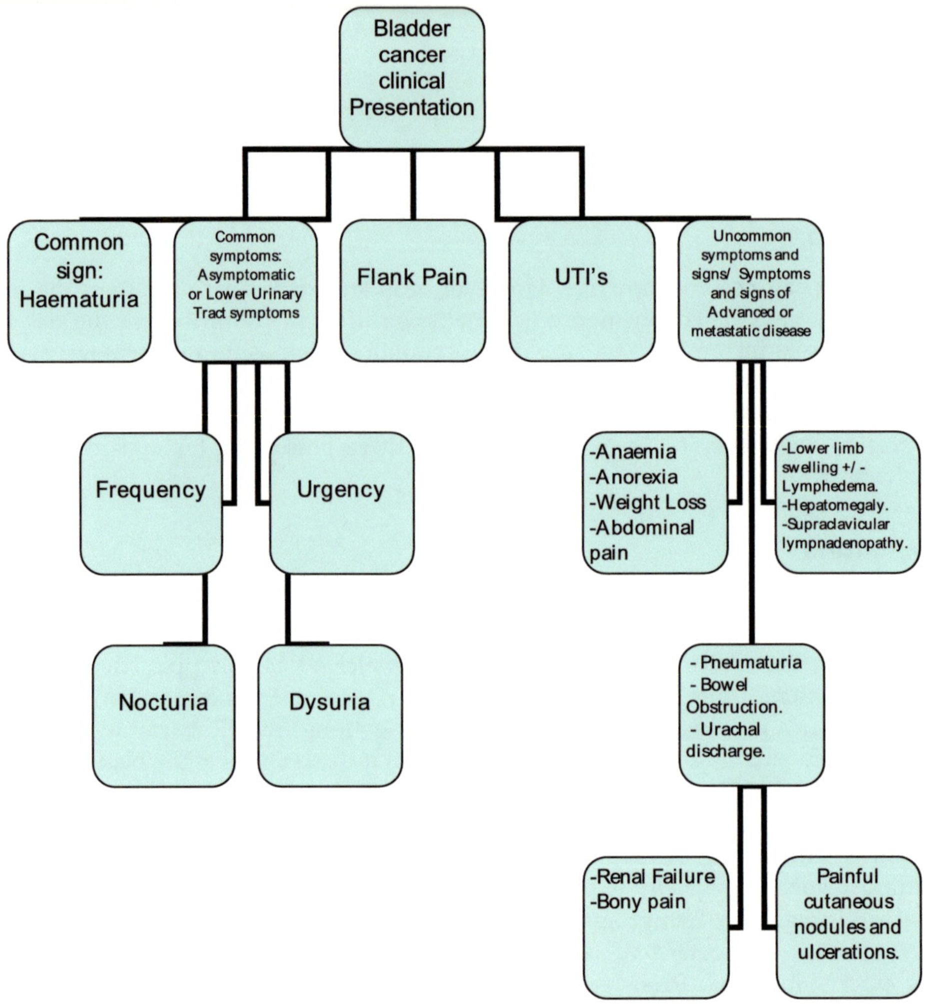

Fig. 1. Diagram showing the common and uncommon presenting symptoms and signs of bladder cancer.

and some evidence is existent that it could well reduce the time to cancer diagnosis and treatment (Katmawi-Sabbagh et al., 2010). Patients will require full history and examination including detailed information abouthaematuria, its duration and any associated symptoms. Smoking, occupation and exposure to chemicals and drugs should be documented. Abdominal, genital, and rectal examinations will be required in men. Vaginal examination is also important as vaginal bleeding is sometimes mistaken as haematuria in women. Details of required investigations will be discussed at different chapter of this book. Common causes of haematuria are listed below in Table 1:

	Infective	Neoplasic	Others
Kidney	-Pylonephritis -Tuberculosis(TB)	-Renal cell carcinoma -Transitional cell carcinoma (TCC). - Squamous cell carcinoma (SCC).	-Trauma -Stones. -Nephrological: IgA nephropathy, diabetes, Alport's syndrome, interstitial nephritis, papillary necrosis.
Ureter	-Ureteritis -Tuberculosis	-TCC -Adenocarcinoma. -SCC	-Trauma. -Stones.
Bladder	-Bacterial cystitis. -TB cystitis. -Schistosomiasis	-TCC -Adenocarcinoma -SCC	-Trauma -Stones -Foreign bodies.
Prostate	-Bacterial prostatitis -Granulomatous prostatitis.	-Prostate cancer. -Benign prostatic hypertrophy.	-Trauma - Iatrogenic: Post biopsy.
Urethra and penis	-Urethritis.	-SCC. -TCC.	-Trauma. -Stricture. -Iatrogenic: catheterization.

Table 1. Common causes of Haematuria based on the anatomical location and the causative factors.

3. Lower urinary tract symptoms

Frequency, nocturia, urgency, and urge incontinence are symptoms of vesical irritability. These could be seen in association with haematuria in bladder cancer patients (with or without the presence of dysuria or suprapubic pain). These symptoms were previously named as irritative symptoms and they have association with diffuse carcinoma in situ (CIS) as well as invasive cancer (Farrow et al., 1977).

4. Flank pain

Flank pain can be a symptom of advanced bladder cancer representing ureteric obstruction due to invasion of bladder muscular wall or the ureter. Tumours cause hydronephrosis as they become invasive (Figure 2). This is usually seen with high grade TCC rather than low grade (Table 2).

Alternatively hydronephrosis with or without pain could happen when there is involvement of the ureteric orifice (Leibovitch et al., 1993).

1973 World Health Organisation (WHO) grading
Grade 1: Well differentiated Grade 2: Moderately differentiated Grade 3: Poorly differentiated
2004 WHO grading - Flat lesions:
Hyperplasia (flat lesion without atypia or papillary) Reactive Atypia (flat lesion with atypia) Atypia of unknown significance Urothelial dysplasia Urothelial Carcinoma in situ (CIS)
2004 WHO grading - Papillary lesions:
Urothelial Papilloma (wich is a completely benign lesion) Papillary urothelial neoplasm of low malignant potential Low-grade papillary urothelial carcinoma High-grade papillary urothelial carcinoma

Table 2. WHO grading in 1973 and in 2004 (Sauter el al.,2004)

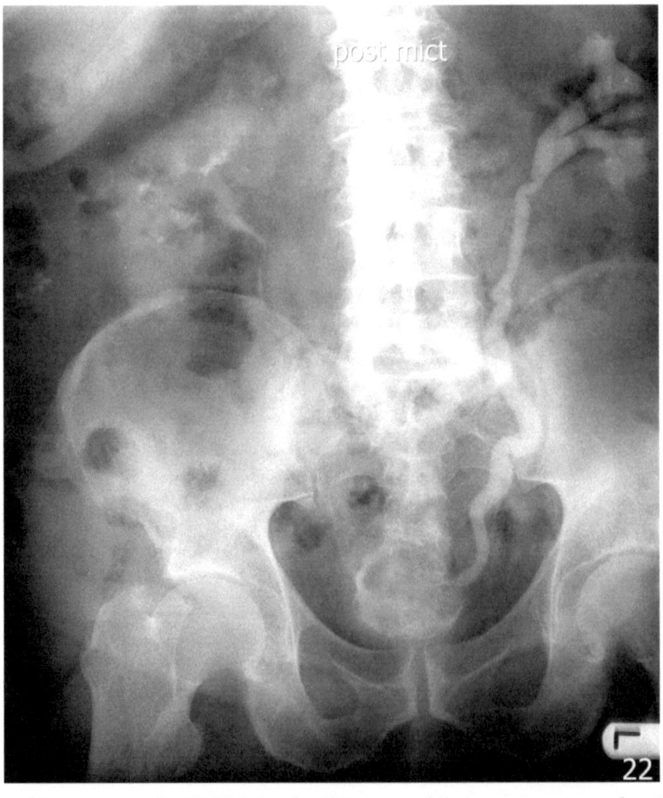

Fig. 2. An Intravenous urography (I.V.U) of a 76 year old man presented with haematuria and left sided loin pain. It shows left sided hydroureteronephrosis and large filling defect in the bladder. Cystoscopy confirmed a bladder tumour and histology revealed invasive G3 pT2 transitional cell carcinoma of the bladder.

Pyelonephritis may result if obstruction is complicated with infection. Flank pain and hydronephrosis could also be seen in cases of retroperitoneal metastasis. Flank pain caused by a bladder tumour is rarely encountered as the obstruction arises gradually. It should be distinguished from the one caused by a urinary stone which could also be associated with a degree of haematuria, but the colicky pain caused by a stone is normally of sudden onset and of higher intensity than that caused by a gradually occurring obstruction. Another differential diagnosis is the flank pain caused by a clot colic related to a bleeding from upper urinary tract transitional cell carcinoma or renal cell carcinoma.

5. Recurrent urinary tract infections (UTI's)

Recurrent urinary tract infections (UTI's) can be the first presentation of patients with necrotic infected bladder tumours. Therefore, it is always recommended to investigate recurrent UTI's with cystoscopic examination to rule out associated bladder tumour. It is also believed that bladder stones, long term catheters, and ova of Schistosoma haematobium (bilharziasis) are all implicated in the development of squamous cell carcinoma of the bladder via the mechanism of chronic inflammation of bladder mucosa.

6. Rare presentation symptoms and signs / symptoms and signs of advanced or complicated disease

The natural history of bladder cancer can be classified as follows:

- No further recurrence following initial presentation, diagnosis and treatment.
- Local recurrence, which can occur on a single occasion or on multiple occasions. The recurrent tumours are usually of the same stage and grade as the primary tumour. Clinically patient may be asymptomatic or represent with haematuria or any other local symptoms.
- Local Progresssion, which represent an increase in the local staging with time, the appearance of distant metastases and subsequent death. It is rare to encounter the symptoms and signs of advanced disease in the first presentation but patients with local recurrence and progression do represent with some of these symptoms and signs that are discussed below.

6.1 Anaemia, Anorexia, weight loss and abdominal mass:

Patients with large volume disease, muscle invasive tumours, or metastatic disease do sometimes present with these symptoms. The mass is properly assessed during bimanual examination under general anaesthesia and if it is immobile, this suggests that it is fixed to adjacent structures. Palpable masses that remain after local resection are likely to be extensive (non organ confined or T3 disease). The Tumour, Node, Metastasis(TNM) classification approved by the Union Internationale Contre le Cancer, which was updated in 2009 is shown in the table 3 (Sobin et al 2009):

T Primary tumour.
TX primary tumour cannot be assessed.
T0 No evidence of primary tumour.
Ta Noninvasive papillary carcinoma.
Tis carcinoma in situ:`Flat tumour`
T1 Tumour invades subepithelial connective tissue.
T2 Tumour invades muscle

T2a Tumour invades superficial muscle (inner half) T2b Tumour invades Deep muscle (outer half) T3 Tumour invades perivesical tissue: T3a Microscopically T3b Macroscopically (extravesical mass) T4 Tumour invades any of the following: Prostate, Uterus, Vagina, Pelvic Wall, abdominal wall. T4a Tumour invades prostate, uterus, or vagina. T4b Tumour invades pelvic wall or abdominal wall.
<u>N Lymph Nodes</u> Nx Regional lymph nodes cannot be assessed. N0 No regional lymph node metastasis N1 Metastasis in a single lymph node in the true pelvis (hypogastric, Obturator, external iliac, or presacral). N2 Metastasis in multiple lymph nodes in the true pelvis (hypogastric, Obturator, external iliac , or presacral). N3 Metastasis in a common iliac lymph node(s).
<u>M Distant metastasis</u> Mx Distant metastasis cannot be assessed. M0 No distant metastasis. M1 Distant metastasis.

Table 3. 2009 TNM classification of urinary bladder cancer

6.2 Lower limb swelling and lymphedema:
This is normally caused by occlusive pelvic lymphadenopathy or venous obstruction in the context of advanced disease.

6.3 Hepatomegaly and supraclavicular lymphadenopathy:
both are signs of metastatic disease.

6.4 Pneumaturia:
uncommon presentation of bladder cancer after enterovesical fistula formation. These type of fistulas are commoner with benign causes such as diverticular and crohn's disease. (Dawam et al.,2004). Nevertheless, pneumaturia warrants further investigations with urine cytology and cystoscopy with bladder biopsy if any neoplastic lesions could be seen.

6.5 Small bowel obstruction:
uncommon and unusual presentation caused by large and advanced disease (Aigen et al.,1983).

6.6 Renal failure:
caused be blocked ureters due to extensive muscle invasive disease or unilateral blockage in case of malfunctioning or absent contralateral kidney. This could also be related to retroperitoneal metastasis.

6.7 Painful cutaneous nodules and ulcerations:
very unusual and rare site of metastasis (Fujita et al., 1994;Block et al.,2006).

6.8 Urachal discharge (mucus or bloody):
a very rare presentation of adenocarcinoma, which is a rare histological subtype of bladder cancer. The tumour could be in the urachus itself or at the dome of the urinary bladder. It could also present with mucosuria.

6.9 Bony pain: a rare symptom that could be seen in cases of bony metastasis (Figure 3).

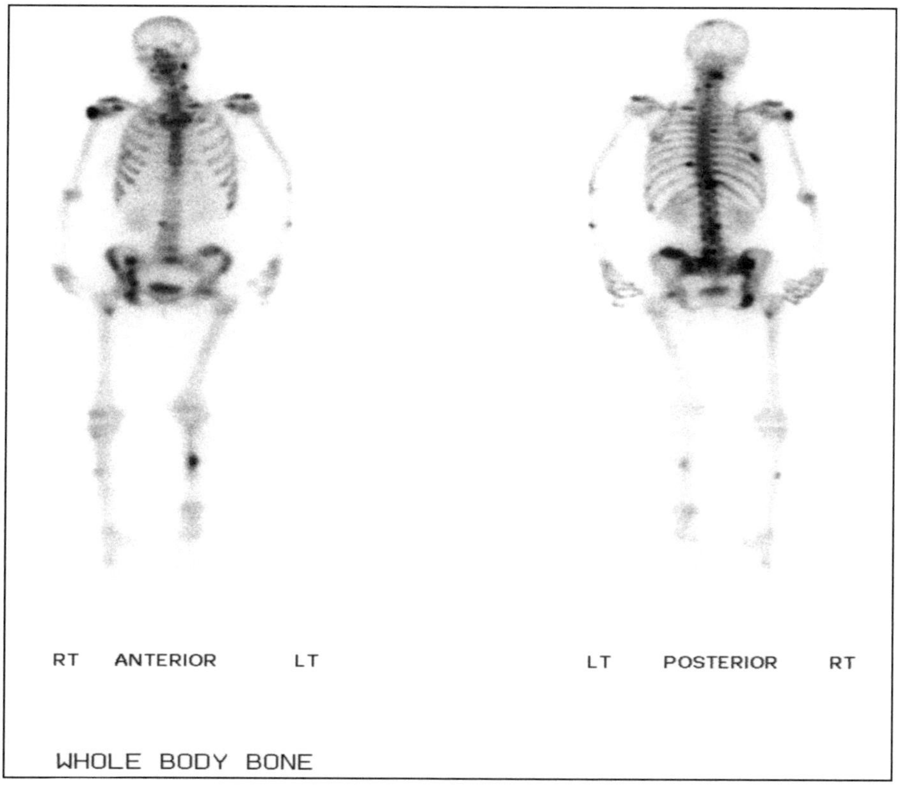

Fig. 3. An isotope bone scan of 38 year-old smoker female patient known to have G3pT2a bladder transitional cell carcinoma. She presented 2 years after radical radiation therapy with left sided hip pain. The bone scan shows wide spread metastasis (Spine, Pelvis, left forearm, left tibia, right femur and tibia).

7. Clinical conditions that could predispose to delayed presentation

7.1 Spina bifida patients

Patients with spinal bifida and bladder cancer present at a young age with variable tumour histology and advanced stage and they also have poor survival. These patients have neuropathic bladder dysfunction in addition to the fact that bladder augmentation is a significant risk factor for developing bladder cancer. Presenting symptoms are often atypical.

Although there has been suggestion of a role for annual serial bladder biopsies (Game et al., 1999) but it is not clear yet if screening would be beneficial for earlier detection and improved outcome. However, bladder cancer should be a consideration in this patient population, even in young adults (Austin et al. 2007).

7.2 Blind and colour blind patients

In a study of 200 bladder cancer patients, we found that those who had colour blindness (21 patients) did present with higher grade and stage disease compared to non colour blind population. The hypothesis is that these patients do not promptly notice the red colour of their urine at earlier stage, However, this is not proven. There is not sufficient evidence for screening of colour blind patients for bladder cancer. However, it is advisable to keep these findings in mind when assessing colour blind patients as they may help in case finding and early diagnosis of bladder cancer in this group of patients (Katmawi-Sabbagh et al., 2009).

8. References

Aigen AB, Schapira HE, Metastatic carcinoma of prostate and bladder. Causing intestinal obstruction. Urology 1983;21: 464-466.

Austin JC, Elliott S, Cooper CS. Patients with Spina bifida and bladder cancer: Atypical presentation, advanced stage and poor survival. J Urol 2007; 178(3): 798-801

Block CA, Dahmoush L, Konety BR. Cutaneous metastases from transitional cell carcinoma of the bladder. Urology 2006.67:846.

Cummings KB, Barone JG, Ward WS. Diagnosis and staging of bladder cancer. Urologic Clinic of N Am 1992;3: 455-465.

Dawam D, Patel S, Kouriefs C, Masood S, Khan O, Sheriff MK. A "Urological" enterovesical fistula. J Urol 2004;172:943-944.

Edwards TJ,Dickson AJ,Natale S,Gosling J,Mcgrath J. A prospective analysis of the diagnostic yield resulting from attendance of 4020 patients at a protocol-driven haematuria clinic.BJU 2006;97:301-305.

Farrow GM, Utz DC, Rife CC, Greene LF. Clinical observations in 69 cases of in situ carcinoma of the urinary bladder. Cancer Res 1977; 37: 2794.

Fujita K, Sakamoto Y, Fujime M, Kitagawa R. Two cases of inflammatory skin metastasis from transitional cell carcinoma of the urinary bladder. Urol Int 1994;53:114-116.

Game X, Villers A, Malavaud B, Sarramon J. Bladder cancer arising in a Spina bifida patient. Urology 1999;54:923.

Katmawi-Sabbagh S, Haq A, Jane S, Subhas G, Turnham H. Impact of colour blindness on recognition of Haematuria in bladder cancer. Urol Int 2009; 83(3): 289-290

Katmawi-Sabbagh S, Hussain T, Al-Sudani M, England R, Khan Z. The role of the one-stop haematuria clinic in reducing time to diagnsis and treatment of Urological cancers. Italian Journal of Urology and Nephrology 2010;62(3):331-332.

Kelly JD,Fawcett D, Goldberg L. Assessment and investigation of non- visible haematuria in the primary care setting. BMJ 2009; 338:a3021

Khadra MH, Pickard RS, Charlton M. A prospective analysis of 1930 patients with hematuria to evaluate current diagnostic practice. J Urol 2000;163:524-527

Leibovitch I, Ben-Chaim J, Ramon J, Madjar I, Engelberg IS, Goldwasser B. The significance of ureteral obstruction in invasive transitional cell Carcinoma of the urinary bladder. J Surg Oncol 1993; 52: 31-35.

Sauter G, Algaba F, Amin M. Tumours of the urinary system: Non - Invasive urothelial neoplasias. In: Eble JN, Sauter G, Epstein JI, Sesterhenn I. WHO classification of tumours of the urinary system And male genital organs. Lyon, France: IARCC Press; 2004.

Sobin LH, Gospodarowicz MK, wittekind C. TNM classification of Malignant tumours (UICC International Union Against Cancer). Ed 7. New York, NY:Wiley-Blackwell;2009. p.262-265.

Part 4

Infectious Agents and Bladder Cancer

9

Role of HPV in Urothelial Carcinogenesis: Current State of the Problem

G.M. Volgareva, V.B. Matveev and D.A. Golovina
N.N. Blokhin Cancer Research Center of the Russian Academy of Medical Sciences, Russia

1. Introduction

Human papillomaviruses (HPV) of the so-called high risk types (HR-HPV) cause cervical cancer (CC). Carcinomas in other organs such as vagina, vulva, penis, oropharynx and rectum are known to be aetiologically heterogeneous with respect to HPV (zur Hauzen, 2000, 2008; Gillison & Shah, 2003; International Agency for Research on Cancer [IARC], 2008). HPV-positive cancer in those organs including cervix uteri differs from HPV-negative one in molecular-genetic profile, morphology as well as in clinical peculiarities (Morrison et al., 2001; Gillison & Shah, 2003).

Carcinogenicity of the HR-HPV is determined by two viral genes, *E6* and *E7*. Their expression is recognized as a necessary condition for conversion of virus-infected cell from normal to malignant state. Viral oncoproteins E6 and E7 can interact with various cellular proteins and thus preclude their normal functioning. Among numerous activities of viral oncoproteins the following two are usually regarded as principal ones. E7 is capable of binding to retinoblastoma protein pRb, and E6 can interact with p53. Therefore both above mentioned tumor suppressors become inactivated and then degraded. Cellular functions such as proliferation, apoptosis, DNA repair etc., controlled by pRb and p53, become disturbed (zur Hauzen, 2000, 2008; IARC, 2008).

Since CC is a frequent female malignancy many research groups were occupied in search of early diagnostic markers for this cancer type. Experience thus obtained extends usually to HPV-associated carcinomas of other organs after necessary validation. Attempts to detect HR-HPV DNA by PCR did not leads in those studies to designing of a reliable diagnostic test because cancer *in situ* and invasive CC developed in a small proportion of women with HR-HPV-positive dysplasia (zur Hauzen, 2000). So specificity of the given approach turned out to be low despite the known very high PCR sensitivity. Current attempts to improve early diagnostics of CC and some other HPV-associated cancers are mostly focused on search of genes in virus-infected host cell whose expression becomes unconvertably altered under the influence of viral oncoproteins (Santin et al., 2005).

One of these genes is *INK4a* encoding $p16^{INK4a}$ protein, an inhibitor of cyclin D-dependent kinases Cdk 4/6 (Serrano et al., 1993). *INK4a* transcription in displastic and cancer cells becomes much more active in comparison with its level in normal epithelium being triggered by HR-HPV oncoprotein E7; the content of $p16^{INK4a}$ in a cell increases correspondingly (Li et al., 1994; Khleif et al., 1996; Sano et al., 1998; Kaneko et al., 1999; Klaes et al., 2001). This phenomenon formed experimental grounds for the immunohistochemical test which is currently widely applied in early CC diagnostics (Klaes et al., 2001, 2002; Milde-Langosch et al., 2001; Volgareva et al., 2002, 2004, 2006). This test is becoming popular in diagnostics of HR-HPV-associated carcinomas of other localizations (Begum et al., 2007; Kim et al., 2007).

Bladder cancer (BC) takes 7-th place in the global cancer incidence making up ~ 2-5% of all neoplasms. BC is 2.5-6 times more frequent in men than in women: 260000 new BC cases are registered annually among men and only 76000 among women. Bladder tumors are rare in people under 35 years old; however BC has become younger recently (Parkin et al., 2003). It seems reasonable to mention in this connection the data of Scandinavian investigators (Litlekalsoy et al., 2007) concerning dynamics of the BC molecular markers. They reported that significant shift in the BC molecular profile occurred during 70 years. This shift possibly reflects some alterations in the set of BC causative factors which might have taken place during these years.

In Russia BC makes up ~ 3 % of all malignant tumors; the trend has been registered for the steady elevation of new cases number (Chissov et al., 2010). Mortality among male BC patients in Russia is higher (> 7 in many regions) than the highest indices for countries from the WHO mortality list; as to female BC patiens, mortality figures do not differ in this group from those in other European countries (Zaridze, 2009).

BC development is a multistage process with unpredictable course. Several risk factors for BC are known (Zaridze et al., 1992; Dinney et al., 2004). Among these factors are: geographic region (BC morbidity may vary worldwide up to tenfold); professional occupation (there are about 40 professions at high risk); smoking; nutritional habits and drinking water quality; use of certain medicines; parasitic diseases caused by some Trematoda (Schistosomas). Possible significance of some other factors is still under discussion including irradiation, hereditary predisposition, some other.

Association of some biological agents with BC development might be suggested from results of one study in ~ 6000 patients cohort (Adami et al., 2003). Various organs had been transplanted to those patients with consequent immunosuppressor treatment. BC incidence in this group turned out to be 2-4 times higher as compared with corresponding index for the population as a whole. Carcinomas with proven causative role of HPV occurred in this group of patients even more frequently. Thus prevalence of vulvar and vaginal cancer was 20 times higher than expected one, and that for rectal and oropharyngeal cancer - 10 and 5 times higher, respectively.

The problem of HPV involvement in urinary bladder carcinogenesis is not novel. Historically one of the first indications to the possible linkage between these viruses and BC was the fact that secondary BC occurrence in women with primary CC was significantly higher (five to six-fold) than its occurrence in general population (Bailar, 1963; Newell et al., 1974, 1975). The interpretation of that data in favor of real HPV involvement in urothelial carcinogenesis became possible later after the discovery of HR-HPV carcinogenicity for cervical epithelium by H. zur Hausen and co-authors (Durst et al., 1983, zur Hauzen, 2000, 2008). However definitive commentary on those results as proving HPV carcinogenicity for urinary bladder is still difficult due to the known fact that both CC and BC are more frequent among smoking women.

One more evidence in favour of HPV involvement into BC development was obtained in observations carried out on immunodeficient patients with benign or malignant bladder

neoplasms where HPV DNA was found (Del Mistro et al., 1988; Kitamura et al, 1988; Querci della Rovere et al., 1988; Maloney et al., 1994).
The International Expert Group on HPV selected over twenty studies dedicated to HPV role in BC which had been published in 1991-2001 worldwide. The authors had detected HPV DNA in BC specimens by PCR, *in situ* hybridization and/or Southern blot hybridization. Percentage of HPV-positive cases in these communications varied from 0 up to 82.6 %. Therefore the experts included BC into the category of cancers for which aetiological role of HPV remains unclear - "inadequate evidence" (IARC, 2008).

2. The recent data warn against HPV underestimation as a risk factor in urinary bladder carcinogenesis

Several researchers have published recently some data proving topicality of the HPV problem in BC aetiology (Barghi et al., 2005; Yang et al., 2005; Helal Tel et al., 2006; Moonen et al., 2007; Badawi et al., 2008).
Thus ~ 36 % of transitional-cell BC specimens from Iran (21 out of 59 studied) harboured HPV DNA (Barghi et al., 2005). HPV 18 predominated over other types of the viruses (it was found in 17 patients out of 21, - 81 %); - viruses of the given type are second most frequent causative agents for CC (the first place belongs to HPV16). Urinary bladder tissues from 20 non-oncological patients were taken for control in this study and HPV18 DNA was detected in 1 patient with heavy cystitis. Possibility of precancerous alterations in the latter case could not be ruled out. The authors concluded that HPV may play role of a causative BC factor.
Similar was the opinion by the researchers from the Netherlands who carried out study of BC specimens from 107 patients and found DNA of various HPV types in ~ 15 %; HR-HPV DNA was detected in ~ 8 % (Moonen et al., 2007). Percentage of HR-HPV DNA-positive specimens increased with progression of clinical stage of BC (Ta, T1 and T2-T4), making 0, 12.5 and 18.2 % respectively
Group of investigators from Egypt and USA presented data on HPV-positivity of 27 Schistosoma-associated BC cases (Yang et al., 2005). All of them harboured HPV16. Highly sensitive variety of PCR was used in the study. The results reported by another group from Egypt (Helal Tel et al., 2006) differ dramatically from the data of H. Yang et al. These authors found HPV 16/18 DNA in a single Schistosoma-associated BC specimen (squamous cancer *in situ*) out of 64 studied. Much lower sensitivity of *in situ* hybridization used in the last study for HPV DNA detection in comparison with the method used by H. Yang et al. may be responsible for such a sharp data discrepancy. The total sum of BC specimens examined by A. Helal Tel et al. was 114 including 67 transitional-cell, 32 squamous and 15 other. The above mentioned case was the only HPV-positive BC in this study. The results obtained enabled the authors to conclude that HPV do not play any significant role in pathogenesis of urinary bladder in Egypt.
The data reported by these two research groups, H. Yang et al. and A. Helal Tel et al. and mutually exclusive inferences made by the investigators warn against underestimation of HPV as a risk factor in BC genesis. Essential in this connection is the fact that results reported by H. Yang et al. were confirmed recently by another research group from Egypt (Badawi et al., 2008). The authors using PCR detected HR-HPV DNA (belonging to types 16,18 and 52) more frequently in BC specimens than in urothelial biopsies from cystitis patients. The PCR data were compared with the data on antibody to HPV16 protein L1

detection in blood serum of the HPV16-positive BC patients; perfect coincidence of these results took place. The association was observed in this study between HPV-positivity of BC and its propensity for relapse. The authors concluded that HPV participates in BC genesis in combination with other risk factors, including Schistosomas which were commonly found in the group of patients examined. The authors recommend detection of antibodies to HPV L1 to optimize the treatment of BC patients and their further follow-up .

3. Aspects of the problem to be addressed

Thus a glimpse into the problem of HPV role in BC gives idea of its complexity. Therefore we rise the following questions:

1. What reasons may be the for conflicting data communicated by different research groups? Are there any ways to optimize the methodology of the study and get uniform data?
2. What is the incidence of HPV-positivity among urothelial dysplasia and BC specimens obtained from Russian patients keeping in mind ethno-geographic BC heterogeneity?
3. Have there been any attempts to investigate the role of papillomaviruses in urothelial carcinogenesis in experimental models?
4. What benefits may it bring to practical oncourology provided that a certain role of HPV in BC is accepted by medical community?

4. What reasons may be for conflicting data communicated by different research groups? Are there any ways to optimize the methodology of the study and get uniform data?

The authors usually explain the conflicting data character by different research groups by either of the following factors:

1. objective ethno-geographic heterogeneity of BC and
2. technical peculiarities of studies.

Concerning the first factor, a relationship seems to be evident between the state of the excretory organ lining, on the one hand, and environmental factors such as drinking water quality, regional and ethnic specificity of food, endemic urinary bladder parasitic diseases, etc., on the other hand. Each of these factors may influence the HPV-BC association rate. This statement could be verified by comparison of HPV-positivity in BC from different regions worldwide done by the same research group with unified technical approaches. Such studies have never been carried out as far as we know .

The second group of factors includes small numbers of specimens tested in some works; application of a single test for viral DNA detection (most commonly PCR or *in situ* hybridization, wherein both techniques have benefits and limitations); detection of only one or two HPV types, usually HPV16 and HPV18, which are most frequent in CC, while other HPV types might be involved in carcinogenesis in urinary bladder. The data by C. De Gaetani et al. prove the latter point (De Gaetani et al., 1999). Using *in situ* hybridization with probe to 31/33/35 viral types the authors detected HPV DNA positivity in 60 % of BC specimens, while the index turned out to be 24 % with probe to the types 16/18 .

In addition, a predominant majority of groups which publish data on high incidence of HR-HPV DNA in BC made no attempts to confirm viral genome expression and in particular *E6/ E7* expression.

Contamination should be mentioned also besides the above-listed factors. It may be either laboratory (admixing of products of viral genome amplification to the samples under study) or patient related. The former is a well-known source of false-positivity of PCR data. Possibility of the latter is to be kept in mind in studies of BC specimens particularly. If any adjacent organ (vulva, penis, urethra) is HPV-infected, casual bladder contamination with HPV-harbouring cell(s) might occur through blood during surgical operation or by endoscope during cystoscopy. False HPV-positivity data may occur both in PCR done to screen materials for viral DNA presence and in reverse-transcription PCR (RT-PCR) study of viral genome expression as well.

Thereby complex approach seems to be reasonable to study possible HPV role in urothelial carcinogenesis. Techniques are reasonable which enable to detect DNA not only of HPV16 and HPV18 but of other types of viruses as well. To check up whether viral oncogenes *E6* and *E7* are expressed in DNA-HPV-positive specimens methods seem to be appropriate of both viral mRNA *E6/E7* detection (by RT-PCR) and viral oncoproteins E6 and E7 revelation (by immunohistochemistry). In female BC cases it may be reasonable to examine patient's cervical epithelium for HPV infection.

5. What is the incidence of HPV-positivity among urothelial dysplasia and BC specimens obtained from Russian patients?

The given section presents data of two independent studies of Russian patients with urinary bladder oncological conditions including results of our own complex approach to HPV detection in BC specimens.

5.1 Attempts to determine occurrence of HPV-positivity in bladder urothelium

DNA of HPV16 and HPV18 was found in ~ 50 % of urinary bladder dysplasia and carcinoma in situ specimens by in situ hybridization; an attempt to detect HPV of other types (6, 11, 31, 33 and 51) gave negative results (Frank et al., 2002).

We have screened 130 transitional BC specimens (1-3 grade) obtained by transurethral resections for HPV DNA using several PCR versions with primers to *L1, E6* and *E7* genes of the viral genome (Volgareva et al., 2007, 2008, 2009; Trofimova et al., 2009). Our tests included application of literary primers My09/11 and GP5-GP6 to *L1* enabling one to detect HPV of various types; these primer sets are commonly used in similar studies (Resnik et al., 1990; van den Brule et al., 1990). HPV16 genetic material was found in ~ 40% of the specimens tested, DNA of other HPV types was not found. Viral genome expression was confirmed at the level of mRNA by RT-PCR in some of the specimens (Volgareva et al., 2009; Trofimova et al., 2009). Viral oncoprotein E7 was spotted by immunohistochemistry in ~30% of DNA HPV16-positive cases (Cheng et al., 2009; Volgareva et al., 2009 a,b). BC specimens stained positively with polyclonal anti-E7 HPV16 serum (done by Fiedler et al., 2004) turned out to be positive also when stained by monoclonal antibodies to HPV16 E6 and E7 from Neodiagnostic (Cheng et al., 2009). Five examples of BC specimens' screening for HPV are presented in Table 1 and Figure 1.

The fact that HPV16 oncoprotein E7 is detected in ~30% of BC specimens means that HPV16 plays some role in urothelial carcinogenesis in Russian patients. However in case of urothelial malignization some deviations there seem to exist from the known role of these viruses in cervical carcinogenesis. Signs testifying to the truth of the given assumption are as follows.

Case No	DNA*	RNA**	Protein E7*** (type of staining)
1	-	not studied	-
2	+	+	+ (diffuse)
3	+	+	+ (diffuse)
4	+	-	+ (focal)
5	+	-	+ (focal)

* HPV DNA was detected by PCR, viral typing carried out either by PCR with type-specific primers or by restriction fragment length polymorphism test (Astori et al.,1997). Specimens 2-5 appeared to harbour DNA of HPV16.

** reverse-transcription PCR was carried out with primers to *E6/E7* HPV16.

*** immunohistochemical staining was performed with polyclonal serum to HPV16 oncoprotein E7 (Fiedler et al., 2004). The type of staining was either diffuse (over 25% of stained cells in a cancer tissue) or focal (less than 25% of stained cancer cells).

Table 1. Data of the complex approach to HPV detection in five BC specimens. Case 1: Transitional BC relapse, focuses of squamous metaplasia, 3-d grade, muscle-invasive. Case 2: Transitional BC, 3-d grade, muscle-invasive. Case 3: Transitional BC, 2-d grade, submucosal invasion, no muscle cells on the slide. Case 4: Transitional BC, focuses of squamous metaplasia, 2-3-d grade, growth within mucous layer, no invasion into muscle. Case 5. Transitional BC, 3-d grade, submucosal invasion, no muscle cells on the slide.

Firstly, along with BC specimens expressing viral oncoprotein E7 in a predominant majority of cancer cells throughout cancer tissue (as was usually the case with CC in our previous studies, - the so-called "diffuse staining"; - Volgareva et al., 2006) we observed some BC cases in which E7 was registered only in certain groups of cancer cells or in separate cells, - the so-called "focal staining" (Table 1, cases 4 and 5; Fig. 1d,e). It should be underlined in this connection that we confirmed HPV16 genome expression at the level of mRNA by RT-PCR for some of such BC specimens. However it was not in every BC specimen studied that the results of RT-PCR and immunohistochemistry coincided: cases 4 and 5 in Table 1 serve as examples of the lack of the data homogeneity. Focal character of HPV16 genome expression registered immunohistochemically may perhaps be responsible for this discrepancy: HPV16-harbouring cells detected by staining in a certain section of a BC specimen might not occur in another section of the same specimen from which mRNA was obtained. It is also important that in all such specimens HPV16 E7-expressing cells were found in the internal layers of cancer tissue but not at its brims (Fig. 1d,e). This observation enables one to rule out the above-mentioned possibility of the urinary bladder intrapatient contamination with cells of some adjacent HPV-infected organ. Focal HPV16 E7 expression in some BC specimens in our study is in a good agreement with the data by C. De Gaetani et al. on HPV DNA detection in BC by *in situ* hybridization (De Gaetani et al., 1999). These investigators had at their disposal several biopsy samples for each of ten patients under study. It was from only one out of ten patients that the test results were permanently positive in all biopsies, while in the rest nine cases only a quota of samples was DNA HPV-positive.

Secondly, in some cases of focal E7 expression BC cells contain this viral oncoprotein only in a cytoplasm (Fig 1e). Its ability to get bound to the nuclear pRb remains under question in such cases.

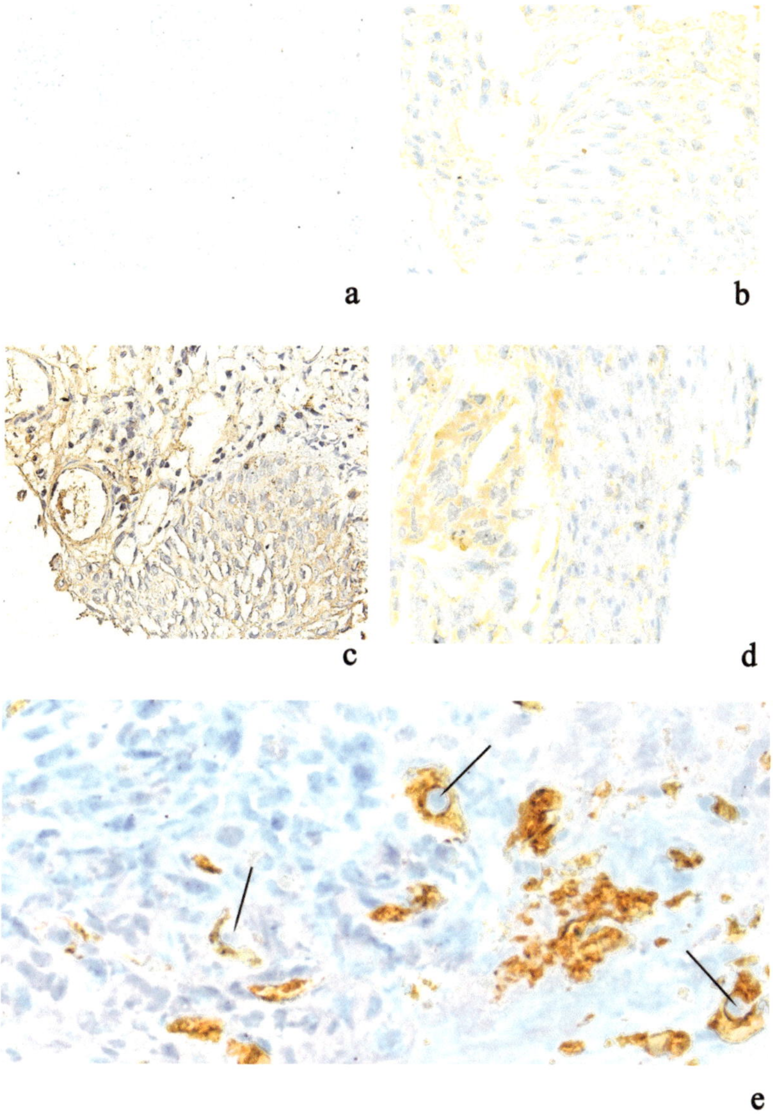

Fig. 1. Results of the HPV16 E7 immunohistochemical detection in BC specimens. Specimens' numbers match to those in Table 1. a Negative reaction with E7-specific serum in specimen N1. b, c Diffuse staining of specimens NN 2 and 3, respectively. d, e Focal staining of specimens NN 4 and 5, respectively. Uncoloured nuclei of three cells expressing E7 in a cytoplasm are indicated with arrows in "e".

Thirdly, the results of our repeated examination of the female patient with relapsing BC turned out to be quite unexpected. In her original tumor removed surgically in 2004 we detected HPV16 DNA, *E7* mRNA as well as protein E7 (the latter spotted independently in two laboratories with different antibodies) (Volgareva et al., 2009 b; Cheng et al., 2009). The patient is a hard smoker. For more than 20 years she had worked at a chemical factory and had been exposed with solvents and aniline dyes. Three BC relapses took place in 2005-2008.

During this period the patient undervent surgery, chemotherapy and BCG treatment. At the next relapse in 2009 we performed repeated study. Neither HPV DNA nor protein E7 were found in BC cells. Colposcopy study was also performed and HPV DNA tested in cervical cells by PCR; the results of both analyses proved absence of HPV in cervical epithelium of the patient (Volgareva et al., 2010a). Could there occur a total clearance from virus-harbouring cells due to surgical and other treatments in this patient? Further observations on similar cases are desirable to answer in the affirmative.

5.2. Study of *INK4a* expression in DNA HPV16-positive bladder cancer specimens

To verify the fact of HPV16 genome expression in 50 DNA HPV16-positive BC specimens we studied cellular *INK4a* expression at the levels of mRNA (Fig. 2) and respective protein $p16^{INK4a}$ (Fig. 3) (Volgareva et al., 2010b). The above mentioned phenomenon of the *INK4a* overexpression indicating to HR-HPV E7 activity in cervical cells served as a rationale. In 12 BC specimens under study the HPV16 *E7* expression had been detected at the mRNA and/or protein level. Five conditionally normal urothelial specimens obtained from the same BC patients were studied as well. In some BC cases associated with HPV16 DNA we detected *INK4a* overexpression at the both levels (Fig. 2, patients A,B and E; Fig. 3c).

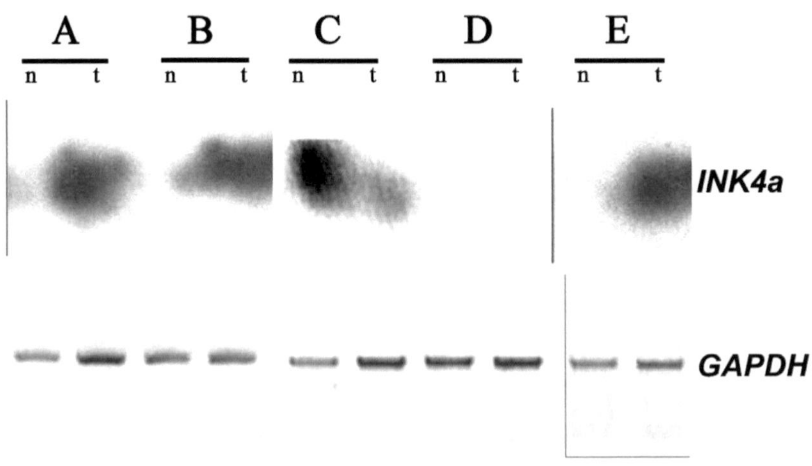

Fig. 2. Analysis of expression of *INK4a* by RT-PCR in BC specimens obtained from five patients (A, B, C, D and E); t - urinary bladder carcinoma, n – morphologically normal tissue adjacent to tumour.
The top-panel electrophoregram developed after Southern blot hybridization with the *INK4a*-specific radio-active probe according to Nguyen and co-authors (Nguyen et al., 2000).
The bottom panel: results with *GAPDH*-specific primers as a control for stability and concentration of RNA; amplification products visualized by staining with ethidium bromide.

Incidence of $p16^{INK4a}$- overexpressing BC specimens was ~ 10% (Fig. 3c), however as opposed to CC in BC it did not correlate with HPV16 E7 expression in any case (Figures 2c and 3d present lack of such correlation for one and the same BC specimen).

We don't regard this result as evidence disproving the role of HPV in urinary bladder carcinogenesis. The point is, according to literature data, that factors determining *INK4a* expression in HPV-associated BC may differ in essence from those in HPV-positive CC. Thus in BC, in contrast to CC, *INK4a* undergoes frequent deletions, point mutations or promoter methylations (Ruas, Peters, 1998; Aveyard, Knowles, 2004; Gallucci et al., 2007). Due to any of these events its expression at the level of protein $p16^{INK4a}$ may become partly or fully lost. For example, homozygous *INK4a* deletions depriving cell of $p16^{INK4a}$ synthesis were found in ~ 30-50 % of BC specimens (Aveyard, Knowles, 2004; Gallucci et al., 2007). Thus our data might prove unsuitability of $p16^{INK4a}$ for role of the HPV-associated BC marker.

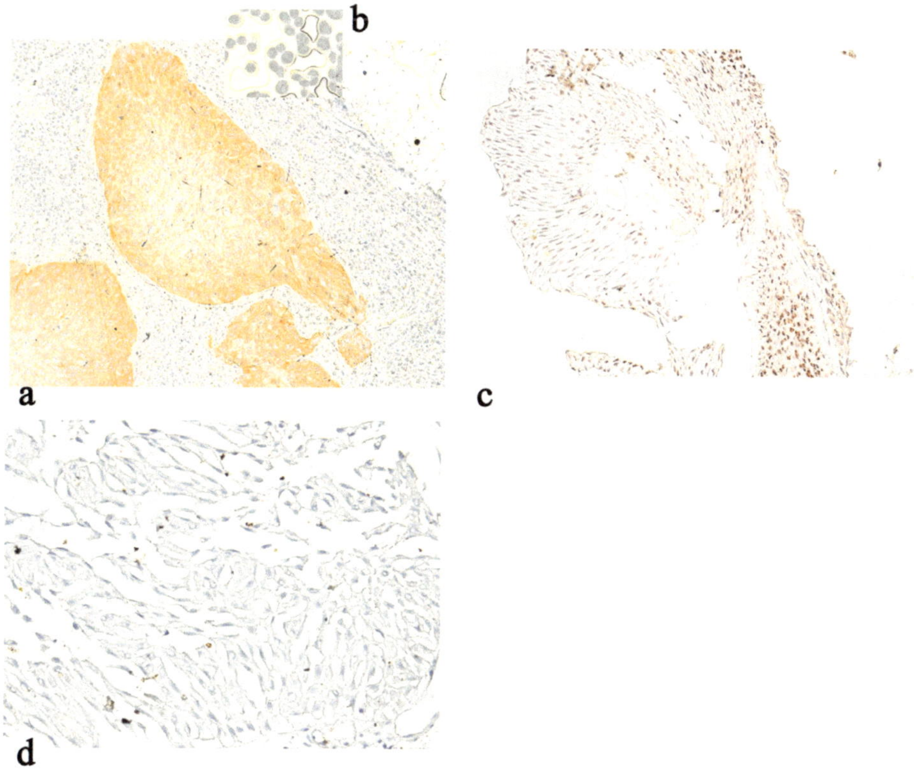

Fig. 3. Results of the immunohistochemical $p16^{INK4a}$ detection in BC specimens.
a. Positive control: HPV16 - harbouring cervical cancer, diffuse staining.
b. Negative control: cells of HCT line (smear), negative reaction with $p16^{INK4a}$-specific antibodies.
c. BC, diffuse staining.
d. BC specimen represented as N3 in Table 1 and "c" in Fig. 1, negative reaction with $p16^{INK4a}$-specific antibodies.

5.3 Summary

The results obtained in two independent samplings of urothelial dysplasia and BC from Russian patients show as a whole that HR-HPV DNA-positivity reaches up to ~ 40-50 %.

Presence of viral DNA in cancer cells is frequently accompanied by expression of viral oncogenes. These results are in agreement with the notion that HR-HPV may take part in BC initiation either solely or in combination with other factors, in particular chemical carcinogens. There are certain reasons still to assume some difference in the action of these viruses in urothelium in comparison with their manifestation in cervical epithelium.

6. Have there been any attempts to investigate the role of papillomaviruses in urothelial carcinogenesis in experimental models?

Urinary bladder similarly to other parts of urinary system (renal pelvis, ureter, etc.) is lined with epithelium of a special kind, the so-called transitional epithelium (Henle epithelium). The question is of particular interest in this connection whether HPV can cause oncogenesis in urinary bladder lining.

M. Campo and co-authors addressed this problem in vivo in cattle (Campo et al., 1992; Campo, 2002). The investigators demonstrated that bovine papillomavirus BPV-2 takes part in BC development under both spontaneous and experimental infection. An important peculiarity of their model is that BPV-associated BC develops commonly in animals being fed with a certain kind of plant, namely bracken fern. Besides BC these animals are affected often with carcinomas in various segments of gastrointestinal tract. When studied particularly bracken fern appeared to contain a number of ingredients which possess mutagenic, carcinogenic and immunosuppressive activities.

The thesis of a species-specific character of papillomavirus infection is well-known (IARC, 2008). In view of this point an exact extrapolation of the data by M. Campo et al. to human papillomaviruses and their possible role in human urothelial oncogenesis seems not quite correct. There are yet some indirect evidences that such extrapolation is not fully groundless. They are as follows. First of all, these researchers found among various histological BC types substantial quota of transitional carcinomas, the type of BC predominating among human patients in many countries including Russia. Secondly, bracken fern similarly to cattle promotes in a human organism carcinogenesis just in gastrointestinal tract. In the regions where it is consumed as food (Brazil in particular) HPV16 is commonly found in dysplasia and carcinoma specimens of esophagus (Campo et al., 1999, as cited in Campo, 2002). Thirdly, transactivation of HPV16 promoter was achieved in experimental model by quercetine, one of the mutagenic ingredients of bracken fern; in such a way it was demonstrated that some types of human cancer in which HPV are being regularly detected may be aetiologically similar to corresponding cancer types of cattle (Campo et al., 1999, as cited in Campo, 2002).

C. Reznikoff and co-authors carried out study on HPV oncogenicity in human urothelial cells in vitro (Reznikoff et al., 1994). The authors transformed isogenic mucosal cells of ureteral uroepithelium obtained from a healthy donor by HPV16 *E6* and/or *E7* gene(s). Cellular immortalization occurred after the integration of either of these viral oncogenes into host chromosomes. Simultaneous integration of both of them led to similar effect. Phenotypic and genotypic alterations were more prominent in cells immortalized by *E6* alone or in combination with *E7* than in cells harbouring sole *E7*. Neither of the transformed cell clones formed tumors when inoculated into nude mice. Some chromosomal alterations found in the transformed cells were identical to karyotype abnormalities found by other researchers in clinical specimens from BC patients. The authors inferred that the phenomena taking place in vitro may correspond to initial stages of urothelial oncogenesis in vivo.

Thus the results obtained in experimental models show that there is no good cause to eliminate papillomaviruses from the list of potential carcinogens in urinary bladder urothelium of Homo sapiens.

7. What benefits may it bring to practical oncourology provided that a certain role of HPV in BC is accepted by medical community?

If this notion is accepted new prospects for BC prevention may come to light. Keeping in mind that efficient vaccines were designed for CC prevention, on the one hand, and that BC is a predominantly male type of cancer, on the other hand, both girls and boys vaccination might become one of such prospects. It is noteworthy in this connection that when the item of reasonability of boys' vaccination is being discussed it is usually being done for the sake of CC prevention in their wives-to-be. Resolution is usually made in the negative in resource-constrained countries. As to the female BC, possibility to prevent women from urothelial carcinogenesis might become an additional convincing argument in favour of their vaccination.

Possible ways of HPV ingress into human urinary bladder lining should be thought over by both clinicians and experimenters. The idea of HPV-associated BC may form grounds for adding of some tests (aimed to detect anogenital HPV) to the currently accepted ways of preoperative check-up of BC patients. This idea may also become the reason to reconsider safety of cystoscope and catheter in treatment of BC patients infected with HPV in anogenital region.

Despite that HPV role in urothelial carcinogenesis is still open-ended question several research groups tried to find an answer to the related one: whether clinical course of BC is affected by HPV presence in urothelial cells.

Y. Andreeva and co-authors studied if papillomaviruses influence relapse incidence in BC patients (Andreeva et al., 2008). The authors preselected 44 BC specimens taken from patients with superficial tumors (stages Ta and T1) on the basis that there occurred koilocytes in these specimens (an indirect morphological sign of viral infection). The specimens were then subdivided into 3 groups: (1) 16 ones from patients with high relapse incidence, (2) 13 - from patients with moderate and (3) 15 - from patients with low relapse incidence. DNA of HPV16 and HPV18 was found by *in situ* hybridization in specimens from patients of the first and second groups only. Seven out of 16 specimens (44%) harboured HPV16 DNA in the first group. Three specimens (23%) were HPV18-positive while HPV16 genetic material was found in neither case in the second group. The authors concluded that HPV occurrence in urothelial cells increases the risk of a superficial BC relapse.

A. Lopes-Beltran and co-authors studied whether HPV DNA presence in cancer cells may influence BC patient survival (Lopes-Beltran et al., 1996). The group of 76 BC patients with transitional BC was formed without any preselection. In materials obtained at transurethral resections the authors detected DNA of HPV6, HPV11, HPV16 and HPV18 using PCR. Follow-up lasted for 5 years. The resultant survival among HPV-positive patients was found to be ~ 29 % (2 out of 7), while among negative ones - 75 % (52 out of 69). The authors concluded that HPV-DNA-positivity serves as a negative predictor of BC patient survival.

The results reported by C. De Gaetani and co-authors (De Gaetani et al., 1999) are in good agreement with those data. The authors found by *in situ* hybridization with the probes to viral types 16/18 and 31/33/35 HPV DNA in 17 out of 43 BC specimens. Follow-up lasted for 72 months. During this time 10 HPV-positive patients died (~59%). Meanwhile 5 out of 26 HPV-negative patients died (~20%).

If HPV contribution to urinary bladder carcinogenesis gains recognition current therapeutic methods might be supplemented in the near future with the administration to the bladder of HPV-positive BC patients of low molecular weight chemical substances inhibiting HPV oncogenes expression. Results of successful studies of such substances in experimental models were presented at the 25-th International papillomavirus conference (Hellner et al., 2009).

8. Conclusion

The problem of HPV involvement in urinary bladder carcinogenesis is still open. In a complex study performed on clinical specimens of dysplasia and carcinoma of urinary bladder from Russian patients with the use of several methods of HPV DNA detection (*in situ* hybridization, PCR with several types of primers) we registered up to 40-50 % of DNA HPV-positive cases. In many cases DNA HPV-positivity was accompanied with expression of viral oncogenes *E6* and *E7* at the levels of mRNA and/or protein. Thus we detected oncoprotein E7 HPV16 known for its ability to interfere with the normal pRb functioning (which leads to unchecked transition of a cell from G1 to S stage of the cell cycle) in every third BC specimen harbouring HPV16 DNA. Results reported by other research groups obtained both in clinical materials and in experimental models *in vivo* and *in vitro* confirm the idea of HPV as a possible causative agent of BC. There are certain signs that role of HPV in urinary bladder carcinogenesis may be somewhat different from their role in CC origination. Their most probable role in urothelial carcinogenesis seems to be partnership in initiation of the process jointly with other agents (such as parasitic helminths, components of cigarette smoke, chemical pollutants of industrial origin, etc.). The notion that HPV in some cases takes part in urinary bladder carcinogenesis may be helpful for BC prevention, prediction of its clinical course and, in prospect, for treatment of HPV-associated BC.

9. Acknowledgements

The authors are grateful to professors V.A. Kobliakov, B.P. Kopnin, B.P. Matveev and A.A. Shtil' for promoting discussions and critical reading of the manuscript and to Dr. V.A. Glazunova for patient assistance in technical work on the manuscript.

10. References

Adami, J., Gabel, H., Lindelof, B., Ekstrom, K., Rydh, B., Glimelius, B., Ekbom, A., Adami, H.O., & Granath, F. (2003). Cancer risk following organ transplantation: a nationwide cohort study in Sweden. *Br. J. Cancer*, Vol. 89, No 7, pp. 1221-1227.

Andreeva, Y.Y., Zavalishina, L.D., Morozov, A.A., Rusakov, I.G., & Frank, G.A. (2008). Localization of HPV DNA in superficial urothelial bladder carcinoma. *Oncourology*, No 1, pp. 34-35, ISSN 1726-9776. (In Russian).

Astori, G., Arzese, A., Pipan, C., de Villiers, E.-M.,& Botta, G.A. (1997). Characterization of a putative new HPV genomic sequence from a cervical lesion using L1 consensus primers and restriction fragment length polymorphism. *Virus Res.*, Vol. 50, No 1, pp. 57-63.

Aveyard, J.S., & Knowles, M.A. (2004). Measurement of relative copy number of CDKN2A/ARF and CDKN2B in bladder cancer by real-time quantitative PCR and multiplex ligation-dependent probe amplification. *J. Mol. Diagnostics,* Vol. 6, No 4, pp. 356-364.

Badawi, H., Ahmed, H., Ismail, A., Diab, M, Moubarak, M, Badawy, A, & Saber, M. (2008). Role of human papillomavirus types 16, 18 and 52 in recurrent cystitis and urinary bladder cancer among Egyptian patients. *Medscape J Med.,* Vol.10 (10), p. 232. Retrieved from: http://www.ncbi.nlm.nih.gov/pmc/articles/PMC2605136/.

Bailar, J.C. (1963). The incidence of independent tumors among uterine cancer patients. *Cancer,* Vol. 16 (Jul.), pp. 842-853.

Barghi, M.R., Hajimohammadmehdiarbab, A., Moghaddam, S.M., & Kazemi B. (2005). Correlation between human papillomavirus infection and bladder transitional cell carcinoma. *BMC Infect. Dis.,* Vol. 5: 102. Retrieved from: http://www.biomedcentral.com/1471-2334/5/102

Begum, S., Gillison, M.L., Nikol, T.L., & Westra W.H. (2007). Detection of human papillomavirus-16 in fine-needle aspirates to determine tumor origin in patients with metastatic squamous cell carcinoma of the head and neck. *Clin Cancer Res.* , Vol. 13, No 4, pp. 1186-1191.

Campo, M.S. (2002). Animal models of papillomavirus pathogenesis. *Virus Res.*, Vol. 89, No 2, pp. 249-261.

Campo, M.S., Jarrett, W.F., Barron, R., O'Neil, B.W., & Smith, K.T. (1992). Association of bovine papillomavirus type 2 and braken fern with bladder cancer in cattle. *Cancer Res.*, Vol. 52, No 24, pp. 6898-6904.

Cheng, S., Hsiao, L., Jung, S., & Volgareva, G.M. (2009). Detection of HPV E6 and E7 oncoproteins in bladder cancers. *Proceedings of the 25-th International Papillomavirus Conference,* Malmo, Sweden, May 2009, P-14.09.

Chissov, V.I, Starinsky, V.V., Petrova, G.V. (Eds.). (2010). *Malignant malformations in Russia (morbidity and mortality).,* P.A. Hertzen Moscow Research Oncological Institute. ISBN 5-85502-024-X, Moscow. (In Russian).

De Gaetani, C., Ferrari, G., Righi, E., Bettelli, S., Migaldi, M., Ferrari, P., & Trentini, G.P. (1999). Detection of human papillomavirus DNA in urinary bladder carcinoma by in situ hybridization. *J. Clin. Pathol.*, Vol. 52, No 2, pp. 103-106.

Del Mistro, A., Koss, L.G., Braunstein, J., Bennett, B., Saccomano, G., & Simons, K.M. (1988). Condyloma acuminata of the urinary bladder. Natural history, viral typing, and DNA content. *Am J Surg Path.*, Vol. 12, No 3, pp.205-212.

Dinney, C.P.N., McConcey, D.J., Millikan, R.E, Wu, X., Bar-Eli, M., Adam, L., Kamat, A.M., SiefkerRadtke, A.O., Tuziak, T., Sabichi, A.L., Grossman, H.B., Benedict, W.F., & Czerniak, B. (2004). Focus on bladder cancer. *Cancer Cell,* Vol.6, No 2, pp.111-116.

Durst, M., Gissmann, L., Ikenberg, H., & zur Hauzen, H. (1983). A papillomavirus DNA from a cervical carcinoma and its prevalence in cancer biopsy samples from different geographic regions. *Proc. Natl Acad. Sci USA*, Vol.80, No 12, pp. 3812-3815.

Fiedler, M., Muller-Holzner, E., Viertler, H.-P., Widschwendter, A., Laich, A., Pfister, G., Spoden, G.A., Jansen-Dürr, P., & Zwerschke, W. (2004). High level HPV-16 E7 oncoprotein expression correlates with reduced pRb-levels in cervical biopsies. *The FASEB Journal*, Vol. 18, No 10; pp 1120-1122. Retrieved from: http://www.fasebj.org/content/early/2004/06/29/fj.03-1332fje.long

Frank, G.A., Zavalishina, L.E., & Andreeva, Iu.Iu. (2002). Immunohistochemical characteristics and a degree of differentiation of urinary bladder cancer. *Arkhiv Patologii*, Vol. 64, No 6, pp. 16-18, ISSN 0004-1955. (In Russian).

Gallucci, M., Vico, E., Merola, R., Leonardo, C, Sperduti, I, Felici, A, Sentinelli, S, Cantiani, R, Orlandi, G, & Cianciulli, A. (2007). Adverse genetic prognostic profiles define a poor outcome for cystectomy in bladder cancer. *Exp. Mol. Pathol.*, Vol. 83, No 3, pp. 385-391.

Gillison, M.L., & Shah, K.V. (2003). Role of mucosal human papillomavirus in nongenital cancers. *J. Natl Cancer Inst. Monographs*, No 31, pp. 57-65.

Helal Tel, A., Fadel, M.T., & El-Sayed, N.K. Human papilloma virus and p53 expression in bladder cancer in Egypt: correlation to schistosomiasis and clinicopathologic factors. (2006). *Pathol. Oncol. Res.*, Vol. 12, No 3, pp. 173-178.

Hellner, K., Baldwin, A., Xian, J., Stein, R., Glicksman, M., & Munger, K. (2009). PAK3 inhibitors identified by high-throughput-screening as therapeutics for HPV-associated cancers. *Proceedings of the 25-th International Papillomavirus Conference*, Malmo, Sweden, May 2009, O-09.05.

IARC Monographs on the Evaluation of Carcinogenic Risks to Humans. Vol. 90. *Human Papillomaviruses*. ISBN 978-92-832-1290-4, Lyon, France, 2007. Retrieved from: http://monographs.iarc.fr/ENG/Monographs/vol90/index.php.

Kaneko, S., Nishioka, J., Tanaka, M., Nakashima, K., & Nobori, T. (1999). Transcriptional regulation of the CDK inhibitor p16^{INK4a} gene by a novel pRb-associated repressor, RBAR1. *Biochem Mol Biol Int*. Vol. 47, No 2, pp.205- 215.

Khleif, S.N., DeGregori, J., Yee, C., Otterson G.A., Kaye F.J., Nevins J.R., & Howley P.M. (1996). Inhibition of cyclin D-CDK4/CDK6 activity is associated with an E2F-mediated induction of cyclin kinase inhibitor activity. *Proc Natl Acad Sci USA*. Vol. 93., No 9, pp. 4350-4354.

Kim, S.H., Koo, B.S., Kang, S., Park, K., Kim, H., Lee, M.J., Kim J.M., Choi, E.C., & Cho, N.H. (2007). HPV integration begins in the tonsillar crypt and leads to the alteration of p16, EGFR and c-myc during tumor formation. *Int J Cancer*, Vol. 120, No 7, pp. 1418-1425.

Kitamura, T., Yogo, Y., Ueki, T., Murakami, S, & Aso, Y. (1988). Presence of human papillomavirus type 16 genome in bladder carcinoma in situ of a patient with mild immunodeficiency. *Cancer Res.*, Vol. 48, No 24, pt.1, pp.7207-7211.

Klaes, R., Friedrich, T., Spitkovsky, D., Ridder, R, Rudy, W., Petry, U., Dallenbach-Hellweg, G., Schmidt, D., & von Knebel Doeberitz, M. (2001). Overexpression of p16(INK4a)

as a specific marker for dysplastic and neoplastic epithelial cells of the cervix uteri. *Int J Cancer*. Vol. 92, No 2, pp. 276-284.

Klaes, R., Benner, A., Friedrich, T., Ridder, R., Herrington, S., Jenkins, D., Kurman, R.J., Shmidt, D., Stoler, M., & von Knebel Doeberitz, M. (2002). p16INK4a immunohistochemistry improves interobserver agreement in the diagnosis of cervical intraepithelial neoplasia. *Am J Surg Pathol.*, Vol. 26, No 11, pp. 1389-1399.

Li, Y., Nichols, M.A., Shay, J.W., & Xiong Y. (1994). Transcriptional repression of the D-type cyclin-dependent kinase inhibitor p16 by the retinoblastoma susceptibility gene product pRb. *Cancer Res.*, Vol. 54, No 23, pp. 6078-6082.

Litlekalsoy, J., Vatne, V., Hostmark, J.G., & Laerum, O.D. (2007). Immunohistochemical markers in urinary bladder carcinomas from paraffin-embedded archival tissue after storage for 5-70 years. *Br J Urol Int*, Vol. 99, No 5, pp. 1013-1119.

Lopes-Beltran, A., Escudero, A.L., Vicioso, L., Munoz, E., & Carrasco, J.C. (1996). Human papillomavirus DNA as a factor determining the survival of bladder cancer patients. *Br. J. Cancer*, Vol. 73, No 1, pp. 124-127.

Maloney, K.E., Wiener, J.S., & Walther, P.J. (1994). Oncogenic human papillomaviruses are rarely associated with squamous cell carcinoma of the bladder: evaluation by differential polymerase chain reaction. *J Urol.*, Vol.151, No 2, pp. 360-364.

Milde-Langosch, K., Riethdorf, S., Kraus-Poppinghaus, A., Riethdorf, L., & Loning, T. (2001). Expression of cyclin-dependent kinase inhibitors p16MTS1, p21WAF1, and p27KIP1 in HPV-positive and HPV-negative cervical adenocarcinomas. *Virchows Arch.*, Vol. 439, No 1, pp. 55-61.

Morrison, C., Catania, F., Wakely, P., Jr., & Nuovo, G.J. (2001) Highly differentiated keratinizing squamous cell cancer of the cervix. A rare, locally aggressive tumor not associated with human papillomavirus or squamous intraepithelial lesions. *Am J Surg Path*, Vol. 25, No 10, pp. 1310-1315.

Moonen, P.M., Bakkers, J.M., Kiemeney, L.A. Schalken, JA, Melchers, WJ, & Witjes JA. (2007). Human papilloma virus DNA and p53 mutation analysis on bladder washes in relation to clinical outcome of bladder cancer. *Eur. Urol.*, Vol. 52, No 2, pp. 468-469.

Newell, G.R., Rawlings, W., Krementz, E.T., & Roberts, J.D. (1974). Multiple primary neoplasms in blacks compared to whites. III. Initial cancers at the female breast and uterus. *J. Natl Cancer Inst.*, Vol. 53, No 2, pp. 369-373.

Newell, G.R., Krementz, E.T., & Roberts, J.D. (1975). Exess occurrence of cancer of the oral cavity, lung, and bladder following cancer of the cervix. *Cancer*, Vol. 36, No 6, pp.2155-2158.

Nguyen, T.T., Nguyen, C.T., Gonsales, F.A., Nichols, P.W., Yu, M.C., & Jones, P.A. (2000). Analysis of cyclin-dependent kinase inhibitor expression and methylation pattern in human prostate cancers. *Prostate*, Vol. 43, No 3, pp. 233-242.

Parkin, D.M., Whelean, S.L., & Ferlai, J. (2003), IARC Press, Lyon, France, No 155.

Querci della Rovere, G., Oliver, R.T., McCance, D.J., & Castro, J.E. (1988). Development of bladder tumor containing HPV type 11 DNA after renal transplantation. *Br J Urol.*, Vol. 62, No 1, pp. 36-38.

Resnick, R.M., Cornekissen, M.T.E., Wright, D.K., Eichinger, G.H., Fox, H.T., ter Schegget, J, & Manos, M. (1990). Detection and typing of human papillomavirus in archival cervical cancer specimens by DNA amplification with consensus primers. *J. Natl Cancer Inst.*, Vol. 82, No 18, pp. 1477-1484.

Reznikoff, C.A., Belair, C., Savelieva, E., Zhai Y., Pfeifer, K., Yeager, T., Thompson, K.J., DeVries, S., Bindley, C., Newton, M.A., Sekhon, G., & Waldman., F. (1994). Long-term genome stability and minimal genotypic and phenotypic alterations in HPV16 E7-, but not E6-, immortalized human uroepithelial cells. *Genes and Dev.*, Vol. 8, No 18, pp. 2227-2240.

Ruas, M., & Peters, G. (1998). The p16INK4a/CDKN2A tumor suppressor and its relatives. *Biochim Biophys Acta*, Vol. 1378, No 2, pp.115- 177.

Sano, T., Oyama, T., Kashiwabara, K., Fukuda, T., & Nakajima, T. (1998). Expression status of p16 protein is associated with human papillomavirus oncogenic potential in cervical and genital lesions. *Am J Pathol.*, Vol.153, No 6, pp.1741- 1748.

Santin, A.D., Zhan, F., Bignotti, E., Siegel, E.R., Cane, S., Bellone, S., Palmieri, M., Anfossi, S., Thomas, M., Burnett, A., Kay, H.H., Roman, J.J., O'Brieb, T.J., Tian, E., Cannon, M.J., Shaughnessy, J. Jr. & Pecorelli, S. (2005). Gene expression profiles of primary HPV16- and HPV18-infected early stage cervical cancers and normal cervical epithelium: identification of novel candidate molecular markers for cervical cancer diagnosis and therapy. *Virology*, Vol. 331, No 2, pp. 269-291.

Serrano, M., Hannon, G. J. & Beach, D. (1993). A new regulatory motif in cell-cycle control causing specific inhibition of cyclin D/CDK4. *Nature*, Vol. 366, No 6456, pp. 704-707.

Trofimova, O., Kuevda, D., Shipulina, O., & Volgareva, G. (2009). Development of HPV genotyping and expression methods and validation on group of urinary bladder cancer. *Proceedings of the 25-th International Papillomavirus Conference*, Malmo, Sweden, May 2009, P-29.58.

van den Brule, A.J.C., Snijders, P.J.F., Gordijn, R.I.J., Bleker, O.P., Meijer, C.J.L.M., & Walboomers, J.M.M. (1990). General primer-mediated polymerase chain reaction permits the detection of sequenced and still unsequenced human papillomavirus genotypes in cervical scrapes and carcinomas. *Int. J. Cancer*, Vol. 45, No 4, pp. 644-649.

Volgareva, G.M., Zavalishina, L.E., Frank, G.A., Andreeva, Yu.Yu., Petrov, A.N., Kisseljov, F.L., & Spitkovsky, D.D. (2002). Expression of protein marker $p16^{INK4a}$ in uterine cervical cancer. *Arkhiv Patologii*; Vol. 64, N1, pp. 22-24, ISSN 0004-1955. (In Russian).

Volgareva, G., Zavalishina, L., Andreeva, Y., Frank, G., Krutikova, E., Golovina, D.,Bliev, A., Spitkovsky, D., Ermilova, V., & Kisseljov, F. (2004). Protein p16 as a marker of dysplastic and neoplastic alterations in cervical epithelial cells. *BMC Cancer*, Aug 31;4:58. Retrieved from:
http://www.pubmedcentral.gov/articlerender.fcgi?tool=pubmed&pubmedid=15339339

Volgareva, G.M., Zavalishina, L.E., Golovina, D.A., Andreeva, Y.Y., Petrov, A.N., Bateva, M.V., Petrenko, A.A., Ermilova, V.D., Kisseljova, N.P., & Frank, G.A. (2006). The protein p16[INK4a] as a reliable indicator of the HPV-induced carcinogenesis, In: *New Research on Cervical Cancer* (Rolland GZ, ed.). Nova Science Publishers, ISBN 13 978-1-60021-300-7 ISBN 10 1-60021—300-6, New York. pp. 129-147.

Volgareva, G., Zavalishina, L., Golovina, D., Andreeva, Y.Y., Cheban, N.L., Ermilova, V.D., Petrov, A.N., Bateva, M.V., Matveev, V.B., Shtil, A.A., & Frank, G.A. (2007). In search of bladder cancer markers: are human papillomaviruses and cellular *INK4a* expression associated? In: *Tumor Markers Research Perspectives* (G.A. Sinise, ed.). Nova Science Publishers, ISBN: 1-60021-423-1,New York, pp. 135-143.

Volgareva, G.M., Kuevda, D.A., Zavalishina, L.E., Shipulina, O.Y.,Trofimova, O.B., Golovina, D.A., Andreeva, Y.Y., Ermilova, V.D., Cheban, N.L., Glazunova, V.A., Bateva, M.V., Petrov, A.N., Matveev, V.B., Shtil, A.A., & Frank, G.A. (2008). Human papillomaviruses: is bladder urothelium a target of their carcinogenic action? *Proceedings of the World Cancer Congress*, UICC, Geneva, Switzerland, August 2008, P216.

Volgareva, G., Trofimova, O., Kuevda, D., Zavalishina, L., Golovina, D., Andreeva, Y., Ermilova, V., Cheban, N., Glazunova, V., Matvejev, V., Shipulina, O., & Frank, G. (2009). HPV and urinary bladder cancer. *Proceedings of the 25-th International Papillomavirus Conference*, Malmo, Sweden, May 2009, P-18.42.

Volgareva, G.M., Zavalishina, L.D., Golovina, D.A., Andreeva, Iu.Iu., Ermilova, V.D., Cheban, N.L., Kuevda, D.A., Trofimova, O.B., Shipulina, O.Iu., Pavlova, L.S., Petrov, A.N., Matveev, V.B., Shtil', A.A., & Frank, G.A. (2009). Detection of oncoprotein E7 HPV16 in the cancer and normal urinary bladder urothelium. *Arkhiv Patologii*, Vol. 71, No 1, pp. 29-30, ISSN 0004-1955. (In Russian).

Volgareva, G.M., Zavalishina, L.É., Trofimova, O.B., Korolenkova, L.I., Khachaturian, A.V., Andreeva, Iu.Iu., Ermilova, V.D., Cheban, N.L., Kuevda, D.A., Shipulina, O.Iu., Glazunova, V.A., Golovina, D.A., Petrov, A.N., Matveev, V.B., & Frank, G.A. (2010a). Are human papillomaviruses responsible for the occurrence of bladder cancer? *Arkhiv Patologii*, Vol.72, No 4, pp. 24-27, ISSN 0004-1955. (In Russian).

Volgareva, G.M., Zavalishina, L.E., Golovina, D.A., Andreeva, Y.Y., Ermilova, V.D., Trofimova, O.B., Kuevda, D.A., Shipulina, O.Y., Glazunova, V.A., Cheng, S., Pavlova, L.S., Cheban, N.L., Matveev, V.B., & Frank, G.A. (2010b). Cellular expression of *INK4a* gene in cells of bladder cancer associated with human papillomavirus-16. *Bulletin of Experimental Biology and Medicine*. Vol. 149, No 2, pp. 242-245, ISSN 0365-9615. (In English, Russian). May be purchased from SpringerLink:
http://www.springerlink.com/openurl.asp?genre=article&id=doi:10.1007/s10517-010-09

Yang, H., Yang, K., Khafagi, A., Tang, Y, Carey, T.E., Opipari, A.W., Lieberman, R., Oeth, P.A., Lancaster, W., Klinger, H.P., Kaseb, A.O., Metwally, A., Khaled, H., & Kurnit, D.M. (2005). Sensitive detection of human papillomavirus in cervical, head/neck, and schistosomiasis-associated bladder malignancies. *Proc. Natl Acad. Sci USA*, Vol. 102, No 21, pp. 7683-7688.

Zaridze, D.G. (2009). *Cancer prevention*. IMA-PRESS, ISBN 978-5-904356-05-7, Moscow. (In Russian).

Zaridze, D.G., Nekrasova, L.I., & Basieva, T.Kh. (1992). Increased risk factors for the occurrence of bladder cancer. *Voprosy. Onkologii (Problems in Oncology),* Vol. 38, No 9, pp. 1066-1073, ISSN 0507-3558. (In Russian).

zur Hauzen, H. (2000) Papillomaviruses causing cancer: evasiom from host-cell control in early events in carcinogenesis. *J. Natl Cancer Inst.,* Vol. 92, No 9, pp. 690-698.

zur Hauzen, H. (2008) Papillomaviruses - to vaccination and beyond. *Biochemistry (Moscow),* Vol.73, No 5, pp. 619-626, ISSN 0006-2979.

10

Bladder Cancer and Schistosomiasis: Is There a Difference for the Association?

Mohamed S. Zaghloul and Iman Gouda
Radiation Oncology and Pathology Departments,
Children's Cancer Hospital and National Cancer Institute,
Cairo University, Cairo,
Egypt

1. Introduction

Bladder cancer represents a significant worldwide health problem with an estimated 386,300 new cases and 150,200 deaths in 2008 worldwide. The majority of bladder cancer occurs in males and there is a 14-fold variation in incidence internationally. The highest incidence rates are found in the countries of Europe, North America, and Northern Africa (Jemal et al.2011). Smoking and occupational exposures are the major risk factors in Western countries, whereas chronic infection with Schistosoma hematobium (SH) in developing countries, particularly in Africa and the Middle East, accounts for about 50% of the total burden. The majority of bladder cancers associated with schistosomiasis are squamous cell carcinoma **(Figure 1)**.

Although the majority of bladder cancers, present with disease confined to the superficial layer of the bladder wall, approximately 20–40% of the patients will present with or subsequently develop invasive cancer. Bladder cancer is morphologically heterogeneous; more than 90 % of bladder cancer cases are urothelial (UC, transitional cell, TCC) carcinoma, whereas primary squamous cell carcinoma (SCC), adenocarcinoma, small cell carcinoma and other rare tumors are less common (Lopez-Beltran and Cheng, 2006). Urothelial cell carcinoma can present mixed with other malignant components (**figure 2**). These mixed forms of bladder histologies include squamous differentiation (present in 20 - 60% of bladder cancer cases), adenocarcinoma or glandular differentiation (10%), sarcomatoid (7%), micropapillary (3.7%) and lymphoepìtelioma-like carcinoma. About 1 in 25 Western men and 1 in 80 women will be diagnosed with bladder cancer (BC) sometime in their life. In many developing countries, life expectancy is much lower than Westerns, which is one of the reasons why overall BC incidence (not age-specific incidence) is lower in these developing countries (Albertson and Pinkel, 2003). It is associated with substantial morbidity and mortality. History of Tobacco smoking not only increases the incidence of BC, but also it can increase the tumor grade, its size and the number of tumor lesions (Muscheck et al, 2000). Chronic schistosomal cystitis was related for a long period to the development of BC in areas endemic for schistosomiasis like Egypt. In these areas, risk factors are many, including exposure to schistosomiasis, increased smoking rate and exposure to carcinogenic chemicals (Kallioniemi et al, 1992).

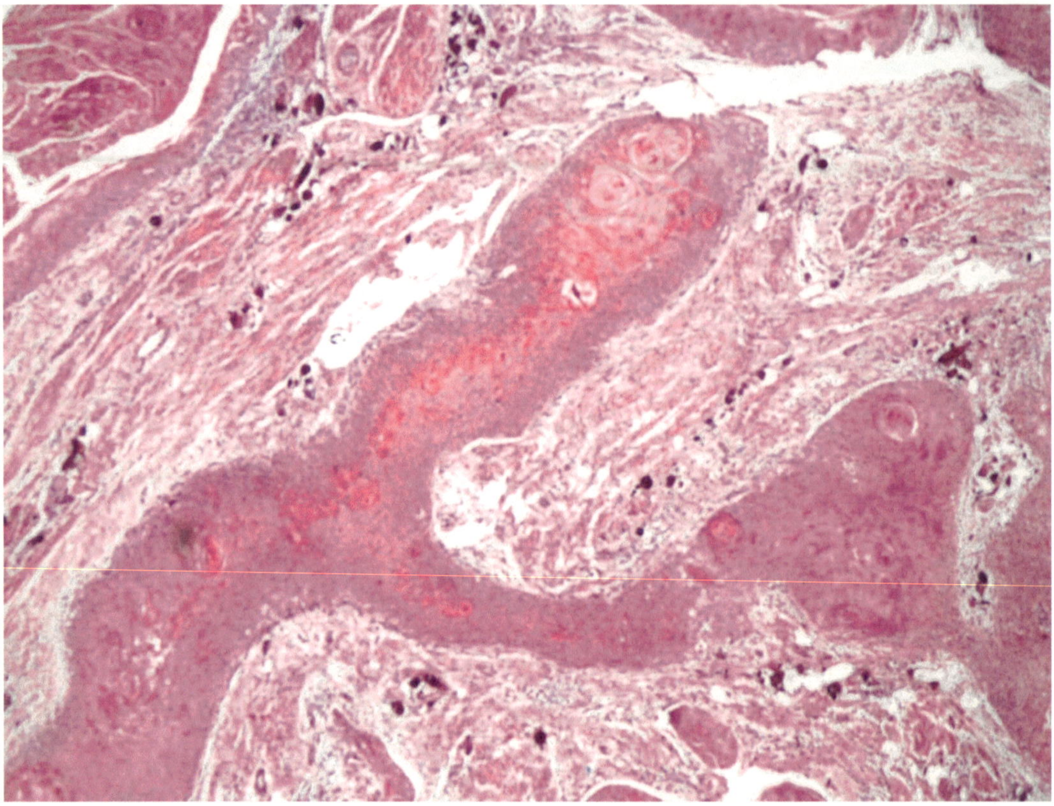

Fig. 1. Squamous cell carcinoma. Groups of malignant squamous cells show central keratin nests formation. Aggregates of calcified bilharzias eggs are seen between groups of malignant cells.

Although smoking is still recognized as a major risk factor of cancers including bladder cancer, the increasing incidence of bladder cancer, despite the reduction in smoking in the United States, suggests that other environmental factors may be playing an increasing role in the development of bladder cancer. Unlike the common belief, risk factors such as positive family history, parent's consanguinity, exposure to pesticides and chronic cystitis seem to play now more important roles than bilharziasis and smoking in the development of this disease in Egypt, yet reports on larger numbers of patients are needed to support this conclusion (Zarzour et al, 2008).

2. Bladder cancer formation

Urothelial tumor is characterized by its multifocality. There have been two theories proposed to explain the frequency of this Urothelial tumor multifocality. One theory, the monoclonal theory, suggests that multiple tumors arise from a single transformed cell that proliferates and spreads throughout the urothelium. The second theory, the field-effect theory, explains tumor multifocality as a development secondary to the field cancerization effect. In the last scenario, carcinogens cause independent transforming genetic alterations at different sites in the urothelial lining leading to multiple genetically defective tumors

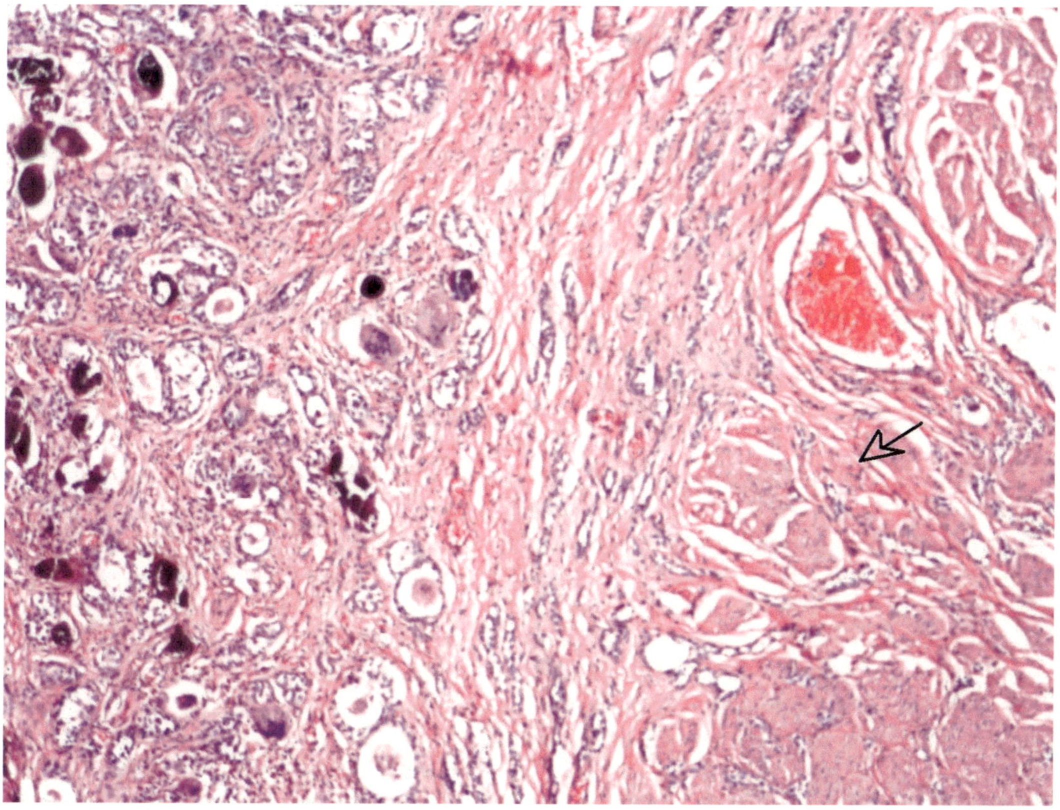

Fig. 2. Invasive urothelial cell carcinoma. Small groups of cells with glandular differentiation on the right are seen infiltrating muscle layer (arrow). Bilharzial granulomas are seen on the left.

(Cheng et al, 2010). That may highlight the existence of different histopathologies in the same specimen. A recent study suggests that both field cancerization and monoclonal tumor spread may coexist in the same patient (Jones et al, 2005). In this study, molecular evidence supported an oligoclonal origin for multifocal Urothelial carcinoma. Field cancerization, which is an important cause of multicenteric squamous cell carcinoma (SCC) of head and neck postulates that multifocal Urothelial carcinoma arises in the same way. The independent transformations are a consequence of external cancer-causing influences. Premalignant changes, such as dysplasia or carcinoma in situ (CIS) are often found in Urothelial mucosa distant from an invasive bladder cancer. Furthermore, various theories have been proposed to combine the two mechanisms. Early or preneoplastic lesions may arise independently with specific clone and pseudomonoclonality (Hafner et al, 2002). The modern carcinogenesis model suggests that malignancy represents clonal expansion of one or a few cancer stem cells that proliferate through asymmetric differentiation and can diversify into heterogeneous cancer cell lineages. Asymmetric differentiation means that following cell division, one daughter cell retains the capacity to divide again and the other daughter cell possesses genetic plasticity, allowing phenotypic variation in the offspring. When tumors arise from Chromosomal Somatic Changes (CSC) of progenitor cells, a specific set of genomics, epigenomic and/ or microenvironment niche alterations is essential for continued clonal expansion. Therefore, each CSC and its pro/zaxgency possess a unique set of genetic, epigenetic and phenotypic features. Genetic alterations of stromal somatic cells assist CSCs in the niche to promote cancer development and progression (Cheng and Zhang, 2008). Since the sixties of the last century, meaningful chromosomal changes were subsequently reported in human cancer. With the establishment of different new methods, detection of these changes became more apparent and allowed better understanding of the process of evolving of different kinds of cancer. Each new method widened the recognition of karyotypic changes, increasing the resolution of cytogenetic details until the limit of microscopic visualization were almost reached. The evolution of cytogenetics encompasses also molecular approaches such as fluorescent in situ hybridization (FISH) and comparative genomic hybridization (CGH) whether metaphasic or array. These techniques have revealed novel and otherwise cryptic rearrangements, as well as providing chromosomal information for cases in which conventional cytogenetic analysis is not possible (Sendberg and Meloni-Ehrg, 2010).

A meta-analysis examining urine markers for surveillance showed that Fluorescence In Situ Hybridization (FISH) test had a median sensitivity of 79% and median specificity of 70% in detecting genetic abnormalities in cells present in urine using FISH (Van Rhijin et al, 2005). The main disadvantages of FISH are the lack of standardization of the criterion for a positive test, the low sensitivity of detecting low-grade tumors, its expense, and the need for specially trained laboratory personnel to perform the test (Degtyar et al, 2004 & Lokeshwar et al, 2005). Combined testing with other assays may improve the effectiveness of this biomarker. Several markers have shown promise as noninvasive biomarkers of bladder cancer, and some may be useful as therapeutic targets. To date, however, none have found a strong niche in clinical care because of the lack of evidence demonstrating that outcomes are altered on a practical basis. In addition, at this time, none of these markers can supplant cystoscopy, and most add little advantage to the combination of cystoscopy and cytology.

3. Schistosomiasis

Schistosomiasis infect 200 million people according to the World Health Organization and is endemic in as much as 76 tropical developing countries. S. hematobium (SH) is associated with bladder cancer. Schistosomes are dioecious parasitic blood flukes, which have a mammalian host and an intermediate invertebrate host: fresh water snails (Kuper et al, 2000). There are four human schistosomes :S. haematobium, S. mansoni, S. japonicum, S. mekonji. The S. haematobium, like other schistosomes is dioecious and the adult female lives in-copulo in the gynecophoral canal of the male; this species of schistosome lives in the venules of the human urinary bladder. Eggs laid in the urinary bladder produce irritation and eventual fibrosis, contributing to the events that lead to human carcinogenicity (Fried et al, 2011).

All schistosoma infections follow direct contact with fresh water that harbors free-swimming larval forms of the parasite known as cercariae. Cercariae penetrate the skin. The cercariae shed their bifurcated tails, and the resulting schistosomula enter capillaries and lymphatic vessels en route to the lungs. After several days, the worms migrate to the portal venous system, where they mature and unite. Pairs of worms then migrate to the vesical plexus and veins draining the ureters. Egg production commences four to six weeks after infection and continues for the life of the worm, usually three to five years. Eggs pass from the lumen of blood vessels into adjacent tissues, and many then pass through the bladder mucosa and are shed in the urine. The life cycle is completed when the eggs hatch, releasing miracidia that, in turn, infect specific freshwater snails (Bulinus species).After two generations - primary and then daughter sporocysts – within the snail, cercariae are released (Ross et al, 2002).

4. Schistosoma-Associated Bladder Cancer (SA-BC)

Schistosomiasis was first linked to urinary bladder cancer in Egypt in 1911 (Ferguson et al, 1911). The incidence of urinary bladder cancer in the Middle East and Africa is greater in areas with high rather than low SH prevalence; the aforementioned study noted that 60% of the Egyptian population was at risk of infection with SH, with rural school children at particular risk because of their proximity to contaminated water. The overall prevalence of SH infection in Egypt was 37–48% that decreased due to the antibilharzial campaign to 3 % (Ministry of Health and Population, 2004). The urinary bladder cancer accounted for about 31% of the total incidence of cancers in Egypt that subsequently decreased to 12% in recent years. However still, it is the most common type of cancer in males and the second most prevalent, after breast cancer, in females (Gouda et al, 2007). In Egypt, Iraq, Zambia, Zimbabwe, Malawi and Sudan, the incidence of SA-BC peaks at 40–49 years of age; the male to female ratio for bladder cancer is 5:1 in endemic and 3:1 in non-endemic areas. This relates to the fact that it is agricultural workers, mainly men, who have daily exposure to water infected with SH cercariae. (Makhyoun et al, 1971). Mechanicaly, there are several factors that may contribute to the oncological potential of schistosomia infection. Schistosoma ova deposited in the bladder provoke an intense inflammatory reaction, associated with the production of oxygen-derived free radicals, which may induce genetic mutations or promote the production of carcinogenic compounds (such as N-nitrosamines and polycyclic aromatic hydrocarbons) (Marletta 1988 & Rosin et al, 1994) ,leading to malignant transformation. Shokeir (2004) showed that schistosomiasis is often accompanied by chronic bacterial super-infection, which may in itself predispose to squamous cell (SC) neoplasia. Bacteria found to accompany schistosomiasis can promote the formation of N-nitrosation of amines, adding to those from other sources such as the diet. A 54–81% incidence of SCC was found in all cases of bladder cancers in endemic areas, opposed to 3–10% in Western countries. The higher incidence of SCC is probably due to exposure to carcinogens such as N-nitroso compounds that are abundantly present in the urine of patients with SH (Tricker et al,1989). International Agency for Research on Cancer (IARC) found that the intensity of infection was determined by urinary egg counts and confounded by smoking, a recognized cause of bladder cancer in non-endemic countries, and the combination was strongly considered. Positive association between bladder cancer and SH infection was detected, with odd ratios ranging from 2 to 14. The more heavily infected individuals were with this schistosome, the more likely they were to develop bladder cancer, and at a younger age (IARC, 1994).

Most of the pathological findings of schistosomiasis are due to an inflammatory and immunological response to egg deposition. Granulomatous areas form around the eggs and induce an exudative cellular response consisting of lymphocytes, polymorphonuclear leukocytes and eosinophil. The early stage of SH infection is characterized by egg deposition in the lower ureters and urinary bladder. Resultant perioval granulomas, fibrosis and muscular hypertrophy are seen histologically. In the ureter, lesions can cause stenosis, leading to hydronephrosis. In the urinary bladder, masses of large granulomatous inflammatory polyps containing eggs are found at the bladder apex, dome, trigone and posterior wall. Polyps may ulcerate and slough, producing haematuria. Hyperplasia of the urothelium occurred in 38% of the autopsied SH cases as opposed to 21% in non-infected cases; also, metaplasia in 31.6% versus 11.5% and dysplasia in 27.2% versus 8.5% cases were found. Late-stage infections were characterized by schistosomal bladder ulcers and sandy patches, and irregularly thickened or atrophic mucosa in the posterior bladder or trigone area. Histologically, fibrosis with some round cell infiltration was seen; old granulomas containing calcified or disintegrating eggs were also seen (Smith and Christie, 1986). The inflammatory and fibrotic response to egg deposition could lead to calcification of the urinary bladder, infection and stone disease and these changes are frequently associated with urinary bladder cancer (EL-Bolkainy et al, 1981). These lesions may be at least partially responsible to the reported clinical picture of SA-BC. Furthermore, the following sequence of events in SH-induced carcinogenesis has been suggested: chronic infection leads to schistosoma eggs being trapped in the bladder wall. Proliferation of cells in the bladder mucosa results from constant irritation and inflammation. Clones of neoplastic cells develop, stimulated by N-nitrosamines and other environmental carcinogens such as cigarette smoke and pesticides (Abdel et al, 2000). The importance of urinary retention, whether from fibrosis and obstruction of the urinary bladder neck or from voluntary causes such as pain on urination, in prolonging the exposure of the bladder mucosa to various exogenous and endogenous carcinogens was documented. Schistosome-induced urinary stasis allows increased absorption of carcinogens and therefore plays an integral role in carcinogenesis. Recurrent bacterial urinary tract infections are associated with squamous cell carcinoma of the urinary bladder, even in the absence of SH infection (Genile et al, 1985). Carcinogenesis of SH involving an initiating and promoting effect has been described. First, the damage occurs to the DNA template which, unless repaired, leads to irreversible changes in the complementary strand of DNA produced during the S-phase of the cell cycle. Somatic mutation results when the altered strand is used as a template. The promotion phase followed by stimulation of cell proliferation. Different cancer-associated genes, notably protoncogenes/oncogenes and tumor suppressor genes, were known to be associated with numerous human cancers; recent efforts have been made to study the specific genes involved in the induction of SA-BC. Cell exposed to SH cell total antigen (warm exttract) was found to divide faster than those not exposed to the parasite and died much less. This was probably due to increased level of bcl2, a protein involved in cancer apoptosis that may lead to SH carcinogenic ability in bladder urothelium (Botelho et al, 2009). The urothelium of mice exposed to SH total antigen showed dysplasia, low grade intra-urothelial neoplasm, non-invasive malignant flat lesions in 70 % of the tested mice after 40 weeks of exposure. Carcinoma of the bladder frequently harbors gene mutations that constitutively activate the receptors tyrosine kinase Ras pathway (Wu, 2005). The Ras gene product is a monometric membrane-localized G protein of 21 Kd that functions as a molecular switch linking receptors and non-receptors tyrosine kinase activation to downstream cytoplasmic or nuclear events. Each mammalian cell contains at least three distinct Ras proto-oncogenes encoding closely related but distinct protein, Kras, Hras and Nras. Activating mutation in these Ras protein, result in constitutive signaling. Thereby stimulating cell proliferation and inhibiting apoptosis. Oncogenic mutations in the Ras gene are present in approximately 30% of all human cancer (Adjer, 2001). Botelho et al (2010) used the dysplastic bladders induced by SH in mice and screened them by sequencing for mutations in Kras codon hotspots gene. They concluded that the parasite abstract has carcinogenic ability possibly through oncogenic mutation of Kras gene.

5. Genetic changes in SA-BC

Among the most common genetic changes in bladder cancer is the loss of heterozygosity (LOH) on chromosomes 9p and 9q, which is found regardless of tumor grade and stage (Jacobs et al,2010 & McConkey et al, 2010). A prospective study stated that there was no evident line of demarcation between schistosomiasis-associated and non schistosomiasis-associated bladder cancer in terms of LOH of microsatellite markers on chromosome 9. This suggests that data obtained from schistosoma-associated bladder cancer can be extrapolated to bladder cancer induced by a schistosomiasis independent mechanism (Abdel Wahab et al, 2005). DNA microsatellites are highly polymorphic repeats found throughout the genome, and microsatellite markers can detect cancer-associated alterations in genetic material, including microsatellite instability and LOH (Nielsen et al, 2006). A more recent analytical tool that has been developed to detect genomic instability in urinary DNA uses small nucleotide polymorphisms (SNPs). SNP chips have a potential advantage over microsatellite analysis in that they can screen more than 300 genetic loci at once compared with 13-20 loci, which leads to a greater sensitivity of the detection of molecular changes (Hoque et al, 2003).

6. Cytogenetics for understanding carcinogenesis

Carcinogenesis is a complex process in which normal cell growth is modified as a result of the interaction of multiple factors, including xenobiotics and endogenous constituents. Carcinogenic process results from the accumulation of both genetic and epigenetic changes that are driven by instability of cellular genome and alterations in inter- or intra-cellular communication, which disrupt the cell proliferation regulation process (Loeb and loeb, 2000). Cytogenetics is concerned with the task of finding recurrent (repeated) or specific abnormalities associated with cancer, and continues to provide crucial diagnostic and prognostic information. In current practice, cytogenetic data often serve as a guide in other studies, ranging from the exploration of cytogenetic findings with various methodologies, singly or in combination, including fluorescence in situ hybridization (FISH), polymerase chain reaction (PCR), or microarray-based technologies such as comparative genomic hybridization (CGH), both metaphasic (mCGH) and array (aCGH), to the use of immunohistochemical techniques by the pathologist. Cytogenetic data also provide key background information for the recognition and identification of genes (and their networks) involved in cancer. Progress in understanding the cytogenetic and molecular basis of neoplastic transformation has strengthened the conception of cancer as a genetic disease. Thus, the finding of apparently normal karyotypes in abnormal cells presents an enigma. It can be assumed that cryptic genetic changes are involved in such cases. Newer technologies highlight the more complicated and perplexing aspects of cancer that have eluded more traditional cytogenetic studies. For example, molecular studies have demonstrated fusion genes associated with many tumors like prostate and lung cancers that are not discernible cytogenetically. These findings raise the strong possibility that more epithelial carcinomas, which are usually associated with numerous or complex karyotypic alterations, will be shown to have cryptic primary genetic alterations (Sandberg et al,2010)

7. Requirements and limitations of cancer cytogenetic studies

Cytogenetic techniques require the presence of dividing cells (preferably in the metaphase stage) for the visualization of chromosomes. Thus, fresh specimens are necessary for establishing either short-term or long-term cultures (Sandberg, 1990, Brigge and Sandberg, 2000, Sandberg and Chen, 2001& Gersen and Keagle, 2005). Nevertheless, useful genetic information can be obtained from fixed specimens with appropriate FISH or other molecular techniques (Gersen and Keagle, 2005). Cytogenetic changes represent genetic mechanisms that are thought to be responsible for the biology of the respective clinical conditions, and have become important components of diagnostic and prognostic criteria. There are two different classes of genetic alterations associated with cancer: activation of oncogenes and inactivation of tumor suppressor genes. Rearrangements are a common source of activating mutations. Another scenario is exemplified by chromosome translocations, inversions, or insertions that lead to formation of fusion oncogenes. The oncogene fusion mechanism has received increased attention, because many of these fusions lead to activation of protein tyrosine kinases (PTKs) in various types of cancer. Most of the cytogenetic changes involve activation of receptor proteins, especially PTKs. Receptor PTKs are a highly regulated family of proteins in normal cells, but may undergo activating mutations or structural alterations to become oncoproteins in human malignancies. As already noted, oncogenic activation of PTKs can result from genetic lesions such as point mutations, deletions, or overexpression by gene amplification. Alternatively, chromosomal rearrangements such as translocations, inversions, and insertions that lead to formation of an oncogenic gene fusion can involve receptor PTK or other PTK encoding genes as fusion partners. Another type of gene rearrangement involves tumor suppressor genes, whose products normally serve as brakes on cell growth and runaway cell proliferation. Inactivation of tumor suppressor genes leads to uncontrolled cell proliferation and downregulation of apoptosis (programmed cell death)(Jones and Baylin, 2002 & Feinberg and Tycko, 2004). The activation of oncogenes sometimes results from complex genetic rearrangements. In each of the fusion genes the kinase domain of the neural-associated receptor tyrosine kinase gene is fused to an activating domain of another gene. The same genes may be altered in a number of different tumors, but apparently at varying chronologies in tumor development and associated with different genetic changes. In many tumors, a specific translocation may be the only alteration present. Many cases, however, display additional structural or numeric karyotypic changes that may be responsible for, or at least are associated with, disease progression(Sandberg, 1990). The relevance of additional abnormalities is also reflected by alterations in the expression of a number of genes apart from those involved in the translocations. The exact cause or causes of these additional alterations is unknown, and it remains uncertain whether the primary translocation per se is responsible for the basic genetic process underlying the tumor genesis. These additional changes usually vary from tumor to tumor, even among tumors with the same diagnosis. Tumors with specific translocations may exhibit a variety of anomalies, with or without additional chromosome changes, at the molecular level. Carcinomas being diagnosed relatively late in their development, thus allow for the genesis of chromosomal rearrangements in addition to the primary genetic event. Although some of the chromosomal changes have been related to prognosis and tumor biology yet, few recurrent or repeated chromosomal anomalies have been identified as characterizing these tumors (Teixeira et al, 2006).

MicroRNAs (miRNAs) constitute a rapidly developing field of study at many levels. The miRNAs are short segments of RNA (~22 bases in length) that affect mRNA functions, most often by suppressing translation of the protein product or by promoting degradation of them. An important value of miRNAs is that they can be detected and quantified in a variety of samples, including plasma and formalin-fixed, paraffin-embedded tissues. This makes them a valuable testing tool, particularly in the clinical arena(Wijnhoven et al, 2007, Grady and Tewari, 2010 & Ferracin et al, 2010)

In cancer, the combination of cytogenetic and molecular studies (FISH, SKY, PCR, CGH, and related methodologies) can more clearly define pathogenetic pathways and the biologic functions of molecular markers than either approach alone. Such a dual approach should lead to less empiric and more biologically oriented approaches to tumor classification and, ultimately, to more efficient clinical use of biomarkers (Wang,2002 & Balsara et al, 2002). Findings based on the combination of cytogenetic and molecular approaches have improved the criteria for diagnosis of cancer. The hypothesis that specific clones of spontaneously evolving aneuploidies or karyotypes, rather than specific mutations, generate the individuality of cancers (Fabarius et al, 2008), may apply to at least some of, if not all, the conditions .Cancer development not only depends on genetic alterations but also on epigenetic changes (Jones and Baylin, 2007). These changes modify gene expression through DNA methylation, histone modifications, chromatin remodeling, and/or the expression of noncoding RNA(Esteller, 2007 & Zaratiegui et al, 2007).

Epigenetic gene silencing in cancer was thought to be restricted to focal events that silenced isolated genes (Smith and Costello, 2006). However, recent findings have indicated that epigenetic silencing can extend to a whole chromosomal region and has been reported to involve DNA methylation and/or histone modification in various cancers (bladder, breast, colorectal, and prostate cancer) (Coolen et al, 2010).

The development of cancer is often a multistage process where the disruption of specific subsets of genes can result in cells expressing a malignant phenotype. However, the series of mutations leading to malignancy has only been elucidated for a small number of human cancers (e.g., polyposis of the colon, retinoblastoma). There has been no entirely specific cytogenetic aberration identified for bladder cancer, but various nonrandom deletions, gains of chromosomes, polyploidisation, and formation of isochromosomes have been observed (Gibas and Gibas, 1997).

8. Bladder cancer cytogenetics and epigenetics

Chromosome 1 has been reported as being the most frequently involved chromosome in rearrangements; other chromosomes commonly reported in bladder cancer include chromosomes 3,5,7, and 9 (Heim and Mitelman, 1995). Yunis and Soreng (1984) suggested that there was a relationship between chromosomal fragile sites and oncogenesis. It is believed that fragile sites provide regions of the genome that are more susceptible to damage and that this contributes to the carcinogenic process because of subsequent changes to gene function or dosage. Bladder cancer is a very heterogenous disease cytogenetically, which suggests that the pathogenesis of the disease may not be consistent for every case. A possible scenario of pathogenesis could be the disruption of a nonconsistent set of cell regulatory genes compounded with disruption to genes that have a phenotypic effect on the bladder. Sustained disruptions to fragile regions as a result of prolonged exposure to clastogens in vivo are likely to lead to enduring chromosomal rearrangements and associated gene alterations. The heterogeneity of cytogenetic findings in bladder cancer hints that there might be different "fingerprints" or accumulations of genetic changes that individually lead to bladder cancer and that fragile sites may be providing a gateway for oncogenesis for some cases. Different combinations of these damaged sites could result in varying cancer phenotypes, depending upon which particular genes were located at the sites susceptible to the mutagens.

Protoncogenes encode proteins that ultimately enhance cell proliferation. Events that convert protoncogenes to oncogenes can lead to uncontrolled cell proliferation and carcinogenesis (Badawi et al, 1995). The RAS oncogene and its potential association with urinary bladder cancer was studied, though still not totally clear. The RAS oncogene encodes a 21-kDa protein that affects signal transmission between the nucleus and tyrosine kinase receptors. H-RAS activation was estimated in bladder cancer to range between 7% and 17%, with its expression being similar with or without concurrent schistosomal infection. The TP53 tumor suppressor gene, located on the short arm of chromosome 17, encodes a protein that regulates DNA damage repair and controls aspects of the cell cycle involving cellular apoptosis and senescence. TP53 mutation results in a reduction of DNA damage surveillance leading to instability of the genome and malignant transformation (Strohmeyer and Slamon, 1994). The overexpression of the BCL-2 gene in SA-BC patients was found to be up-regulated in squamous but not transitional cell cancers of the urinary bladder. Therefore, this BCL-2 overexpression is consistent with the predominance of SCC in SA-BC. Upregulation of this gene overrides programmed cell apoptosis increasing the risk of genomic instability and may interact with various proto-oncogenes facilitating tumorigenesis. Mutations of TP53 were found in 73% of tumors, BCL-2 expression in 32% and abnormalities of both TP53 and BCL-2 in 13%. Loss of the normal reciprocal control mechanism for apoptosis was suggested in the subset of patients with overexpression of both TP53 and BCL-2 (Chaudhary et al, 1997).

Furthermore, cyclooxygenase-2 is overexpressed in SA-BC. The quantitative relationship between cyclooxygenase-2 expression and tumor grade was statistically significant. The cyclooxygenase-2 role in the complex multi-stage process of SA-BC carcinogenesis was proposed: pro-inflammatory cytokines such as interleukin-1, tumor growth factor-β and tumor necrosis factor-alpha, are generated by activated macrophages in the inflammatory lesions. These cytokines and growth factors are potent inducers of cyclooxygenase-2 production. By-products of uncontrolled cyclooxygenase activity together with endogenous genotoxins produce oxidative and nitrosative stress creating lipid peroxidation by-products. Additional mutations are induced: TP53, H-RAS, deletion of p16 and p15, increased epidermal growth factor receptor, c-erb-2 and tumor necrosis factor-alpha. Increased prostaglandin production up-regulates cyclooxygenase-2, decreases killer T-cell activity, increases BCL-2 and glutathione-S-transferase. These changes increase tumorgenicity by decreasing cell apoptosis, creating immunosupression. Prostaglandin products of cyclooxygenase-2 cause tumor progression and eventual metastasis by down-regulating adhesion molecules, increasing the degradation of extracellular matrix and increasing angiogenesis (El-Sheikh et al, 2001).

9. Natural history of SA-BC

The association between SA-BC and SH was established through case-controlled studies and through the close correlation of the incidence of bladder cancer with the prevalence of SH within different geographic areas. Moreover, the association was based on the frequent association of tumors with the presence of parasitic eggs and egg-induced granulomatous pathology involving bladder tissues *(Figure 2)*. Despite that linkage between SH and bladder cancer, only limited data are available on cytopathologic findings in SA-BC. The cellular mechanisms linking SH infestation with bladder cancer formation are not yet defined. In some cases, severe metaplasia in bladder urothelium may represent a precancerous transformation, whereas in others it may merely serve as a marker of prolonged inflammation, which is associated with high cancer risk (Hodder et al, 2000). Keratinizing or adenomatous metaplasia per se has a strong association with cancer formation in patients with chronic irritation due to bladder stones, chronic infection, or prolonged catheterization.

SA-BC was defined by characteristic pathology (i.e., squamous carcinoma, transitional cell carcinoma, or adenocarcinoma, rather than mainly transitional) and cellular and molecular biology that differ from non-Schistosoma-associated bladder cancer (NSA-BC). Few studies have analysed the cytogenetic and molecular genetic abnormalities in SA-BC and some compared DNA copy number changes in SA-BC and NSA-BC (Kallioniemi et al, 1992,Tsutumi et al, 1998, Muscheck et al,2000, Fadl-Elmula et al, 2002 & Albertson and Pinkel, 2003). Further future studies are needed to characterize the genetic alterations in schistosomal bladder tumors and their role in bladder cancer induction.

These studies used metaphase CGH to obtain overview of chromosomal alterations in SA-BC. The value of pooled DNA in aCGH was shown to be advantageous in detecting recurrent changes associated with specific histopathologic or clinical features (Kendziorski et al, 2005). Two more recent studies used aCGH, rather than metaphase CGH (Armengol et al, 2007 & Vauhkonen et al, 2007). Array CGH provides higher density region-specific coverage and direct mapping of aberrations to the genome sequence, as well as higher throughput (Albertson and Pinkel, 2003). This ensures greater accuracy in comparing two groups of tumors (e.g., SA-BC and NSA-BC). Muscheck et al. (2000) demonstrated deletion similarities in Schistosoma-associated transitional cell carcinoma (SA-TCC) and Schistosoma-associated squamous cell carcinoma (SA-SCC), compared to what has been previously reported by Kallioniemi et al. (1992) on NSA-TCC and Tsutsumi et al. (1998) on NSA-SCC. The previous investigators (Kallioniemi et al,1992,Tsutsumi et al,1998, Muscheck et al, 2000, Fadl-Elmula et al, 2002 & Albertson and Pinkel, 2003) used the technique of CGH on individual tumor tissues, not pooled tissues of similar pathologies. Armengol et al. (2007) used an excellent technique of combining similar pathological types into pools of tissue arising from patients having similar pathological subtypes. These pooled DNAs revealed recurrent primary changes covering secondary changes that vary from case to case. The pooled specimens of SA-BC tumors showed no schistosomiasis specific changes, compared with pools of NSA tumors. The comparison between SA-TCC and NSA-TCC and that between SA-SCC and NSA-SCC gave similar results. DNA copy number profiles of urinary bladder SA adenocarcinoma revealed similarities to that of SA-TCC and SA-SCC reported by Vauhkonen et al. (2007). The results in these two publications showed that the detailed analysis of individual genes revealed a set of genes with the same copy number changes in all bladder carcinomas, including both SA and NSA tumors. Armengol et al. (2007) concluded that there are no major cytogenetic differences among different urinary bladder epithelial tumors, regardless of the suspected carcinogen. All the detected imbalances in SA-BC have been repeatedly reported in NSA-BC that suggested that cytogenetic profiles of chemical- and Schistosoma-induced carcinoma are largely similar in the reports of Muscheck et al. (2000) and Fadl-Elmula et al. (2002). Patients having SA-BC usually present late with more advanced stage, due to the repeated SH infestations having similar symptoms. The decreased intensity of schistosomal infestation in Egypt led to a changing pattern of the clinicoepidemiologic features of SA-BC. A decreased SCC/TCC ratio (increase in the percentage of TCC and decrease in that of SCC), lowering of the tumor stage and increase in the mean age incidence and percentage of pelvic nodal involvement have been reported. The reported clinicoepidemiologic differences between SA-BC and SNA-BC are now continuously decreasing and the features of SA-BC is slowly approaching that of NSA-BC as reported by Koraitim et al. (1995) and Zaghloul et al. (2008). These changing features were attributed to the decreased intensity of schistosomal infestation in the urinary bladder, as a higher degree of schistosomal infestation and egg deposition was found more frequently with SCC and a lower with TCC (Zaghloul et al, 2008 & Zaghloul, 2010). Furthermore, these changes are repeatedly evident with the predominance of TCC over the SCC type, and a decrease of male predominance. If these changes continue with the same rate, bladder cancer in Egypt is expected to become identical in features to that of Western countries in the near future (Gouda et al, 2007).

10. Clinical presentation

Clinical presentations in SA-BC and SNA-BC are similar with few minor differences. Hematuria, dysuria and necroturia are the main symptoms in both situations. However, SA-BC patients usually had experienced these symptoms beforehand as a result of simple schistosomal cystitis. This may be the reason of their relatively late presentation. Table (1) showed the postcystectomy pathological staging in SA-BC and SNA-BC large studies. The early stages (Pa, Pis, P1) were fewer in SA-BC than that in SNA-BC in both the Urothelial and non-urothelial pathology. The pelvic nodal involvement was nearly similar in SA-BC (range: 16.7% - 25.5%) , Urothelial SNA-BC (range: 16.3% - 45%) and non-urothelial SNA-BC (21.8% - 23%). The clincopathologic differences between SA-BC and SNA-BC were previously summarized as late presentation, with younger median age and a higher percentage of squamous cell carcinoma category (Zaghloul, 1994).

11. Treatment of non-muscle invasive (superficial) bladder cancer

Treatment of superficial bladder cancer remains to be transurethral resection and bladder biopsy (TURBT) with and without intravesical BCG or chemotherapy instillation. Although this treatment type is very popular in Urothelial cancer, it is less popular in non-urothelial SNA-BC and SA-BC, probably due to the rarity of the non-invasive stages and the presence of many lesions either precancerous or cancerous in the bladder mucosa.

12. Treatment of muscle-invasive bladder cancer

Radical cystectomy

Muscle-invasive bladder cancer is mostly treated with radical cystectomy in many parts of the world. Radical cystectomy procedure includes removal of the bladder, seminal vesicles and prostate together with perivesical fat and peritoneal coverage, in addition to bilateral

Author	Number of Patients	PTa,is,1 %	PT2 %	PT3 %	PT4 %	Nodal involvement
Pure Urothelial Carcinoma (SNA-BC)						
Bassi et al (1999)	338	32.8	19.8	42.0	19.8	NM
Stein et al, (2001)	1057	39.9	23.5	23.5	13	23.3
Cheng et al, (2003)	303	36.1	28.6	25.5	9.9	16.3
Shariat et al, (2006)	958	22	35	31	12	23
Urothelial & Non-urothelial (SNA-BC)						
Rogers et al, (2006)	955	21	33	32	14	23
Lughezzani et al, (2010)	12003	13.4	38.9	28.1	19.6	21.8
Scosyrev et al,(2009)	1422	14.8	29	29.3	26.8	
Urothelial & Non-urothelial (SA-BC)						
El Said et al, (1997)	420	1	3.8	70.7	24.5	16.7
Zaghloul, (1996)	357	0	33.3	47.9	18.8	24.4
El Makresh et al,(1998)	185	7	25	64	7	16
Zaghloul et al, (2006)	192	3.6	28.1	51.6	16.7	25.5
Ghoneim et, (2008)	2720	10.5	63.9	16.6	9.0	20.4
Zaghloul et al, (2008)	5071	1.9	30.1	54.9	13.1	21.9
Khaled et al, (2005)	180	1.2	5.8	14.1	11.5	16.6
Ali-El-Dein, (2009)	180	10.0	62.8	25.0	2.2	18.3

Table 1. Postcystectomy pathological stages and nodal involvement in pure Urothelial and mixed Urothelial and non-urothelial schistosoma-non associated and schistosoma associated bladder cancer in large series.

endopelvic lymphadenectomy (with varying level of dissection) in male patients. In females, it includes removal of the bladder, its perivesical fat and peritoneal coverage, urethra, uterus, ovary and anterior wall of the vagina (anterior pelvic excentration) (Ghoneim et al, 1997 & Stein et al, 2001). A review of recent literature of treatment results of different types of bladder cancer showed that applying the same treatment yielded nearly the same level of results if comparing the same pathological stage (Zaghloul, 2006 & Zaghloul et al, 2006). Similar 5-year overall survival rates were found in SA-BC, pure Urothelial and combined

Urothelial and non-urothelial SNA-BC types (Table 2). The results were slightly higher in Stein et al. (2001) (NSA-BC) and Zaghloul et al.(2006) (SA-BC) as both studies reported neoadjuvant or adjuvant radiotherapy and /or chemotherapy as a part of treatment in more than one third of their patients. Furthermore, this conclusion applies for comparison of disease-free survival, overall survival, or local control rates for radical cystectomy or even in adjuvant and neoadjuvant radiotherapy types of treatment for SA-BC and NSA-BC (Zaghloul, 2006 & 2010). The treatment end-results of radical cystectomy was not affected by

Author	Patients #	PT1	PT2	PT3	PT4	Nodal involvement
Pure Urothelial Carcinoma (SNA-BC)						
Cheng et al, (2003)	218	---	50	28	17	11
Stein et al, (2001)	1054	74	81/68*	47	44	35
Medersbacher et al, (2003)	507	76	62	40	49	26
Takahashi et al, (2004)	466	81	74	47	38	50
Dhar et al, (2006)	385	---	63	19	NM	9
Ho et al, (2009)	148	77	68	65	11	37
Manoharan et al, (2009)	432	79	60	43	17	22
Urothelial & Non-urothelial (SNA-BC)						
Nishiyama et al, (2004)	1113	82	84/69*	59	43	35
Niu et al, (2008)	356	---	73/44*	22	0	8
Gupta et al, (2008)	502	90	78	70/58*	46	NM
Urothelial & Non-urothelial (SA-BC)						
Ghoneim et al, (1997)	1026	73	66	47/31*	19	23
El Mekresh et al, (1985)	185	83		41		21
Khaled et al, (2005)	180	55		12		6
Zaghloul et al, (2006)	192	100	100/47	40	44	31
Zaghloul et al, (2007)	216	100	51	40	30	31
Ghoneim et al, (2008)	2720	82	75/53	40	30	27

*= a/b, NM = not mentioned

Table 2. The 5-y survival of each pathological stage in Schistosoma-non associated and schistosoma associated bladder cancer patients in large radical cystectomy patients.

the association with schistosomiasis, nor tumor cell type (Urothelial or non-urothelial) in most of the recently published literatures (Ghoneim et al, 1997, Stein et al, 2001, Zaghloul et al, 2006) (Table 2). Favorable end-results were reported for patients with pathologically organ confined disease. These results were constant for both SA-BC (ranged from 47% to 83%), and SNA-BC (ranged from 50% to84%). However, the results were significantly worse when reporting upon locally advanced tumors (PT3N0M0, PT4aN0M0 or Any N). Again, these worse results were experienced by both SA-BC and SNA-BC patients (Ghoneim et al, 1997 & 2008,Stein et al, 2001,Gschwend et al, 2002, Chang et al, 2003, Medersbacher et al, 2003, Nishiyama et al, 2004, Takahashi et al, 2004, Rogers et al, 2006 & Lughezzani et al, 2010). Regardless of the old belief that aberrant differentiation leads to worse results, yet many authors reported similar results of these aberrant variants to UC when comparing stage to stage. Rogers et al (2006) reported a 5-year progression-free survival rate of 60±2% after radical cystectomy for UC and 55±11% for SCC. This difference was statistically insignificant. Patients with UC or SCC had statistically significant higher progression-free survival rates than non-UC non-SCC patients including those having adenocarcinoma. Another study containing considerable number of adenocarcinoma patients was conducted using 17 Surveillance, Epidemiology and End Results (SEER) and it showed a difference of statistical significance in adenocarcinoma patients who underwent RC at a more advanced disease stage than their UC counterparts. Another recent study using a similar SEER database demonstrated that SCC was more aggressive than Urothelial cancer after adjusting for common prognostic factors, such as stage and grade (Scosyrev et al, 2009). Scosyrev et al (2009) concluded that SCC was an independent predictor of mortality among patients with stage III and IV disease, and among patients with stage I and II disease who did not undergo cystectomy as part of their treatment. Therefore, squamous histology was not associated with increased mortality among patients with stage I and II disease when treated with cystectomy. Moreover, Ploeg et al (2010) studied all invasive bladder cancer cases treated in The Netherlands during a 12 year period of (1995-2006). They concluded that the relative survival of muscle-invasive adenocarcinoma patients were equal to that of UC patients. For stage II and III disease, adenocarcinoma patients had even better outcome. Muscle-invasive SCC patients showed worse survival regardless of stage. In SA-BC, Ghoneim et al (2008) demonstrated that SCC (1345 patients) had 10 year overall survival rate (OS) of 53.05% (95% CI: 51-57) compared to 48.49% (44-53 for pure UC (705 patients) and 51.18 % (CI: 45-58) for adenocarcinoma (262 patients). Those patients who had UC with squamous or adenomatous metaplasia (286 patients) showed a lower 10-year OS of 42.78% (CI: 36-49). The lowest 10-year OS was experienced by those patients who had undifferentiated pathology (122 patients) having 10-year OS of 34.23 (CI: 24-45). It is clear from this large-number single institution study that the OS of SCC, UC and adenocarcinoma were similar and having the same profile. They demonstrated that although the univariate analysis was significant (Undifferentiated carcinoma had much lower OS), the multivariate analysis proved that tumor cell type is not an independent working factor determining the OS. The only significant prognostic factors were stage, grade and pelvic nodal involvement. Many authors cautiously concluded that RC treatment end-results were not affected by tumor histology or etiology but affected by other prognostic factors like stage, grade, nodal involvement, lymphovascular invasion, angiogenesis, P53, P21, Retinoblastoma genes (Rb) and other biological factors. These prognostic and predictor factors were shown in many SA-BC and SNA-BC studies to have varying weight effect (Ghoneim et al, 2008,Scosyrev et al, 2009,Ploeg et al, 2010 & Zaghloul, 2010).

13. Preoperative and postoperative radiotherapy

The rationale of preoperative radiotherapy is to prevent intraoperative seeding of tumor cells in the operative field and to sterilize microscopic extensions in the perivesical tissues. In the English literature, there are 6 randomized trials addressing the issue of adding preoperative radiotherapy to RC. Two of these 6 studies were on SABC (Awwad et al, 1979 & Ghoneim et al, 1985). Only one (Awwad et al, 1979) showed the benefit of adding preoperative radiotherapy. Most of the other 5 studies showed this effect on high stage and high grade tumors. On the other hand, there were no differences in statistical values in earlier cases. Meta-analysis of these randomized studies showed a corrected odd ratio of 0.94 (95% CI: 0.57-1.55), indicating no benefit for adding preoperative radiotherapy in BC (Huncharek et al,1998).

Postoperative radiotherapy (PORT) has the advantage of dealing with microscopic cells that are easier to sterilize. It allows better identification of the group of patients that may benefit from this adjuvant therapy. One large prospective randomized trial proved the benefit of PORT in locally advanced SA-BC. The 5-year disease-free survival (DFS) rate was 49 and 44 % for hyperfractionated (HF) and conventional fractionation (CF) PORT, respectively compared with 25% for cystectomy alone patients (Zaghloul et al,1992). This effect was constant across all tumor cell type, all muscle-invasive stages and grades in SA-BC. These results were replicated in a non-randomized prospective controlled Radiation Therapy Oncology Group (RTOG) trial on SNA-BC (Reisinger et al,1992). The results ot the 2 studies were nearly identical when compared stage by stage (Zaghloul, 1994). The only difference was the high GIT late complication rate reported by Reisinger et al study. They reported 37% (15 out of 40 patients) developed intestinal obstruction after PORT. Nine out of these 15 patients required surgery and 3 died. On the contrary, Zaghloul et al (1992) reported 5% and 18% all grades of late GIT complications for the HF and CF respectively. Only 4% and 5% out of the HF and CF group respectively necessitated surgical interference. Similar low levels of late GIT complications were experienced by other retrospective studies reported on SA-BC and SNA-BC (Cozzarini et al,1999, Zaghloul et al,2002, Zaghloul et al, 2006).

Abdel Moneim et al (2011) compared, in a prospective randomized trial, preoperative and postoperative radiotherapy in SA-BC. They administered the same dose of 50 Gy in 5 weeks to both groups. The study reported both similar treatment end-results and late complication rates for the two randomized pre- and postoperative groups.

14. Neoadjuvant and adjuvant chemotherapy

Neoadjuvant and adjuvant chemotherapy have been utilized in bladder cancer, in an attempt to improve the outcome for patients with high risk muscle-invasive disease. At least 50% of these patients developed distant metastasis after radical cystectomy. Several meta-analysis of prospective, randomized trials indicated that patients undergoing neoadjuvant chemotherapy with methotrexate, vinblastine, doxorubicin and cisplatin (MVAC) prior to cystectomy have an approximate 5.0 – 6.5 % survival advantage over those who underwent surgery alone (Winquist et al, 2004 & Vaughn et al, 2005). However, some investigators still argue that this neoadjuvant advantage is small and chemotherapy might be better targeted to those at highest risk of relapse after surgery. Furthermore, many elderly patients or who have comorbidities will not tolerate MVAC chemotherapy. Therefore, many investigators tried adjuvant chemotherapy in a supposed more favorable situation. In reality, adjuvant

chemotherapy yielded a modest, statistically significant improvement in survival over cystectomy alone (Vale, 2006 & Ruggeri et al, 2006).
The Egyptian bladder cancer cooperative group compared Neoadjuvant chemotherapy using gemcitabine-cisplatin regimen to cystectomy alone in 109 SA-BC patients, in a prospective controlled randomized study. The one-year survival rate was 54% for the cystectomy alone patients compared to 69% for the neoadjuvant chemotherapy patients (Khaled et al, 2003).

15. Bladder preservation trimodality treatment

Since the late 1980s, many centers investigated the bladder preservation strategy as an alternative to radical cystectomy. The rationale of this strategy depends on 3 goals: first, eradication of the local disease, second, elimination of potential micrometastasis and third, maintenance of the best possible quality of life (QoL) through organ preservation (Rodel, 2004). Several treatment protocols were carried out by different investigators. However, they all characterized 3 main and essential procedures with varying timing and varying minute details. The first main procedure is maximal TURBT. This is to be followed by neoadjuvant chemotherapy or radiochemotherapy (second procedure) and then after cystoscopic assessment, followed by either radical radiotherapy or consolidation radiochemotherapy for the complete responders (third procedure). There was another group treated with radiochemotherapy after TURBT. Cystoscopic assessment will segregate the complete responder (CR) for bladder-conserving management and those showing less than CR to undergo salvage cystectomy (Zaghloul and Mousa,2010). The 5-year OS rates ranged between 39% and 58% and the 5-year survival with native bladder preservation ranged from 36% to 43% (Tester et al, 1993,Kachnic et al, 1997, Shipley et al, 1998, Sauer et al, 1998 & Arias et al, 2000). Saba et al (2010) reported similar results for UC (SA-BC and SNA-BC) in Egypt using a trimodality treatment. Complete remission was achieved in 79% of cases after initial radiochemotherapy using gemcitabine- cisplatin regimen. The 5-year OS rate for patients with initial CR was 68% which is comparable to the results in SNA-BC in the western countries treated with trimodality therapy. Moreover, Sabba et al (2010) found that the association with schistosomiasis had no significant impact on the results of therapy for their patients.

16. References

Abdel MM, Hassan A, El-Sewedy S. Human bladder cancer, schistosomiasis, N-nitroso compounds and their precursors,International Journal of Cancer 2000; 88: 682–683.

Abdel Wahab AH, Abo-Zeid HI, El-Husseini MI, Ismail M, El-Khor AM. Role of loss of heterozygosity on chromosomes 8 and 9 in the development and progression of cancer bladder. J Egypt Natl Canc Inst. 2005; 17(4):260-9.

Adjei AA. Blocking oncogenic Ras signaling for cancer therapy. J Natl Cancer Inst 2001; 93: 1062-1074.

Albertson DG, Pinkel D. Genomic microarrays in human genetic disease and cancer. Hum Mol Genet 2003;12: 145-152.

Ali-El-Dein B. Oncological outcome after radical cystectomy and orthotopic bladder substitution in women. Eur J Surg Oncol. 2009 ;35(3):320-5.

Arias F, Domínguez MA, Martínez E, et al. Chemoradiotherapy for muscle invading bladder carcinoma. Final report of a single institutional organ-sparing program. Int J Radiat Oncol Biol Phys. 2000 ;47(2):373-8

Armengol G, Eissa S, Lozano JJ, Shoman S, Sumoy L, Caballı´n MR, Knuutila S. Genomic imbalances in Schistosoma-associated and non Schistosoma-associated bladder carcinoma: an array comparative genomic hybridization analysis. Cancer Genet Cytogenet 2007;177: 16-19.

Awwad HK, Baki HA, El Bolkainy *et al.*: Preoperative irradiation of T3 carcinoma in Bilharzial bladder. *Int. J. Radiat. Oncol. Biol.Phys. 1979;* 5: 787–794.

Badawi AF, Mostafa MH, Prober tA,. O'ConnorPJ. Role of schistosomiasis in human bladder cancer: evidence of association, aetiological factors, and basic mechanisms of carcinogenesis, European Journal of Cancer Prevention 1995;4: 45–49.

Balsara BR, Pei J, -Testa JR. Comparative genomic hybridization analysis. Methods Mol Med 2002;68:45-57.

Bassi P, Ferrante GD, Piazza N *et al.* Prognostic factors of outcome after radical cystectomy for bladder cancer, a retrospective study of homogenous patient cohort. *J. Urol.* 1999; 161, 1494–1497

Botelho M, FerreiaAC, Olivieira MJ, Domingues A, Machado JC, de Costa JM. Schistosoma haematobium total antigen and decreased apoptosis of normal epithelial cells. Int. J Parasitol 2009;39: 1083-1091.

Botelho MC, Machado JC, deCosta JM. Schistosoma hematobium and bladder cancer. Virulence 2010; 1: 2, 84-87.

Bridge JA, Sandberg AA. Cytogenetic and molecular genetic techniques as adjunctive approaches in the diagnosis of bone and soft tissue tumors. Skeletal Radiol 2000;29: 249-58.

Chaudhary KS, Lu KS, Abel PD, et al. Expression of bcl-2 and p53 oncoproteins in schistosomiasis-associated transitional and squamous cell carcinoma of the urinary bladder, British Journal of Urology 1997;79: 78–84.

Cheng L, Weaver AL, Leibovich BC et al. Predicting the survival of bladder carcinoma patients treated with radical cystectomy. Cancer 2000;88: 2326-2332.

Cheng L , Zhang D. Molecular genetic pathology. Humana Press/Sprnger, NY, USA 2008.

Cheng L, Davidson D, Mac Lennan GT, et al. The origin of Urothelial cancer. Exp Review Anticancer Ther 2010; 10 (6): 865-880.

Coolen MW, Stirzaker C, Song JZ, et al. Consolidation of the cancer genome into domains of repressive chromatin by long-range epigenetic silencing (LRES) reduces transcriptional plasticity. Nat Cell Biol 2010;12(3):235–246.

Cozzarini C, Pelegrini D, Fallini M *et al.*: Reappraisal of the role of adjuvant radiotherapy in muscle-invasive transitional cell carcinoma of the bladder.Int. J. Radiat. Oncol. Biol. Phys.*1999;* 45:221.

Degtyar P, Neulander E, Zirkin H, et al. Fluorescence in situ hybridization performed on exfoliated urothelial cells in patients with transitional cell carcinoma of the bladder. Urology. 2004;63:398-401.

Dhar NB, Campbell SC, Zippe CD *et al.* Outcomes in patients with Urothelial carcinoma of the bladder with limited pelvic lymph node dissection. BJU Int. 2006; 98(6), 1172–1175.

El-Bolkainy MN, Mokhtar NM,. Ghonim MA, HusseinMH. The impact of schistosomiasis on the pathology of bladder carcinoma, Cancer; 1981;48: 2643–2648.

El-Mekresh MM, el-Baz MA, Abol-Enein H, Ghoneim MA. Primary adenocarcinoma of the urinary bladder: a report of 185 cases. Br J Urol. 1998 ;82(2):206-12.

El-Moneim HA, El-Baradie MM, Younis A, Ragab Y, Labib A, El-Attar I. A prospective randomized trial for postoperative vs. preoperative adjuvant radiotherapy for muscle-invasive bladder cancer. Urol Oncol 2011 Feb 24 [Epub ahead of print]

El-Said A, Omar S, Ibrahim AS. et al. Bilharzial bladder cancer in Egypt. A review of 420 cases of radical cystectomy. Jap J Clin Oncol 1979; 9: 117-122.

El-Sheikh SS, Madaan S, Alhasso A, Abel P, Stamp G, Lalani EN. Cyclooxygenase-2: a possible target in Schistosomaassociated bladder cancer, British Journal of Urology 2001;88:921–927.

Esteller M. Cancer epigenomics: DNA methylomes and histone-modification maps. *Nat Rev Genet.* 2007;8(4):286–298.

Fabarius A, Li R, Yerganian G, Hehlmann R, Duesberg P. Specific clones of spontaneously evolving karyotypes generate the individuality of cancer. Cancer Genet Cytogenet 2008;180: 89-99.

Fadl-Elmula I, Kytola S, Leithy ME, et al. Chromosomal aberrations in benign and malignant bilharzia-associated bladder lesions analyzed by comparative genomic hybridization. BMC Cancer 2002; 2:5.

Feinberg AP, Tycko B. The history of cancer epigenetics. Nat Rev Cancer 2004;4:143-53.

Ferguson A.R., Associated bilharziasis and primary malignant disease of the urinary bladder with observations on a series of forty cases, Journal of Pathology and Bacteriology 1911; 16:76–94.

Ferracin M, Veronese A, Negrini M. Micromarkers: miRNAs in cancer diagnosis and prognosis. Expert Rev Mol Diagn 2010;10:297-308.

Fried B, Reddy A, Mayer D. Helminths in human carcinogenesis. Cancer letters 2011; 305 (2): 239-249.

Gentile JM. Schistosome related cancers: a possible role for genotoxins, Environmental Mutagenesis 1985;7: 775–785.

Gersen SL, Keagle MB. Editors. The principles of clinical cytogenetics. 2nd ed. Totowa. NJ; Humama Press. 2005: 42-43.

Ghoneim MA, Ashamalla AG, Awwad HK, Whitmore WF Jr: Randomized trial of cystectomy with or without preoperative radiotherapy for carcinoma of the bilharzial bladder. J. Urol.1985; 134, 266–268.

Ghoneim MA, El-Mekresh MM, El-Baz MA, El-Attar IA, Ashamallah A. Radical cystectomy for carcinoma of the bladder: critical evaluation of the results in 1,026 cases. J Urol 1997;158:393-399.

Ghoneim MA, Abdel-Latif M, el-Mekresh M *et al.*: Radical cystectomy for carcinoma of the bladder: 2,720 consecutive cases 5 year later. *J. Urol.2008;* 180(1), 121–127.

Gibas Z, Gibas L. Cytogenetics of bladder cancer. Cancer Genetics Cytogenetics 1997;95:108–15.

Gouda I, Mokhtar N, Bilal D, El-Bolkainy T, El-Bolkainy NM. Bilharziasis and bladder cancer: a time trend analysis of 9843 patients. J Egypt Natl Canc Inst. 2007; 19(2):158-62.

Grady WM, Tewari M. The next thing in prognostic molecular markers: microRNA signatures of cancer. Gut 2010; 59:706-8.

Gschwend JE, Dahm P, Fair WR. Disease specific survival as endpoint of outcome for bladder cancer patients following radical cystectomy.Eur Urol. 2002 ; 41(4):440-8.

Gupta NP, Kolla SB, Seth A et al. Radical cystectomy for bladder cancer: A single center experience. Indian J Urol 2008; 24 (1): 54-59.

Hafner C, Knuechel R, Hartmann A, Clonality and multifocal Urothelial carcinoma: 10 years of molecular genetic studies. Int J Cancer 2002; 101: 1-5.

Heim S, Mitelman F. Cancer cytogenetics. 2nd edition. New York: Wiley-Liss Inc., 1995.

Ho CH, Huang CY, Lin WC *et al.*: Radical cystectomy in the treatment of bladder cancer: oncological outcome and survival predictors. J. Formos. Med. Assoc. 2009; 108(11), 872–878.

Hodder SL, Mahmoud AA, Sorenson K, et al. Predisposition to urinary tract epithelial metaplasia in Schistosoma haematobium infection. Am J Trop Med Hyg 2000;63:133-138.

Hoque MO, Lee CC, Cairns P, Schoenberg M, Sidransky D. Genome-wide geneticcharacterization of bladder cancer: a comparison of high-density single-nucleotide polymorphism arrays and PCR-based microsatellite analysis. *Cancer Res.* 2003;63:2216-2222.

Huncharek M, Muscat J, Geschwind JF: Planned preoperative radiation therapy in muscle invasive bladder cancer. Results of metaanalysis. Anticancer Res.1998: 18: 1931–1934.

IARC, Monograph on the evaluation of carcinogenic risks to humans: schistosomes, liver flukes and Helicobacter pylori, WHO: International Agency for Research on Cancer 1994; 61: 9-175.

Jacobs BL, Lee CT, Montie JE. Bladder cancer in 2010: how far have we come? CA Cancer J Clin. 2010;60(4):244-72.

Jemal A, Bray F, Center MM, Ferlay J, Ward E, Forman D. Global cancer statistics. CA Cancer J Clin 2011; 61: 69-90.

Jones PA, Baylin SB. The fundamental role of epigenetic events in cancer. Nat Rev Genet 2002;3:415-28.

Jones PA, Baylin SB. The epigenomics of cancer. *Cell.* 2007;128(4):683–692.

Jones TD, Wang M, Eble JN, et al Molecular evidence supporting field effect in urothelial carcinogenesis. Clin Cancer Res. 2005; 11(18):6512-9.

Kallioniemi A, Kallioniemi OP, Sudar D, Rutovitz D, Gray JW, Waldman F, Pinkel D. Comparative genomic hybridization for molecular cytogenetic
analysis of solid tumors. Science 1992;258: 818-821.

Kachnic LA, Kaufman DS, Heney NM, et al. Bladder preservation by combined modality therapy for invasive bladder cancer.J Clin Oncol. 1997 ; 15(3):1022-9.

Kendziorski C, Irizarry RA, Chen KS, Haag JD, Gould MN. On the utility of pooling biological samples in microarray experiments.Proc Natl Acad Sci U S A. 2005;102(12):4252-4257.

Khaled H, Zaghloul M, Ghoneim M, et al: Gemcitabine and cisplatin as neoadjuvant chemotherapy for invasive bladder cancer: Effect on bladder preservation and survival. Proc Am Soc Clin Oncol 2003; 22:411, (abstr 1652).

Khaled H, El-Hattab O, Moneim DA, Kassem HA, Morsi A, Sherif G: A prognostic index (bladder prognostic index) for bilharzial-related invasive bladder cancer. Urol. Oncol. 2005; 23, 254–260.

Koraitim MM, Metwalli NE, Atta MA, El-Sadr. Changing age incidence and pathological types of schistosoma-associated bladder carcinoma. J Urol 1995;154: 1714-1716.

Kuper H, Adami HO, Trichopoulos D. Infections as a major preventable cause of human cancer. J Intern Med 2000; 248: 171-83

Loeb K and Loeb I. The significance of multiple mutation in tumor. Carcinogenesis. 2000;21: 379-385.

Lokeshwar VB, Habuchi T, Grossman HB, et al. Bladder tumor markers beyond cytology: International Consensus Panel on bladder tumor markers. Urology. 2005; 66:35-63.

Lopez-Beltran A, Cheng L. Histologic variants of Urothelial carcinoma: differential diagnosis and clinical implications. Hum Paththol 2006; 37: 1371-1388.

Lughezzani G, Sun M, Jeldres C *et al.*: Adenocarcinoma versus urothelial carcinoma of the urinary bladder: comparison between pathologic stage at radical cystectomy and cancer-specific mortality. *Urology 2010;* 75(2):376–381.

Madersbacher S, Hochreiter W, Burkhard F, et al. Radical cystectomy for bladder cancer today: a homogeneous series without neoadjuvant therapy. J Clin Oncol 2003;21:690-696.

Makhyoun NA., El-Kashlan KM, Al-Ghorab MM, Mokhles AS. Aetiological factors in bilharzial bladder cancer, Journal of Tropical Medicine and Hygiene 1971; 74: 73–78.

Manoharan M, Ayyathurai R, Soloway MS: Radical cystectomy for urothelial carcinoma of the bladder: an analysis of perioperative and survival outcome. BJU Int. 2009; 104(9), 1227–1232.

Marletta MA. Mammalian synthesis of nitrite, nitrate, nitric oxide, and nnitrosating agents. *Chem Res Toxicol* 1988; 1: 249–57.

McConkey DJ, Lee S, Choi W, et al. Molecular genetics of bladder cancer: Emerging mechanisms of tumor initiation and progression. Urol Oncol. 2010; 28(4):429-40.

Ministry of Health and Population, Egypt, Department of Endemic Diseases, Prevalence of schistosomiasis in Egypt over time, 2004.

Muscheck M, Abol-Enein H, Chew K, Moore D 2nd, Bhargava V, Ghoneim MA, Carroll PR, Waldman FM. Comparison of genetic changes in schistosome-related transitional and squamous bladdercancers using comparative genomic hybridization. Carcinogenesis 2000; 21:1721-1726.

Nielsen ME, Gonzalgo ML, Schoenberg MP, Getzenberg RH. Toward critical evaluation of the role(s) of molecular biomarkers in the management of bladder cancer. *World J Urol.* 2006; 24:499-508.

Nishiyama H, Habuchi T, Watanabe J, Teramukai S, Tada H, Ono Y, Ohshima S, Fujimoto K, Hirao Y, Fukushima M, Ogawa O. Clinical outcome of a large-scale multi-institutional retrospective study for locally advanced bladder cancer: a survey including 1131 patients treated during 1990-2000 in Japan. Eur Urol 2004;45: 176-181.

Niu HT, Xu T, Zhang YB et al.: Outcomes for a large series of radical cystectomies for bladder cancer. Eur. J. Surg. Oncol. 2008; 34(8), 911–915.

Ploeg M, Aben KK, Hulsbergen-van de Kaa CA *et al.*: Clinical epidemiology of nonurothelial bladder cancer: analysis of The Netherlands Cancer Registry. *J. Urol.*2010; 183(3), 915–920.

Reisinger S, Mohiuddin M, Mulholland S: Combined pre- and post-operative adjuvant radiation therapy for bladder cancer - a ten year experience. Int. J. Radiat. Oncol. Biol.Phys. 1992; 24: 463–468.

Rödel C. Current status of radiation therapy and combined-modality treatment for bladder cancer. Strahlenther Onkol. 2004 ;180(11):701-9.

Rogers CG, Palapattu GS, Shariat SF *et al.*: Clinical outcomes following radical cystectomy for primary nontransitional cell carcinoma for the bladder compared with transitional cell carcinoma of the bladder. *J. Urol.*2006; 175: 2048–2053

Rosin MP, Saad el Din Zaki S, Ward AJ, Anwar WA. Involvement of inflammatory reactions and elevated cell proliferation in the development of bladder cancer in schistosomiasis patients. *Mutat Res* 1994; 305 : 83– 92.

Ross AGP, BartlyPB, Sleigh AC, et al. Schistosomiasis. N Engl J Med, 2002; 346(16): 1212-1220.

Ruggeri EM, Giannarelli D, Bria E et al. Adjuvant chemotherapy in muscle-invasive bladder cancer: a pooled analysis from phase III studies. Cancer 2006; 106:783-788.

Sabaa MA, El-Gamal OM, Abo-Elenen M, Khanam A. Combined modality treatment with bladder preservation for muscle invasive bladder cancer. Urol. Oncol. 2010; 28, 14–20.

Sandberg AA. The chromosomes in human cancer and leukemia. 2nd ed. New York. Elsevier, 1990.

Sandberg AA, Chen Z. Cytogenetic analysis. Methods Mol Med 2001; 55: 3-41

Sandberg AA, Meloni-Ehrig AM. Cytogenetics and genetics of human cancer: methods and accomplishments.Cancer Genet Cytogenet. 2010;203(2):102-26.

Sauer R, Birkenhake S, Kühn R, Wittekind C, Schrott KM, Martus P. Efficacy of radiochemotherapy with platin derivatives compared to radiotherapy alone in organ-sparing treatment of bladder cancer. Int J Radiat Oncol Biol Phys. 1998 ;40(1):121-7

Scosyrev E, Yao J, Messing E: Urothelial carcinoma versus squamous cell carcinoma of bladder: is survival different with stage adjustment? *Urology 2009;* 73: 822–827.

Shokeir AA. Squamous cell carcinoma of the bladder: pathology, diagnosis and treatment. *BJU Int* 2004; 93: 216–20.

Shariat SF, Karakiewicz PI, Palapattu GS. Outcomes of radical cystectomy for transitional cell carcinoma of the bladder: a contemporary series from the Bladder Cancer Research Consortium. J Urol. 2006 ;176(6):2414-22;

Shipley WU, Winter KA, Kaufman DS, et al. Phase III trial of neoadjuvant chemotherapy in patients with invasive bladder cancer treated with selective bladder preservation by combined radiation therapy and chemotherapy: initial results of Radiation Therapy Oncology Group 89-03. J Clin Oncol. 1998 ;16(11):3576-83

Smith JH, Christie JD. The pathobiology of Schistosoma haematobium infection in humans, Human Pathology 1986; 17: 333–345.

Smith JS, Costello JF. A broad band of silence. *Nat Genet.* 2006; 38(5):504–506.

Stein JP, Lieskovsky G, Cote R, et al. Radical cystectomy in treatment of invasive bladder cancer: long-term results in 1,054 patients. J Clin Oncol 2001; 19: 666-675.

Strohmeyer TG, Slamon DJ. Proto-oncogenes and tumor suppressor genes in human urological malignancies, Journal of Urology 1994;151: 479–1497.

Takahashi A, Tsukamoto T, Tobisu K *et al.*:Radical cystectomy for invasive bladdercancer, results of multi-institutional pooled analysis. *Jpn. J. Clin. Oncol. 2004;* 34: 14–19.

Teixeira MR. Recurrent fusion oncogenes in carcinomas. Crit Rev Oncogenesis 2006;12:257-71.

Tsutsumi M, Tsai YC, Gonzalgo ML, Nichols PW, Jones PA. Early acquisition of homozygous deletions of p16/p19 during squamous cell carcinogenesis and genetic mosaicism in bladder cancer. Oncogene 1998;17:3021-3027.

Tricker AR, Mostafa MH, Spiegelhalder B, Preussmann R. Urinary excretion of nitrate, nitrite and N-nitroso compounds in schistosomiasis and bilharzial bladder cancer patients, Carcinogenesis1989; 10 : 547–552.

Tester W, Porter A, Asbell S *et al.* Combined modality program with possible organ preservation for invasive bladder carcinoma: results of RTOG protocol 85–12. Int. J. Radiat. Oncol. Biol. Phys.1993; 25(5), 783–790.

Vale CL. Advanced Bladder Cancer Meta-analysis Collaboration. Adjuvant chemotherapy for invasive bladder cancer. Cochrane Database Syst Rev2006:CD006018.

van Rhijn BW, van der Poel HG, van der Kwast TH. Urine markers for bladder cancer surveillance: a systematic review. *Eur Urol.* 2005;47:736-748.

Vaughn DJ, Malkowicz SB. Neoadjuvant chemotherapy in patients with invasive bladder caner. Urol Clin North Am. 2005; 32: 231-237.

Vauhkonen H, Bohling T, Eissa S, Shoman S, Knuutila S. Can bladder adenocarcinomas be distinguished from schistosomiasisassociated bladder cancer by using comparative genomic hybridization analysis? Cancer Genet Cytogenet 2007;177:153-157.

Wang N. Methodologies in cancer cytogenetics and molecular cytogenetics. Am J Med Genet 2002;115:118-24.

Wijnhoven BPL, Michael MZ, Watson DI. MicroRNAs and cancer.Br J Surg 2007;94:23-30Winquist E, Kichner TS, Segal R et al. Neoadjuvant chemotherapy for transitional cell carcinoma of the bladder: a systematic review and meta-analysis. J Urol 2004; 171: 561-569.

Wu XR. Urothelial tumorigenesis: a tale of divergent pathway. Nat Rev Cancer 2005;5: 713-725.

Yunis JJ, Soreng AL. Constitutive fragile sites and cancer. Science 1984;226:1199–204.

Zaratiegui M, Irvine DV, Martienssen RA. Noncoding RNAs and gene silencing. *Cell.* 2007;128(4):763–776.

Zarzour AH, Selim M, Abd-Elsayed AA, Hameed DA, Abdelaziz MA. Muscle invasive bladder cancer in Upper Egypt: the shift in risk factors and tumor characteristics. BMC Cancer 2008; 8: 250-255.

Zaghloul MS: Radiation as adjunctive therapy to cystectomy for bladder cancer.Is there a difference for bilharzial association? *Int. J. Radiat. Oncol. Biol. Phys.*1994; 28: 783.

Zaghloul, M.S.,: Distant metastasis from bilharzial bladder cancer. Cancer 77: 743-749, 1996.

Zaghloul MS : Adjuvant radiation therapy for locally advanced bladder cancer. Touchbriefings, US oncological disease 2006 issue 2, 86-9.

Zaghloul MS. Adjuvant and neoadjuvant radiotherapy for bladder cancer: revisited. Future Oncol. 2010; 6(7):1177-1191.

Zaghloul MS, Mousa AG. Trimodality treatment for bladder cancer: does modern radiotherapy improve the end results? Expert Rev Anticancer Ther. 2010 ;10(12):1933-44

Zaghloul MS, Awwad HK, Omar S *et al.*: Postoperative radiotherapy of carcinoma in bilharzial bladder. Improved disease-free survival through improving local control. Int.J. Radiat. Oncol. Biol. Phys.1992; 22: 511–517.

Zaghloul MS, Mohran TZ, Saber RA, Agha N: Postoperative radiotherapy in bladder cancer. J. Egypt. Nat. Cancer Inst.2002; 14: 161–168.

Zaghloul MS, Nouh A, Nazmy M, Ramzy S, Zaghloul A, Sedira MA, Khalil E. Long-term results of primary adenocarcinoma of the urinary bladder: a report on 192 patients. Urol Oncol 2006; 24:13-20.

Zaghloul MS, El Baradie Nouh MA, Abdel-Fatah S, Taher A and Shalaan M. Prognostic index for primary adenocarcinoma of the urinary bladder. Gulf J Oncol 2007. 1 (2), 47- 54.

Zaghloul MS, Nouh A, Moneer M, El-Baradie M, Nazmy M, Younis A. Time-trend in epidemiological and pathological features of schistosoma-associated bladder cancer. J Egypt Natl Canc Inst. 2008 ;20(2):168-74..

Part 5

Non-Muscle Invasive Disease

11

Hemocyanins in the Immunotherapy of Superficial Bladder Cancer

Sergio Arancibia[1], Fabián Salazar[1] and María Inés Becker[1,2]
[1]*Fundación Ciencia y Tecnología para el Desarrollo (FUCITED)*
[2]*Biosonda Corporation*
[1,2]*Chile*

1. Introduction

Chemo- and immunotherapeutic approaches have been used to prevent recurrence of transitional cell carcinoma (TCC), the most common type of superficial bladder cancer (SBC). The bacillus Calmette-Guérin (BCG) vaccine for tuberculosis, which consists of an attenuated form of *Mycobacterium bovis*, is the most commonly used immunotherapeutic agent (Morales et al., 1976). Despite the successful results achieved with BCG, its serious side effects have led researchers to investigate other immunostimulatory substances. In the early 1970s, Olsson and collaborators reported that subcutaneous stimulation with keyhole limpet hemocyanin (KLH) from the Californian marine gastropod *Megathura crenulata* significantly reduced SBC recurrence frequency in TCC patients without any toxic side effects, making it ideal for long-term repetitive treatments (Olsson et al., 1974). These results provided promising support for the use of mollusk hemocyanins as alternative agents in SBC immunotherapy.

Hemocyanins, blue respiratory glycoproteins that were discovered in 1878 by Léon Fredericq (Ghiretti-Magaldi & Ghiretti, 1992), are found freely dissolved in the blood of some mollusks and arthropods. These proteins are giant structures with molecular weights between 4 and 8 MDa, and they exhibit some of the most complex and sophisticated quaternary structures known. Hemocyanins are part of the type-3 group of copper proteins that includes phenoloxidases and tyrosinases (Decker & Tuczek, 2000). These proteins contain active copper-containing sites in which the Cu(I,I) state is oxidized to the Cu(II,II) state, thus accounting for their distinctive deep blue color. Because of these properties, the biochemistry of hemocyanins has been intensively studied (van Holde & Miller, 1995). The pioneering work of Weigle in the 1960s on the immunochemical properties of KLH demonstrated its remarkable immunostimulatory properties in an experimental animal model (Weigle, 1964). These results were quickly incorporated into clinical studies to evaluate its immunological effects.

Because the primary amino acid sequences of mollusk hemocyanins are highly divergent from mammalian sequences, they are strongly recognized by the immune system, resulting in potent immunogenicity; these proteins can be used therapeutically as non-specific immunostimulants with beneficial clinical outcomes. Moreover, hemocyanins have been extensively used as carriers to generate antibodies against diverse hapten molecules and peptides and to induce antigen-specific CD8+ and CD4+ T cell responses (Harris & Markl, 1999). Currently, hemocyanins are used as carrier-adjuvants for several tumor-associated antigens (TAAs), such as glycolipid and glycoprotein (mucin-like) antigens, in experimental therapeutic vaccines against certain cancers, including melanomas, sarcomas, breast, prostate, ovary and lung (Musselli et al., 2001; Schumacher, 2001; Zhu et al., 2009; Del Campo et al., 2011). Other therapeutic strategies that use hemocyanins include dendritic cell (DC) vaccines pulsed with tumor lysates to enhance interferon gamma (IFN-γ) production by tumor-reactive T cells (Timmerman & Levy, 2000; Shimizu et al., 2001; Millard et al., 2003; Lopez et al., 2009; Jacobs et al., 2010; Lesterhuis et al., 2011) and anti-idiotype vaccines for some types of B cell malignancies (Leitch & Connors, 2005; Kafi et al., 2009). KLH has been the gold standard for these applications for over 40 years simply because it was used in earlier studies instead of other hemocyanins (Harris & Markl, 1999). The first studies used a research-grade KLH (non-GMP) containing different levels of endotoxin (Vandenbark et al., 1981); since then, several companies have produced clinical-grade KLH.

The versatile properties of KLH in biomedical and biotechnological applications have led to increasing commercial demand and growing interest in finding new, alternative hemocyanins with similar or more potent immunomodulatory properties. Although the KLH gene has been cloned, and its amino acid sequence is known, it has not been possible to express a heterologous protein, mainly because of its complex structure (Lieb et al., 2001; Markl et al., 2001; Altenhein et al., 2002). Therefore, this protein can be obtained only from its natural source. Several hemocyanins from other species of mollusks have been studied biochemically and immunologically, including *Haliotis tuberculata* (HtH, Abalon) (Markl et al., 2001); *Helix vulgarix* (HpH, Vineyard snail), *Rapana venosa* (RvH, Asian rapa whelk), and *Rapana thomasiana* (RtH, Black sea murex) (Dolashka-Angelova et al., 2003; 2008; 2010); and *Concholepas concholepas* (CCH, Loco), which is found on the pacific Chilean coast (De Ioannes et al., 2004). Only CCH has been pre-clinically evaluated in a murine experimental model of SBC and may be considered a safe alternative therapy (Moltedo et al., 2006; Atala, 2006). Although KLH and CCH have different origins and structure they have similar immunostimulatory capacities, suggesting that a conserved pattern common to both hemocyanins induces an ancient immunological mechanism (Moltedo et al., 2006). Interestingly, we have described a new hemocyanin from *Fissuerella latimarginata* (FLH) that exhibits higher immunogenicity than either CCH or KLH, opening a new avenue for research on the use of hemocyanins (Espinoza et al., 2006; Arancibia et al., 2010).

Notwithstanding the biomedical interest in mollusk hemocyanins, the molecular and cellular bases of their adjuvant/immunostimulatory capacity in SBC remain poorly understood. Currently, we know that hemocyanins are able to drive the differentiation of T helper (Th) cells toward a Th1 phenotype, characterized by increased secretion of IFN-γ and the production of IgG2a isotype antibodies (Moltedo et al., 2006).

In this chapter, we will review what is currently known about the experimental and clinical uses of mollusk hemocyanins as non-specific immunostimulants to prevent SBC recurrence, including the details of their intricate structure and the immunologic mechanisms that have been proposed to explain their antitumor activity.

2. Structure of the mollusk hemocyanins

Because of their enormous size, mollusk hemocyanins are easily observed by transmission electron microscopy (TEM) using negative staining. These molecules have a cylindrical form with an external diameter of approximately 350 nm and length of approximately 400 nm. Fig. 1 shows the characteristic appearance of gastropod hemocyanins under TEM.

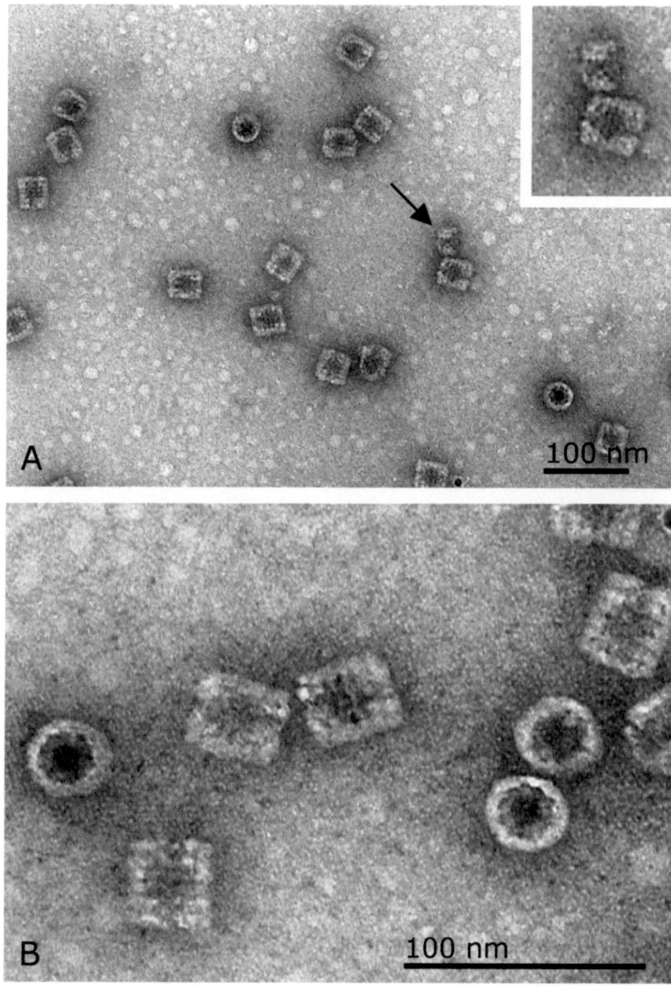

Fig. 1. Electron microscopy of negatively stained *C. concholepas* hemocyanin molecules. **A.** Low magnification micrographs of a preparation of the protein showing their characteristic hollow cylinder form. The images show the top (circles) and lateral (rectangles) views of the molecule. The arrow shows a decamer. **B.** High magnification images of hemocyanin molecules showing their intricate structure. The side views show the proteins' characteristic didecameric form with subunits arranged in layers.

Many experimental studies on hemocyanins, using different dissociation and association conditions and physicochemical and biochemical methods, have helped to elucidate their hierarchically organized structure (van Holde & Miller, 1995; Harris & Markl, 1999). As shown in Fig. 2, the basic structure of hemocyanins is composed of ten subunits that are self-assembled into a hollow cylinder, a structure known as a decamer, with a lumen that is narrowed by a complex collar (Harris et al., 1993; Cuff et al., 1998; Decker et al., 2007). In gastropods, the decamers can self-associate face-to-face to form stable dimers or didecamers, which display an intricate internal arrangement and result in the formation of extremely large structures with approximate D5 symmetry (Orlova et al., 1997). Hemocyanin subunits have a molecular weight ranging from 350 to 450 kDa and are composed of a string of seven or eight globular domains called functional units (FUs), each with a molecular weight between 35 and 50 kDa. These FUs are connected by a short flexible linker peptide strand of 10 to 15 amino acid residues. Each FU has two well-separated copper atoms that reversibly capture O_2 molecules; one is called the A site, which is located towards the N-terminus, and the other is called the B site and is located downstream of the polypeptide (van Holde et al., 2001).

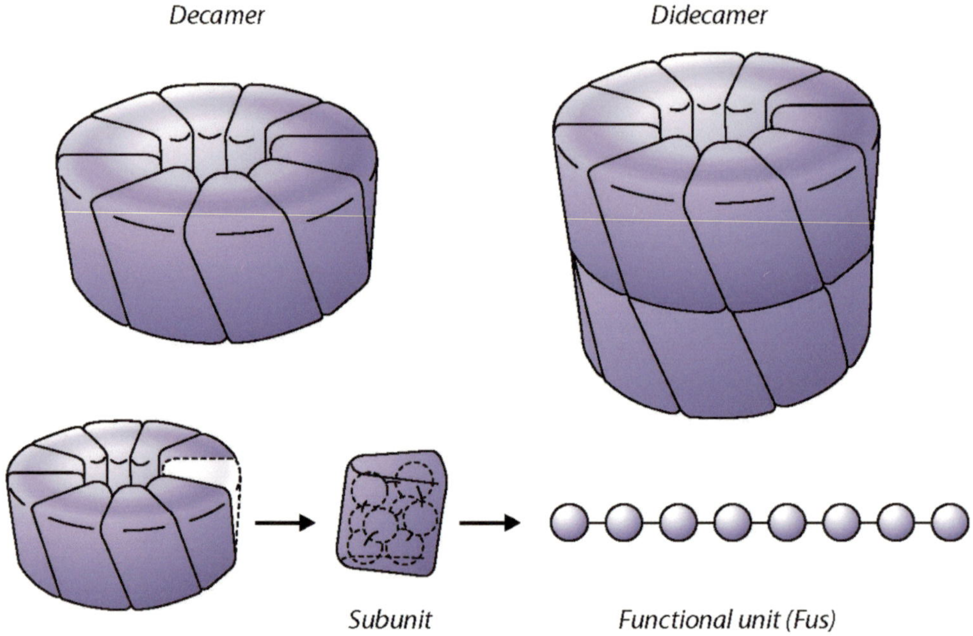

Fig. 2. Model of the structure of mollusk hemocyanin. The basic structure of a mollusk hemocyanin is a decamer, which is formed by the association of 10 polypeptides or subunits. In hemocyanins from some species of mollusk, such as gastropods, including KLH and CCH, the decamers are associated in pairs to form very large molecules called didecamers. The subunit consists of seven or eight globular domains linked by a peptide spacer consisting of 10 to 15 amino acid residues, similar to a pearl necklace. Each of these globular domains has a pair of copper atoms that reversibly bind one oxygen molecule, which is why they are called functional units.

Knowledge of the carbohydrate moieties present in mollusk hemocyanins has been essential for understanding their organization, antigenicity and biomedical properties (Paccagnella et al., 2004; Siddiqui et al., 2007). In fact, several authors have reported that hemocyanin carbohydrates may play a role in their immunostimulatory effects. The high carbohydrate content of hemocyanins, up to 9% (w/w), has been measured by different methods, including the use of lectins and high-pressure liquid chromatography-tandem mass spectrometry (HPLC-MS/MS). The presence of numerous N-glycosylation sites and a reduced number of O-glycosylation sites has been established (Dolashka-Angelova et al., 2003; Gielens et al., 2004; Idakieva et al., 2004; Gatsogiannis & Markl, 2009; Dolashka et al., 2010). Mollusk hemocyanins contain diverse sugar moieties, including mannose, D-galactose, fucose, N-acetyl-D-galactosamine and N-acetyl-glucosamine residues, with mannose being the most abundant (Harris & Markl, 1999). Hemocyanins also contain monosaccharides that are not usually found in animal proteins, such as xylose (Lommerse et al., 1997).

2.1 KLH and CCH

Although KLH and CCH each have two subunits that constitute the basic structure known as a decamer, closer analysis revealed unique differences. Native gel electrophoresis has shown that KLH is made up of two different non-covalently linked subunits called KLH1 (350 KDa) and KLH2 (350 KDa) that do not display shared epitopes (Swerdlow et al., 1996). Using the same approach, it was demonstrated that CCH is also made up of two different subunits, CCHA (405 kDa) and CCHB (350 kDa), that contain common and specific epitopes (Oliva et al., 2002; De Ioannes et al., 2004). In KLH, the subunits form homodidecamers (i.e., the molecules are formed from either KLH1 or KLH2 subunits). However, in CCH the subunits form heterodidecamers (i.e., the molecules are formed by pairing the two different subunits). In addition, purified KLH requires divalent cations in storage buffers to maintain the stability of its quaternary structure, whereas CCH does not (De Ioannes et al., 2004); this is probably a consequence of the higher hydrophobicity of CCH (Leyton et al., 2005). Despite these differences, the immunogenic properties of CCH and KLH are similar. CCH has been successfully used as a carrier protein to generate antibodies against hapten molecules and peptides (Becker et al., 1998; Torres et al., 1999; Mura et al., 2002; Duvillie et al., 2003; Manosalva et al., 2004; Cancino et al., 2007; Gravotta et al., 2007; Matus et al., 2007; Grenegard et al., 2008); as a carrier in vaccines (Miller et al., 2006; Mauldin & Miller, 2007; Pilon et al., 2007) and as an experimental antigen (Becker et al., 2007; Moltedo et al., 2009).
Several studies have demonstrated that KLH contains approximately 3.2% (w/w) carbohydrate residues, displaying specific structural motifs on N-glycans, such as Fuc(alpha1-3)GalNAc, Gal-(beta1-6)Man-, Gal(beta1-4)Fuc-, and Gal(beta1-4)Gal(beta(1-4)Fuc-, which are thought to contribute to its non-specific immunostimulatory capacities in SBC (Wuhrer et al., 2004). Our knowledge of the corresponding oligosaccharide composition of CCH is very limited. However, we have demonstrated using selective glycosidase treatments and electrophoretic analysis that sugar moieties account for 3.1% (w/w) of the mass of CCH. A comparative analysis using lectin staining indicated that mannose is the only exposed carbohydrate common to CCH and KLH (Becker et al., 2009). It is important to note that, despite the differences in carbohydrate composition between KLH and CCH, both proteins have similar immunogenicity and immunotherapeutic capacity in SBC, suggesting that other factors are responsible for this effect. We assume that the primary structure of these proteins contains the determining factor because they share regions of high sequence homology (van Holde et al., 2001; Manubens et al., 2010). These regions were confirmed in antibody cross-reactivity experiments that revealed the presence of common or mimetic epitopes in CCH and KLH (Oliva et al., 2002).

3. Use of hemocyanins in experimental SBC

Rats and various strains of mice have been used as *in vivo* SBC models to evaluate therapeutic agents because bladder tumors in these rodents have similarities with human tumors. In addition, tumor cells can be established subcutaneously (heterotopically) or in the bladder (orthotopically) by either transplantation or chemical induction, allowing the investigation of clinical aspects such as pharmacokinetics and toxicity (Gunther et al., 1999; Linn et al., 2000; Arentsen et al., 2009).

The first controlled study of a hemocyanin as immunotherapy in the treatment of superficial bladder cancer was published in the 1980s by the Lamm group (Lamm et al., 1981). They developed the mouse bladder tumor-2 cell (MBT-2) transplantable murine model of SBC and demonstrated that pre-immunization with 200 µg of KLH three weeks prior to subcutaneous injection with MBT-2, followed by intralesional immunotherapy with 50 µg one and seven days after inoculation, resulted in a significant reduction in tumor growth and a prolongation of animal survival. Later, other studies by the same researchers evaluated non-specific immunotherapeutic regimens (Lamm et al., 1982). Animals received an intradermal MBT-2 inoculation, and the immunotherapy was administered intralesionally one day after tumor transplantation. Tumors were excised at a volume of 400 mm^3, and the animals were re-challenged with tumor cells, treated again, and followed for tumor incidence, growth rate and survival. This study demonstrated that KLH had a weak antitumor effect compared with the response to BCG. In 1986, Lau and collaborators studied the same response, this time comparing intraperitoneal and intralesional administration of the agents. C3H/He mice were injected subcutaneously with 5×10^4 tumor cells. After that, the mice received either intraperitoneal or intralesional treatments (50 µg KLH); these experiments demonstrated that the intralesional route was more effective than intraperitoneal administration for tumor growth inhibition (Lau et al., 1986).

Lamm´s group also evaluated the possible additive and/or synergistic effects of KLH immunotherapy in the MBT-2 model in conjunction with other treatments, such as IFN-α. Tumor cells were transplanted subcutaneously without prior immunization. Treatment was given intraperitoneally twice weekly for three weeks, except for BCG, which was administered once a week. Significant reductions in tumor incidence relative to the controls were observed in groups receiving KLH (42%), IFN-α (42%) and KLH + IFN-α (17%) (Riggs et al., 1992). The following year, the same group compared two alternative immunotherapies in the MBT-2 model: crude KLH and Immucothel, a clinical-grade KLH from Biosyn Arzneimittel GmbH. Mice were sensitized with 50 or 100 µg KLH, and 21 days later, 10^3 tumor cells were injected. Intralesional treatment with 50 or 100 µg KLH was performed on days 1, 7 and 13 or 14. Crude KLH required either immunization before tumor transplant or frequent therapy after transplantation to be effective. In addition, Immucothel required pre-immunization to be effective, even with an increased frequency and dosage of the post-transplant immunizations. In a subsequent study, the endotoxin contamination of KLH was demonstrated to be partly responsible for the antitumor activity because treatment with endotoxin alone resulted in a significant reduction of tumor growth and mortality (50% survival) (Lamm et al., 1993). Moreover, KLH + 100 Endotoxin Units (EU) resulted in complete inhibition of tumor growth and 100% survival. KLH + 1000 EU appeared to reduce the antitumor response (50% survival), suggesting that endotoxin may interfere with the response to purified KLH. Finally, endotoxin-free KLH induced antitumor responses (50% survival). However, pre-immunization was required for KLH to exert a significant (75% survival) antitumor effect (Lamm et al., 1993).

Walsh and collaborators studied KLH immunotherapy in two different models with no promising results. First, they transplanted 2.5×10^6 MBT-2 tumor cells subcutaneously after pre-immunization 20 days prior. Treatment was given on days 1, 8 and 18 in the form of subcutaneous or intralesional injection of 50 μg KLH. The results showed no difference between the control and treated groups in terms of either tumor growth or animal survival. Alternatively, they transplanted 2.1 x 10^6 MBT-2 tumor cells into the bladder of C3H/He mice. The bladder was irrigated with 1.5 mg N-methyl-N-nitrosourea 48 hours prior. The treatment group was injected with 50 μg KLH on day 1, and the bladders were instilled with 200 μg KLH on days 14 and 21. There was no significant difference from the control group (Walsh et al., 1983). Using a similar model, Marsh and collaborators demonstrated that intravesical immunotherapy with *Corynebacterium parvum* and *Allium sativum* was more effective than KLH and slightly more effective than BCG. MBT-2 cells were delivered into the bladder transurethrally using a small catheter, and the immunotherapy was administered directly into the bladder via this catheter on day 1 or day 6, or both. The authors associated the lack of a significant effect with inappropriate dosage or insufficient stimulation of the immune system (Marsh et al., 1987). Later, the antitumor activity and potential toxicity of a clinical grade KLH preparation named KLH-Immune Activator (KLH-IA) was examined. Mice were immunized subcutaneously with KLH-IA two weeks prior to intravesical implantation with 2 x 10^4 MB-49 tumor cells. Treatment consisted of intravesical KLH-IA (10 or 100 μg) 1, 4, 7, 14 and 21 days after implantation. By four weeks after implantation, tumor outgrowth in the treated groups was significantly decreased. Prior subcutaneous immunization was required to elicit the antitumor activity of KLH-IA. Animals treated with a dissociated form of KLH showed decreased tumor outgrowth, but this was not significant. A separate toxicity study in which KLH-IA was given subcutaneously (4 mg/kg), intraperitoneally (40 mg/kg) or intravesically (40 mg/kg) reported no significant gross or histopathological abnormalities, except for mild to moderate papillary hyperplasia in all catheterized animals (Swerdlow et al., 1994).

A third model developed by Recker and collaborators also showed the effectiveness of KLH. Bladder carcinoma was induced in Wistar rats using N-butyl-N-(4-hydroxybutyl) nitrosamine (BBN). Stimulation of the rats with 12.5 mg of KLH administered intravesically and 0.5 mg administered subcutaneously twice weekly after sensitization with 1 mg subcutaneous KLH resulted in a reduction in BBN-induced bladder tumors. These results confirmed that effective induction of an immune response is important for the control of tumor development because immune-suppressed rats treated with cyclosporine A (CsA) showed enhanced bladder tumor expansion compared with rats treated with 0.05% BBN alone (Recker & Rubben, 1989). A subsequent study distinguished between intravesical and subcutaneous application to determine the most effective treatment regime. Five weeks after the completion of tumor induction with 0.05% BBN solution, exophytic bladder tumors appeared in all control animals. In group 2, which was given KLH via intravesical instillation, tumors developed in 73.5% of cases. In group 1, with subcutaneous administration, tumors developed in only 50% of cases. The tumor growth was significantly slower in group 1 than group 2 (Linn et al., 2000).

The results described above demonstrated promising potential for the use of KLH in SBC therapy. More recently, preclinical studies have proven hemocyanin from *Concholepas concholepas* (CCH) to be a reliable alternative to KLH (Moltedo et al., 2006). C3H/He mice were primed with CCH before subcutaneous implantation of MBT-2 cells. Treatment consisted of a subcutaneous dose of CCH (1 mg or 100 μg) at different intervals after implantation. The results demonstrated a significant antitumor effect, as indicated by decreased tumor growth and incidence, prolonged survival and a lack of toxic effects. These results were similar to those achieved with KLH.

Model	Priming[1]	Via Administration	Therapeutic Dosage and Schedule[2]	Results	Reference
Mouse, MBT-2	Yes 200 µg	Intralesional	50 µg Days: 1 and 7.	Significant reduction of tumor growth and survival with KLH.	Lamm et al.1981
	No	Intralesional	Day: 1	KLH presented a minor antitumor effect compared with BCG.	Lamm et al. 1982
	Yes	Subcutaneous or intralesional	50 or 200 µg Days: 1, 8 and 18 or 1, 14 and 21.	KLH do not show difference with controls in tumor growth or animal survival.	Walsh et al. 1983
	No	Intraperitoneal v/s intralesional	50 µg	Intralesional route of inoculation of KLH was more effective.	Lau et al. 1986
	No	Intravesical	50 µg Days: 1 or 6, or both.	Immunotherapy with *C. parvum* and *A. sativum* was more effective than KLH.	Marsh et al.1987
	No	Intraperitoneal	50 µg Twice weekly for 3 weeks.	Better response in the animals treated with KLH more INF-α.	Riggs et al. 1992
	Yes 50 or 100 µg	Intralesional	50 or 100 µg Days: 1, 7 and 13 or 14.	Required pre-immunization of KLH and Immucothel to be effective.	Lamm et al. 1993a
	Yes 50 or 100 µg	Intralesional	50 or 100 µg Days: 1, 7 and 13 or 14.	Endotoxin contamination of KLH was responsible in part for the antitumor activity.	Lamm et al. 1993b
	Yes 200 to 400 µg	Subcutaneous	1 mg Days: 1 to 6 or 100 µg Days: 1, 3, 5, 7 and 9.	Significant reduction of tumor growth and survival with CCH.	Moltedo et al. 2006
	Yes 200 µg	Subcutaneous	100 µg Days: 1, 3, 5, 7 and 9.	Better antitumor effect with CCHA subunit than CCHB subunit.	Becker et al. 2009
Mouse, MB-49	Yes 100 µg	Intravesical	10 or 100 µg Days: 1, 4, 7, 14 and 21.	Prior immunization of KLH-IA was required to elicit antitumor activity.	Swerdlow et al. 1994
Rats, tumor induction with BBN[3]	Yes 1 mg	Intravesical and subcutaneous	12.5 mg and 500 µg Twice weekly.	Reduction of bladder tumors with KLH.	Recker et al. 1989
	Yes 1 mg	Intravesical v/s subcutaneous	500 µg Twice weekly for 8 weeks.	Subcutaneous route of KLH was more effective than intravesical route.	Linn et al. 2000

[1] Priming: Usually, around two weeks prior to tumor challenge. [2] Immunotherapy after tumor transplantation. [3] BNN: N-butyl-N-(4-hydroxybutyl) nitrosamine

Table 1. Preclinical studies in different animal models of SBC with KLH or CCH as an immunotherapeutic agent.

Later, the individual contributions of the CCHA and CCHB subunits of CCH as immunotherapeutic agents in the same bladder cancer model were studied. C3He/He mice were subcutaneously primed with CCHA or CCHB; whole CCH and PBS were used as positive and negative controls, respectively. After day 15, mice were challenged with a subcutaneous injection of 2 x 10^5 MBT-2 cells, and the antitumor treatment was started; treatment consisted of a subcutaneous dose of either subunit or a control on alternate days for 9 days. Surprisingly, either subunit alone showed an antitumor effect in the MBT-2 model. However, the tumor incidence was lower in animals treated with CCHA (44% incidence) than with CCHB (60% incidence) or whole CCH (62.5% incidence). Moreover, the survival probability increased in mice under immunotherapy with CCHA (69.5%) compared with CCHB- (64%), CCH- (60%) and PBS-treated (46.5%) mice. In conclusion, this study indicated that the CCHA subunit accounts for the most important immunogenic effects of CCH (Becker et al., 2009). Together, these preclinical studies (summarized in Table 1) demonstrated that hemocyanins have beneficial effects in animal models of SBC that resemble human disease without the negative side effects of BCG (Schenkman & Lamm, 2004).

4. Use of hemocyanins in clinical studies of SBC

Surgical procedures such as transurethral resection (TUR) are commonly used as the first option to treat SBC. However, there are some tumors that must be treated by other strategies, due to the difficulties of fully removing them and the high risk of recurrence. Thus, intravesical administration of chemotherapeutic and biological agents has been demonstrated to be an effective method in the early stages of the disease, either to treat an existing tumor or to prevent recurrence and tumor progression after TUR (Perabo & Muller, 2004). BCG is one biological therapy that is used as a non-specific immunostimulant to treat several malignant tumors (Edwards & Whitwell, 1974; Milas & Withers, 1976), including SBC (Morales et al., 1976). BCG has become the first-line treatment and the most effective intravesical immunotherapy, lowering the risk of recurrence to an average of 27% of cases (Nseyo & Lamm, 1997). Despite these successful results, BCG therapy causes numerous side effects, such as dysuria, urinary frequency, cystitis (90% of cases), hematuria and, in rare cases, sepsis, indicating the need for new approaches that provide the same or a better response without toxic effects (Lamm, 2003).

In a 1974 delayed-type hypersensitivity (DTH) experiment to measure the immune competence of patients with TCC, Olson and collaborators reported the unexpected result that patients subcutaneously primed with 5 mg of KLH and then subcutaneous immunized with 200 μg of KLH had a significantly diminished tumor recurrence rate over a study period of two years. Those patients that were DTH positive to KLH, and therefore immune competent, had almost no recurrences (Olsson et al., 1974). This outstanding effect was confirmed many years later in a controlled study of patients in stages Ta and T1 who had previously been subject to TUR. In this study, the ability of KLH to prevent tumor recurrence was compared to mitomycin C (MMC). The patients were subcutaneously immunized with 1 mg of KLH and then received monthly intravesical administrations of 10 mg of KLH. Only 14% of the patients treated with KLH had recurrences, in contrast to the MMC patients, 39% of whom reported recurrences, demonstrating that KLH was significantly more effective than MMC (Jurincic et al., 1988).

A prospective randomized trial compared the effects of ethoglucid and KLH in patients who were unresponsive to the chemotherapeutic treatments, doxorubicin or MMC. The recurrence rate and the tumor progression rate for the two therapies showed no statistical differences (Flamm et al., 1990). Wishahi et al., reported that the incidence of recurrence in patients with TCC associated with urinary schistosomiasis was 15% after KLH treatment compared with 77% before therapy (Wishahi et al., 1995). This result was similar to the results obtained by Olson et al., (1974) and Jurincic et al., (1998) confirming the outstanding immunotherapeutic properties of KLH (Olsson et al., 1974; Jurincic et al., 1988). The efficacy of this treatment in patients with carcinoma *in situ* (CIS) grade 3 was studied in a long-term follow-up. The patients received an intravesical instillation of KLH weekly for 6 weeks, monthly for 1 year and bimonthly for the following 2 years. Patients who were unresponsive to KLH were treated with BCG. CIS long-term remission was observed only in a limited number of cases, and most cases progressed over time, indicating the aggressiveness of this disease (Jurincic-Winkler et al., 1995a). In Table 2, we summarize the clinical studies previously described.

Currently, Immucothel, a clinical-grade KLH preparation, is being evaluated in a Phase III clinical trial in Germany for its efficacy in SBC treatment (Biosyn). The Food and Drug Administration (FDA) has also authorized another Phase III trial to evaluate the efficacy and safety of KLH BCI-Immune Activator (Intracell, USA) versus doxorubicin in BCG refractory or intolerant patients with carcinoma *in situ*, with or without resected SBC. However, this study has been suspended.

The mechanism associated with the immunotherapeutic effect of KLH in this disease is still poorly understood. However, there are immunohistological studies on biopsies of TCC patients treated with KLH that show strong cellular activation characterized by the infiltration of large numbers of mononuclear cells and CD4+ lymphocytes, and to a lesser extent, CD8+ T cells and granulocytes, nine months after the beginning of therapy (Jurincic-Winkler et al., 1995b). This result suggests that the effect of KLH might be strongly related to a non-specific immunostimulation of the immune system leading to the development of an antitumor response.

5. Immunologic mechanisms involved in the immunotherapy of SBC with hemocyanins

Although hemocyanins are widely used as thymus-dependent model antigens, the relationship between the structure of hemocyanins and the molecular and cellular basis of their immunostimulatory capacity is still largely unknown. Investigations into the antitumor effect of hemocyanins in human and murine models of SBC have demonstrated a systemic activation of the immune response. In these experiments, priming with hemocyanins is crucial for the induction of antitumor activity (Lamm et al., 2000; Moltedo et al., 2006). This could partially explain why hemocyanins stimulate the immune system. In patients with TCC under intravesical KLH therapy, DTH reactions occur. As mentioned previously, studies on biopsies of TCC patients treated with KLH showed a higher increase in CD4+ cell infiltration than CD8+ T lymphocytes in the submucosa and urothelial cells (Jurincic-Winkler et al., 1995b). Currently, we know that such responses are characteristic of Th1 type responses, which mediate inflammatory functions critical for the development of cell-mediated immune responses (Szabo et al., 2003). Other investigations demonstrated that during immunization with KLH, the T CD4+ lymphocyte response showed a mixed profile of IL-4 and IFN-γ with an increase in T CD8+ cells in the lymphatic nodules (Doyle et al., 1998).

Patients	Control Group	Priming	Therapeutic Dosage and Schedule	Recurrence Rate	Reference
19	10	5 mg subcutaneous	200 μg Subcutaneous	11%	Olsson et al. 1974
44	23	1 mg subcutaneous	10 mg Intravesical, monthly for 21 months, approximately.	14%	Jurincic et al. 1988
84	46	1 mg subcutaneous	30 mg Intravesical, weekly for six weeks and then monthly for one year.	55%	Flamm et al. 1990
13	Own controls	1 mg subcutaneous for five days until DTH	10 mg Intravesical, for seven days.	15%	Wishashi et al. 1995
21	Own controls	No	20 mg Intravesical, weekly for six weeks and then monthly for one year or bimonthly for two years.	43% of patients presented long-term remission 57% had to be cystectomized because of CIS progression	Jurincic-Winkler et al. 1995a

Table 2. Clinical studies using KLH as an immunotherapeutic agent in SBC patients.

The fact that the non-specific immunotherapeutic effects of hemocyanins are not due to any super-antigen-like activity, but rather rely on adequate priming, strongly suggests that their therapeutic properties could be attributable to a bystander effect on the tumor due to either a loss of tolerance toward tumor antigens or an enhancement of the immune response to the tumor. This kind of response would favor a milieu that augments the antigen-specific activity of cytotoxic T lymphocytes (CTLs) and natural killer (NK) cell responses. These hypotheses are supported by the observation that IFN-γ and IL-2 are secreted in the regional lymph nodes in response to hemocyanin treatment (Gilliet et al., 2003; Verdijk et al., 2009). NK cells are strongly stimulated by IL-2 secreted by T lymphocytes, leading to their differentiation into lymphokine-activated killer cells (LAK) and increasing the destructive elements acting on tumor cells. It has been reported that

MBT-2 cells do not grow when they are injected into the bladders of mice treated with a combination of IL-2 and the cytotoxic agent cyclophosphamide (Ikemoto et al., 1997). Moreover, KLH has been shown to enhance NK cell activity and stimulate IFN-γ secretion in SBC patients (Molto et al., 1991). Our later results confirm these observations; mice treated with KLH or CCH increase NK cell activity and serum levels of IFN-γ (Moltedo et al., 2006). This is a very important result because, in primary tumors, IFN-γ is a tumor suppressor cytokine that coordinates T and NK cell activities (Kaplan et al., 1998). Indeed, it has been demonstrated that the depletion of NK cells abolishes the immunotherapeutic effect of BCG on bladder cancer in mice, confirming that these cells play a key role in the destruction of primary tumors (Brandau & Bohle, 2001).

In addition to the antitumor effect provided by the secretion of IFN-γ, NK cells can delay tumor growth by means of antibody-dependent cell-mediated cytotoxicity (ADCC), which induces effector cells to kill bladder tumor target cells. We have observed that, in the MBT-2 model, intralesional CCH or KLH induce an increase in the humoral immune response against cell surface tumor antigens in addition to the CCH or KLH antibody response. Biopsies taken from the surrounding bladder tissues in SBC patients treated with KLH showed an increase in the B lymphocyte population in the lymph follicles, suggesting that humoral mechanism are also involved in the immune response induced by hemocyanins (Jurincic-Winkler et al., 1995b).

Finally, the fact that the immunotherapeutic effects of KLH and CCH on bladder cancer do not require an adjuvant raises intriguing questions regarding the means by which hemocyanins initiate the non-specific anti-tumor immune response and which cells are involved. It is possible that hemocyanins interact with a putative receptor on the cell surface of antigen presenting cells, leading to their internalization and processing. A promising candidate was the mannose receptor because of the high levels of this sugar residue in KLH and CCH and the fact that this receptor is highly expressed in antigen presenting cells. However, experiments on endocytosis inhibition performed in human DCs cultured *in vitro* with an anti-mannose receptor antibody and KLH showed that while KLH incorporation by DCs was partially inhibited, KLH still promoted the activation and maturation of DCs as assessed by the up-regulation of the cell surface expression of Major Histocompatibility Complex (MHC) class II and co-stimulatory molecules (Presicce et al., 2008). In contrast, Teitz-Tennenbaum and collaborators (2008) demonstrated that murine DCs pulsed with KLH for 18 hours *in vitro* did not undergo DC maturation, a result that is consistent with *in vivo* experiments (Teitz-Tennenbaum et al., 2008; Moltedo et al., 2009) and our current results. We observed that DCs internalized (Fig. 3) but did not mature within 72 hours of culture *in vitro* with this protein

It is not known whether hemocyanins might be processed and presented by bladder tumor cells themselves, leading to the stimulation of the cytotoxic killer cell antitumor activity. Murine bladder tumor cells have been shown to be able to present BCG antigens to specific CD4+ T lymphocytes in a classic MHC Class II (Ia)-dependent fashion (Lattime et al., 1992). Experiments performed in our laboratory demonstrated that primary cultures of mouse bladder epithelial cells and MBT-2 cells cultured *in vitro* incorporate hemocyanin; however, we did not observe any changes in the expression pattern of MHC I and MHC II antigens (Del Campo et al., 2007). In addition, *in vitro* anti-cancer effects of KLH against breast, esophageal, prostate and pancreas cancer has been reported (Riggs et al., 2002), also in melanoma (Somasundar et al., 2005), however if this effect have an *in vivo* implication is unknown.

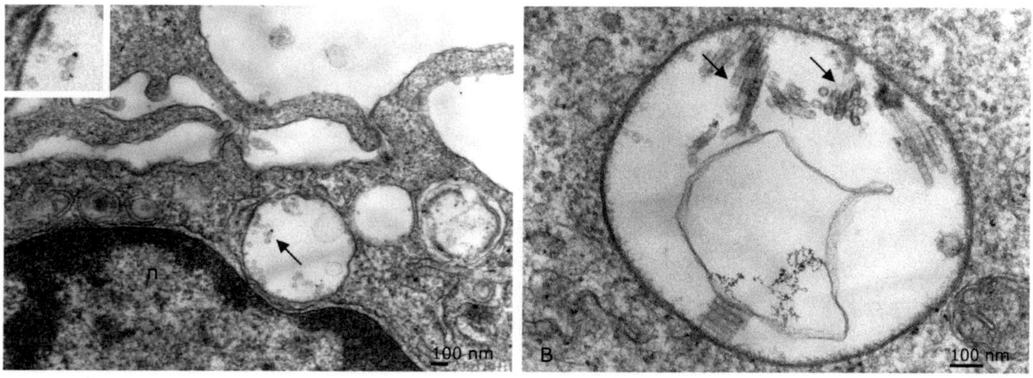

Fig. 3. Incorporation of *Concholepas* hemocyanin by mouse myeloid dendritic cells cultured *in vitro*, analyzed by transmission electron microscopy. Mouse myeloid DCs of 5th day of culture *in vitro* as described (Inaba et al., 1992), previously isolated by positive selection with immunomagnetic beads, and later culture with CCH during different times. **A.** Dendritic cell cultured during 30 minutes with CCH. The photograph shows its characteristic superficial membrane process, the nucleus (n), and hemocyanin molecules inside a clear vacuole (arrow) that resemble a primary lysosome. **B.** Because of the large size of CCH, and because of its peculiar structure as a hollow cylinder, we were able to identify the presence of whole hemocyanin molecules inside secondary lysosome like vesicles (arrows) containing membrane debris (Del Campo et al., 2007).

Macrophages are another potential cell type through which hemocyanins could initiate anti-tumor immune responses. Indeed, IL-1α, a pro-inflammatory cytokine produced by activated macrophages, has been shown to be increased in the urine after intravesical instillation with KLH in patients with SBC (Jurincic-Winkler et al., 1995c). Similarly, this cytokine, in addition to other pro-inflammatory cytokines, has been detected in the urine after BCG instillation along with an influx of mononuclear cells into the bladder (Teppema et al., 1992; Brandau & Bohle, 2001; Brandau et al., 2001).
In summary, considering that BCG is a whole organism, whereas KLH or CCH are single molecules, it is amazing that it induces a similar response. In both cases, however, it is not clear which cytokines and cells contribute directly to the anti-tumor activity and which represent a secondary phenomenon.

6. Conclusions

Hemocyanins have proven to be safe and useful in the immunotherapy and prophylaxis of patients with superficial bladder cancer who have failed or are intolerant to the current BCG therapy. Moreover, KLH has been shown to produce a more predictable reaction than BCG, eliminating the risk of further infections. Despite the fact that biomedical interest in mollusk hemocyanins goes back more than 40 years, the precise molecular and cellular mechanisms underlying the non-specific immunostimulatory capacities of KLH and, more recently, CCH, are poorly understood. The current evidence shows that these huge proteins can induce an inflammatory milieu and activate innate immunity, driving a vigorous antitumor adaptive immune response characterized by long-lasting HLA-DR+ cell infiltration into the bladder and the secretion of a Th1-type cytokine profile.

7. Acknowledgments

We thank Alfredo De Ioannes, Cristóbal Dünner and Augusto Manubens (Biosonda Corporation) and Miguel Del Campo, Pablo De Ioannes and Bruno Moltedo (Fundación Ciencia y Tecnología para el Desarrollo, FUCITED) for their valuable discussions during the course of this work. The authors are grateful to Gabriel De Ioannes for the mollusk hemocyanin structure model.
This study was partially supported by FONDECYT grant 1110651 (to María Inés Becker). Sergio Arancibia is a CONICYT (National Commission for Sciences and Technology of Chile) doctoral fellow.

8. References

Altenhein, B., Markl, J. & Lieb, B. (2002). Gene structure and hemocyanin isoform HtH2 from the mollusc *Haliotis tuberculata* indicate early and late intron hot spots. *Gene*, Vol.301, No.1-2: pp. 53-60, 0378-1119

Arancibia, S., Espinoza, C., Del Campo, M., Salazar, F. & Becker, M.I. (2010). Exceptional immunological and anticancer properties of a new hemocyanin from *Fissurella Latimarginata* (FLH). *Proceedings of International Society for Biological Therapy of Cancer*. Washington, USA. October, 2010

Arentsen, H.C., Hendricksen, K., Oosterwijk, E. & Witjes, J.A. (2009). Experimental rat bladder urothelial cell carcinoma models. *World J Urol*, Vol.27, No.3: pp. 313-317, 1433-8726

Atala, A. (2006). This month in investigative urology. *J Urol* 2006. *J Urol*, Vol.176, No.6 Pt 1: pp. 2335-2336, 0022-5347

Becker, M.I., Carrasco, I., Beltran, C., Torres, M., Jaureguiberry, B. & De Ioannes, A.E. (1998). Development of monoclonal antibodies to gizzerosine, a toxic component present in fish meal. *Hybridoma*, Vol.17, No.4: pp. 373-381, 0272-457X

Becker, M.I., De Ioannes, A.E., Leon, C. & Ebensperger, L.A. (2007). Females of the communally breeding rodent, *Octodon degus*, transfer antibodies to their offspring during pregnancy and lactation. *J Reprod Immunol*, Vol.74, No.1-2: pp. 68-77, 0165-0378

Becker, M.I., Fuentes, A., Del Campo, M., Manubens, A., Nova, E., Oliva, H., Faunes, F., Valenzuela, M.A., Campos-Vallette, M., Aliaga, A., Ferreira, J., De Ioannes, A.E., De Ioannes, P. & Moltedo, B. (2009). Immunodominant role of CCHA subunit of *Concholepas* hemocyanin is associated with unique biochemical properties. *Int Immunopharmacol*, Vol.9, No.3: pp. 330-339, 1878-1705

Biosyn. In: *Vacmune Immucothel*, July 2011, Available from: http://www.biosyncorp.com/bc_downloads/vacmune.pdf.

Brandau, S. & Bohle, A. (2001). Activation of natural killer cells by Bacillus Calmette-Guerin. *Eur Urol*, Vol.39, No.5: pp. 518-524, 0302-2838

Brandau, S., Riemensberger, J., Jacobsen, M., Kemp, D., Zhao, W., Zhao, X., Jocham, D., Ratliff, T.L. & Bohle, A. (2001). NK cells are essential for effective BCG immunotherapy. *Int J Cancer*, Vol.92, No.5: pp. 697-702, 0020-7136

Cancino, J., Torrealba, C., Soza, A., Yuseff, M.I., Gravotta, D., Henklein, P., Rodriguez-Boulan, E. & Gonzalez, A. (2007). Antibody to AP1B adaptor blocks biosynthetic and recycling routes of basolateral proteins at recycling endosomes. *Mol Biol Cell*, Vol.18, No.12: pp. 4872-4884, 1059-1524

Cuff, M.E., Miller, K.I., van Holde, K.E. & Hendrickson, W.A. (1998). Crystal structure of a functional unit from *Octopus* hemocyanin. *J Mol Biol*, Vol.278, No.4: pp. 855-870, 0022-2836

De Ioannes, P., Moltedo, B., Oliva, H., Pacheco, R., Faunes, F., De Ioannes, A.E. & Becker, M.I. (2004). Hemocyanin of the molluscan *Concholepas concholepas* exhibits an unusual heterodecameric array of subunits. *J Biol Chem*, Vol.279, No.25: pp. 26134-26142, 0021-9258

Decker, H. & Tuczek, F. (2000). Tyrosinase/catecholoxidase activity of hemocyanins: structural basis and molecular mechanism. *Trends Biochem Sci*, Vol.25, No.8: pp. 392-397, 0968-0004

Decker, H., Hellmann, N., Jaenicke, E., Lieb, B., Meissner, U. & Markl, J. (2007). Minireview: Recent progress in hemocyanin research. *Integr Comp Biol*, Vol.47, No.4: pp. 631-644, 1540-7063

Del Campo, M., Lagos, L., Manubens, A., Ioannes, A., Moltedo, B. & Becker, M.I. (2007). Efecto de la hemocianina de *C. Concholepas* (CCH) en la maduración de células dendríticas. *Proceedings of XXX Reunión Anual de la Sociedad de Bioquímica y Biología Molecular de Chile*. Chillán, Chile. September, 2007.

Del Campo, M., Arancibia, S., Nova, E., Salazar, F., Gonzalez, A., Moltedo, B., De Ioannes, P., Ferreira, J., Manubens, A. & Becker, M.I. (2011). Hemocyanins as immunostimulants. *Rev. méd. Chile*, Vol.139, No.2: pp. 236-246

Dolashka-Angelova, P., Beck, A., Dolashki, A., Beltramini, M., Stevanovic, S., Salvato, B. & Voelter, W. (2003). Characterization of the carbohydrate moieties of the functional unit RvH1-a of *Rapana venosa* haemocyanin using HPLC/electrospray ionization MS and glycosidase digestion. *Biochem J*, Vol.374, No.Pt 1: pp. 185-192, 0264-6021

Dolashka-Angelova, P., Stefanova, T., Livaniou, E., Velkova, L., Klimentzou, P., Stevanovic, S., Salvato, B., Neychev, H. & Voelter, W. (2008). Immunological potential of *Helix vulgaris* and *Rapana venosa* hemocyanins. *Immunol Invest*, Vol.37, No.8: pp. 822-840, 1532-4311

Dolashka, P., Velkova, L., Shishkov, S., Kostova, K., Dolashki, A., Dimitrov, I., Atanasov, B., Devreese, B., Voelter, W. & Van Beeumen, J. (2010). Glycan structures and antiviral effect of the structural subunit RvH2 of *Rapana* hemocyanin. *Carbohydr Res*, Vol.345, No.16: pp. 2361-2367, 1873-426X

Doyle, A.G., Ramm, L. & Kelso, A. (1998). The CD4+ T-cell response to protein immunization is independent of accompanying IFN-gamma-producing CD8+ T cells. *Immunology*, Vol.93, No.3: pp. 341-349, 0019-2805

Duvillie, B., Attali, M., Aiello, V., Quemeneur, E. & Scharfmann, R. (2003). Label-retaining cells in the rat pancreas: location and differentiation potential in vitro. *Diabetes*, Vol.52, No.8: pp. 2035-2042, 0012-1797

Edwards, F.R. & Whitwell, F. (1974). Use of BCG as an immunostimulant in the surgical treatment of carcinoma of the lung. *Thorax*, Vol.29, No.6: pp. 654-658, 0040-6376

Espinoza, C., De Ioannes, A.E. & Becker, M.I. (2006). Caracterización bioquímica e inmunoquímica de la hemocianina de tres especies de lapas chilenas de la Familia

Fissurellidae. Proceedings of XXIX Reunión Anual de la Sociedad de Bioquímica y Biología Molecular de Chile. Pucón, Chile. November, 2006.

FDA. In: *ClinicalTrials.gov*, July 2011, Available from: http://clinicaltrials.gov/ct2/results?tem=KLH

Flamm, J., Bucher, A., Holtl, W. & Albrecht, W. (1990). Recurrent superficial transitional cell carcinoma of the bladder: adjuvant topical chemotherapy versus immunotherapy. A prospective randomized trial. *J Urol*, Vol.144, No.2 Pt 1: pp. 260-263, 0022-5347

Gatsogiannis, C. & Markl, J. (2009). Keyhole limpet hemocyanin: 9-A CryoEM structure and molecular model of the KLH1 didecamer reveal the interfaces and intricate topology of the 160 functional units. *J Mol Biol*, Vol.385, No.3: pp. 963-983, 1089-8638

Ghiretti-Magaldi, A. & Ghiretti, F. (1992). The pre-history of hemocyanin. The discovery of copper in the blood of molluscs. *Experientia*, Vol.48: pp. 971-972

Gielens, C., De Geest, N., Compernolle, F. & Preaux, G. (2004). Glycosylation sites of hemocyanins of *Helix pomatia* and *Sepia officinalis*. *Micron*, Vol.35, No.1-2: pp. 99-100, 0968-4328

Gilliet, M., Kleinhans, M., Lantelme, E., Schadendorf, D., Burg, G. & Nestle, F.O. (2003). Intranodal injection of semimature monocyte-derived dendritic cells induces T helper type 1 responses to protein neoantigen. *Blood*, Vol.102, No.1: pp. 36-42, 0006-4971

Gravotta, D., Deora, A., Perret, E., Oyanadel, C., Soza, A., Schreiner, R., Gonzalez, A. & Rodriguez-Boulan, E. (2007). AP1B sorts basolateral proteins in recycling and biosynthetic routes of MDCK cells. *Proc Natl Acad Sci U S A*, Vol.104, No.5: pp. 1564-1569, 0027-8424

Grenegard, M., Vretenbrant-Oberg, K., Nylander, M., Desilets, S., Lindstrom, E.G., Larsson, A., Ramstrom, I., Ramstrom, S. & Lindahl, T.L. (2008). The ATP-gated P2X1 receptor plays a pivotal role in activation of aspirin-treated platelets by thrombin and epinephrine. *J Biol Chem*, Vol.283, No.27: pp. 18493-18504, 0021-9258

Gunther, J.H., Jurczok, A., Wulf, T., Brandau, S., Deinert, I., Jocham, D. & Bohle, A. (1999). Optimizing syngeneic orthotopic murine bladder cancer (MB49). *Cancer Res*, Vol.59, No.12: pp. 2834-2837, 0008-5472

Harris, J.R., Gebauer, W. & Markl, J. (1993). Immunoelectron Microscopy od Hemocyanin from the Keyhole Limpet (*Megathura crenulata*): A Parallel Subunit Model. *J Struct Biol*, Vol.111: pp. 96-104

Harris, J.R. & Markl, J. (1999). Keyhole limpet hemocyanin (KLH): a biomedical review. *Micron*, Vol.30, No.6: pp. 597-623, 0968-4328

Idakieva, K., Stoeva, S., Voelter, W. & Gielens, C. (2004). Glycosylation of *Rapana thomasiana* hemocyanin. Comparison with other prosobranch (gastropod) hemocyanins. *Comp Biochem Physiol B Biochem Mol Biol*, Vol.138, No.3: pp. 221-228, 1096-4959

Ikemoto, S., Kamizuru, M., Wada, S., Asai, Y. & Kishimoto, T. (1997). Changes in lymphocyte subsets following administration of interleukin 2 and cyclophosphamide in mice with transitional cell carcinoma. *Oncol Res*, Vol.9, No.2: pp. 71-75, 0965-0407

Inaba, K., Inaba, M., Romani, N., Aya, H., Deguchi, M., Ikehara, S., Muramatsu, S. & Steinman, R.M. (1992). Generation of large numbers of dendritic cells from mouse bone marrow cultures supplemented with granulocyte/macrophage colony-stimulating factor. *J Exp Med*, Vol.176, No.6: pp. 1693-1702, 0022-1007

Jacobs, J.F., Punt, C.J., Lesterhuis, W.J., Sutmuller, R.P., Brouwer, H.M., Scharenborg, N.M., Klasen, I.S., Hilbrands, L.B., Figdor, C.G., de Vries, I.J. & Adema, G.J. (2010). Dendritic cell vaccination in combination with anti-CD25 monoclonal antibody treatment: a phase I/II study in metastatic melanoma patients. *Clin Cancer Res*, Vol.16, No.20: pp. 5067-5078, 1078-0432

Jurincic-Winkler, C., Metz, K.A., Beuth, J., Sippel, J. & Klippel, K.F. (1995a). Effect of keyhole limpet hemocyanin (KLH) and bacillus Calmette-Guerin (BCG) instillation on carcinoma in situ of the urinary bladder. *Anticancer Res*, Vol.15, No.6B: pp. 2771-2776, 0250-7005

Jurincic-Winkler, C., Metz, K.A., Beuth, J., Engelmann, U. & Klippel, K.F. (1995b). Immunohistological findings in patients with superficial bladder carcinoma after intravesical instillation of keyhole limpet haemocyanin. *Br J Urol*, Vol.76, No.6: pp. 702-707, 0007-1331

Jurincic-Winkler, C.D., Gallati, H., Alvarez-Mon, M., Sippel, J., Carballido, J. & Klippel, K.F. (1995c). Urinary interleukin-1 alpha levels are increased by intravesical instillation with keyhole limpet hemocyanin in patients with superficial transitional cell carcinoma of the bladder. *Eur Urol*, Vol.28, No.4: pp. 334-339, 0302-2838

Jurincic, C.D., Engelmann, U., Gasch, J. & Klippel, K.F. (1988). Immunotherapy in bladder cancer with keyhole-limpet hemocyanin: a randomized study. *J Urol*, Vol.139, No.4: pp. 723-726, 0022-5347

Kafi, K., Betting, D.J., Yamada, R.E., Bacica, M., Steward, K.K. & Timmerman, J.M. (2009). Maleimide conjugation markedly enhances the immunogenicity of both human and murine idiotype-KLH vaccines. *Mol Immunol*, Vol.46, No.3: pp. 448-456, 0161-5890

Kaplan, D.H., Shankaran, V., Dighe, A.S., Stockert, E., Aguet, M., Old, L.J. & Schreiber, R.D. (1998). Demonstration of an interferon gamma-dependent tumor surveillance system in immunocompetent mice. *Proc Natl Acad Sci U S A*, Vol.95, No.13: pp. 7556-7561, 0027-8424

Lamm, D.L., Reyna, J.A. & Reichert, D.F. (1981). Keyhole-limpet haemacyanin and immune ribonucleic acid immunotherapy of murine transitional cell carcinoma. *Urol Res*, Vol.9, No.5: pp. 227-230, 0300-5623

Lamm, D.L., Reichert, D.F., Harris, S.C. & Lucio, R.M. (1982). Immunotherapy of murine transitional cell carcinoma. *J Urol*, Vol.128, No.5: pp. 1104-1108, 0022-5347

Lamm, D.L., DeHaven, J.I., Riggs, D.R. & Ebert, R.F. (1993a). Immunotherapy of murine bladder cancer with keyhole limpet hemocyanin (KLH). *J Urol*, Vol.149, No.3: pp. 648-652, 0022-5347

Lamm, D.L., DeHaven, J.I., Riggs, D.R., Delgra, C. & Burrell, R. (1993b). Keyhole limpet hemocyanin immunotherapy of murine bladder cancer. *Urol Res*, Vol.21, No.1: pp. 33-37, 0300-5623

Lamm, D.L., Dehaven, J.I. & Riggs, D.R. (2000). Keyhole limpet hemocyanin immunotherapy of bladder cancer: laboratory and clinical studies. *Eur Urol*, Vol.37 Suppl 3: pp. 41-44, 0302-2838

Lamm, D.L. (2003). Laboratory and Clinical Experience with Keyhole limpet hemocyanin (Immunocothel) in superficial bladder cancer. *J. Urol.*, Vol.10, No.2: pp. 18-21

Lattime, E.C., Gomella, L.G. & McCue, P.A. (1992). Murine bladder carcinoma cells present antigen to BCG-specific CD4+ T-cells. *Cancer Res*, Vol.52, No.15: pp. 4286-4290, 0008-5472

Lau, B.H., Woolley, J.L., Marsh, C.L., Barker, G.R., Koobs, D.H. & Torrey, R.R. (1986). Superiority of intralesional immunotherapy with *Corynebacterium parvum* and *Allium sativum* in control of murine transitional cell carcinoma. *J Urol*, Vol.136, No.3: pp. 701-705, 0022-5347

Leitch, H.A. & Connors, J.M. (2005). Vaccine therapy for non-Hodgkin's lymphoma and other B-cell malignancies. *Curr Opin Investig Drugs*, Vol.6, No.6: pp. 597-604, 1472-4472

Lesterhuis, W.J., Schreibelt, G., Scharenborg, N.M., Brouwer, H.M., Gerritsen, M.J., Croockewit, S., Coulie, P.G., Torensma, R., Adema, G.J., Figdor, C.G., de Vries, I.J. & Punt, C.J. (2011). Wild-type and modified gp100 peptide-pulsed dendritic cell vaccination of advanced melanoma patients can lead to long-term clinical responses independent of the peptide used. *Cancer Immunol Immunother*, Vol.60, No.2: pp. 249-260, 1432-0851

Leyton, P., Lizama-Vergara, P.A., Campos-Vallete, M.M., Becker, M.I., Clavijo, E., Cordova Reyes, I., Vera, M. & Jerez, C.A. (2005). Surface enhanced Raman spectrum of nanometric molecular systems. *J. Chile. Chem. Soc.*, Vol.50, No.4: pp. 725-730, 0717-9707

Lieb, B., Altenhein, B., Markl, J., Vincent, A., van Olden, E., van Holde, K.E. & Miller, K.I. (2001). Structures of two molluscan hemocyanin genes: significance for gene evolution. *Proc Natl Acad Sci U S A*, Vol.98, No.8: pp. 4546-4551, 0027-8424

Linn, J.F., Black, P., Derksen, K., Rubben, H. & Thuroff, J.W. (2000). Keyhole limpet haemocyanin in experimental bladder cancer: literature review and own results. *Eur Urol*, Vol.37 Suppl 3: pp. 34-40, 0302-2838

Lommerse, J.P., Thomas-Oates, J.E., Gielens, C., Preaux, G., Kamerling, J.P. & Vliegenthart, J.F. (1997). Primary structure of 21 novel monoantennary and diantennary N-linked carbohydrate chains from alphaD-hemocyanin of *Helix pomatia*. *Eur J Biochem*, Vol.249, No.1: pp. 195-222, 0014-2956

Lopez, M.N., Pereda, C., Segal, G., Munoz, L., Aguilera, R., Gonzalez, F.E., Escobar, A., Ginesta, A., Reyes, D., Gonzalez, R., Mendoza-Naranjo, A., Larrondo, M., Compan, A., Ferrada, C. & Salazar-Onfray, F. (2009). Prolonged survival of dendritic cell-vaccinated melanoma patients correlates with tumor-specific delayed type IV hypersensitivity response and reduction of tumor growth factor beta-expressing T cells. *J Clin Oncol*, Vol.27, No.6: pp. 945-952, 1527-7755

Manosalva, H., De Ioannes, A.E. & Becker, M.I. (2004). Development of monoclonal antibodies bearing the internal image of the gizzerosine epitope and application in a competitive ELISA for fish meal. *Hybrid Hybridomics*, Vol.23, No.1: pp. 45-54, 1536-8599

Manubens, A., Salazar, F., Haussmann, D., Figueroa, J., Del Campo, M., Pinto, J.M., Huaquin, L., Venegas, A. & Becker, M.I. (2010). *Concholepas* hemocyanin biosynthesis takes place in the hepatopancreas, with hemocytes being involved in its metabolism. *Cell Tissue Res*, Vol.342, No.3: pp. 423-435, 1432-0878

Markl, J., Lieb, B., Gebauer, W., Altenhein, B., Meissner, U. & Harris, J.R. (2001). Marine tumor vaccine carriers: structure of the molluscan hemocyanins KLH and HtH. *J Cancer Res Clin Oncol*, Vol.127 Suppl 2: pp. R3-9, 0171-5216

Marsh, C.L., Torrey, R.R., Woolley, J.L., Barker, G.R. & Lau, B.H. (1987). Superiority of intravesical immunotherapy with *Corynebacterium parvum* and *Allium sativum* in control of murine bladder cancer. *J Urol*, Vol.137, No.2: pp. 359-362, 0022-5347

Matus, S., Burgos, P.V., Bravo-Zehnder, M., Kraft, R., Porras, O.H., Farias, P., Barros, L.F., Torrealba, F., Massardo, L., Jacobelli, S. & Gonzalez, A. (2007). Antiribosomal-P autoantibodies from psychiatric lupus target a novel neuronal surface protein causing calcium influx and apoptosis. *J Exp Med*, Vol.204, No.13: pp. 3221-3234, 1540-9538

Mauldin, R.E. & Miller, L.A. (2007). Wildlife contraception: targeting the oocyte. Managing Vertebrate Invasive Species: Proceedings of an International Symposium. G.W. Witmer, W.C. Pitt&K.A. Fagerstone. National Wildlife Research Center, Fort Collins, CO.

Milas, L. & Withers, H.R. (1976). Nonspecific immunotherapy of malignant tumors. *Radiology*, Vol.118, No.1: pp. 211-218, 0033-8419

Millard, A.L., Ittelet, D., Schooneman, F. & Bernard, J. (2003). Dendritic cell KLH loading requirements for efficient CD4+ T-cell priming and help to peptide-specific cytotoxic T-cell response, in view of potential use in cancer vaccines. *Vaccine*, Vol.21, No.9-10: pp. 869-876, 0264-410X

Miller, L.A., Talwar, G.P. & Killian, G.J. (2006). Contraceptive effect of a recombinant GnRH vaccine in adult female pigs. Proc. 22nd Vertebr. Pest. Conf. O.B.J. Timm RM, Univ. of Calif: pp. 106-109.

Moltedo, B., Faunes, F., Haussmann, D., De Ioannes, P., De Ioannes, A.E., Puente, J. & Becker, M.I. (2006). Immunotherapeutic effect of *Concholepas* hemocyanin in the murine bladder cancer model: evidence for conserved antitumor properties among hemocyanins. *J Urol*, Vol.176, No.6 Pt 1: pp. 2690-2695, 0022-5347

Moltedo, B., Lopez, C.B., Pazos, M., Becker, M.I., Hermesh, T. & Moran, T.M. (2009). Cutting edge: stealth influenza virus replication precedes the initiation of adaptive immunity. *J Immunol*, Vol.183, No.6: pp. 3569-3573, 1550-6606

Molto, L.M., Carballido, J., Jurincic, C., Lapena, P., Manzano, L., Salmeron, I., Klippel, K.F. & Alvarez-Mon, M. (1991). Keyhole limpet hemocyanine can enhance the natural killer activity of patients with transitional cell carcinoma of the bladder. *Eur Urol*, Vol.19, No.1: pp. 74-78, 0302-2838

Morales, A., Eidinger, D. & Bruce, A.W. (1976). Intracavitary Bacillus Calmette-Guerin in the treatment of superficial bladder tumors. *J Urol*, Vol.116, No.2: pp. 180-183, 0022-5347

Mura, C.V., Becker, M.I., Orellana, A. & Wolff, D. (2002). Immunopurification of Golgi vesicles by magnetic sorting. *J Immunol Methods*, Vol.260, No.1-2: pp. 263-271, 0022-1759

Musselli, C., Livingston, P.O. & Ragupathi, G. (2001). Keyhole limpet hemocyanin conjugate vaccines against cancer: the Memorial Sloan Kettering experience. *J Cancer Res Clin Oncol*, Vol.127 Suppl 2: pp. R20-26, 0171-5216

Nseyo, U.O. & Lamm, D.L. (1997). Immunotherapy of bladder cancer. *Semin Surg Oncol*, Vol.13, No.5: pp. 342-349, 8756-0437

Oliva, H., Moltedo, B., De Ioannes, P., Faunes, F., De Ioannes, A.E. & Becker, M.I. (2002). Monoclonal antibodies to molluskan hemocyanin from *Concholepas concholepas* demonstrate common and specific epitopes among subunits. *Hybrid Hybridomics*, Vol.21, No.5: pp. 365-374, 1536-8599

Olsson, C.A., Chute, R. & Rao, C.N. (1974). Immunologic reduction of bladder cancer recurrence rate. *J Urol*, Vol.111, No.2: pp. 173-176, 0022-5347

Orlova, E.V., Dube, P., Harris, J.R., Beckman, E., Zemlin, F., Markl, J. & van Heel, M. (1997). Structure of keyhole limpet hemocyanin type 1 (KLH1) at 15 A resolution by electron cryomicroscopy and angular reconstitution. *J Mol Biol*, Vol.271, No.3: pp. 417-437, 0022-2836

Paccagnella, M., Bologna, L., Beccaro, M., Micetic, I., Di Muro, P. & Salvato, B. (2004). Structural subunit organization of molluscan hemocyanins. *Micron*, Vol.35, No.1-2: pp. 21-22, 0968-4328

Perabo, F.G. & Muller, S.C. (2004). Current and new strategies in immunotherapy for superficial bladder cancer. *Urology*, Vol.64, No.3: pp. 409-421, 1527-9995

Pilon, J., Loiacono, C., Okeson, D., Lund, S., Vercauteren, K., Rhyan, J. & Miller, L. (2007). Anti-prion activity generated by a novel vaccine formulation. *Neurosci Lett*, Vol.429, No.2-3: pp. 161-164, 0304-3940

Presicce, P., Taddeo, A., Conti, A., Villa, M.L. & Della Bella, S. (2008). Keyhole limpet hemocyanin induces the activation and maturation of human dendritic cells through the involvement of mannose receptor. *Mol Immunol*, Vol.45, No.4: pp. 1136-1145, 0161-5890

Recker, F. & Rubben, H. (1989). Variation of the immunosystem by ciclosporin and keyhole-limpet hemocyanin--are there effects on chemically induced bladder carcinoma? *Urol Int*, Vol.44, No.2: pp. 77-80, 0042-1138

Riggs, D.R., Tarry, W.F., DeHaven, J.I., Sosnowski, J. & Lamm, D.L. (1992). Immunotherapy of murine transitional cell carcinoma of the bladder using alpha and gamma interferon in combination with other forms of immunotherapy. *J Urol*, Vol.147, No.1: pp. 212-214, 0022-5347

Riggs, D.R., Jackson, B., Vona-Davis, L. & McFadden, D. (2002). *In vitro* anticancer effects of a novel immunostimulant: keyhole limpet hemocyanin. *J Surg Res*, Vol.108, No.2: pp. 279-284, 0022-4804

Schenkman, E. & Lamm, D.L. (2004). Superficial bladder cancer therapy. *ScientificWorldJournal*, Vol.4 Suppl 1: pp. 387-399, 1537-744X

Schumacher, K. (2001). Keyhole limpet hemocyanin (KLH) conjugate vaccines as novel therapeutic tools in malignant disorders. *J Cancer Res Clin Oncol*, Vol.127 Suppl 2: pp. R1-2, 0171-5216

Shimizu, K., Thomas, E.K., Giedlin, M. & Mule, J.J. (2001). Enhancement of tumor lysate- and peptide-pulsed dendritic cell-based vaccines by the addition of foreign helper protein. *Cancer Res*, Vol.61, No.6: pp. 2618-2624, 0008-5472

Siddiqui, N.I., Idakieva, K., Demarsin, B., Doumanova, L., Compernolle, F. & Gielens, C. (2007). Involvement of glycan chains in the antigenicity of *Rapana thomasiana* hemocyanin. *Biochem Biophys Res Commun*, Vol.361, No.3: pp. 705-711, 0006-291X

Somasundar, P., Riggs, D.R., Jackson, B.J. & McFadden, D.W. (2005). Inhibition of melanoma growth by hemocyanin occurs via early apoptotic pathways. *Am J Surg*, Vol.190, No.5: pp. 713-716, 0002-9610

Swerdlow, R.D., Ratliff, T.L., La Regina, M., Ritchey, J.K. & Ebert, R.F. (1994). Immunotherapy with keyhole limpet hemocyanin: efficacy and safety in the MB-49 intravesical murine bladder tumor model. *J Urol*, Vol.151, No.6: pp. 1718-1722, 0022-5347

Swerdlow, R.D., Ebert, R.F., Lee, P., Bonaventura, C. & Miller, K.I. (1996). Keyhole limpet hemocyanin: structural and functional characterization of two different subunits and multimers. *Comp Biochem Physiol B Biochem Mol Biol*, Vol.113, No.3: pp. 537-548, 1096-4959

Szabo, S.J., Sullivan, B.M., Peng, S.L. & Glimcher, L.H. (2003). Molecular mechanisms regulating Th1 immune responses. *Annu Rev Immunol*, Vol.21: pp. 713-758, 0732-0582

Teitz-Tennenbaum, S., Li, Q., Davis, M.A. & Chang, A.E. (2008). Dendritic cells pulsed with keyhole limpet hemocyanin and cryopreserved maintain anti-tumor activity in a murine melanoma model. *Clin Immunol*, Vol.129, No.3: pp. 482-491, 1521-7035

Teppema, J.S., de Boer, E.C., Steeremberg, P.A. & van der Meijden, A.P. (1992). Morphological aspects of the interaction of Bacillus Calmette-Guérin with urothelial bladder cells *in vivo* and *in vitro*: relevance for antitumor activity. *Urol. Res.*, Vol.20: pp. 219-228

Timmerman, J.M. & Levy, R. (2000). Linkage of foreign carrier protein to a self-tumor antigen enhances the immunogenicity of a pulsed dendritic cell vaccine. *J Immunol*, Vol.164, No.9: pp. 4797-4803, 0022-1767

Torres, M., Manosalva, H., Carrasco, I., De Ioannes, A.E. & Becker, M.I. (1999). Procedure for radiolabeling gizzerosine and basis for a radioimmunoassay. *J Agric Food Chem*, Vol.47, No.10: pp. 4231-4236, 0021-8561

van Holde, K.E. & Miller, K.I. (1995). Hemocyanins. *Adv Protein Chem*, Vol.47: pp. 1-81, 0065-3233

van Holde, K.E., Miller, K.I. & Decker, H. (2001). Hemocyanins and invertebrate evolution. *J Biol Chem*, Vol.276, No.19: pp. 15563-15566, 0021-9258

Vandenbark, A.A., Yoshihara, P., Carveth, L. & Burger, D.R. (1981). All KLH preparations are not created equal. *Cell Immunol*, Vol.60, No.1: pp. 240-243, 0008-8749

Verdijk, P., Aarntzen, E.H., Lesterhuis, W.J., Boullart, A.C., Kok, E., van Rossum, M.M., Strijk, S., Eijckeler, F., Bonenkamp, J.J., Jacobs, J.F., Blokx, W., Vankrieken, J.H., Joosten, I., Boerman, O.C., Oyen, W.J., Adema, G., Punt, C.J., Figdor, C.G. & de Vries, I.J. (2009). Limited amounts of dendritic cells migrate into the T-cell area of lymph nodes but have high immune activating potential in melanoma patients. *Clin Cancer Res*, Vol.15, No.7: pp. 2531-2540, 1078-0432

Walsh, W.G., Tomashefsky, P., Olsson, C.A. & deVere White, R. (1983). Keyhole-limpet haemocyanin (KLH) immunotherapy of murine transitional cell carcinoma. *Urol Res*, Vol.11, No.6: pp. 263-265, 0300-5623

Weigle, W.O. (1964). Immunochemical Properties of Hemocyanin. *Immunochemistry*, Vol.1: pp. 295-302, 0019-2791

Wishahi, M.M., Ismail, I.M., Ruebben, H. & Otto, T. (1995). Keyhole-limpet hemocyanin immunotherapy in the bilharzial bladder: a new treatment modality? Phase II trial: superficial bladder cancer. *J Urol*, Vol.153, No.3 Pt 2: pp. 926-928, 0022-5347

Wuhrer, M., Robijn, M.L., Koeleman, C.A., Balog, C.I., Geyer, R., Deelder, A.M. & Hokke, C.H. (2004). A novel Gal(beta1-4)Gal(beta1-4)Fuc(alpha1-6)-core modification attached to the proximal N-acetylglucosamine of keyhole limpet haemocyanin (KLH) N-glycans. *Biochem J*, Vol.378, No.Pt 2: pp. 625-632, 1470-8728

Zhu, J., Wan, Q., Lee, D., Yang, G., Spassova, M.K., Ouerfelli, O., Ragupathi, G., Damani, P., Livingston, P.O. & Danishefsky, S.J. (2009). From synthesis to biologics: preclinical data on a chemistry derived anticancer vaccine. *J Am Chem Soc*, Vol.131, No.26: pp. 9298-9303, 1520-5126

12

The Potential Role of Chemoprevention in the Management of Non-Muscle Invasive Bladder Urothelial Carcinoma

Unyime O. Nseyo[1], Katherine A. Corbyons[2] and Hari Siva Gurunadha Rao Tunuguntla[3]
[1]North Florida-South Georgia Veterans Health System, Gainesville, Florida,
[2]University of Florida, Gainesville, Florida,
[3]Robert Wood Johnson Medical School, New Brunswick, New Jersey,
USA

1. Introduction

1.1 Epidemiology and bladder carcinogenesis

Cancer represents phenotypic manifestations of abnormal gene expression. Genetic mutations, dysregulation, and gene losses can influence cell proliferation and differentiation, and eventually lead to formation of cancer. Risk factors and etiologic agents involved in the genetic abnormalities influence the distribution of cancer worldwide. This chapter aims at highlighting the epidemiologic significance of urothelial bladder cancer; reviewing its natural history, the roles of industrial and environmental carcinogens and life style factors in urothelial carcinogenesis; and framing possible strategies for chemoprevention in the management of human urothelial cancer of the urinary bladder.

Bladder cancer remains a serious public health problem worldwide, and accounts for 5-10% of all malignancies annually in western countries (*Cancer Treatment of America*). Though the age-adjusted incidence varies in the different parts of the world, the highest rates are found in men from North America (23.3/100,000), North Africa (23.3/100,000) and Southern Europe (22.0/100,000), while the corresponding rates are 5.4, 4.8, and 3.2 per 100000 for women (*Cancer Treatment of America*). These high rates may be influenced by increased industrialization, cigarette smoking, and infection of schistosomiasis (primarily of concern in North Africa). The lowest rates for both sexes have been reported for the Melanesia region of South Pacific and Middle Africa (*Cancer Treatment of America*; Prout, Barton et al. 1992; Grasso 2008; *American Cancer Society* 2010).

Bladder cancer, which is immensely impacted by environmental carcinogens and tobacco smokes, remains a common disease in the United States, and it is estimated that 70, 530 persons (52,760 men and 17,770 women) were diagnosed with cancer of the urinary bladder in 2010, (*Cancer Treatment of America; American Cancer Society* 2010) and an estimated 14, 680 died of the disease accounting for 3% and 2% of all cancer deaths in men and women, respectively (*Cancer Treatment of America; American Cancer Society* 2010). Estimates of new cancer cases classify *urothelial bladder cancer* (UBC) as the fourth most common in men and the eighth most common in women. The prevalence of UBC in the US is estimated at about one million cases annually, and worldwide, UBC ranks as the ninth most frequent cancer (*Cancer Treatment of America;* Prout, Barton et al. 1992; Grasso 2008; American Cancer Society 2010).

Bladder cancer is a disease of aging; the incidence of UBC rises with age with an average of onset at 69 for men and 67 for women (*Cancer Treatment of America;* Prout, Barton et al. 1992; Dalbagni and Herr 2000; Grasso 2008; *American Cancer Society* 2010). Bladder cancer that occurs at ages 40 or younger tends to be low grade Ta cancer with almost negligible recurrence potential. Given sufficient time, however 50-70% of UBC patients will develop recurrent disease. Recurrences tend to be characterized by multiplicity in time and space, primarily if the initial tumors occurred early in life and were large or multiple in numbers. A majority, 70-75%, of UBC are superficial, that is, non-muscle invasive, and non-lethal, but they are characterized by frequent recurrences. However, the remaining 25-30% of the annual cases of UBC invades into the muscular propria, making them life threatening, because approximately 50% harbor micro-metastases that often manifest within three years out from diagnosis (Droller 2006).

The non-muscle invasive UBC (NMIUBC) that are confined to the mucosa/urothelium Ta, remain non-lethal with a progression rate of less than 5%, and occur often as large or multiple tumors. Ten to twenty percent of the superficially-invasive UBC that is confined to the lamina propria, T1, converts to muscle invasive disease on repeat resection (Dalbagni and Herr 2000).

Variable morphology, natural history, and prognosis demonstrate that transitional cell carcinoma (TCC) or urothelial carcinoma (UC) of the bladder is not a single disease, but occurs in three distinct forms, each possessing characteristic features that include low grade papillary, noninvasive; carcinoma in situ (CIS); and high grade, invasive (Grasso 2008). Seventy to eighty-five percent of new bladder cancer cases, are superficial or *non-muscle invasive* UBC, which include disease confined to the mucosa in CIS: CIS (10%), and Ta (70%), or lamina propria in T1 (20%) (Prout, Barton et al. 1992; Dalbagni and Herr 2000; Droller 2006; Grasso 2008). These types of tumors are considered to have variable invasive potential with a progression rate to invasive cancer of 15% to 50% (Prout, Barton et al. 1992; Dalbagni and Herr 2000; Grasso 2008). However, more than 70% of patients with NMIUBC have one or more recurrences within 5 years of initial diagnosis (Prout, Barton et al. 1992; Dalbagni and Herr 2000; Droller 2006; Grasso 2008). Further analysis shows that approximately 50% of patients diagnosed with solitary bladder cancer will experience recurrences within 4 years, while 70% of multiple bladder tumors reoccur within one year (Prout, Barton et al. 1992; Dalbagni and Herr 2000; Droller 2006; Grasso 2008).

The fact that the bladder serves as a reservoir for urine and its waste product contents predisposes it to the constant cumulative exposure to carcinogens which include industrial toxins and cigarette smoke chemicals. The multiple-step process of carcinogenesis includes induction/activation, promotion and progression, which exists as a continuum in the bladder environment. Consequently, preventive intervention can be difficult to implement under these conditions of cumulative exposures, and the definitive strategy will be to minimize constant cumulative exposure of carcinogenic agents from smoking and industrial sources. Increased carcinogenic exposure by itself cannot explain the 40% increase in bladder cancer incidence in the last 15 years in the US. The explanation certainly includes increased smoking that has added a large population of women, cumulative industrial exposure, and host factors. These host characteristics are likely to influence racial differences in the incidence of bladder cancer. Caucasians have overall bladder cancer risk of 3.9% versus 0.8% overall chance in African Americans: 2.8% in men and 1.5% in women (Droller 2006).

Earliest reported association of industrial carcinogenic exposure and development of bladder cancer was by Rehn (Dietrich and Dietrich 2001). Observations have also documented associations between carcinogen ingestion in animals and development of bladder cancer (Okey, Harper et al. 1998; Sporn and Lippman 2003). Several legislative measures have been implemented in an attempt to decrease the intensity and cumulative nature of the carcinogen exposure. However, cigarette smoking trumps all considerations of environmental and industrial exposure and is the major factor underlying the spread and occurrence of bladder cancer around the globe.

It is estimated that 30% of bladder cancer mortality is attributable to a history of tobacco abuse/dependence (*American Cancer Society*), and studies have tried to characterize the different carcinogenic agents in cigarette smoke that define the causal relationship between smoking and development of urothelial cancer (*American Cancer Society*; Droller 2006). Investigators have tried to correlate bladder cancer risk with the manufacturing processes such as the type of filter used, type of tobacco used, and the curing technique: black versus blonde (Droller 2006). The curing technique determines the concentration of the carcinogens in the cigarette. The smoke of black (air-cured) versus blonde (flue-cured) has been analyzed to show higher concentration of carcinogens in black tobacco. How these commercial practices influence urothelial carcinogenesis remains to be elucidated.

Several specific carcinogens in cigarette smoke have been implicated in the development of urothelial cancer, including polycyclic aromatic hydrocarbons, aromatic and aryl amines (including 4-amino biphenyl), unsaturated aldehydes (e.g. acrolein) and oxygen-free radicals (*American Cancer Society*; Sabichi and Lippman; Droller 2006). Aromatic amines were the first carbon compounds of industrial by-products that were suspected in work- related urothelial cancer, found primarily in those workers who were exposed to the dye, rubber, and plastic manufacturing. These epidemiological data suggest up to 100-fold increased risk that is mediated by cumulative intensity and duration of exposure. Regulatory and legislative efforts to retard the work place risk contributed to the birth of occupational safety and health administration in the industrialized countries around the world.

In spite of extensive efforts since then to curb workplace exposure to industrial carcinogens, textile, dry cleaning, hair dressing, and coal gasification continue to generate the carcinogens in the manufacturing process. The culprit agents are per-chloroethylene (an organic solvent used in dry cleaning), chemical dyes, aromatic amines (used in textile industry), and hair dyes that contain chemical carcinogens. These agents have been associated with bladder cancer development. Other carcinogens, outside of the workplace, that have been associated with the development of urothelial cancer include arsenic in ground water in southeastern Michigan in the US and southwestern Taiwan (Haack, Treccani et al. 2000; Kim, Nriagu et al. 2000; Welch, Westjohn et al. 2000; Droller 2006); ingestion of fang chi (Chinese herb used in weight control); ingestion of ochratoxin A in the Balkan countries resulting indirectly from animals that consumed blackened fern (Droller 2006). Several medications and medical therapies have also been associated with urothelial cancer development including phenacetin used to treat headaches, cyclophosphamide (cytoxan) used to treat pediatric and adult hematologic malignancies (lymphoma and leukemia), and pelvic radiation for cervical and prostate cancer.

In parts of the world with endemicity, there are reports of association between *Schistosoma haematobium* infection and the development of urothelial cancer, primarily squamous cell carcinoma, and some cases of transitional cell cancer (Sabichi and Lippman; Okey, Harper et al. 1998; Sporn and Lippman 2003; Droller 2006). The inciting factors include an inflammatory response to the deposited parasitic ova of *Schistosoma haematobium* in the periurethral areas of the bladder ,as well as conversion of nitrates to nitrites with the nitrosamines mediating the development of urothelial cancer. Other carcinogenic exposures such as fertilizers and cigarette smoke may also play putative roles in the urothelial carcinogenesis in these patients.

In urothelial carcinogenesis, several host factors have been recognized as playing either permissive or protective roles. Acetylation of aromatic amines remains an important mechanism of carcinogenic inactivation in urothelial carcinogenesis. The detoxification of carcinogens is mediated by genes namely NAT1 and NAT2 which are responsible for generating the detoxifying enzymes N-acetyl transferase, and NAT2 remains the predominant gene involved. Individuals who are homozygous for NAT2 are classified as slow acylators and they detoxify carcinogens quite slowly allowing prolonged contact with DNA to induce mutations and carcinogenesis (Sabichi and Lippman; Weber 1987; Droller 2006). These individuals have a two- to four-fold increased risk for the development of urothelial cancer. On the other hand, the heterozygous fast acylators are able to rapidly detoxify these aromatic amines that lower their risk of developing urothelial cancer. Researchers have suggested that the potential differences in racial and ethnic risk of urothelial cancer development are attributable to the difference in the expression of these two genes (Sabichi and Lippman; Weber 1987; Droller 2006; Lattouf 2009).The P450 cytochrome oxidase system is also important in metabolism and detoxification of urothelial carcinogens. The CYP1A2 might be particularly important in metabolizing aromatic amines (Sabichi and Lippman; Okey, Harper et al. 1998; Sporn and Lippman 2003; Droller 2006). Also, individuals deficient in the enzyme glutathione transferase may be at risk for deficient metabolism of polycyclic aromatic amines, which could put them at a 30-50% risk of developing bladder cancer (Okey, Harper et al. 1998; Sporn and Lippman 2003; Droller 2006).

2. Molecular biology of carcinogenesis and chemoprevention

The classic multistep process of carcinogenesis which has been widely accepted includes initiation, promotion, and progression. A clear-cut sequential compartmentalization probably does not always occur, but the multistep structure could be exploited strategically for chemopreventative measures. The first step, initiation, depends upon three cellular functions, namely carcinogen metabolism, DNA repair, and cell proliferation. Cell damage can occur by activation/deactivation mediated by the carcinogen; this cell can cycle through DNA repair or exists as an altered gene (no tumor development) and can be propagated as such, or go through cell proliferation. In the promotion phase, the altered cell continues to undergo repeated bombardment by the promoter agent (initiator or not) leading to additional genomic damage and subsequent clonal expansion into a tumor. In the progression phase, the tumor acquires multicellular defective mutations enhanced by acquired or inherited mutations in the control genes such as p53, Rb, or DNA mismatch repairs (Okey, Harper et al. 1998; Sporn and Lippman 2003; Droller 2006). Consequently a tumor is born that lacks cellular growth controls, and has proliferative autonomy. The challenge in designing a preventive strategy is selecting whether to target genomic or cellular events as well as determining the order of subsequent sequential targeting.

Genotoxic carcinogens can be enzymatically bioactivated and converted into water soluble metabolites to be excreted in urine or bile. These carcinogens can also be inadvertently transformed into electrophiles which react with DNA. Metabolism of carcinogens or broadly biotransformation may depend upon genetic and environmental factors in an individual who is exposed to the carcinogens. The drug metabolizing enzymes are classified into Phase I and Phase II enzymes, with Phase I enzyme being primarily typified by cytochrome P450 mono-oxygenase (CYP) super family. These enzymes function by unmasking the parent substrates (Okey, Harper et al. 1998; Sporn and Lippman 2003; Droller 2006). The Phase II enzymes including sulfotransferase, glutathione transferase (GST), and acetyltransferase primarily detoxify reactive metabolites. They catalyze the conjugation of bulky water insoluble components into hydroxyl groups which can easily be excreted.

As discussed above, carcinogenesis is a multistep process; therefore chemopreventive agents could affect different mechanisms. In practice chemoprevention would require continuous administration of a non-toxic compound over a long period or lifetime of the at-risk individual. However, the chemoprevention strategy would begin with the population approach that advocates a dietary program of increased consumption of fruits and vegetables which have been reported to reduce general cancer risk (Sabichi and Lippman; Sporn and Lippman 2003; Lattouf 2009). At the individual level, the approach would be to reduce the intensity of cumulative exposure through programs that include reduction/elimination of exposure to the carcinogens, dilution and elimination of bladder content by drinking plenty of water and urinating frequently, followed by introduction of the at-risk individual to the chemopreventive agent(s). The potential chemoprevention agents can be broadly classified into two categories: (a) agents that decrease bioactivation or increase detoxification of carcinogens, and (b) agents that alter promotion and progression (Okey, Harper et al. 1998; Sporn and Lippman 2003).

2.1 Agents that decrease bioactivation or increase detoxification of carcinogens

The cytochrome P450 enzyme family, which typifies the Phase I enzymes, acts bidirectionally by bioactivating procarcinogens into reactive metabolites that bind to DNA, but also enhances overall clearance of both the procarcinogens and carcinogens from the body. The first pass clearance of the carcinogen by the high activity of P450 enzymes in the human liver exposes the susceptible peripheral organ/ tissue to reduced concentrations of the carcinogens (Okey, Harper et al. 1998; Sporn and Lippman 2003)..

In bladder cancer, the Phase II enzymes include the detoxifier glutathione transferases which conjugate reactive metabolites with glutathione. These Phase II enzymes can be induced by plant products such as sulforaphane from broccoli. This induction can be highly protective in animals against major carcinogens. However, they can also act bidirectionally to favor Phase I class of enzymes (Okey, Harper et al. 1998; Sporn and Lippman 2003).

Interestingly, oltipraz, an anti-schistosomiasis drug, functions bidirectionally to inhibit the predominant activating enzyme CYPIA2, and also induces a glutathione S-transferase Phase II enzyme that detoxifies carcinogens by conjugation. Another cytochrome P450 modulator is indole-3-carbinole (I3C) which is abundant in broccoli, brussels sprouts, and cruciferous vegetables (Okey, Harper et al. 1998; Sporn and Lippman 2003).

The phytochemicals that reduce adduct formation include vitamin E (α-tocopherol) and vitamin C (ascorbic acid). These act as scavengers of the reactive metabolites, or act as antioxidants (Okey, Harper et al. 1998; Sporn and Lippman 2003). However, they have not been found to decrease the risk of cancer in high-risk populations.

2.2 Agents that alter promotion and progression

Inflammation, increased cell proliferation/decreased differentiation, deficiency of apoptosis, and cumulative genetic instability constitute putative molecular and cellular events that induce promotion and progression during carcinogenesis (Okey, Harper et al. 1998; Sporn and Lippman 2003; Droller 2006). These cellular events are attractive potential targets for chemopreventative intervention.

Synthetic retinoids have been shown to alter gene expression and stimulate apoptosis. However, these have failed as primary chemopreventive agents, but have been shown to delay the appearance of secondary primary cancers of head and neck (Sabichi and Lippman; Okey, Harper et al. 1998; Sporn and Lippman 2003). However, natural retinoids such as β-carotene have shown a paradoxical increase in lung cancer in smokers and asbestos-exposed workers.

Targeting inflammation has become an attractive approach in chemoprevention as scientists gain better understanding of the association between inflammation and increased cancer risk, particularly colon cancer. Both the older-generation non-specific inhibitors of cyclooxygenase including: aspirin and non-steroidal anti-inflammatory agents (NSAIDS) and the newer synthetic selective COX-2 inhibitors such as Celecoxib have shown promising results in preventing colon cancer in rodent models and in humans(Sporn and Lippman 2003).

3. Conventional strategies in preventing recurrence/occurrence and progression

Approaches to bladder cancer prevention include primary prevention which aims at avoiding cancer development in healthy populations, secondary prevention, which aims at preventing premalignant lesions from undergoing promotion and progression into cancer under conducive conditions during carcinogenesis; and tertiary prevention, which aims at aborting cancer progression in patients who have been treated for the cancer. In bladder cancer, primary prevention is widely regarded as impractical. Even if good chemopreventive agents were available the risk-benefit ratio would have to be low in such a large at risk population. The other challenges to primary intervention strategy are discussed in the sections above about the uncertainty of appropriate molecular/cellular targets to prevent tumor initiation. In practice techniques of secondary and tertiary prevention are indistinguishable.

Following the initial diagnosis with transurethral resection of bladder tumor (TURBT), there are several interventions that may be undertaken to retard cancer recurrence and progression: selected patients may undergo repeat TURBT to better delineate the nature of their disease (Prout, Barton et al. 1992; Oosterlinck, Kurth et al. 1993; Lamm, Blumenstein et al. 1995; Dalbagni and Herr 2000), approximately 20% will receive intravesical chemotherapy to potentially eradicate residual disease (Prout, Barton et al. 1992;

Oosterlinck, Kurth et al. 1993; Lamm, Blumenstein et al. 1995; Dalbagni and Herr 2000) and the majority will be placed on some type of endoscopic surveillance schedule. The necessity for early adjuvant treatment, mainly intravesical instillation of immunotherapeutic or chemotherapeutic agents in the management of high-risk CIS, Ta/high grade and T1/any grade is recognized globally (Prout, Barton et al. 1992; Oosterlinck, Kurth et al. 1993; Lamm, Blumenstein et al. 1995; Dalbagni and Herr 2000). The hope is that this treatment, by altering the neoplastic potential of the urothelium, will reduce the risk for recurrence and progression. The subsets of the patients with NMIUBC who fail the conventional intravesical therapies will ultimately be subjected to radical cystectomy with resultant loss of bladder function, body image and sexual function (Prout, Barton et al. 1992; Oosterlinck, Kurth et al. 1993; Lamm, Blumenstein et al. 1995; Dalbagni and Herr 2000). The newest strategy in the management of NMIUBC is Photodynamic Diagnosis (PDD) with Hexvix® (*PhotoCure ASA, Oslo, Norway*) to minimize recurrences/occurrences and progression. PPD uses Hexvix which is an ester derivative of 5-Aminolevulinic Acid (ALA) (Jichlinski, Guillou et al. 2003; Fradet, Grossman et al. 2007) was recently approved by the US Food and Drug Administration (FDA) for management of NMIUBC primarily to improve the diagnostic and staging accuracy of cystoscopy leading to improvement in survival. Photodynamic diagnosis occurs when a photosensitizing agent is first concentrated in malignant or abnormal tissue, and then activated by light (Henderson 1992). The activated photosensitizer either returns to ground state, and releases energy as fluorescence, which can be used in detection (PDD), or the photosensitizer enters into its triplet state, and causes physico-chemical reactions to generate reactive oxygen species (ROS), for therapy as in Photodynamic therapy (PDT). Hexvix-PDD has been reported to improve the diagnostic rate of Ta and T1 papillary bladder cancers by 16.4% and the detection of CIS by 31% (as compared to white light cystoscopy) (Jichlinski, Guillou et al. 2003). Recently, Karl et al., reported that PDD during initial TURBT for T1G3 NMBIC exhibited a significant reduction in recurrence rate; led to detection of additional 35.4% CIS versus 21.8% in the control group (standard white light TURBT).The authors concluded that the initial use of PDD-directed TURBT could provide a superior cancer control and effective treatment of patients with T1G3 NMIBC (Karl 2010).

Bacillus Calmette-Guerin (BCG), an immunotherapy, remains the most effective and widely used intravesical agent to prevent recurrence and progression (Oosterlinck, Kurth et al. 1993; Lamm, Blumenstein et al. 1995; Dalbagni and Herr 2000). Mitomycin, thiotepa and epirubicin are the commonly used intravesical chemotherapeutic agents. while intravesical Valrubicin is FDA-approved as an alternative intravesical therapy to radical cystectomy for BCG refractory CIS patients (Dalbagni and Herr 2000). Administering Mitomycin or epirubicin immediately following TURBT has been reported as effective in preventing tumor implant; however, this approach has failed to ultimately prevent disease progression or mortality (Oosterlinck, Kurth et al. 1993). Of course, each intravesical agent is associated with both local and systemic side effects. Despite current treatment strategies, 30-80% of these patients develop recurrences within 5 years, and this high rate of recurrence of NMIBC invariably leads to a high economic impact (Hedelin, Holmang et al. 2002; Botteman, Pashos et al. 2003; Uchida, Yonou et al. 2007; Hong and Loughlin 2008; Sievert, Amend et al. 2009). The disease progression rate to muscle invasiveness is 42-83% in BCG-treated patients who have concomitant CIS and papillary NMIUBC, and 30-50% in those BCG-treated patients with primary CIS (Oosterlinck, Kurth et al. 1993; Lamm, Blumenstein et al. 1995; Dalbagni and Herr 2000). Frequent follow ups and re-treatment of patients due to the recurrences exert heavy untold burden on the affected patients; eventually leading to morbidity as well as increased expenditure because of continuous treatment (Hedelin, Holmang et al. 2002; Botteman, Pashos et al. 2003; Uchida, Yonou et al. 2007; Hong and Loughlin 2008; Sievert, Amend et al. 2009).

3.1 Chemoprevention in the armamentarium of management of NMIUBC

Early detection and advances in treatments over the last two decades have resulted in an overall reduction in bladder cancer mortality (Cancer Treatment of America; American Cancer Society 2010). The public health and socioeconomic burden of bladder cancer could be reduced through practice of systematic prevention measures including elimination/minimization of exposure to carcinogens, hydration for dilution and frequent urination to expulse potential carcinogens; and practice of active dietary and/or pharmacologic preventative interventions. Unfortunately, in bladder cancer there are still no definite interventions that have been shown to be effective, and research in this area has yielded no evidence-based data to inform on strategies for systematic practice of bladder cancer prevention. Bladder urothelial cancer has biologic and clinical characteristics that favor it as an ideal cancer for chemoprevention. These special features include its susceptibility; carcinogenesis; frequent recurrences, and clinical presentation.

3.2 Cessation of smoking

The most cost-effective measure in bladder cancer prevention strategy would certainly be smoking cessation. This, of course, would be very difficult because of the addictive nature of the current cadre of manufactured cigarettes. In the meantime therapeutic intervention is needed to complement and perhaps even supplant the current socio-cultural as well as the legislative strategies to reduce the economic burden, suffering and death from bladder cancer through tobacco control. In the following section we will review the available evidence for the various chemotherapeutic agents.

4. Bladder cancer chemoprevention strategies: Non-pharmacologic and dietary approach (see also Table 1)

4.1 Fluid intake

The Health Professional Follow Up Study validated the concept that increased fluid intake could substantially lower the risk of UBC due to lowered intensity and cumulative exposure of carcinogens (Michaud, Spiegelman et al. 1999). The study involved mailing questionnaires to 47,903 men; and analysis of their responses regarding daily fluid intake. The data showed inverse association between total daily fluid intake and risk of urothelial cancer (UC) with a relative risk of 0.51 (0.32-0.81, 95% confidence interval: CI) in those who consumed the largest amount of fluid. Daily water consumption offered the best protection when compared with other fluids. However, Geoffrey-Perez and colleagues countered by reporting that there was an absence of association between bladder cancer risk and fluid consumption (Geoffroy-Perez and Cordier 2001). Intuitively it remains logical that dilution of bladder carcinogenic contents with frequent urination would be beneficial and less expensive practice.

4.2 Fat and caloric intake

In the Spanish study, Riboli and associates reported an association between fat consumption and urothelial cancer that showed a 2-fold increase in cancer incidence (Riboli, Gonzalez et al. 1991). Surveillance Epidemiology and End Results (SEER) population-based study data provided further evidence that fat rich diets are associated with an increase in incidence of UC (OR 2.24 for the highest quartile, 95% CI, 1.25-4.03, P=0.006) (Bruemmer, White et al. 1996). A Swedish study suggests a dose dependent effect of fat diet on the incidence of UC (Steineck, Hagman et al. 1990). In a meta-analysis of 36 studies evaluating 6 dietary variables in relation to UC, Steinmaus and group reported a positive association between intake of fat and UC (Relative ratio, RR 1.37, 95% CI, 1.16-1.62), but not with meat consumption (RR 1.08, 95% CI, 0.82-1.42) (Steinmaus, Nunez et al. 2000). However, there was no positive association between total caloric intake and UC over 12 years in the Health Professional Follow-Up Study (Michaud, Spiegelman et al. 2000). The traditional flaws of epidemiologic studies certainly affect the results of these studies including recall bias and lack of prospective randomized data. Other confounding factors include concomitant increased in caloric intake with increased fat intake. Despite these drawbacks of the reports, decreased fat intake should be a recommendation for prevention strategy of UC.

4.3 Green tea

Drinking tea has been reported to confer protective health benefits which include prevention of human cancers including prostate and bladder cancers (Trevisanato and Kim 2000).

The polyphenols found in green tea are potent antioxidants; they also inhibit ornithine decarboxylase which is an enzyme that promotes tumor proliferation via nucleic acid regulation (Steele, Kelloff et al. 2000). The incidence of UC in Asian populations with increased tea consumption is lower than in North America; a weak inverse relationship between tea intake and UC has been reported in one epidemiological study (Kemberling, Hampton et al. 2003). In order to settle the ongoing controversy, NCI-sponsored phase 2 and 3 clinical trials are in progress (National Cancer Institute).

4.4 Soy

Soy products have potential apoptotic and anti-angiogenic actions attributable to their high isoflavone content (Su, Yeh et al. 2000).Their role in UC chemoprevention, unlike in prostate cancer, has yet to be elucidated. Contrary Su and group reported in a Singapore-based population study an increased UC incidence associated with high consumption of soy food (95% CI, 1.1-5.1) (Su, Yeh et al. 2000).This risk was independent of smoking. There is no data yet favoring recommendation of soy for chemoprevention in UC.

5. Bladder cancer chemoprevention strategies: Pharmacologic agents

5.1 Vitamins and supplements

Researchers have long regarded vitamins and the so-called micronutrients as ideal agents for primary chemoprevention for human cancer. For the reasons discussed earlier primary chemoprevention in human bladder cancer lacks an effective agent as well as evidence-based data to encourage wide clinical practice.

5.1.1 Vitamin A and analogues

Epidemiologic data in humans regarding the efficacy of Vitamin A are inconsistent. Many reports have suggested a therapeutic benefit from retinoid supplements. Data includes the SEER database controlled study, which compared 1592 UC participants to a matched neighborhood controls (Castelao, Yuan et al. 2004). Carotenoids were found to be beneficial in previous or current smokers. Authors using fenretinide in a randomized study failed to demonstrate the difference in tumor detection by flow cytometry between treatment and placebo arms in a sample of 99 participants (Decensi, Torrisi et al. 2000). Fenretinide is a synthetic derivative of Vitamin A which is FDA approved for the treatment of macular degeneration, and cystic fibrosis; and it has been investigated for use in cancer chemoprevention. Studer and group treated 90 Ta and T1 patients after transurethral resection with etretinate (Studer, Jenzer et al. 1995). They observed that time to first tumor occurrence was the same in both treatment and placebo groups, however, time to second tumor occurrence was lower for treatment group versus placebo (20.3 v 12.7 months, $P>0.006$). The data suggests that the agent acts not on established bladder cancer, but acts to prevent new cancer. Vitamin A overdose is known to cause low blood pressure, fever, and pulmonary insufficiency. Synthetic formulations of vitamin A are reported to show less significant adverse events (Sporn and Lippman 2003).
Sabichi and colleagues reported on a negative Phase III chemoprevention trial that showed that Fenretinide was well tolerated but failed to show a significant reduction in high incidence of recurrent non-muscle invasive urothelial bladder cancer (Sabichi, Lerner et al. 2008). The authors speculated that variable of dosing and scheduling could have affected the clinical results. However, data from other randomized clinical studies in contralateral breast cancer, ovarian cancer and oral premalignancy suggested preventative benefit of fenretinide in these malignancies (Sporn and Lippman 2003). In another clinical prevention trial in bladder cancer, this agent was reported as being less toxic and more efficacious than the retinoid etretinate (Sabichi, Lerner et al. 2008).

5.1.2 Vitamin B6 (Pyridoxine)

Vitamin B6 has been evaluated in patients with history of recurrent UC. The Veterans Administration Study by Byar and group showed that Pyridoxine provided the best benefit ($P=0.03$) in a 3-ARM trial of intravesical thiotepa, Pyridoxine and placebo in 121 patients with history of recurrent NMIUBC (Byar and Blackard 1977). The authors also showed that the efficacy of Pyridoxine was equivalent to that of thiotepa. The theory was that Pyridoxine would correct the abnormalities of Tryptophan metabolism often found in patients with bladder cancer. This data was not supported in a large study of 291 patients in the EORTC trial of Pyridoxine versus placebo with neither treatment showing any benefit in preventing occurrence or recurrence of UC (Newling, Robinson et al. 1995).

5.1.3 Vitamin C

Ascorbic acid (Vitamin C) is a potent antioxidant reported in human epidemiological studies to prevent UC (Shibata, Paganini-Hill et al. 1992; Michaud, Spiegelman et al. 2000). The effect is also thought to be dose dependent, with improved benefit associated with higher consumption (Shibata, Paganini-Hill et al. 1992; Michaud, Spiegelman et al. 2000). Favorable reports are inconsistent in large cohorts.

5.1.4 Vitamin E

Vitamin E is another antioxidant and is capable of reducing the carcinogenic N-nitroso compounds. Vitamin E has been reported in multiple studies to show benefit in reducing incidence of UC (Bruemmer, White et al. 1996; Michaud, Spiegelman et al. 2000). However, a meta-analysis by Miller and associates showed a potential increased in all-cause mortality associated with Vitamin E consumption (Miller, Pastor-Barriuso et al. 2005). This finding has dampened enthusiasm in the use of Vitamin E in chemoprevention for UC.

5.1.5 Selenium

There is no data yet suggesting a chemopreventive role for this oligoelement in UC.

5.1.6 Mega dose vitamins

Vitamins and dietary supplements/modifications have received slightly skewed publicity as alternative protective strategies against bladder cancer (Kamat and Lamm 2002). Individual vitamins including Vitamin A, and its analogues, Vitamin B6 (pyridoxine), Vitamin C, Vitamin E have been studied individually, reported and proposed as dietary supplements to prevent bladder cancer.as discussed above (Byar and Blackard 1977; Shibata, Paganini-Hill et al. 1992; Newling, Robinson et al. 1995; Studer, Jenzer et al. 1995; Decensi, Torrisi et al. 2000; Kamat and Lamm 2002; Castelao, Yuan et al. 2004; Miller, Pastor-Barriuso et al. 2005; Sabichi, Lerner et al. 2008). However, Lamm et al. combined mega doses of Vitamins A(40,000U), B6(100mg), C(2000 mg), E(400U) and Zinc (90mg) in a randomized 2x2 factorial design study in which 65 patients were randomized to receive intraderrmal BCG (Lamm, Riggs et al. 1994). Participants who demonstrated a response to induction intravesical BCG, were randomized to receive either Megadose vitamins or recommended daily allowance (RDA).The use of intradermal BCG did not appear to affect the clinical outcome. The Mega-dose vitamins treatment group showed a 50% reduction in overall NMIUBC recurrence at 4 years, The fact that there was no reduction in tumor recurrence rate in the Megadose vitamins group in the first 10 months, would suggest that these supplements/agents do not affect existing tumors but hinder the formation of new tumors.

5.2 Difluoromethylornithine

Difluoromethylornithine (DFMO) is a competitive inhibitor of ornithine decarboxylase (ODC) which is an enzyme that induces polyamine production necessary for tumor growth. A negative study was reported by Messing and associates who observed that daily oral supplementation of difluoromethylornithine (DFMO) compared with placebo, did not prevent frequent recurrence and progression of low grade NMIBC in patients who had been completely resected at enrollment (Messing, Kim et al. 2006).

5.3 COX Inhibitors

NSAID inhibit the cyclooxygenase (COX) enzyme, which breaks down arachidonic acid into leukotrienes and prostaglandins. Prostaglandin-2 can enhance cell proliferation, angiogenesis, and inhibit apoptosis (Sabichi and Lippman; Okey, Harper et al. 1998; Sporn and Lippman 2003). In vitro evidence suggests that there is an over expression of COX 2 isoform in UC (Okey, Harper et al. 1998; Sporn and Lippman 2003). Theoretically, COX 2 isoform inhibitors could be used in chemoprevention of UC. Castelao and colleagues reported on a population-based, case-control study, in which they evaluated non-steroidal anti-inflammatory drugs (NSAIDs) in NMIUBC (Castelao, Yuan et al. 2000). This study found a 19% decrease in UC risk in those patients treated with oral agents, except those patients treated with phenacetine and pyrazolone derivatives (Castelao, Yuan et al. 2000). Therefore, COX-2 remains a very viable target for future evaluation in bladder cancer chemoprevention.

Preventive Strategy	**Methodology**	**Mechanism**	**Published studies**	**Significance**	**Current status**
Fluid intake	Mailing Questionnaires	Increased fluid intake results in lowered cumulative exposure of urothelium to carcinogens with *reduced risk*	The Health Professional Follow up Study (n = 47,903)	High	Recommended (Level 4 evidence; Grade C recommendation)
Fat and calorie intake	Population based study (SEER) and meta-analysis of 36 studies evaluating 6 dietary variables in relation to UC	2-fold increase in cancer with increased fat consumption	Riboli et al & SEER studies: positive correlation; Health Professionals follow up study: no correlation	Intermediate	Recommended (Level 2 evidence; Grade B recommendation)
Green Tea	Epidemiological	Polyphenols contents of green tea are potent antioxidants; also inhibit ornithine decarboxylase which is an enzyme that promotes tumor proliferation via nucleic acid regulation; a *weak inverse relationship between tea intake and UC*	NCI-sponsored phase 2 and 3 clinical trials are in progress	Low	Recommended (Level 4 evidence; Grade C recommendation)

Preventive Strategy	Methodology	Mechanism	Published studies	Significance	Current status
Soy	Popublation based	potential apoptotic and action attributable to the high isoflavone content; *no data yet favoring recommendation*	Singapore-based population study	Very low	Not recommended
Smoking	Population based	Smoking cessation correlates with decreased incidence	Population based	High - most cost-effective measure in bladder cancer prevention strategy	Highly recommended (Level 3 evidence; Grade B recommendation)
Vitamin A	compared 1592 UC participants to a matched neighborhood controls	Agent does act not on established bladder cancer, but *prevents new cancer*	SEER database controlled study	Low - lacks an effective agent as well as evidence-based data to encourage wide clinical practice	Recommended (Level 3 evidence; Grade B recommendation)
Vitamin B6	3-arm trial; placebo controlled trial	Pyridoxine provided the best benefit (P=0.03) in a 3-Arm trial of intravesical thiotepa, placebo, and Pyridoxine; however, this data was not supported in EORCT trial (n=291) of Pyridoxine versus placebo, *both showing no benefit in preventing occurrence or reoccurrence*	The Veterans Administrati on Study (Byar et al)	Intermediate	Not recommended
Vitamin C	Human epidemiological studies	potent antioxidant; *effect dose dependent, better with higher consumption*	Large cohort studies	Inconsistent	Not recommended

Preventive Strategy	Methodology	Mechanism	Published studies	Significance	Current status
Vitamin E	meta-analysis	antioxidant capable of reducing carcinogenic N-nitroso compounds in urothelium	Miller et al.	Potential increase in all-cause mortality with Vitamin E consumption	Not recommended
Selenium	No data	no data yet suggesting a chemopreventive role for this oligoelement in UC	No data	N/A	Not recommended
Megadose vitamins	randomized 2x2 design study in which 65 patients were randomized to received intraderrmal BCG or not, and also randomized after response to induction intravesical BCG to receive Megadose vitamins versus daily recommended daily allowance	Possible anti-oxidant role	Small trial from a single institution	Mega-dose vitamins-treated group showed a 50% reduction in overall NMIBC recurrence at 4 years	Not recommended
Difluoromethylornithine (DFMO)	Messing et al	DFMO is a competitive inhibitor of *ornithine decarboxylase* that induces polyamine production necessary for tumor growth	Negative study	daily oral supplementation vs. placebo, did not prevent recurrence and progression of low grade NMIBC following prior TUR-BT	Not recommended

Preventive Strategy	Methodology	Mechanism	Published studies	Significance	Current status
COX inhibitors	Castelao et al.	Prostaglandin-2 can enhance cell proliferation, angiogenesis, and inhibit apoptosis. In vitro evidence suggests over expression of COX 2 isoform in UC	a population-based, case-control study - NSAIDs in NMIUBC showed a19% decrease in UC risk in those treated with oral NSAIDs (except phenacetine and pyrazolone derivatives)	COX-2 remains a very viable target in bladder cancer chemopreventi on	Recommended (non-evidence based)

Table 1. Summary of Reports (discussed above) of various Chemopreventative Strategies (refs:28-51)

6. Future research and experimental cancer chemoprevention

Research continues intensely in the evaluation of pharmaceutical agents for chemoprevention in bladder cancer. However, dietary supplement, multivitamins and phytochemicals/botanical agents are being evaluated in the prevention of many human cancers (Byar and Blackard 1977; Shibata, Paganini-Hill et al. 1992; Lamm, Riggs et al. 1994; Newling, Robinson et al. 1995; Studer, Jenzer et al. 1995; Castelao, Yuan et al. 2000; Decensi, Torrisi et al. 2000; Michaud, Spiegelman et al. 2000; Kamat and Lamm 2002; Castelao, Yuan et al. 2004; Miller, Pastor-Barriuso et al. 2005; Messing, Kim et al. 2006; Sabichi, Lerner et al. 2008). Investigators have reported on results of screening strategies for synthetic pharmaceuticals in an experimental bladder cancer prevention model using the chemically-induced rat bladder tumor model (Sindhwani, Hampton et al. 2001; Lubet, You et al. 2006; Park, Kim et al. 2006; Tian, Wang et al. 2008; Parada, Reis et al. 2011). They reported that low dose aspirin and resveratrol were least effective in preventing large tumor formation, while naproxen and Iressa were most effective (Lubet, You et al. 2006).

In recent years there has been a substantial interest in the application of botanically derived phytochemicals to reduce the incidence of variety of human tumors. Intense research is ongoing to provide evidence-based recommendations to incorporate plant foods or botanical products or dietary modifications into the practice of clinical cancer chemoprevention. There is the salient speculation that Curcumin, a very popular Indian food spice, derived from the rhizome plant called curcuma longa Linn (Zingiberaceae), has been responsible for lower incidence of urothelial malignancies (Sindhwani, Hampton et al. 2001; Tian, Wang et al. 2008)and lower rate of colorectal cancer (Tian, Wang et al. 2008) in the populations that consume Curcumin as a staple part of their diet (Sindhwani, Hampton et al. 2001; Tian, Wang et al. 2008). Investigators have reported on Curcumin induced apoptosis in MBT-2 cells[56] G2/M cell cycle arrest in T-24 cells (Sindhwani, Hampton et al. 2001; Tian, Wang et al. 2008). Curcumin inhibition of intravesical tumor implant in mouse model (Sindhwani, Hampton et al. 2001) and prevention of OH-BBN induced bladder carcinogenesis in rodent, as well as inhibition of tumor development and growth in an intravesical murine bladder model (Sindhwani, Hampton et al. 2001; Tian, Wang et al. 2008).

Seventy-five percent of all pharmaceuticals were discovered by studying the use of plants in traditional medicine. Of the 92 antitumor drugs approved by the FDA between 1983 and 1994, 62 (67%) were either of natural origin or based on a natural compound (Chung, Anscher et al. 2001).

7. Conclusions and clinical practice suggestions

Bladder cancer is a common, but serious health problem globally. It is immensely impacted by environmental carcinogens, tobacco smokes, and infectious etiologies in endemic areas. The bladder urothelial cancer special features which include its susceptibility; carcinogenesis; frequent recurrences, and clinical presentation favor it as an ideal cancer for chemoprevention. Unfortunately, in bladder cancer there are still no definite interventions that have been shown to be effective, and research in this area has yielded no evidence-based data to inform on strategies for systematic practice of bladder cancer prevention. The positive data from the clinical trials with vitamins individually or in combinations suggest that these agents might act not on established bladder cancer, but act to prevent occurring of new cancers, probably by hindering promotion of altered cells to overt cancer. Cessation of smoking will always remain the lofty but impractical goal of prevention strategies in urothelial bladder cancer; however, a plausible paradigm would suggest a chemoprevention strategy that should begin with the population approach that advocates a dietary program of increased consumption of fruits and vegetables which have been reported to reduce general cancer risk. The at-risk individual would embark on additional programs to reduce/eliminate the intensity of cumulative exposure to the carcinogens, dilution and elimination of bladder content by drinking plenty of water and urinating frequently, followed by introduction of the specific chemopreventive agent(s), probably in combination with the vitamins.

8. References

American Cancer Society. "Global Cancer Facts and Figures." Retrieved July 22, 2011, from http://www.acscan.org/tobaccoreports.

American Cancer Society. (2010). "Cancer Facts and Figures 2010." Retrieved July 15, 2010, from http://www.seer.cancer.gov/statfacts/html/urinb.html.

Botteman, M. F., C. L. Pashos, et al. (2003). "The health economics of bladder cancer: a comprehensive review of the published literature." *Pharmacoeconomics* 21(18): 1315-1330.

Bruemmer, B., E. White, et al. (1996). "Nutrient intake in relation to bladder cancer among middle-aged men and women." *Am J Epidemiol* 144(5): 485-495.

Byar, D. and C. Blackard (1977). "Comparisons of placebo, pyridoxine, and topical thiotepa in preventing recurrence of stage I bladder cancer." *Urology* 10(6): 556-561.

Cancer Treatment of America. "World-Class Cancer Center." Retrieved January, 2011, from http://www.cancercenter.com/carethatneverquits.

Castelao, J. E., J. M. Yuan, et al. (2004). "Carotenoids/vitamin C and smoking-related bladder cancer." *Int J Cancer* 110(3): 417-423.

Castelao, J. E., J. M. Yuan, et al. (2000). "Non-steroidal anti-inflammatory drugs and bladder cancer prevention." *Br J Cancer* 82(7): 1364-1369.

Chung, T., M. Anscher, et al. (2001). The role of Hypericum Perforatum in Cancer Research. *Global Science Books*. 5.

Dalbagni, D. and H. Herr (2000). Current clinical questions concerning intravesical bladder cancer. *Urologic Clinic of North America*. Loughlin. 27.

Decensi, A., R. Torrisi, et al. (2000). "Randomized trial of fenretinide in superficial bladder cancer using DNA flow cytometry as an intermediate end point." *Cancer Epidemiol Biomarkers Prev* 9(10): 1071-1078.

Dietrich, H. and B. Dietrich (2001). "Ludwig Rehn (1849-1930)--pioneering findings on the aetiology of bladder tumours." *World J Urol* 19(2): 151-153.

Droller, M. (2006). Introduction. *Textbook of bladder cancer*. S. P. Lerner and M. P. Schoenberg.

Fradet, Y., H. B. Grossman, et al. (2007). "A comparison of hexaminolevulinate fluorescence cystoscopy and white light cystoscopy for the detection of carcinoma in situ in patients with bladder cancer: a phase III, multicenter study." *J Urol* 178(1): 68-73; discussion 73.

Geoffroy-Perez, B. and S. Cordier (2001). "Fluid consumption and the risk of bladder cancer: results of a multicenter case-control study." *Int J Cancer* 93(6): 880-887.

Grasso, M. (2008). "Bladder cancer: a major public health issue." *European Urology Supplements* 7(7): 510-515.

Haack, S., S. Treccani, et al. (2000). *Arsenic concentration and selected geochemical characteristics for ground water and aquifer materials in southeastern Michigan*, US Department of the Interior, US Geological Survey.

Hedelin, H., S. Holmang, et al. (2002). "The cost of bladder tumour treatment and follow-up." *Scand J Urol Nephrol* 36(5): 344-347.

Henderson, B. D., TJ (1992). "How does photodynamic therapy work?" *Photochem Photobiol* 55(1): 145-157.

Hong, Y. M. and K. R. Loughlin (2008). "Economic impact of tumor markers in bladder cancer surveillance." *Urology* 71(1): 131-135.

Jichlinski, P., L. Guillou, et al. (2003). "Hexyl aminolevulinate fluorescence cystoscopy: new diagnostic tool for photodiagnosis of superficial bladder cancer--a multicenter study." *J Urol* 170(1): 226-229.

Kamat, A. and D. L. Lamm (2002). Chemoprevention of bladder cancer. *Urologic Clinics of North America*. Loughlin. 29.

Karl, A. Z., D; Staddler, T. (2010). Influence of photodynamic diagnosis on recurrence rates of T1G3 bladder cancer. *American Urological Association*. San Francisco, CA.

Kemberling, J. K., J. A. Hampton, et al. (2003). "Inhibition of bladder tumor growth by the green tea derivative epigallocatechin-3-gallate." *J Urol* 170(3): 773-776.

Kim, M.-J., J. Nriagu, et al. (2000). "Carbonate ions and arsenic dissolution by groundwater." *Environmental Science and Technology* 34(15): 3094-3100.

Lamm, D. L., B. A. Blumenstein, et al. (1995). "Randomized intergroup comparison of bacillus calmette-guerin immunotherapy and mitomycin C chemotherapy prophylaxis in superficial transitional cell carcinoma of the bladder a southwest oncology group study." *Urol Oncol* 1(3): 119-126.

Lamm, D. L., D. R. Riggs, et al. (1994). "Megadose vitamins in bladder cancer: a double-blind clinical trial." *J Urol* 151(1): 21-26.

Lattouf, J. B. (2009). "Chemoprevention in bladder cancer: What's new?" *Can Urol Assoc J* 3(6 Suppl 4): S184-187.

Lubet, R., M. You, et al. (2006). Chemopreventive effects of Iressa against methylnitrosourea (MNU) induced mammary cancers and 4-hydroxybutyl*butyl)-nitrosamine (OH-BBN) induced urinary bladder cancers. *American Association of Cancer Research*

Messing, E., K. M. Kim, et al. (2006). "Randomized prospective phase III trial of difluoromethylornithine vs placebo in preventing recurrence of completely resected low risk superficial bladder cancer." *J Urol* 176(2): 500-504.

Michaud, D. S., D. Spiegelman, et al. (1999). "Fluid intake and the risk of bladder cancer in men." *N Engl J Med* 340(18): 1390-1397.

Michaud, D. S., D. Spiegelman, et al. (2000). "Prospective study of dietary supplements, macronutrients, micronutrients, and risk of bladder cancer in US men." *Am J Epidemiol* 152(12): 1145-1153.

Miller, E. R., 3rd, R. Pastor-Barriuso, et al. (2005). "Meta-analysis: high-dosage vitamin E supplementation may increase all-cause mortality." *Ann Intern Med* 142(1): 37-46.

National Cancer Institute. "Clinical Trials." Retrieved July 18, 2011, from http://www.cancer.gov/CLINICALTRIALS.

Newling, D. W., M. R. Robinson, et al. (1995). "Tryptophan metabolites, pyridoxine (vitamin B6) and their influence on the recurrence rate of superficial bladder cancer. Results of a prospective, randomised phase III study performed by the EORTC GU Group. EORTC Genito-Urinary Tract Cancer Cooperative Group." *Eur Urol* 27(2): 110-116.

Okey, A., P. Harper, et al. (1998). Chemical and radiation carcinogenesis. *The basic science of oncology*. I. Tannock and R. P. Hill. New York, McGraw-Hill, Health Professions Division: xii, 539 p.

Oosterlinck, W., K. H. Kurth, et al. (1993). "A prospective European Organization for Research and Treatment of Cancer Genitourinary Group randomized trial comparing transurethral resection followed by a single intravesical instillation of epirubicin or water in single stage Ta, T1 papillary carcinoma of the bladder." *J Urol* 149(4): 749-752.

Parada, B., F. Reis, et al. (2011). "Inhibition of bladder tumour growth by sirolimus in an experimental carcinogenesis model." *BJU Int* 107(1): 135-143.

Park, C., G. Y. Kim, et al. (2006). "Induction of G2/M arrest and inhibition of cyclooxygenase-2 activity by curcumin in human bladder cancer T24 cells." *Oncol Rep* 15(5): 1225-1231.

Prout, G. R., Jr., B. A. Barton, et al. (1992). "Treated history of noninvasive grade 1 transitional cell carcinoma. The National Bladder Cancer Group." *J Urol* 148(5): 1413-1419.

Riboli, E., C. A. Gonzalez, et al. (1991). "Diet and bladder cancer in Spain: a multi-centre case-control study." *Int J Cancer* 49(2): 214-219.

Sabichi, A. L., S. P. Lerner, et al. (2008). "Phase III prevention trial of fenretinide in patients with resected non-muscle-invasive bladder cancer." *Clin Cancer Res* 14(1): 224-229.

Sabichi, A. L. and S. M. Lippman Chemoprevention of superficial bladder cancer. *Chemoprevention strategies.*

Shibata, A., A. Paganini-Hill, et al. (1992). "Intake of vegetables, fruits, beta-carotene, vitamin C and vitamin supplements and cancer incidence among the elderly: a prospective study." *Br J Cancer* 66(4): 673-679.

Sievert, K. D., B. Amend, et al. (2009). "Economic aspects of bladder cancer: what are the benefits and costs?" *World J Urol* 27(3): 295-300.

Sindhwani, P., J. A. Hampton, et al. (2001). "Curcumin prevents intravesical tumor implantation of the MBT-2 tumor cell line in C3H mice." *J Urol* 166(4): 1498-1501.

Sporn, M. and S. M. Lippman (2003). Chemoprevention in cancer. *Cancer medicine 6*. D. W. Kufe, J. F. Holland, E. Frei and American Cancer Society. Hamilton, Ont.; Lewiston, NY, BC Decker: 377-388.

Steele, V. E., G. J. Kelloff, et al. (2000). "Comparative chemopreventive mechanisms of green tea, black tea and selected polyphenol extracts measured by in vitro bioassays." *Carcinogenesis* 21(1): 63-67.

Steineck, G., U. Hagman, et al. (1990). "Vitamin A supplements, fried foods, fat and urothelial cancer. A case-referent study in Stockholm in 1985-87." *Int J Cancer* 45(6): 1006-1011.

Steinmaus, C. M., S. Nunez, et al. (2000). "Diet and bladder cancer: a meta-analysis of six dietary variables." *Am J Epidemiol* 151(7): 693-702.

Studer, U. E., S. Jenzer, et al. (1995). "Adjuvant treatment with a vitamin A analogue (etretinate) after transurethral resection of superficial bladder tumors. Final analysis of a prospective, randomized multicenter trial in Switzerland." *Eur Urol* 28(4): 284-290.

Su, S. J., T. M. Yeh, et al. (2000). "The potential of soybean foods as a chemoprevention approach for human urinary tract cancer." *Clin Cancer Res* 6(1): 230-236.

Tian, B., Z. Wang, et al. (2008). "Effects of curcumin on bladder cancer cells and development of urothelial tumors in a rat bladder carcinogenesis model." *Cancer Lett* 264(2): 299-308.

Trevisanato, S. I. and Y. I. Kim (2000). "Tea and health." *Nutr Rev* 58(1): 1-10.

Uchida, A., H. Yonou, et al. (2007). "Intravesical instillation of bacille Calmette-Guerin for superficial bladder cancer: cost-effectiveness analysis." *Urology* 69(2): 275-279.

Weber, W. W. (1987). *The acetylator genes and drug response*. New York, Oxford University Press.

Welch, A., D. Westjohn, et al. (2000). "Arsenic in ground water of the United States--occurrence and geochemistry." *Ground Water* 38(4): 589-604.

Part 6

Metastatic Disease

13

The Molecular Basis of Cisplatin Resistance in Bladder Cancer Cells

Beate Köberle and Andrea Piee-Staffa
Institute of Toxicology, University of Mainz Medical Center, Mainz, Germany

1. Introduction

Bladder cancer is one of the most common cancers among men and women, with men being twice as likely affected from the disease (Jemal et al., 2005). The most common type of bladder cancer is transitional cell carcinoma (TCC), which is derived from the urothelium and constitutes more than 90 % of all bladder cancers (Bischoff & Clark, 2009). Cisplatin-based combination therapy is the standard therapy for the treatment of advanced or metastatic bladder cancers (Cohen et al., 2006, Kaufman, 2006). However, the outcome of patients with metastatic bladder cancer remains poor, as tumors become resistant to cisplatin therapy. It is still not entirely known, which factors influence the response of bladder cancers to the drug and how this cancer acquires cisplatin resistance. Cisplatin is a neutral planar complex (Figure 1A).

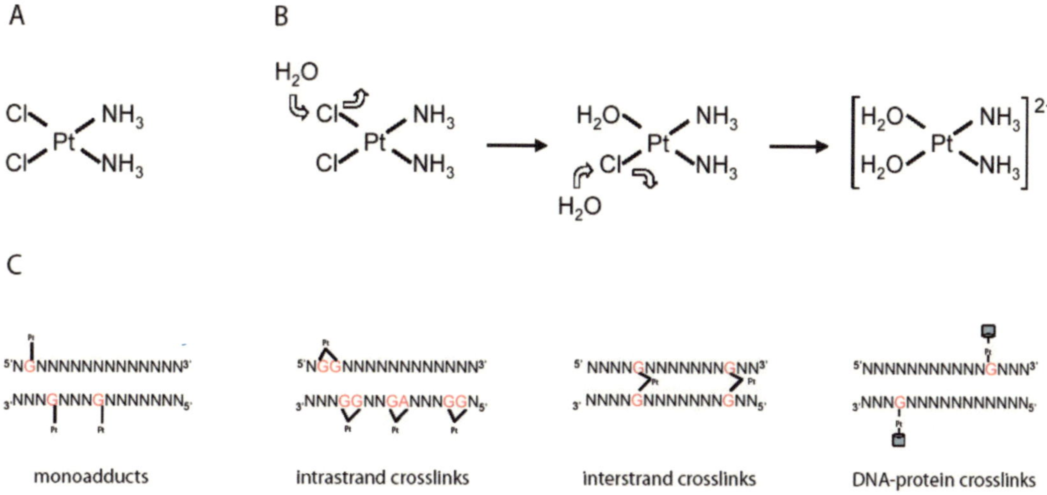

Fig. 1. **A:** The chemical structure of cisplatin. **B:** After entering the cells, cisplatin is transformed to a positively charged molecule that reacts with DNA **C:** Cisplatin induced lesions. Cisplatin preferably binds to the nucleophilic N7 position of the purine bases guanine or adenine, leading to different types of lesions including monoadducts, intrastrand crosslinks, interstrand crosslinks and DNA-protein crosslinks

After entering the cell, it is activated through a series of aquation reactions, in which the chloro ligands are replaced by water molecules (Figure 1B). The resulting positively charged molecule can react with nucleophilic sites on macromolecules, leading to DNA, RNA and protein adducts. It preferably binds to the nucleophilic N7 position of the purine bases guanine or adenine, which leads to different types of lesions (Figure 1C) (Jamieson & Lippard, 1999). In a first reaction, cisplatin binds to DNA, leading to monoadducts, which in a second reaction lead to the formation of DNA crosslinks. The most frequently observed cisplatin DNA lesions are DNA intrastrand crosslinks between adjacent guanines (65 % of all lesions) or intrastrand crosslinks between guanine and adenine (25 %). Interstrand crosslinks between two guanines on the opposite strands of DNA account for less than 5% of all cisplatin-induced lesions. It is still unknown, which of the various DNA lesions ultimately results in cell death (Chu, 1994, Jordan & Carmo-Fonseca, 2000, Kartalou & Essigmann, 2001).

The efficacy of cisplatin in cancer chemotherapy, however, is limited by resistance. While cancers of the bladder, lung and ovary respond initially in 50 % or more of cases, they will almost inevitably relapse with drug-resistant disease. The mechanisms of cisplatin resistance have been studied in numerous cell culture models of cisplatin sensitive and resistant cancer cells lines. It has been shown that a cancer cell can develop cisplatin resistance through different mechanisms (Figure 2). Cisplatin resistance can be due to (i) changes in drug transport, leading to reduced cellular cisplatin accumulation, (ii) increased drug detoxification, also resulting in reduced cellular cisplatin accumulation, (iii) changes in DNA repair mechanisms including nucleotide excision repair, interstrand crosslink repair and mismatch repair, (iv) changes in DNA tolerance mechanisms, and finally (v) alterations in the apoptotic cell death pathways (Köberle et al., 2010, Rabik & Dolan, 2007, Siddik, 2003). In this chapter we describe and discuss the contribution of these mechanisms for the development of cisplatin resistance in bladder cancer cells *in vitro* and compare the preclinical findings to data obtained in clinical studies. A better understanding of the molecular basis of cisplatin resistance may lead to new anticancer strategies that will sensitize unresponsive bladder cancers to cisplatin-based chemotherapy.

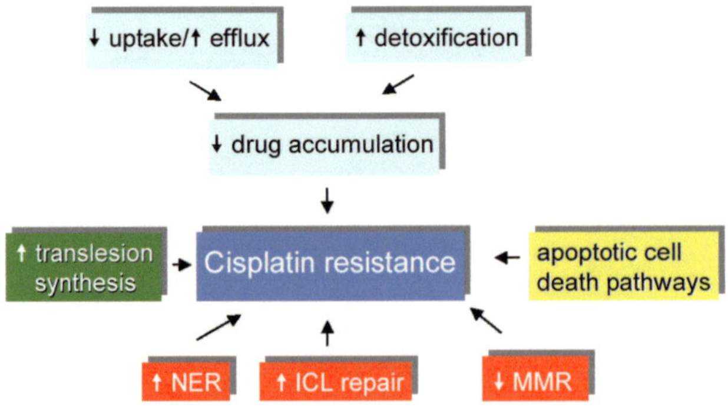

Fig. 2. Mechanisms of resistance towards cisplatin include: Reduced drug accumulation due to changes in drug uptake, efflux or detoxification. Alterations in DNA repair such as increased removal of the damage by nucleotide excision repair (NER) or interstrand crosslink repair (ICL repair) as well as decreased mismatch repair (MMR). Enhanced translesion synthesis (TLS) to tolerate unrepaired cisplatin lesions. Alterations in apoptosis pathways: changes in expression levels of pro- and anti-apoptotic proteins.

2. Intracellular drug accumulation as a determinant of cellular cisplatin sensitivity

2.1 Cellular uptake and efflux of cisplatin

Reduced intracellular cisplatin accumulation has been associated with cisplatin resistance in numerous cancer cell lines (Siddik, 2003). A correlation between intracellular cisplatin accumulation and cisplatin resistance was observed in a series of seven bladder cancer cell lines displaying different sensitivities to cisplatin (Koga et al., 2000). Similarly, using a bladder cancer cell line and its cisplatin-resistant subline, we found reduced accumulation of cisplatin in the resistant subline when compared to its parental cells (Köberle et al., 1996). Reduced accumulation may result from changes in drug transport or increased drug detoxification. Even though the exact mechanism by which cisplatin is taken up by the cells is not fully understood, both passive diffusion and active transport appear to be involved. For active transport the copper transporter 1 (Ctr1), which controls intracellular copper homeostasis, seems to play an important role (Kuo et al., 2007, Safaei, 2006). It has been reported that loss of Ctr1 lead to cisplatin resistance in various cell lines (Holzer et al., 2006, Ishida et al., 2002, Song et al., 2004). However, no data as to Ctr1 expression in bladder cancer cell lines or tumor tissue have been reported to date. Therefore, no conclusion about the importance of uptake for cisplatin response can be drawn for bladder cancer cells (Table 1).

Increased efflux of cisplatin from the cell may also lead to resistance. Efflux pumps such as MRP1/2 (multidrug resistance associated protein) and p-glycoprotein/multidrug resistance 1 (MDR1) are implicated as efflux pumps for cisplatin (Taniguchi et al., 1996, Yeh et al., 2005). Tada and co-workers investigated the relationship between expression of p-glycoprotein expression or MRP1/2 and drug sensitivity in 47 clinical samples of bladder cancer. They showed that expression of p-glycoprotein and MRP1/2 was higher in samples of recurrent tumors than in untreated primary tumors (Tada et al., 2002), indicating that increased efflux can contribute to the development of drug resistance and poor clinical outcome in bladder cancers (Table 1).

2.2 Detoxification of cisplatin by intracellular thiol molecules

Cisplatin resistance can be the result of increased inactivation of the drug by intracellular thiol-containing molecules such as glutathione and metallothionein. Glutathione is a tripeptide that plays an important role for the detoxification of xenobiotic substances by scavenging free radicals. Cisplatin can be conjugated with glutathione, which will inhibit its binding to DNA and other cellular molecules. This reaction is catalyzed by the glutathione-S-transferase (GST) (Mannervik, 1987). Extensive studies about the role of the glutathione system for cisplatin resistance have been carried out in cell lines and in cancer tissue. A correlation between expression of the glutathione system and cisplatin resistance has been reported for ovarian, cervical and lung cancer cell lines (Jansen et al., 2002, Meijer et al., 1992, Mellish et al., 1993). Attempts to correlate expression of the glutathione system with cisplatin resistance in bladder cancer cell lines showed inconsistent findings. Bedford and co-workers investigated the expression of the glutatione system in different bladder cancer cells lines and reported higher levels of glutathione and GST in the less sensitive cells (Bedford et al., 1987). Similarly, using a model system of a bladder cancer cell line and two derived sublines with acquired cisplatin resistance, Kotoh and co-workers observed an increased glutathione content and elevated GST activity in the sublines (Kotoh et al., 1997). Buthionine sulphoximine (BSO), which depletes glutathione, or indomethacin, which blocks

GST, significantly decreased the cisplatin resistance in T24 bladder cancer cells, which is yet another indication that the glutathione-based detoxification system is involved in cisplatin resistance in bladder cancer cells (Byun et al., 2005). However, no correlation between glutathione content and resistance to cisplatin was observed in a study by Koga and co-workers (Koga et al., 2000). In this study, the expression of GST was also not significantly related to cisplatin resistance. In another study with bladder cancer cells, which were either sensitive or progressively resistant to cisplatin, it was observed that expression of GST was increased in the cisplatin resistant cells, however, the increase in glutathione contents did not reach statistical significance (Hour et al., 2000). In conclusion, bladder cancer cells may gain cisplatin resistance through up-regulation of GST, while glutathione contents seems to play a less important role for the development of cisplatin resistance.

Metallothioneins (MT) belong to a family of low molecular weight, thiol-rich proteins that play a role in metal homeostasis and detoxification (Kagi & Schaffer, 1988). MTs can bind to cisplatin, leading to the inactivation of the drug. For numerous cancer cell lines (derived from prostate, lung, ovary and cervical cancer), a correlation between MT expression and cisplatin resistance has been observed (Kasahara et al., 1991, Kondo et al., 1995, Mellish et al., 1993, Surowiak et al., 2007). For bladder cancer cell lines cisplatin resistance, was also correlated with increased levels of MT (Siegsmund et al., 1999, Singh et al., 1995). A role of MT for cisplatin resistance in bladder cancer has been proposed by Satoh and co-workers (Satoh et al., 1994). The authors investigated the effect of modulation of the MT levels for the antitumor activity of cisplatin in nude mice inoculated with human bladder cancer cells. While increasing MT levels reduced the antitumor activity of cisplatin, decreased levels of MT diminished the resistance to the drug (Satoh et al., 1994). Using a different bladder tumor model in mice, it was also suggested that MT might play a role for acquired resistance towards cisplatin (Saga et al., 2004). The clinical relevance of MT levels for cisplatin chemotherapy in bladder cancers has been investigated in a number of studies. In an investigation involving 118 patients with bladder cancer, it was observed that overexpression of MT was associated with a poorer outcome from cisplatin-based chemotherapy (Siu et al., 1998). Similarly, for intrinsic cisplatin resistance of urinary tract TCCs, an involvement of MT has been suggested (Kotoh et al., 1994), and MT overexpression was proposed to be a mechanism for cisplatin resistance in bladder cancer tissue (Wood et al., 1993). In line with this observations are more recent studies, which also reported that high levels of MT expression in bladder cancer tissue were correlated with poor survival after cisplatin chemotherapy (Hinkel et al., 2008, Wülfing et al., 2007). Taken together, the data indicate that high levels of MT in bladder cancers might be a major problem for effective cisplatin-based chemotherapy. In our opinion, expression of MT is one of the main cellular factors for both intrinsic and acquired cisplatin resistance in bladder cancers (Table 1).

3. DNA repair and cisplatin resistance

The contribution of DNA repair for cisplatin resistance has been investigated for many years. In model systems of tumor cell lines and sublines with acquired cisplatin resistance, increased removal of cisplatin induced lesions has been observed in the sublines. For example, ovarian cancer cells with acquired resistance towards cisplatin show an increased removal of cisplatin induced lesions in comparison with their cisplatin sensitive counterparts (Johnson et al., 1994a, Johnson et al., 1994b, Parker et al., 1991). Similarly, colon

Molecular mechanism	Preclinical evidence	Clinical evidence
Intracellular cisplatin accumulation		
Decreased uptake	no data reported	no data reported
Increased efflux	no data reported	observed in resistant tumors
Increased glutathione/ GST levels	conflicting results	Conflicting results
Increased metallothioneine levels	Observed in resistant cancer cell lines	correlated with poor clinical outcome
DNA repair		
Nucleotide excision repair (NER)	High levels of ERCC1 in resistant cancer cells	Conflicting results
ICL repair	Proficiency in resistant bladder cancer cell lines	no data reported
Translesion synthesis (TLS)	no data reported	no data reported
Mismatch repair (MMR)	No association with acquired resistance	Conflicting results
DNA damage response		
p53	Conflicting results	Conflicting results
Bcl-2, Bcl-xL	Overexpression in cisplatin resistant cancer cells	Low levels correlate with better prognosis
Survivin	High levels in bladder cancer cells	Expression as a marker for clinical outcome
XIAP	High expression in bladder cancer cells	High levels correlate with poor prognosis

Table 1. Mechanisms of cisplatin resistance in bladder cancers: preclinical findings and clinical evidence (Table adapted from Köberle et al., 2010)

carcinoma cell lines with acquired cisplatin resistance showed a higher extent of removal of DNA platination compared to the parental cells (Oldenburg et al., 1994), indicating that the acquired resistance to cisplatin might be related to the increased DNA repair capacity. In contrast, when we investigated DNA damage removal in a bladder cancer cell line with acquired cisplatin resistance, we observed no enhanced repair compared to the parental cell line, suggesting that this bladder cancer cell line did not acquire resistance to cisplatin by increasing the DNA repair capacity (Köberle et al., 1996). However, when we compared bladder cancer cell lines with cisplatin sensitive testis tumor cells, we observed that bladder cancer cells are proficient in removing cisplatin damage from the DNA, while testis tumor cells were repair deficient (Köberle et al., 1997), supporting the hypothesis that susceptibility to cisplatin might be related to the repair capacity.

3.1 Nucleotide excision repair

Cisplatin-induced GpG and GpA DNA intrastrand crosslinks are repaired by nucleotide excision repair (NER). NER is a multistep mechanism, which deals with bulky helix-distorting lesions such as UV-induced cyclobutane pyrimidine dimers and 6-4 photoproducts, and DNA lesions induced by many chemotherapeutic drugs (Gillet & Schärer, 2006, Shuck et al., 2008, Wood et al., 2000). The repair of the lesions begins with recognition of the damage and incision on both sides of the lesion, followed by DNA synthesis to replace the excised fragment. The core incision reaction requires the protein factors XPA, RPA, XPC-HR23B, TFIIH, ERCC1-XPF and XPG (Aboussekhra et al., 1995). It is possible to carry out the core NER reaction in a cell free system using cellular protein extracts (Shivji et al., 1999, Shivji et al., 2005). Using this system, it could be confirmed that the increased removal of cisplatin lesions, which has been observed in cisplatin resistant ovarian cancer cells, is in fact due to enhanced NER (Ferry et al., 2000). We found that cellular protein extracts of a bladder cancer cell line were proficient for NER (Köberle et al., 1999). Furthermore, the core NER proteins are expressed to a similar extent in bladder cancer cell lines compared to normal non-cancerous cells (Köberle et al., 1999, Welsh et al., 2004). The removal of cisplatin induced DNA platination, which we previously observed in bladder cancer cell lines (Köberle et al., 1997), is therefore, at least in part, due to NER proficiency in these cells.

Conclusive evidence for functionally increased NER in cisplatin-resistant cancers, however, has not yet been presented. This is due to the lack of methods to easily and reliably measure NER activities in tissue samples. For example, even in protein extracts prepared from cell lines, a significant variability in NER capacity is observed. Even more, in protein extracts prepared from biopsies of human ovarian carcinoma, Jones and co-workers found that the NER capacity varied significantly by as much as ten-fold (Jones et al., 1994). This could be due to either inter-individual variations or to technical problems to obtain active extracts from tissue material. Therefore, as measuring NER capacity in tissue samples is a challenging task, a different approach is to investigate the expression of NER factors on the mRNA or protein level and attempt to correlate these with response to chemotherapy. In these studies, special emphasis was given to ERCC1, the first human DNA repair gene cloned (Westerveld et al., 1984). In preclinical studies, a correlation between ERCC1 expression and cisplatin resistance has been presented (Li et al., 1998, Li et al., 2000, Metzger et al., 1998). By demonstrating that down-regulation of ERCC1 by siRNA sensitized bladder cancer cell lines to cisplatin, we could confirm the importance of ERCC1 for cisplatin resistance in bladder cancer cells (Usanova et al., 2010).

In cancer tissues, ERCC1 mRNA or protein levels show an inverse correlation with the response to platinum therapy or overall survival. High ERCC1 mRNA levels are associated with resistance to cisplatin-based chemotherapy in ovarian, cervical, gastric, colorectal, head and neck, esophageal and lung cancer (Dabholkar et al., 1992, Dabholkar et al., 1994, Gossage & Madhusudan, 2007, Handra-Luca et al., 2007, Jun et al., 2008, Kim et al., 2008, Metzger et al., 1998, Olaussen et al., 2006, Weberpals et al., 2009). Based on these findings, it was suggested that ERCC1 can be used as a predictive and prognostic marker for the outcome of cisplatin-based chemotherapy. For patients with advanced bladder cancer, a significantly higher survival rate was reported when ERCC1 levels in the tumor tissue were low (Bellmunt et al., 2007). However, in another study, no significant difference in overall survival between bladder cancer patients with ERCC1 negative tumors and ERCC1 positive tumors was observed (Kim et al., 2010). On the other hand, the authors reported that progression free survival was longer in patients with ERCC1 negative bladder cancers compared to ERCC1 positive cancers (Kim et al., 2010). Based on these conflicting results, it is difficult to conclude that ERCC1 expression in bladder cancer negatively contributes to the clinical outcome. Furthermore, even though ERCC1 positive tumors would be expected to have a high NER capacity, and ERCC1 negative tumors would be expected to have low NER capacity, these conclusions must be drawn with caution, as functional NER assays for tissue material are still missing. It therefore remains speculative whether altered ERCC1 levels have an impact on NER in tumor tissue. Therefore, the question about the contribution of enhanced NER for cisplatin resistance in cancers, especially in bladder cancers, remains to be solved (Table 1).

3.2 Interstrand crosslink repair

Besides intrastrand adducts, cisplatin induces interstrand crosslinks (ICLs), which are removed by ICL repair, a process less understood than NER (McHugh et al., 2001). Repair of ICLs is a challenging problem for cells. In bacteria and lower eukaryotes, NER and homologous recombination are involved in ICL repair (Cole, 1973, Jachymczyk et al., 1981). In mammalian cells, these both pathways may also operate (De Silva et al., 2000). Besides that, mammalian cells have additional pathways of ICL repair involving DNA polymerases that can bypass the lesion (Sarkar et al., 2006, Shen et al., 2006, Zheng et al., 2005). A contribution of increased ICL repair for acquired resistance to cisplatin has been described for ovarian cancer cells in culture (Zhen et al., 1992). It also seems to play a role for clinical cisplatin resistance, as in paired tumor samples obtained prior to treatment and at relapse following platinum chemotherapy, increased repair of cisplatin ICLs in cells of relapsed ovarian cancer was observed (Wynne et al., 2007). We found that bladder cancer cell lines, which are relatively resistant to cisplatin, are proficient in repairing ICLs (Usanova et al., 2010). Biochemical and cell biological data implicate that ERCC1 is not only involved in NER, but also in ICL repair (Kuraoka et al., 2000, Niedernhofer et al., 2004, Sijbers et al., 1996). Our own experiments revealed that down-regulation of ERCC1 by siRNA affected ICL repair in the bladder cancer cell lines and rendered the cells more sensitive to cisplatin supporting the notion about the importance of ICL repair for cisplatin resistance in cancer cells. However, to date there is no information as to ICL repair in bladder cancer tissue (Table 1).

3.3 Translesion synthesis (TLS)

As described in 3.1 and 3.2, cisplatin damage is removed by NER and ICL repair. However, some lesions may remain. A mechanism, by which cells can tolerate unrepaired DNA lesions, is translesion synthesis (TLS). TLS is carried out by a group of specialized DNA polymerases, which are capable of bypassing unrepaired DNA lesions. For mammalian cells pol η (POLH), pol ι (POLI), pol κ (POLK), REV1 and pol ζ (REV3 and REV7) are the main TLS polymerases, which have been shown to possess different substrate specificity. Depending on the type of damage, different combinations of TLS polymerases act in concert to bypass the DNA lesions (Shachar et al., 2009). Cisplatin GpG intrastrand crosslinks seem to be bypassed by pol η and pol ζ (Alt et al., 2007, Shachar et al., 2009). For pol κ conflicting results have been reported. While an in vitro assay suggests that pol κ is unable to bypass a GpG intrastrand crosslink, in vivo TLS assays implicated pol κ in combination with pol η for TLS across cisplatin GpG intrastrand crosslinks (Ohashi et al., 2000, Shachar et al., 2009). The importance of TLS in the tolerance towards cisplatin has been shown in cell lines deficient in TLS polymerase activity (Cruet-Hennequart et al., 2008, Cruet-Hennequart et al., 2009, Albertella et al., 2005a, Roos et al., 2009, Wittschieben et al., 2006). Similarly, TLS polymerases may play a role for cisplatin resistance in tumor samples (Albertella et al., 2005b, Ceppi et al., 2009, Wang et al., 2009). However, no data have been reported as to the expression of TLS polymerases in bladder cancer cell lines and tumor specimens. We therefore can neither include nor exclude TLS polymerases as a factor determining efficacy of cisplatin therapy in the clinic (Table 1).

3.4 DNA mismatch repair (MMR)

Mismatch repair (MMR) is the pathway that removes mispaired nucleotides or insertion/deletion loops, which arise during DNA replication or as a result of damage to DNA. MMR consists of following steps: (1) recognition of the mismatch, (2) identification and excision of the mispairs or looped intermediates, and (3) resynthesis of the excised strand (Kunkel & Erie, 2005). In early investigations it has been observed that loss of MMR led to resistance to cisplatin and other platinating agents (Aebi et al., 1996, Fink et al., 1996). A possible explanation for the association of absence of a repair mechanism with increased drug resistance was the observation that MMR proteins can bind to cisplatin damage possibly leading to futile repair and therefore increased drug lethality. The mismatch repair complex MutSα (which is a heterodimer containing MSH2 and MSH6) binds to cisplatin DNA lesions in vitro (Duckett et al., 1996, Mello et al., 1996). Binding of MutSα to cisplatin crosslinks could start the MMR process by recruiting the mismatch repair complex MutLα (consisting of MLH1 and PMS2). It is assumed that lethal intermediates arise by the attempt of the MMR machinery to remove cisplatin lesions, and these lethal intermediates might set off a futile MMR cycle, similar to what has been reported for methylating agents (Dunkern et al., 2001). An alternative model suggests that binding of the MMR complex to cisplatin DNA damage might cause direct activation of the DNA damage response (DDR). A third model is based on the finding that TLS polymerases can bypass of 1,2-intrastrand crosslinks (Alt et al., 2007, Shachar et al., 2009). Since TLS polymerases are error prone causing mis-incorporation of bases, mismatches will be generated that are recognised by the MutSα complex. This in turn causes a futile repair cycle that triggers DDR. New data suggest that mitochondrial pro-death signaling involving cytochrome c and caspases-9 and -3 is required for the execution of MMR protein-mediated induction of cell death by cisplatin (Topping et al., 2009). The importance of MMR for cisplatin resistance has been investigated in a number of cancer cell lines, however, with conflicting results. On the one hand it was observed that

MMR deficient cell lines were more tolerant to cisplatin (Bignami et al., 2003, Fink et al., 1996, Papouli et al., 2004). This was explained by the hypothesis that cisplatin lesions are not processed into lethal intermediates. In other studies, however, it was shown that defective MMR is only a minor contributor for the cisplatin resistance phenotype or is not involved at all (Branch et al., 2000, Claij & te Riele, 2004, Massey et al., 2003). We found that the MMR protein MSH2 was expressed at lower levels in bladder cancer cells compared to cisplatin sensitive testis tumor cells. However, no difference was observed in the expression level of the MMR proteins hMLH1 and PMS2 in this model system of cisplatin resistant and sensitive cell lines. Even more, no difference in the levels of MSH2, MLH1 and PMS2 was observed in parental RT112 bladder cancer cells and the subline with acquired cisplatin resistance (Köberle, unpublished results), suggesting that MMR may not be of importance for cisplatin resistance in our model system.
The clinical relevance of loss of MMR for cisplatin chemotherapy has been investigated in a number of clinical studies, and it was concluded that MMR deficiency is associated with chemotherapy resistance in ovarian and testicular germ cell tumors (Gifford et al., 2004, Helleman et al., 2006, Wei et al., 2002). In 115 patients with bladder cancers, the expression pattern of hMSH2 protein was investigated and a reduced expression of hMSH2 was significantly more frequent in high grade tumors (Jin et al., 1999). Similarly, Catto and co-workers reported that reduced expression of hMLH1 and hMSH2 was seen more commonly in muscle invasive and high grade bladder cancer (Catto et al., 2003). In contrast, in a set of 130 urothelial carcinomas of the bladder, hMSH2 and hMSH6 negative tumors were found to have a favorable impact on overall patient survival (Mylona et al., 2008). In a number of studies, the degree of microsatellite instability (MSI) was investigated in different cancer tissues, such as colorectal-, ovarian- and gastric carcinoma (Dietmaier et al., 1997, Ichikawa et al., 1999, Ottini et al., 1997). MSI is the result from inactivating mutations in MMR genes and suggests MMR deficiency (Parsons et al., 1993, Strand et al., 1993). However, MSI has been observed only infrequently in bladder cancer tissues (Bonnal et al., 2000, Gonzalez-Zulueta et al., 1993, Hartmann et al., 2002). Furthermore, reduced expression of hMLH1 and hMSH2 was not correlated with MSI in bladder cancer (Catto et al., 2003). Based on these conflicting data, a conclusion as to whether MMR impacts the development of cisplatin resistance in bladder cancer in the clinic cannot be drawn to date (Table 1).

4. DNA damage response and apoptosis pathways in cisplatin resistance

It is known that cisplatin treatment induces apoptosis in cells, thereby killing the cells (Chu, 1994). The apoptotic pathways, which are induced following cisplatin treatment, were extensively studied, hence not yet fully understood. Cisplatin-induced apoptosis may be triggered through the extrinsic death receptor pathway, which is mediated through the JNK signaling cascade. Alternatively, the intrinsic mitochondrial pathway may be induced, mediated through p53 and anti- or pro-apoptotic members of the Bcl-2 family proteins (Brozovic et al., 2004, Pabla et al., 2008, Siddik, 2003). Decreased expression or loss of pro-apoptotic proteins may result in cisplatin resistance, similarly may increased expression of anti-apoptotic proteins lead to cisplatin resistance (Brozovic & Osmak, 2007). The contribution of these mechanisms for preclinical and clinical cisplatin resistance of bladder cancer cells will be discussed in the following section.

4.1 p53 and cisplatin resistance of bladder cancer cells

The tumor suppressor protein p53 is activated in cancer cells after treatment with chemotherapeutic drugs and has a central role for the induction of apoptosis. The influence of the p53 status for cisplatin resistance has been studied in numerous cancer cell lines, however, with contradictory results. While no correlation between cisplatin resistance and p53 status was observed in testis and ovarian cancer cell lines (Burger et al., 1997, De Feudis et al., 1997), other studies using breast, lung, colon, kidney, ovarian, leukaemia, melanoma and prostate cancer cell lines showed that p53 mutated cell lines were more resistant to cisplatin compared to p53 wild-type cell lines (Branch et al., 2000, O'Connor et al., 1997).
Contradictory results about the importance of p53 status for cisplatin resistance are also reported for bladder cancer cells. Comparing the cisplatin sensitivity in bladder cancer cell lines with different p53 status revealed that p53 wild type bladder cancer cells were more susceptible to cisplatin, while mutant cell lines were resistant (Kawasaki et al., 1996, Konstantakou et al., 2009). In line with these findings, it was also shown that cisplatin resistance in bladder cancer cells was enhanced by overexpression of mutant p53 protein (Miyake et al., 1999). Our own studies revealed that cisplatin resistant bladder cancer cell lines were mutated for p53, while cisplatin sensitive testis tumor cells showed functional p53 activity after cisplatin treatment (unpublished results). Contrary to these observations, Chang and co-workers investigated the effect of p53 mutations for drug sensitivity and found that bladder cancer cell lines expressing various human mutated p53 proteins displayed enhanced cisplatin sensitivity (Chang & Lai, 2001). Even more, when cisplatin sensitivity was measured in a series using 89 bladder cancer cell lines with different p53 status, it was found that p53 heterozygous cells were most susceptible to cisplatin (Chang & Lai, 2000). Altogether, we therefore conclude that, at least in bladder cancer cell lines, p53 mutations do not always lead to the development of cisplatin resistance.
In a number of studies it has been investigated whether the p53 status can be a predictor for the response to platinum-based chemotherapy in the clinic. Gadducci and co-workers reported that ovarian cancer patients with tumors harbouring p53 mutations experience a lower chance to achieve a complete response following cisplatin therapy, while patients with wild-type p53 tumors have a good chance to respond (Gadducci et al., 2002). In bladder cancers, mutations in the p53 gene are a frequent event (Esrig et al., 1994). However, there are conflicting results whether the p53 status can be used to predict the responsiveness to cisplatin treatment in bladder cancers (Nishiyama et al., 2008). On the one hand, it was shown that in a cohort of patients with TCC only the patients with altered p53 in the tumor would benefit from adjuvant cisplatin chemotherapy (Cote et al., 1997). On the other hand, p53 immunoreactivity could not be used to predict tumor response and patient survival in a cohort of 83 patients (Qureshi et al., 1999). Similarly, no clear conclusion as to whether p53 wild type was related to increased resistance or increased responsiveness could be drawn by Watanabe and co-workers in a study investigating 75 tumor specimens (Watanabe et al., 2004). Therefore, it cannot be concluded to date that the p53 status influences cisplatin responsiveness in bladder cancers (Table 1).

4.2 Anti-apoptotic proteins and cisplatin resistance

Cisplatin resistance has been associated with the expression of a number of anti-apoptotic proteins, both in cell cultures and in clinical samples. Expression of the anti-apoptotic proteins Bcl-2 and Bcl-x_L resulted in cisplatin resistance in ovarian cancer cell lines (Yang et al., 2004). In bladder cancer cell lines, which were resistant to cisplatin and etoposide, Chresta and co-workers also observed high levels of Bcl-2 (Chresta et al., 1996). In addition, levels of the pro-apoptotic protein Bax were very low in the three bladder cancer cell lines under investigation (Chresta et al., 1996). We also observed low endogenous levels of Bax in cisplatin resistant bladder cancer cells compared to cisplatin sensitive testis tumor cell lines (unpublished observations). Furthermore, cisplatin treatment lead to translocation of Bax to the mitochondrial membrane in testis tumor cells, which was not observed in bladder cancer cell lines (unpublished observations). An association between cisplatin resistance, Bcl-2 expression and Bax translocation has also been proposed by Cho and co-workers who observed in cisplatin resistant bladder cancer sublines that Bcl-2 was up-regulated, which resulted in inhibition of Bax translocation to the mitochondrial membrane and reduced cell death (Cho et al., 2006). To elucidate the role of Bcl-2 for cisplatin resistance in bladder cancer cells, Miake and co-workers transfected the human bladder transitional cell carcinoma line KoTTC-1 with an expression plasmid for Bcl-2 and observed that overexpression conferred resistance to cisplatin (Miyake et al., 1998). Stably expressing Bcl-2 cells were then injected subcutaneously into nude mice to determine whether the Bcl-2 status can affect the efficacy of cisplatin treatment. Using this tumor cell implantation model, the authors could show that mice with tumors expressing Bcl-2 have an inferior prognosis compared to mice with tumors with no detectable Bcl-2 protein (Miyake et al., 1998). Altogether, the data suggest that Bcl-2 might be one of the factors influencing cisplatin resistance in bladder cancer cells. In proof of principle experiments, Bcl-2 levels in bladder cancer cells were decreased using Bcl-2 antisense oligonucleotides. These studies revealed that down-regulation of Bcl-2 expression resulted in a significant increase in toxicity of cisplatin in various bladder cancer cell lines (Bolenz et al., 2007, Hong et al., 2002), supporting the notion that expression of Bcl-2 may be associated with cisplatin resistance in bladder cancer cells (Table 1).

Expression levels of the anti-apoptotic factors Bcl-2 and Bcl-xL were determined in tumor samples from a diverse range of tissue to investigate for a possible involvement in clinical resistance, however, with contradictory results. While in ovarian carcinoma patients, expression of Bcl-xL was correlated with a decreased response to platinum chemotherapy (Williams et al., 2005), no association between response and Bcl-2 expression was observed in breast cancer patients (Parton et al., 2002). For bladder cancers, the clinical relevance of Bcl-2 expression for cisplatin resistance has been shown by Cooke and co-workers. The authors observed in a cohort of 51 patients with bladder cell carcinoma who received neo-adjuvant cisplatin chemotherapy that patients with Bcl-2 negative tumors had a significantly better prognosis (Cooke et al., 2000). An improved survival of patients with Bcl-2 negative tumors was also observed in a cohort of 89 patients with invasive bladder cancers who received cisplatin-based chemotherapy (Kong et al., 1998). In conclusion, expression of the anti-apoptotic factor Bcl-2 appears to affect the efficacy of cisplatin therapy for bladder cancers and might be used as a prognostic marker to predict the response to treatment.

The inhibitor of apoptosis (IAP) gene family encodes proteins, which have been reported to play an important role in cellular drug resistance. These proteins have been shown to be endogenous inhibitors of caspases, thus resulting in inhibition of cell death. Survivin, one of the members of the IAP family, is activated by cisplatin, which in part protects cells from cisplatin-induced apoptosis (Belyanskaya et al., 2005). An associated between survivin levels and cisplatin resistance has been reported for a number of cell lines derived from various cancer tissues including thyroid, lung and colon (Tirro et al., 2006) (Belyanskaya et al., 2005,

Hopkins-Donaldson et al., 2006, Pani et al., 2007). Bladder cancer cell lines showed a high expression of survivin compared to non-cancerous uro-epithelial cells (Yang et al., 2010).
In clinical studies it has been investigated whether survivin might serve as a prognostic marker to predict clinical outcome. In tumor material of 30 patients with advanced bladder cancer, survivin expression has been identified as a marker for poor clinical outcome (Als et al., 2007). Similarly, Shariat and co-workers identified survivin as an independent predictor for recurrence of the disease in a cohort of 726 patients (Shariat et al., 2009).
The X-linked inhibitor of apoptosis (XIAP) is another member of the family of IAP proteins. Preclinical studies indicate that XIAP expression may be associated with cisplatin resistance. In ovarian carcinoma cell lines, for example, enhanced expression of XIAP was connected to the acquisition of cisplatin resistance (Mansouri et al., 2003). Bilim and co-workers reported considerable levels of XIAP in a panel of 4 bladder cancer cell lines, which are known to be cisplatin resistant (Bilim et al., 2003). The clinical relevance of XIAP for the efficacy of cisplatin treatment has been studied in a number of studies. Parton and co-workers found no association between XIAP expression and response to chemotherapy in ovarian cancer tissue (Parton et al., 2002). An inverse correlation between XIAP expression in the cancer tissue and pathological response was observed for patients with advanced bladder cancer (Pinho et al., 2009). The correlation, however, was not statistically significant. This study also demonstrated that bladder cancer patients with high levels of XIAP-associated factor 1 protein (XAF1) in the cancer tissue had a better prognosis after cisplatin based chemotherapy (Pinho et al., 2009). XAF1 inhibits the anti-caspase activity of XIAP, therefore antagonizing the anti-apoptotic action (Liston et al., 2001). Most likely, this resulted in increased sensitivity towards cisplatin. Another study investigated the expression of XIAP in bladder tumor specimens of 108 patients and found that XIAP was expressed at significantly higher levels in tumors compared to normal urothelium (Bilim et al., 2003). Unfortunately, it was not investigated, whether XIAP positivity was correlated with clinical response to cisplatin. However, it was suggested that XIAP upregulation might play a role in early TCC carcinogenesis (Bilim et al., 2003).
Altogether, information about expression of factors involved in cisplatin-induced apoptotic cell death pathways and its relation to cisplatin resistance is still emerging (Table 1). More information about the clinical relevance of apoptosis-related factors for the clinical outcome is needed, as this may identify new targets for pharmacological intervention.

5. Strategies for overcoming cisplatin resistance

As cisplatin resistance influences the clinical outcome, strategies are needed to circumvent the resistance phenotype. In a number of preclinical studies, modulators of cisplatin resistance were specifically targeted, and it was investigated whether this would influence cisplatin sensitivity. For example, the glutathione system may be modulated by glutathione depletion or GST blocking agents. Using these approaches, Buyn and co-workers could significantly enhance the cisplatin toxicity in bladder cancer cell lines (Byun et al., 2005). Similarly, inhibition of DNA repair has the potential to enhance the cytotoxicity of anticancer agents, as preclinical studies have confirmed that modulation of repair pathways can enhance the sensitivity to DNA damaging agents (Damia & D'Incalci, 2007, Ding et al., 2006). We found that siRNA-mediated down-regulation of the repair factor ERCC1-XFP decreased the repair of cisplatin-induced ICLs in bladder cancer cells and subsequently resulted in reduced cisplatin resistance (Usanova et al., 2010). In a number of studies, the effect of down-regulation of anti-apoptotic proteins for cisplatin resistance was studied. Down-regulation of Bcl-2 and Bcl-xL with antisense oligonucleotides enhanced the cisplatin sensitivity in four human bladder cancer cell lines (Bolenz et al., 2007). Antisense oligonucleotides against Bcl-2 were also used by Schaaf and co-workers who also observed an synergistic effect on cisplatin sensitivity (Schaaf et al., 2004). These findings show that reducing anti-apoptotic proteins positively influences cisplatin efficacy in bladder cancer cell lines and imply that targeting these factors may be a new therapeutic strategy for the treatment of bladder cancer.

6. Novel therapeutic strategies for bladder cancer treatment

Gemcitabine (2´,2´-difluorodeoxycytidine) is a deoxycytidine analogue, which can inhibit the ribonucleotide reductase or may be incorporated into DNA as a false base. Both mechanisms result in inhibition of DNA synthesis thereby leading to induction of apoptosis (Mini et al., 2006). Gemcitabine is used either as a single agent or in combination with other chemotherapeutic drugs for the treatment of cancer. For patients with locally advanced and metastatic bladder cancer, combination treatment of cisplatin or carboplatin and gemcitabine is the current standard chemotherapy regimen (von der Maase et al., 2005). Even though drug resistance is a major clinical problem, the resistance phenotype of bladder cancer cells to gemcitabine has not been investigated in great detail. An increase in expression of the anti-apoptotic protein clusterin has been described as a mechanism for acquired gemcitabine resistance in bladder cancer cells (Muramaki et al., 2009). Knock-down of clusterin sensitized gemcitabine-resistant bladder cancer cells indicating clinical significance (Muramaki et al., 2009). Gemcitabine resistance in bladder cancer cells might differ from cisplatin resistance as gemcitabine has been used for the treatment of cisplatin-refractory metastatic bladder cancer (Soga et al., 2010). The beneficial effect of gemcitabine for the treatment of cisplatin-refractory urothelial carcinoma, however, was not observed in the study of Lin and co-workers who reported that gemcitabine and ifosfamide showed insufficient clinical activity in patients with cisplatin-refractory bladder cancer (Lin et al., 2007). More promising approaches to increase the activity of cisplatin plus gemcitabine for treating metastatic bladder cancer have been reported in a number of recent studies. Addition of vitamin D3 increased the antitumor activity of cisplatin plus gemcitabine in bladder cancer cells and enhanced the antitumor activity in a xenograft model (Ma et al., 2010). The antibody Bevacizumab, which is directed against vascular endothelial growth factor (VEGF), has been shown to have a beneficial effect on cisplatin plus gemcitabine in patients with metastatic bladder cancer (Hahn et al., 2011). More clinical trials combining novel agents with cisplatin and gemcitabine, however, are needed to improve the treatment of bladder cancers.

7. Conclusion

Cisplatin-based combination therapy is the standard therapy for the treatment of advanced or metastatic cancer of the bladder. However, the efficacy of cisplatin is limited by intrinsic or acquired resistance to the drug. Mechanisms determining cisplatin resistance include drug transport, detoxification, DNA repair and expression of pro- and anti-apoptotic proteins. The clinical significance of these mechanisms for bladder cancers is not yet fully understood and still evolving. A better understanding about resistance mechanisms in bladder cancers is essential for developing therapeutic strategies aimed at circumventing cisplatin resistance for improving cancer therapy.

8. References

Aboussekhra, A.; Biggerstaff, M.; Shivji, M. K. K.; Vilpo, J. A.; Moncollin, V.; Podust, V. N.; Protic', M.;Hübscher, U.; Egly, J.-M. & Wood, R. D. (1995). Mammalian DNA nucleotide excision repair reconstituted with purified protein components. *Cell,* Vol. 80, pp. 859-868.

Aebi, S.; Kurdihaidar, B.; Gordon, R.; Cenni, B.; Zheng, H.; Fink, D.; Christen, R. D.; Boland, C. R.; Koi, M.; Fishel, R. & Howell, S. B. (1996). Loss of DNA mismatch repair in acquired-resistance to cisplatin. *Cancer Res,* Vol. 56, pp. 3087-3090.

Albertella, M. R.; Green, C. M.; Lehmann, A. R. & O'Connor, M. J. (2005a). A role for polymerase eta in the cellular tolerance to cisplatin-induced damage. *Cancer Res,* Vol. 65, pp. 9799-9806.

Albertella, M. R.; Lau, A. & O'Connor, M. J. (2005b). The overexpression of specialized DNA polymerases in cancer. *DNA Repair (Amst),* Vol. 4, pp. 583-593.

Als, A. B.; Dyrskjot, L.; von der Maase, H.; Koed, K.; Mansilla, F.; Toldbod, H. E.; Jensen, J. L.; Ulhoi, B. P.; Sengelov, L.; Jensen, K. M. & Orntoft, T. F. (2007). Emmprin and survivin predict response and survival following cisplatin-containing chemotherapy in patients with advanced bladder cancer. *Clin Cancer Res,* Vol. 13, pp. 4407-4414.

Alt, A.; Lammens, K.; Chiocchini, C.; Lammens, A.; Pieck, J. C.; Kuch, D.; Hopfner, K. P. & Carell, T. (2007). Bypass of DNA lesions generated during anticancer treatment with cisplatin by DNA polymerase eta. *Science,* Vol. 318, pp. 967-970.

Bedford, P.; Walker, M. C.; Sharma, H. L.; Perera, A.; McAuliffe, C. A.; Masters, J. R. W. & Hill, B. T. (1987). Factors influencing the sensitivity of two human bladder carcinoma cell lines to cis-diamminedichloro-platinum(II). *Chem-Biol Interactions, Vol. 61,* pp. 1-15.

Bellmunt, J.; Paz-Ares, L.; Cuello, M.; Cecere, F. L.; Albiol, S.; Guillem, V.; Gallardo, E.; Charles, J.; Mendez, P.; de la Cruz, J. J.; *et al.* (2007). Gene expression of ERCC1 as a novel prognostic marker in advanced bladder cancer patients receiving cisplatin-based chemotherapy. *Annals of Oncology,* Vol. 18, pp. 522-528.

Belyanskaya, L. L.; Hopkins-Donaldson, S.; Kurtz, S.; Simoes-Wust, A. P.; Yousefi, S.; Simon, H. U.; Stahel, R. & Zangemeister-Wittke, U. (2005). Cisplatin activates Akt in small cell lung cancer cells and attenuates apoptosis by survivin upregulation. *Int J Cancer,* Vol. 117, pp. 755-763.

Bignami, M.; Casorelli, I. & Karran, P. (2003). Mismatch repair and response to DNA-damaging antitumour therapies. *Eur J Cancer,* Vol. 39, pp. 2142-2149.

Bilim, V.; Kasahara, T.; Hara, N.; Takahashi, K. & Tomita, Y. (2003). Role of XIAP in the malignant phenotype of transitional cell cancer (TCC) and therapeutic activity of XIAP antisense oligonucleotides against multidrug-resistant TCC in vitro. *Int J Cancer, Vol. 103,* pp. 29-37.

Bischoff, C. J. & Clark, P. E. (2009). Bladder cancer. *Curr Opin Oncol,* Vol. 21, pp. 272-277.

Bolenz, C.; Becker, A.; Trojan, L.; Schaaf, A.; Cao, Y.; Weiss, C.; Alken, P. & Michel, M. S. (2007). Optimizing chemotherapy for transitional cell carcinoma by application of bcl-2 and bcl-xL antisense oligodeoxynucleotides. *Urol Oncol,* Vol. 25, pp. 476-482.

Bonnal, C.; Ravery, V.; Toublanc, M.; Bertrand, G.; Boccon-Gibod, L.; Henin, D. & Grandchamp, B. (2000). Absence of microsatellite instability in transitional cell carcinoma of the bladder. *Urology,* Vol. 55, pp. 287-291.

Branch, P.; Masson, M.; Aquilina, G.; Bignami, M. & Karran, P. (2000). Spontaneous development of drug resistance: mismatch repair and p53 defects in resistance to cisplatin in human tumor cells. *Oncogene,* Vol. 19, pp. 3138-3145.

Brozovic, A.; Fritz, G.; Christmann, M.; Zisowsky, J.; Jaehde, U.; Osmak, M. & Kaina, B. (2004). Long-term activation of SAPK/JNK, p38 kinase and fas-L expression by cisplatin is attenuated in human carcinoma cells that acquired drug resistance. *Int J Cancer,* Vol. 112, pp. 974-985.

Brozovic, A. & Osmak, M. (2007). Activation of mitogen-activated protein kinases by cisplatin and their role in cisplatin-resistance. *Cancer Letters,* Vol. 251, pp. 1-16.

Burger, H.; Nooter, K.; Boersma, A. W.; Kortland, C. J. & Stoter, G. (1997). Lack of correlation between cisplatin-induced apoptosis, p53 status and expression of Bcl-2 family proteins in testicular germ cell tumour cell lines. *Int J Cancer,* Vol. 73, pp. 592-599.

Byun, S.-S.; Kim, S. W.; Choi, H.; Lee, C. & Lee, E. (2005). Augmentation of cisplatin sensitivity in cisplatin-resistant human bladder cancer cells by modulating glutathione concentrations and glutathione- related enzyme activities. *Brit J Urol,* Vol. 95, pp. 1086-1090.

Catto, J. W.; Xinarianos, G.; Burton, J. L.; Meuth, M. & Hamdy, F. C. (2003). Differential expression of hMLH1 and hMSH2 is related to bladder cancer grade, stage and prognosis but not microsatellite instability. *Int J Cancer,* Vol. 105, pp. 484-490.

Ceppi, P.; Novello, S.; Cambieri, A.; Longo, M.; Monica, V.; Lo Iacono, M.; Giaj-Levra, M.; Saviozzi, S.; Volante, M.; Papotti, M. & Scagliotti, G. (2009). Polymerase eta mRNA expression predicts survival of non-small cell lung cancer patients treated with platinum-based chemotherapy. *Clin Cancer Res,* Vol. 15, pp. 1039-1045.

Chang, F. L. & Lai, M. D. (2000). The relationship between p53 status and anticancer drugs-induced apoptosis in nine human bladder cancer cell lines. *Anticancer Res,* Vol. 20, pp. 351-355.

Chang, F. L. & Lai, M. D. (2001). Various forms of mutant p53 confer sensitivity to cisplatin and doxorubicin in bladder cancer cells. *J Urol,* Vol. 166, pp. 304-310.

Cho, H. J.; Kim, J. K.; Kim, K. D.; Yoon, H. K.; Cho, M. Y.; Park, Y. P.; Jeon, J. H.; Lee, E. S.; Byun, S. S.; Lim, H. M. *et al.* (2006). Upregulation of Bcl-2 is associated with cisplatin-resistance via inhibition of Bax translocation in human bladder cancer cells. *Cancer Lett,* Vol. 237, pp. 56-66.

Chresta, C. M.; Masters, J. R. & Hickman, J. A. (1996). Hypersensitivity of human testicular tumors to etoposide-induced apoptosis is associated with functional p53 and a high Bax:Bcl-2 ratio. *Cancer Res,* Vol. 56, pp. 1834- 1841.

Chu, G. (1994). Cellular-responses to cisplatin - the roles of DNA-binding proteins and DNA-repair. *J Biol Chem,* Vol. 269, pp. 787-790.

Claij, N. & te Riele, H. (2004). Msh2 deficiency does not contribute to cisplatin resistance in mouse embryonic stem cells. *Oncogene,* Vol. 23, pp. 260-266.

Cohen, S. M.; Goel, A.; Phillips, J.; Ennis, R. D. & Grossbard, M. L. (2006). The role of perioperative chemotherapy in the treatment of urothelial cancer. *Oncologist,* Vol. 11, pp. 630-640.

Cole, R. S. (1973). Repair of DNA containing interstrand crosslinks in *Escherichia coli*: sequential excision and recombination. *Proc Natl Acad Sci USA,* Vol. 70, pp. 1064-1068.

Cooke, P. W.; James, N. D.; Ganesan, R.; Burton, A.; Young, L. S. & Wallace, D. M. (2000). Bcl-2 expression identifies patients with advanced bladder cancer treated by radiotherapy who benefit from neoadjuvant chemotherapy. *BJU Int,* Vol. 85, pp. 829-835.

Cote, R. J.; Esrig, D.; Groshen, S.; Jones, P. A. & Skinner, D. G. (1997). p53 and treatment of bladder cancer. *Nature,* Vol. 385, pp. 123-125.

Cruet-Hennequart, S.; Glynn, M. T.; Murillo, L. S.; Coyne, S. & Carty, M. P. (2008). Enhanced DNA-PK-mediated RPA2 hyperphosphorylation in DNA polymerase eta-deficient human cells treated with cisplatin and oxaliplatin. *DNA Repair (Amst),* Vol. 7, pp-582-596.

Cruet-Hennequart, S.; Villalan, S.; Kaczmarczyk, A.; O'Meara, E.; Sokol, A. M. & Carty, M. P. (2009). Characterization of the effects of cisplatin and carboplatin on cell cycle progression and DNA damage response activation in DNA polymerase eta-deficient human cells. *Cell Cycle,* Vol. 8, pp. 3039-3050.

Dabholkar, M.; Bostick-Bruton, F.; Weber, C.; Bohr, V. A.; Egwuagu, C. & Reed, E. (1992). ERCC1 and ERCC2 expression in malignant tissues from ovarian cancer patients. *J Natl Cancer Inst,* Vol. 84, pp. 1512-1517.

Dabholkar, M.; Vionnet, J.; Bostick-Bruton, F.; Yu, J. J. & Reed, E. (1994). Messenger RNA levels of XPAC and ERCC1 in ovarian cancer tissue correlate with response to platinum-based chemotherapy. *J Clin Invest,* Vol. 94, pp. 703-708.

Damia, G. & D'Incalci, M. (2007). Targeting DNA repair as a promising approach in cancer therapy. *Eur J Cancer,* Vol. 43, pp. 1791-1801.

De Feudis, P.; Debernardis, D.; Beccaglia, P.; Valenti, M.; Graniela, S. E.; Arzani, D.; Stanzione, S.; D'Incalci, M.; Russo, P. & Broggini, M. (1997). DDP-induced cytotoxicity is not influenced by p53 in nine human ovarian cancer cell lines with different p53 status. *Br J Cancer,* Vol. 76, pp. 474-479.

De Silva, I. U.; McHugh, P. J.; Clingen, P. H. & Hartley, J. A. (2000). Defining the roles of nucleotide excision repair and recombination in the repair of DNA interstrand cross-links in mammalian cells. *Mol Cell Biol,* Vol. 20, pp. 7980-7990.

Dietmaier, W.; Wallinger, S.; Bocker, T.; Kullmann, F.; Fishel, R. & Ruschoff, J. (1997). Diagnostic microsatellite instability: definition and correlation with mismatch repair protein expression. *Cancer Res,* Vol. 57, pp. 4749-4756.

Ding, J.; Miao, Z.-H.; Meng, L.-H. & Geng, M.-Y. (2006). Emerging cancer therapeutic opportunities target DNA repair systems. *Trends Pharmacol Scl,* Vol. 27, pp. 338-344.

Duckett, D. R.; Drummond, J. T.; Murchie, A. I. H.; Reardon, J. T.; Sancar, A.; Lilley, D. M. & Modrich, P. (1996). Human MutS-alpha recognizes damaged DNA-base pairs containing O-6-methylguanine, O-4-methylthymine, or the cisplatin-d(GpG) adduct. *Proc Natl Acad Sci U S A,* Vol. 93, pp. 6443-6447.

Dunkern, T. R.; Fritz, G. & Kaina, B. (2001). Cisplatin-induced apoptosis in 43-3B and 27-1 cells defective in nucleotide excision repair. *Mutat Res,* Vol. 486, pp. 249-258.

Esrig, D.; Elmajian, D.; Groshen, S.; Freeman, J. A.; Stein, J. P.; Chen, S. C.; Nichols, P. W.; Skinner, D. G.; Jones, P. A. & Cote, R. J. (1994). Accumulation of nuclear p53 and tumor progression in bladder cancer. *N Engl J Med,* Vol. 331, pp. 1259-1264.

Ferry, K. V.; Hamilton, T. C. & Johnson, S. W. (2000). Increased nucleotide excision repair in cisplatin-resistant ovarian cancer cells: role of ERCC1-XPF. *Biochem Pharmacol,* Vol. 60, pp. 1305-1313.

Fink, D.; Nebel, S.; Aebi, S.; Zheng, H.; Cenni, B.; Nehme, A.; Christen, R. D. & Howell, S. B. (1996). The role of DNA mismatch repair in platinum drug-resistance. *Cancer Res,* Vol. 56, pp. 4881-4886.

Gadducci, A.; Cosio, S.; Muraca, S. & Genazzani, A. R. (2002). Molecular mechanisms of apoptosis and chemosensitivity to platinum and paclitaxel in ovarian cancer: biological data and clinical implications. *Eur J Gynaecol Oncol,* Vol. 23, pp. 390-396.

Gifford, G.; Paul, J.; Vasey, P. A.; Kaye, S. B. & Brown, R. (2004). The acquisition of hMLH1 methylation in plasma DNA after chemotherapy predicts poor survival for ovarian cancer patients. *Clin Cancer Res,* Vol. 10, pp. 4420-4426.

Gillet, L. C. & Schärer, O. D. (2006). Molecular mechanisms of mammalian global genome nucleotide excision repair. *Chem Rev,* Vol. 106, pp. 253-276.

Gonzalez-Zulueta, M.; Ruppert, J. M.; Tokino, K.; Tsai, Y. C.; Spruck, C. H.; 3rd, Miyao, N.; Nichols, P. W.; Hermann, G. G.; Horn, T.; Steven, K. & et al. (1993). Microsatellite instability in bladder cancer. *Cancer Res,* Vol. 53, pp. 5620-5623.

Gossage, L. & Madhusudan, S. (2007). Current status of excision repair cross complementation-group 1 (ERCC1) in cancer. *Cancer Treatment Reviews,* Vol. 33, pp. 565-577.

Hahn, N. M.; Stadler, W. M.; Zon, R. T.; Waterhouse, D.; Picus, J.; Nattam, S.; Johnson, C. S.; Perkins, S. M.; Waddell, M. J. & Sweeney, C. J. (2011). Phase II trial of cisplatin, gemcitabine, and bevacizumab as first-line therapy for metastatic urothelial carcinoma: Hoosier Oncology Group GU 04-75. *J Clin Oncol,* Vol. 29, pp. 1525-1530.

Handra-Luca, A.; Hernandez, J.; Mountzios, G.; Taranchon, E.; Lacau-St-Guily, J.; Soria, J.-C. & Fouret, P. (2007). Excision repair cross complementation group 1 immunohistochemical expression predicts objective response and cancer-specific survival in patients treated by cisplatin-based induction chemotherapy for locally advanced head and neck squamous cell carcinoma. *Clin Cancer Res,* Vol. 13, pp. 38553859.

Hartmann, A.; Zanardo, L.; Bocker-Edmonston, T.; Blaszyk, H.; Dietmaier, W.; Stoehr, R.; Cheville, J. C.; Junker, K.; Wieland, W.; Knuechel, R.; *et al.* (2002). Frequent microsatellite instability in sporadic tumors of the upper urinary tract. *Cancer Res,* Vol. 62, pp. 6796-6802.

Helleman, J.; van Staveren, I. L.; Dinjens, W. N. M.; van Kuijk, P. F.; Ritstier, K.; Ewing, P. C.; van cer Burg, M. E. L.; Stoter, G. & Berns, E. M. J. J. (2006). Mismatch repair and treatment resistance in ovarian cancer. *BMC Cancer,* Vol. 6, pp. 201.

Hinkel, A.; Schmidtchen, S.; Palisaar, R. J.; Noldus, J. & Pannek, J. (2008). Identification of bladder cancer patients at risk for recurrence or progression: an immunohistochemical study based on the expression of metallothionein. *J Toxicol Environ Health A,* Vol. 71, pp. 954-959.

Holzer, A. K.; Manorek, G. H. & Howell, S. B. (2006). Contribution of the major copper influx transporter CTR1 to the cellular accumulation of cisplatin, carboplatin, and oxaliplatin. *Mol Pharmacol,* Vol. 70, pp. 1390-1394.

Hong, J. H.; Lee, E.; Hong, J.; Shin, Y. J. & Ahn, H. (2002). Antisense Bcl2 oligonucleotide in cisplatin-resistant bladder cancer cell lines. *BJU Int,* Vol. 90, pp. 113-117.

Hopkins-Donaldson, S.; Belyanskaya, L. L.; Simoes-Wust, A. P.; Sigrist, B.; Kurtz, S.; Zangemeister-Wittke, U. & Stahel, R. (2006). p53-induced apoptosis occurs in the absence of p14(ARF) in malignant pleural mesothelioma. *Neoplasia,* Vol. 8, pp. 551-559.

Hour, T. C.; Chen, J.; Huang, C. Y.; Guan, J. Y.; Lu, S. H.; Hsieh, C. Y. & Pu, Y. S. (2000). Characterization of chemoresistance mechanisms in a series of cisplatin-resistant transitional carcinoma cell lines. *Anticancer Res,* Vol. 20, pp. 3221-3225.

Ichikawa, Y.; Lemon, S. J.; Wang, S.; Franklin, B.; Watson, P.; Knezetic, J. A.; Bewtra, C. & Lynch, H. T. (1999). Microsatellite instability and expression of MLH1 and MSH2 in normal and malignant endometrial and ovarian epithelium in hereditary nonpolyposis colorectal cancer family members. *Cancer Genet Cytogenet,* Vol. 112, pp. 2-8.

Ishida, S.; Lee, J.; Thiele, D. J. & Herskowitz, I. (2002). Uptake of the anticancer drug cisplatin mediated by the copper transporter Ctr1 in yeast and mammals. *Proc Natl Acad Sci,* Vol. 99, pp. 14298-14302.

Jachymczyk, W. J.; von Borstel, R. C.; Mowat, M. R. & Hastings, P. J. (1981). Repair of interstrand cross-links in DNA of Saccharomyces cerevisiae requires two systems for DNA repair: the RAD3 system and the RAD51 system. *Mol Gen Genet,* Vol. 182, pp. 196-205.

Jamieson, E. R. & Lippard, S. J. (1999). Structure, recognition and processing of cisplatin-DNA adducts. *Chem Rev,* Vol. 99, pp. 2467-2498.

Jansen, B. A. J.; Brouwer, J. & Reedijk, J. (2002). Glutathione induces cellular resistance against cationic dinuclear platinum anticancer drugs. *J Inorg Biochem,* Vol. 89, pp. 197-202.

Jemal, A.; Murray, T.; Ward, E.; Samuels, A.; Tiwari, R. C.; Ghafoor, A.; Feuer, E. J. & Thun, M. J. (2005). Cancer statistics, 2005. *CA Cancer J Clin,* Vol. 55, pp. 10-30.

Jin, T. X.; Furihata, M.; Yamasaki, I.; Kamada, M.; Liang, S. B.; Ohtsuki, Y. & Shuin, T. (1999). Human mismatch repair gene (hMSH2) product expression in relation to recurrence of transitional cell carcinoma of the urinary bladder. *Cancer,* Vol. 85, pp. 478-484.

Johnson, S. W.; Perez, R. P.; Godwin, A. K.; Yeung, A. T.; Handel, L. M.; Ozols, R. F. & Hamilton, T. C. (1994a). Role of platinum-DNA adduct formation and removal in cisplatin resistance in human ovarian cancer cell lines. *Biochem Pharmacol,* Vol. 47, pp. 689-697.

Johnson, S. W.; Swiggard, P. A.; Handel, L. M.; Brennan, J. M.; Godwin, A. K.; Ozols, R. F. & Hamilton, T. C. (1994b). Relationship between platinum-DNA adduct formation and removal and cisplatin cytotoxicity in cisplatin-sensitive and cisplatin-resistant human ovarian-cancer cells. *Cancer Res,* Vol. 54, pp. 5911-5916.

Jones, S. L.; Hickson, I. D.; Harris, A. L. & Harnett, P. R. (1994). Repair of cisplatin-DNA adducts by protein extracts from human ovarian-carcinoma. *Int J Cancer,* Vol. 59, pp. 388-393.

Jordan, P. & Carmo-Fonseca, M. (2000). Molecular mechanisms involved in cisplatin cytotoxicity. *Cell Mol Life Sci*, Vol. 57, pp. 1229-1235.

Jun, H. J.; Ahn, M. J.; Kim, H. S.; Sy, S. Y.; Han, J.; Lee, S. K.; Ahn, Y. C.; Jeong, H.-S.; Son, Y.-I.; Baek, J. H. & Park, K. (2008). ERCC1 expression as a predictive marker of squamous cell carcinoma of the head and neck treated with cisplatin-based concurrent chemotherapy. *Br J Cancer*, Vol. 99, pp. 167-172.

Kagi, J. H. & Schaffer, A. (1988). Biochemistry of metallothionein. *Biochemistry*, Vol. 27, pp. 8509-8515.

Kartalou, M. & Essigmann, J. M. (2001). Recognition of cisplatin adducts by cellular proteins. *Mutat Res*, Vol. 478, pp. 1-21.

Kasahara, K.; Fujiwara, Y.; Nishio, K.; Ohmori, T.; Sugimoto, Y.; Komiya, K.; Matsuda, T. & Saijo, N. (1991). Metallothionein content correlates with the sensitivity of human small cell lung cancer cell lines to cisplatin. *Cancer Res*, Vol. 51, pp. 3237-3242.

Kaufman, D. S. (2006). Challenges in the treatment of bladder cancer. *Ann Oncol*, Vol. 17 Suppl 5, pp. 106-112.

Kawasaki, T.; Tomita, Y.; Bilim, V.; Takeda, M.; Takahashi, K. & Kumanishi, T. (1996). Abrogation of apoptosis induced by DNA-damaging agents in human bladder-cancer cell lines with p21/WAF1/CIP1 and/or p53 gene alterations. *Int J Cancer*, Vol. 68, pp. 501-505.

Kim, K. H.; Do, I. G.; Kim, H. S.; Chang, M. H.; Kim, H. S.; Jun, H. J.; Uhm, J.; Yi, S. Y.; Lim do, H.; Ji, S. H.; *et al.* (2010). Excision repair cross-complementation group 1 (ERCC1) expression in advanced urothelial carcinoma patients receiving cisplatin-based chemotherapy. *Apmis*, Vol. 118, pp. 941-948.

Kim, M. K.; Cho, K.-J.; Kwon, G. Y.; Park, S.-I.; Kim, Y. H.; Kim, J. H.; Song, H.-Y.; Shin, J. H.; Jung, H. Y.; Lee, G. H.; *et al.* (2008). Patients with ERCC1-negative locally advanced esophageal cancers may benefit from preoperative chemotherapy. *Clin Cancer Res*, Vol. 14, pp. 4225-4231.

Köberle, B.; Grimaldi, K. A.; Sunters, A.; Hartley, J. A.; Kelland, L. R. & Masters, J. R. (1997). DNA repair capacity and cisplatin sensitivity of human testis tumour cells. *Int J Cancer*, Vol. 70, pp. 551-555.

Köberle, B.; Masters, J. R.; Hartley, J. A. & Wood, R. D. (1999). Defective repair of cisplatin-induced DNA damage caused by reduced XPA protein in testicular germ cell tumours. *Curr Biol*, Vol. 9, pp. 273-276.

Köberle, B.; Payne, J.; Grimaldi, K. A.; Hartley, J. A. & Masters, J. R. W. (1996). DNA-repair in cisplatin-sensitive and resistant human cell-lines measured in specific genes by quantitative polymerase chain- reaction. *Biochem Pharmacol*, Vol. 52, pp. 1729-1734.

Köberle, B.; Tomicic, M.; Usanova, S. & Kaina, B. (2010). Cisplatin resistance: preclinical findings and clinical implications BBA *Reviews on Cancer*, Vol. 1806, pp. 172-182.

Koga, H.; Kotoh, S.; Nakashima, M.; Yokomizo, A.; Tanaka, M. & Naito, S. (2000). Accumulation of intracellular platinum is correlated with intrinsic cisplatin resistance in human bladder cancer cell lines. *Int J Oncol*, Vol. 16, pp. 1003-1007.

Kondo, Y.; Kuo, S.-M.; Watkins, S. C. & Lazo, J. S. (1995). Metallothionein localization and cisplatin resistance in human hormone-independent prostatic tumor cell lines. *Cancer Res*, Vol. 1995, pp. 474-477.

Kong, G.; Shin, K. Y.; Oh, Y. H.; Lee, J. J.; Park, H. Y.; Woo, Y. N. & Lee, J. D. (1998). Bcl-2 and p53 expressions in invasive bladder cancers. *Acta Oncol*, Vol. 37, pp. 715-720.

Konstantakou, E. G.; Voutsinas, G. E.; Karkoulis, P. K.; Aravantinos, G.; Margaritis, L. H. and Stravopodis, D. J. (2009). Human bladder cancer cells undergo cisplatin-induced apoptosis that is associated with p53- dependent and p53-independent responses. *Int J Oncol,* Vol. 35, pp. 401-416.

Kotoh, S.; Naito, S.; Sakamoto, N.; Goto, K. & Kumazawa, J. (1994). Metallothionein expression is correlated with cisplatin resistance in transitional cell carcinoma of the urinary tract. *J Urology,* Vol. 152, pp. 1267- 1270.

Kotoh, S.; Naito, S.; Yokomizo, A.; Kohno, K.; Kuwano, M. & Kumazawa, J. (1997). Enhanced expression of gamma-glutamylcysteine synthetase and glutathione S-transferase genes in cisplatin-resistant bladder cancer cells with multidrug resistance phenotype. *J Urol,* Vol. 157, pp. 1054-1058.

Kunkel, T. A. & Erie, D. A. (2005). DNA mismatch repair. *Annu Rev Biochem,* Vol. 74, pp. 681-710.

Kuo, M. T.; Chen, H. H. W.; Song, I.-S.; Savaraj, N. & Ishikawa, T. (2007). The roles of copper transporters in cisplatin resistance. *Cancer Metastasis Rev,* Vol. 26, pp. 71-83.

Kuraoka, I.; Kobertz, W. R.; Ariza, R. R.; Biggerstaff, M.; Essigmann, J. M. & Wood, R. D. (2000). Repair of an interstrand DNA crosslink initiated by ERCC1-XPF repair/recombination nuclease. *J Biol Chem,* Vol. 275, pp. 26632-26636.

Li, Q.; Gardner, K.; Zhang, L.; Tsang, B.; Bostick-Bruton, F. & Reed, E. (1998). Cisplatin induction of ERCC-1 mRNA expression in A2780/CP70 human ovarian cancer cells. *J Biol Chem,* Vol. 273, pp. 23419-23425.

Li, Q.; Yu, J. J.; Mu, C.; Yunmbam, M. K.; Slavsky, D.; Cross, C. L.; Bostick-Bruton, F. & Reed, E. (2000). Association between the level of ERCC-1 expression and the repair of cisplatin-induced DNA damage in human ovarian cancer cells. *Anticancer Res,* Vol. 20, pp. 645-652.

Lin, C. C.; Hsu, C. H.; Huang, C. Y.; Keng, H. Y.; Tsai, Y. C.; Huang, K. H.; Cheng, A. L. & Pu, Y. S. (2007). Gemcitabine and ifosfamide as a second-line treatment for cisplatin-refractory metastatic urothelial carcinoma: a phase II study. *Anticancer Drugs,* Vol. 18, pp. 487-491.

Liston, P.; Fong, W. G.; Kelly, N. L.; Toji, S.; Miyazaki, T.; Conte, D.; Tamai, K.; Craig, C. G.; McBurney, M. W. & Korneluk, R. G. (2001). Identification of XAF1 as an antagonist of XIAP anti-Caspase activity. *Nat Cell Biol,* Vol. 3, pp. 128-133.

Ma, Y.; Yu, W. D.; Trump, D. L. & Johnson, C. S. (2010). 1,25D3 enhances antitumor activity of gemcitabine and cisplatin in human bladder cancer models. *Cancer,* Vol. 116, pp. 3294-3303.

Mannervik, B. (1987). The enzymes of glutathione metabolism: an overview. *Biochem Soc Trans,* Vol. 15, pp. 717- 718.

Mansouri, A.; Zhang, Q.; Ridgway, L. D.; Tian, L. & Claret, F. X. (2003). Cisplatin resistance in an ovarian carcinoma is associated with a defect in programmed cell death control through XIAP regulation. *Oncol Res,* Vol. 13, pp. 399-404.

Massey, A.; Offman, J.; Macpherson, P. & Karran, P. (2003). DNA mismatch repair and acquired cisplatin resistance in *E. coli* and human ovarian carcinoma cells. *DNA Repair (Amst),* Vol. 2, pp. 73-89.

McHugh, P. J.; Spanswick, V. J. & Hartley, J. A. (2001). Repair of DNA interstrand crosslinks: molecular mechanisms and clinical relevance. *The Lancet Oncology,* Vol. 2, pp. 483-490.

Meijer, C.; Mulder, N. H.; Timmer-Bosscha, H.; Sluiter, W. J.; Meersma, G. J. & de Vries, E. G. E. (1992). Relationship of cellular glutathione to the cytotoxicity and resistance of seven platinum compounds. *Cancer Res, Vol. 52*, pp. 6885-6889.

Mellish, K. J.; Kelland, L. R. & Harrap, K. R. (1993). In vitro drug chemosensitivity of human cervical squamous cell carcinoma cell lines with intrinsic and acquired resistance to cisplatin. *Br J Cancer,* Vol. 68, pp. 240- 250.

Mello, J. A.; Acharya, S.; Fishel, R. & Essigmann, J. M. (1996). The mismatch-repair protein hMSH2 binds selectively to DNA-adducts of the anticancer drug cisplatin. *Chem Biol,* Vol. 3, pp. 579-589.

Metzger, R.; Leichman, C. G.; Danenberg, K. D.; Danenberg, P. V.; Lenz, H. J.; Hayashi, K.; Groshen, S.; Salonga, D.; Cohen, H.; Laine, L.; *et al.* (1998). ERCC1 mRNA levels complement thymidylate synthase mRNA levels in predicting response and survival for gastric cancer patients receiving combination cisplatin and fluorouracil chemotherapy. *J Clin Oncol,* Vol. 16, pp. 309-316.

Mini, E.; Nobili, S.; Caciagli, B.; Landini, I. & Mazzei, T. (2006). Cellular pharmacology of gemcitabine. *Ann Oncol,* Vol. 17 Suppl 5, v7-12.

Miyake, H.; Hanada, N.; Nakamura, H.; Kagawa, S.; Fujiwara, T.; Hara, I.; Eto, H.; Gohji, K.; Arakawa, S.; Kamidono, S. & Saya, H. (1998). Overexpression of Bcl-2 in bladder cancer cells inhibits apoptosis induced by cisplatin and adenoviral-mediated p53 gene transfer. *Oncogene,* Vol. 16, pp. 933-943.

Miyake, H.; Hara, I.; Yamanaka, K.; Arakawa, S. & Kamidono, S. (1999). Synergistic enhancement of resistance to cisplatin in human bladder cancer cells by overexpression of mutant-type p53 and Bcl-2. *J Urol,* Vol. 162, pp. 2176-2181.

Muramaki, M.; So, A.; Hayashi, N.; Sowery, R.; Miyake, H.; Fujisawa, M. & Gleave, M. E. (2009). Chemosensitization of gemcitabine-resistant human bladder cancer cell line both in vitro and in vivo using antisense oligonucleotide targeting the anti-apoptotic gene, clusterin. *BJU Int,* Vol. 103, pp. 384- 390.

Mylona, E.; Zarogiannos, A.; Nomikos, A.; Giannopoulou, I.; Nikolaou, I.; Zervas, A. & Nakopoulou, L. (2008). Prognostic value of microsatellite instability determined by immunohistochemical staining of hMSH2 and hMSH6 in urothelial carcinoma of the bladder. *Apmis,* Vol. 116, 59-65.

Niedernhofer, L. J.; Odijk, H.; Budzowska, M.; van Drunen, E.; Maas, A.; Theil, A. F.; de Wit, J.; Jaspers, N. G.; Beverloo, H. B.; Hoeijmakers, J. H. & Kanaar, R. (2004). The structure-specific endonuclease Ercc1-Xpf is required to resolve DNA interstrand cross-link-induced double-strand breaks. *Mol Cell Biol,* Vol. 24, pp. 5776- 5787.

Nishiyama, H.; Watanabe, J. & Ogawa, O. (2008). p53 and chemosensitivity in bladder cancer. *Int J Clin Oncol,* Vol. 13, pp. 282-286.

O'Connor, P. M.; Jackman, J.; Bae, I.; Myers, T. G.; Fan, S.; Mutoh, M.; Scudiero, D. A.; Monks, A.; Sausville, E. A.; Weinstein, J. N.; *et al.* (1997). Characterization of the p53 tumor suppressor pathway in cell lines of the National Cancer Institute anticancer drug screen and correlations with the growth-inhibitory potency of 123 anticancer agents. *Cancer Res,* Vol. 57, pp. 4285-4300.

Ohashi, E.; Ogi, T.; Kusumoto, R.; Iwai, S.; Masutani, C.; Hanaoka, F. & Ohmori, H. (2000). Error-prone bypass of certain DNA lesions by the human DNA polymerase kappa. *Genes Dev,* Vol. 14, pp. 1589-1594.

Olaussen, K. A.; Dunant, A.; Fouret, P.; Brambilla, E.; Andre, F.; Haddad, V.; Taranchon, E.; Filipits, M.; Pirker, R.; Popper, H. H.; *et al.* (2006). DNA repair by ERCC1 in non-small-cell lung cancer and cisplatin- based adjuvant chemotherapy. *N Engl J Med,* Vol. 355, pp. 983-991.

Oldenburg, J.; Begg, A. C.; van Vugt, M. J.; Ruevekamp, M.; Schornagel, J. H.; Pinedo, H. M. & Los, G. (1994). Characterization of resistance mechanisms to cis-diamminedichloroplatinum(II) in three sublines of the CC531 colon adenocarcinoma cell line in vitro. *Cancer Res,* Vol. 54, pp. 487-493.

Ottini, L.; Palli, D.; Falchetti, M.; D'Amico, C.; Amorosi, A.; Saieva, C.; Calzolari, A.; Cimoli, F.; Tatarelli, C.; De Marchis, L.; *et al.* (1997). Microsatellite instability in gastric cancer is associated with tumor location and family history in a high-risk population from Tuscany. *Cancer Res,* Vol. 57, pp. 4523-4529.

Pabla, N.; Huang, S.; Mi, Q.-S.; Daniel, R. & Dong, Z. (2008). ATR-Chk2 signaling in p53 activation and DNA damage response during cisplatin-induced apoptosis. *J Biol Chem,* Vol. 283, pp. 6572-6583.

Pani, E.; Stojic, L.; El-Shemerly, M.; Jiricny, J. & Ferrari, S. (2007). Mismatch repair status and the response of human cells to cisplatin. *Cell Cycle,* Vol. 6, pp. 1796-1802.

Papouli, E.; Cejka, P. & Jiricny, J. (2004). Dependence of the cytotoxicity of DNA-damaging agents on the micmatch repair status of human cells. *Cancer Res,* Vol. 64, pp. 3391-3394.

Parker, R. J.; Eastman, A.; Bostick-Bruton, F. & Reed, E. (1991). Acquired cisplatin resistance in human ovarian cancer cells is associated with enhanced repair of cisplatin-DNA lesions and reduced drug accumulation. *J Clin Invest,* Vol. 87, pp. 772-777.

Parsons, R.; Li, G. M.; Longley, M. J.; Fang, W. H.; Papadopoulos, N.; Jen, J.; Delachapelle, A.; Kinzler, K. W.; Vogelstein, B. & Modrich, P. (1993). Hypermutability and mismatch repair deficiency in rer+ tumor- cells. *Cell,* Vol. 75, pp. 1227-1236.

Parton, M.; Krajewski, S.; Smith, I.; Krajewska, M.; Archer, C.; Naito, M.; Ahern, R.; Reed, J. & Dowsett, M. (2002). Coordinate expression of apoptosis-associated proteins in human breast cancer before and during chemotherapy. *Clin Cancer Res,* Vol 8, pp. 2100-2108.

Pinho, M. B.; Costas, F.; Sellos, J.; Dienstmann, R.; Andrade, P. B.; Herchenhorn, D.; Peixoto, F. A.; Santos, V. O.; Small, I. A.; Guimaraes, D. P. & Ferreira, C. G. (2009). XAF1 mRNA expression improves progression- free and overall survival for patients with advanced bladder cancer treated with neoadjuvant chemotherapy. *Urol Oncol.* Vol. 27, pp. 382-390.

Qureshi, K. N.; Griffiths, T. R.; Robinson, M. C.; Marsh, C.; Roberts, J. T.; Hall, R. R.; Lunec, J. & Neal, D. E. (1999). TP53 accumulation predicts improved survival in patients resistant to systemic cisplatin-based chemotherapy for muscle-invasive bladder cancer. *Clin Cancer Res,* Vol. 5, pp. 3500-3507.

Rabik, C. A. & Dolan, M. E. (2007). Molecular mechanisms of resistance and toxicity associated with platinating agents. *Cancer Treat Rev,* Vol. 33, pp. 9-23.

Roos, W. P.; Tsaalbi-Shtylik, A.; Tsaryk, R.; Guvercin, F.; de Wind, N. & Kaina, B. (2009). The translesion polymerase Rev3L in the tolerance of alkylating anticancer drugs. *Mol Pharmacol,* Vol. 76, pp. 927-934.

Safaei, R. (2006). Role of copper transporters in the uptake and efflux of platinum containing drugs. *Cancer Letters,* Vol. 234, pp. 34-39.

Saga, Y.; Hashimoto, H.; Yachiku, S.; Iwata, T. & Tokumitsu, M. (2004). Reversal of acquired cisplatin resistance by modulation of metallothionein in transplanted murine tumors. *Int J Urol*, Vol. 11, pp. 407-415.

Sarkar, S.; A.A.; D.; H.D.; U. & McHugh, P. J. (2006). DNA interstrand crosslink repair during G1 involves nucleotide excision repair and DNA polymerase ζ. *The EMBO J*, Vol. 25, pp. 1285-1294.

Satoh, M.; Cherian, M. G.; Imura, N. & Shimizu, H. (1994). Modulation of resistance to anticancer drugs by inhibition of metallothionein synthesis. *Cancer Res*, Vol. 54, pp. 5255-5257.

Schaaf, A.; Sagi, S.; Langbein, S.; Trojan, L.; Alken, P. & Michel, M. S. (2004). Cytotoxicity of cisplatin in bladder cancer is significantly enhanced by application of bcl-2 antisense oligonucleotides. *Urol Oncol*, Vol. 22, pp. 188-192.

Shachar, S.; Ziv, O.; Avkin, S.; Adar, S.; Wittschieben, J.; Reissner, T.; Chaney, S.; Friedberg, E. C.; Wang, Z.; Carell, T.; *et al.* (2009). Two-polymerase mechanisms dictate error-free and error-prone translesion DNA synthesis in mammals. *Embo J*, Vol. 28, pp. 383-393.

Shariat, S. F.; Karakiewicz, P. I.; Godoy, G.; Karam, J. A.; Ashfaq, R.; Fradet, Y.; Isbarn, H.; Montorsi, F.; Jeldres, C.; Bastian, P. J.; *et al.* (2009). Survivin as a prognostic marker for urothelial carcinoma of the bladder: a multicenter external validation study. *Clin Cancer Res*, Vol. 15, pp. 7012-7019.

Shen, X.; Jun, S.; O"Neal, L. E.; Sonoda, E.; Bemark, M.; Sale, J. E. & Li, L. (2006). REV3 and REV1 play major roles in recombination-independent repair of DNA interstrand cross-links mediated by monoubiquitinated proliferating cell nuclear antigen (PCNA). *J Biol Chem*, Vol. 281, pp. 13869-13872.

Shivji, M. K.; Moggs, J. G.; Kuraoka, I.; & Wood, R. D. (1999). Dual-incision assays for nucleotide excision repair using DNA with a lesion at a specific site. In *DNA Repair Protocols: Eukaryotic Systems, D. S. Henderson, ed. (Totowa, NJ, Humana Press)*, pp. 373-392.

Shivji, M. K.; Moggs, J. G.; Kuraoka, I. & Wood, R. D. (2005). Assaying for the dual incisions of nucleotide excision repair using DNA with a lesion at a specific site. In *DNA Repair Protocols: Eukaryotic Systems, Second Edition, D. S. Henderson, ed. (Totowa, NJ, Humana Press)*, pp. 435-456.

Shuck, S. C.; Short, E. A. & Turchi, J. J. (2008). Eukaryotic nucleotide excision repair: from understanding mechanisms to influencing biology. *Cell Research*, Vol. 18, pp. 64-72.

Siddik, Z. H. (2003). Cisplatin: mode of action and molecular basis of resistance. *Oncogene*, Vol. 22, pp. 7265- 7279.

Siegsmund, M. J.; Marx, C.; Seemann, O.; Schummer, B.; Steidler, A.; Toktomambetova, L.; Kohrmann, K. U.; Rassweiler, J. & Alken, P. (1999). Cisplatin-resistant bladder carcinoma cells: enhanced expression of metallothioneins. *Urol Res*, Vol. 27, pp. 157-163.

Sijbers, A. M.; de Laat, W. L.; Ariza, R. R.; Biggerstaff, M.; Wei, Y.-F.; Moggs, J. G.; Carter, K. C.; Shell, B. K.; Evans, E.; de Jong, M. C.; *et al.* (1996). Xeroderma pigmentosum group F caused by a defect in a structure- specific DNA repair endonuclease. *Cell*, Vol. 86, pp. 811-822.

Singh, S. V.; Xu, B. H.; Jani, J. P.; Emerson, E. O.; Backes, M. G.; Rihn, C.; Scalamogna, D.; Stemmler, N.; Specht, S.; Blanock, K. & et al. (1995). Mechanism of cross-resistance to cisplatin in a mitomycin C-resistant human bladder cancer cell line. *Int J Cancer,* Vol. 61, pp. 431-436.

Siu, L. L.; Banerjee, D.; Khurana, R. J.; Pan, X.; Pflueger, R.; Tannock, I. F. & Moore, M. J. (1998). The prognostic role of p53, metallothionein, P-glycoprotein, and MIB-1 in muscle-invasive urothelial transitional cell carcinoma. *Clin Cancer Res,* Vol. 4, pp. 559-565.

Soga, N.; Kise, H.; Arima, K. & Sugimura, Y. (2010). Third-line gemcitabine monotherapy for platinum-resistant advanced urothelial cancer. *Int J Clin Oncol,* Vol. 15, pp. 376-381.

Song, I.-S.; Savaraj, N.; Siddik, Z. H.; Liu, P.; Wei, Y.; Wu, C. J. & Kuo, M. T. (2004). Role of human copper transporter Ctr1 in the transport of platinum-based antitumor agents in cisplatin-sensitive and cisplatin-resistant cells. *Molec Cancer Therapeutics,* Vol. 3, pp. 1543-1549.

Strand, M.; Prolla, T. A.; Liskay, R. M. & Petes, T. D. (1993). Destabilization of tracts of simple repetitive DNA in yeast by mutations affecting DNA mismatch repair. *Nature,* Vol. 365, pp. 274-276.

Surowiak, P.; Materna, V.; Maciejczyk, A.; Pudelko, M.; Markwitz, E.; Spaczynski, M.; Dietel, M.; Zabel, M. & Lage, H. (2007). Nuclear metallothionein expression correlates with cisplatin resistance of ovarian cancer cells and poor clinical outcome. *Virchows Arch,* Vol. 450, pp. 279-285.

Tada, Y.; Wada, M.; Migita, T.; Nagayama, J.; Hinoshita, E.; Mochida, Y.; Maehara, Y.; Tsuneyoshi, M.; Kuwano, M. & Naito, S. (2002). Increased expression of multidrug resistance-associated proteins in bladder cancer during clinical course and drug resistance to doxorubicin. *Int J Cancer,* Vol. 98, pp. 630- 635.

Taniguchi, K.; Wada, M.; Kohno, K.; Nakamura, T.; Kawabe, T.; Kawakami, M.; Kagotani, K.; Okumura, K.; Akiyama, S. & Kuwano, M. (1996). A human canalicular multispecific organic anion transporter (cMOAT) gene is overexpressed in cisplatin-resistant human cancer cell lines with decreased drug accumulation. *Cancer Res,* Vol. 56, pp. 4124-4129.

Tirro, E.; Consoli, M. L.; Massimino, M.; Manzella, L.; Frasca, F.; Sciacca, L.; Vicari, L.; Stassi, G.; Messina, L.; Messina, A. & Vigneri, P. (2006). Altered expression of c-IAP1, survivin, and Smac contributes to chemotherapy resistance in thyroid cancer cells. *Cancer Res,* Vol. 66, pp. 4263-4272.

Topping, R. P.; Wilkinson, J. C. & Drotschmann Scarpinato, K. (2009). Mismatch repair protein deficiency compromises cisplatin-induced apoptotic signaling. *J Biol Chem,* Vol. 284, pp. 14029-14039.

Usanova, S.; Piee-Staffa, A.; Sied, U.; Thomale, J.; Schneider, A.; Kaina, B. & Köberle, B. (2010). Cisplatin sensitivity of testis tumour cells is due to deficiency in interstrand-crosslink repair and low ERCC1- XPF expression. *Mol Cancer,* Vol. 9, pp. 248.

von der Maase, H.; Sengelov, L.; Roberts, J. T.; Ricci, S.; Dogliotti, L.; Oliver, T.; Moore, M. J.; Zimmermann, A. & Arning, M. (2005). Long-term survival results of a randomized trial comparing gemcitabine plus cisplatin, with methotrexate, vinblastine, doxorubicin, plus cisplatin in patients with bladder cancer. *J Clin Oncol,* Vol. 23, pp. 4602-4608.

Wang, H.; Zhang, S. Y.; Wang, S.; Lu, J.; Wu, W.; Weng, L.; Chen, D.; Zhang, Y.; Lu, Z.; Yang, J.; *et al.* (2009). REV3L confers chemoresistance to cisplatin in human gliomas: the potential of its RNAi for synergistic therapy. *Neuro Oncol,* Vol. 11, pp. 790-802.

Watanabe, J.; Nishiyama, H.; Okubo, K.; Takahashi, T.; Toda, Y.; Habuchi, T.; Kakehi, Y.; Tada, M. & Ogawa, O. (2004). Clinical evaluation of p53 mutations in urothelial carcinoma by IHC and FASAY. *Urology,* Vol. 63, pp. 989-993.

Weberpals, J.; Garbuio, K.; O'Brien, A.; Clark-Knowles, K.; Doucette, S.; Antoniouk, O.; Goss, G. & Dimitroulakos, J. (2009). The DNA repair proteins BRCA1 and ERCC1 as predictive markers in sporadic ovarian cancer. *Int J Cancer,* Vol. 124, pp. 806-815.

Wei, S. H.; Chen, C. M.; Strathdee, G.; Harnsomburana, J.; Shyu, C. R.; Rahmatpanah, F.; Shi, H.; Ng, S. W.; Yan, P. S.; Nephew, K. P.; *et al.* (2002). Methylation microarray analysis of late-stage ovarian carcinomas distinguishes progression-free survival in patients and identifies candidate epigenetic markers. *Clin Cancer Res,* Vol. 8, pp. 2246-2252.

Welsh, C.; Day, R.; McGurk, C.; Masters, J. R.; Wood, R. D. & Köberle, B. (2004). Reduced levels of XPA, ERCC1 and XPF DNA repair proteins in testis tumor cell lines. *Int J Cancer,* Vol. 110, pp. 352-361.

Westerveld, A.; Hoeijmakers, J. H. J.; van Duin, M.; de Wit, J.; Odijk, H.; Pastink, A.; Wood, R. & Bootsma, D. (1984). Molecular cloning of a human DNA repair gene. *Nature,* Vol. 310, pp. 425-429.

Williams, J.; Lucas, P. C.; Griffith, K. A.; Choi, M.; Fogoros, S.; Hu, Y. Y. & Liu, J. R. (2005). Expression of Bcl-xL in ovarian carcinoma is associated with chemoresistance and recurrent disease. *Gynecol Oncol,* Vol. 96, pp. 287-295.

Wittschieben, J. P.; Reshmi, S. C.; Gollin, S. M. & Wood, R. D. (2006). Loss of DNA polymerase zeta causes chromosomal instability in mammalian cells. *Cancer Res,* Vol. 66, pp. 134-142.

Wood, D. P. J.; Klein, E.; Fair, W. R. & Chaganti, R. S. (1993). Metallothionein gene expression in bladder cancer exposed to cisplatin. *Modern Pathology,* Vol. 6, pp. 33-35.

Wood, R. D.; Araújo, S. J.; Ariza, R. R.; Batty, D. P.; Biggerstaff, M.; Evans, E.; Gaillard, P.-H.; Gunz, D.; Köberle, B.; Kuraoka, I.; *et al.* (2000). DNA damage recognition and nucleotide excision repair in mammalian cells. *Cold Spring Harbor Sym Quant Biol,* Vol. 65, pp. 173-182.

Wülfing, C.; van Ahlen, H.; Eltze, E.; Piechota, H.; Hertle, L. & Schmid, K. W. (2007). Metallothionein in bladder cancer: correlation of overexpression with poor outcome after chemotherapy. *World J Urol,* Vol. 25, pp. 199-205.

Wynne, P.; Newton, C.; Ledermann, J. A.; Olaitan, A.; Mould, T. A. & Hartley, J. A. (2007). Enhanced repair of DNA interstrand crosslinking in ovarian cancer cells from patients following treatment with platinum-based chemotherapy. *Br J Cancer,* Vol. 97, pp. 927-933.

Yang, D.; Song, X.; Zhang, J.; Ye, L.; Wang, S.; Che, X.; Wang, J.; Zhang, Z.; Wang, L. & Shi, W. (2010). Therapeutic potential of siRNA-mediated combined knockdown of the IAP genes (Livin, XIAP, and Survivin) on human bladder cancer T24 cells. *Acta Biochim Biophys Sin (Shanghai),* Vol. 42, pp. 137-144.

Yang, X.; Zheng, F.; Xing, H.; Gao, Q.; Wei, W.; Lu, Y.; Wang, S.; Zhou, J.; Hu, W. & Ma, D. (2004). Resistance to chemotherapy-induced apoptosis via decreased caspase-3 activity and overexpression of antiapoptotic proteins in ovarian cancer. J *Cancer Res Clin Oncol,* Vol. 130, pp. 423-428.

Yeh, J. J.; Hsu, N. Y.; Hsu, W. H.; Tsai, C. H.; Lin, C. C. & Liang, J. A. (2005). Comparison of chemotherapy response with P-glycoprotein, multidrug resistance-related protein-1, and lung resistance-related protein expression in untreated small cell lung cancer. *Lung,* Vol. 183, pp. 177-183.

Zhen, W.; Link, C. J.; Jr.; O'Connor, P. M.; Reed, E.; Parker, R.; Howell, S. B. & Bohr, V. A. (1992). Increased gene-specific repair of cisplatin interstrand cross-links in cisplatin-resistant human ovarian cancer cell lines. *Mol Cell Biol,* Vol. 12, pp. 3689-3698.

Zheng, H.; Tomschik, M.; Zlatanova, J. & Leuba, S. H. (2005). Evanescent field fluorescence microscopy (EFFM) for analysis of protein/DNA interactions at the single-molecule level. In *Protein-protein interactions, a molecular cloning manual, 2nd edition, E. Golemis, & P. Adams, eds.* (Cold Spring Harbor, NY, Cold Spring Harbor Laboratory Press), pp. 1-19 Chapter 20.

14

Chemotherapy for Metastatic Disease

Takehiro Sejima, Shuichi Morizane, Akihisa Yao,
Tadahiro Isoyama and Atsushi Takenaka
Division of Urology, Department of Surgery, Tottori University Faculty of Medicine
Japan

1. Introduction

Bladder cancer occurs with a relatively high incidence in industrial nations. For example, bladder cancer is the fourth most common type of cancer in American men. The estimated U.S. incidence in 2008 was 68,810 cases and the mortality was 14,100 cases (Jemal et al., 2008). Of newly diagnosed bladder cancer cases, approximately 70% - 80% will present with non muscle-invasive disease. Among such cases, 50% - 70% will recur, and 10% - 30% will progress to muscle-invasive disease (Soloway et al., 2002; Saad et al., 2002). Radical cystectomy with or without chemotherapy is the standard therapy for muscle-invasive disease; however, some patients will experience metastatic relapse after radical surgery. A few patients present with metastatic disease upon their initial presentation at the hospital. Such advanced bladder cancer remains an incurable terminal disease, and accounts for 3% of the cancer-related mortality in the United States. Deaths from bladder cancer are mainly related to distant spread; hence, prevention of metastatic disease remains a crucial goal in this disease. Systemic chemotherapy achieves palliation, survival benefit, and occasional long-term remissions. For the last two decades, cisplatin-based combination therapies have evolved as the standard. The MVAC regimen (Sternberg et al., 1988) was reported to demonstrate an impressive complete remission rate of 37% in advanced urothelial carcinoma (UC), and in a subsequent comparative study was found to be superior to the single agent cisplatin (Saxman et al., 1997). In this chapter, we review the recent progress in chemotherapeutic regimens not only for advanced bladder cancer, but also for advanced UC in the upper urinary tract. We also show current data on the efficacy of combination therapy with gemcitabine and platinum anti-cancer drugs, which is mainly used as a second-line treatment in our institution.

2. The first successful chemotherapeutic regimen for advanced Urothelial Carcinoma (UC)

Despite recent developments in anti-cancer drugs, advanced UC remains an incurable disease, with a median survival time of only 12 to 14 months (Jemal et al., 2003). The most reliable treatment option for advanced UC is considered to be combination chemotherapy including a platinum anti-cancer drug. The combination chemotherapy regimen of methotrexate / vinblastine / doxorubicin / cisplatin (MVAC) as reported originally by Sternberg (Sternberg et al., 1988) is currently being used worldwide with superior efficacy. However, MVAC treatment is associated with substantial toxicities and has a toxic death rate of approximately

3 - 4% (Sternberg et al., 1989; Loehrer et al., 1992). Therefore, the need for an alternative less toxic combination chemotherapy that can provide efficacy similar or superior to the MVAC regimen has been identified. Gemcitabine, a nucleoside analogue, has demonstrated activity against a range of solid tumors, including metastatic UC (Gatzemeier et al., Moore, 1996; Stadler et al., 1997). In particular, gemcitabine alone has yielded a response rate of 23 - 29%, with a complete response rate of 4 - 13%, in both previously treated and untreated metastatic UC patients (Sternberg, 2000). The good activity and toxicity profiles of single-agent gemcitabine treatment and its synergism with cisplatin in pre-clinical models (Peters et al., 1995) led to the development of this combination for the treatment of advanced UC. After obtaining results from phase 2 trials of combination therapy comprising gemcitabine plus cisplatin (GC) as first- or second-line treatment for UC, von der Maase et al. published a large multinational phase 3 trial comparing MVAC with GC therapy, with a total of 405 patients accrued (von der Maase et al., 2000). The final results show that the two regimens are similar in terms of response rate, time to progression and survival. However, the GC combination showed a better safety profile and tolerability than MVAC. The representative randomized trials on MVAC and GC are summarized in Table 1. Carboplatin shares a common mechanism of action with cisplatin, but the two have different pharmacokinetic and dose-limiting toxicities (Van Echo et al., 1989). Patients with UC are often elderly, and frequently have clinical or subclinical renal function impairment. Thus, the substitution of carboplatin for cisplatin offers a promising alternative for these patients. There have been several phase 2 reports showing that gemcitabine / carboplatin achieved clinical results equivalent to those of GC (Xu et al., 2007; Dogliotti et al., 2007). It can thus be speculated that the combination of gemcitabine plus a platinum anti-cancer drug (cisplatin or carboplatin) is currently being used worldwide in the treatment of advanced UC.

Therapy	No. of Patients	Response Rate/PFS	Median Survival	Hazard Ratio/*P* value
MVAC (Sternberg)	263 (MVAC + High dose MVAC)	50 % (CR 9 %) Med PFS 8.1 months	14.9 months (2 year survival 26.2 %) (5 year survival 13.5 %)	HR = 0.76 *P* = 0.042
High dose MVAC (Sternberg)		64 % (CR 21 %) Med PFS 9.5 months	15.1 months (2 year survival 36.7 %) (5 year survival 21.8 %)	
Cisplatin (Saxman)	122	PR 12 % Med TTP 10 months	8.2 months	*P* = 0.0002
MVAC (Saxman)	133	PR 39 % Med TTP 4.3 months	12.5 months	
MVAC (Von der Maase)	202	46 % Med PFS 8.3 months	15.2 months	*P* = 0.75 HR = 0.042
GC (Von der Maase)	203	49 % Med. PFS 7.7 months	14.0 months	

Table 1. Summary of representative randomized trials exploring chemotherapy in metastatic urothelial cancer

3. The efficacy and safety of combination chemotherapy with gemcitabine and a platinum anti-cancer drug. A regimen mainly used as second-line chemotherapy for patients with advanced UC at Tottori university hospital

Our original data regarding the effects of combination therapy with gemcitabine plus platinum anti-cancer drug as second-line chemotherapy for cases of advanced UC are described below. These data were gathered mainly as a result of limitations in the Japanese insurance system, which until recently did not cover the use of gemcitabine for the treatment of UC. That is, before February 2009, the use of gemcitabine was not allowed for general use in Japan, and thus only referral academic institutions such as ours were able to conduct gemcitabine therapy. Because the incurable rate is still high in advanced UC patients to date in spite of the medical progress of many anti cancer drugs in Japan and other countries, physicians often encounter patients with advanced UC who need to undergo more than one kind of chemotherapy. Therefore sequential data of second-line chemotherapy like ours is considered to be useful for urological oncologists worldwide. In this paragraph, the therapeutic data for cases of upper urinary tract UC are also included. This book is of course about bladder cancer; however, it is often difficult to isolate the therapeutic data for bladder cancer from the data for all cases of UC. Therefore, we regret that we cannot describe the results for bladder cancer data specifically.

3.1 Patients' characteristics

From December 2004 until September 2011, 30 patients received the combination chemotherapy of gemcitabine plus a platinum anti-cancer drug (cisplatin or carboplatin) at

Characteristics	No. of patients (%)	
No. of patients	30	(100%)
Median age, yr (range)	72	(52-83)
Gender		
Male	23	(76.7%)
Female	7	(23.3%)
Previous therapy		
None	4	(13.3%)
Methotrexate/Epirubicin/Cisplatin (MEC)	14	(46.7%)
Methotrexate/Epirubicin/Carboplatin (modified MEC)	9	(30.0%)
Etoposide/ Cisplatin	1	(3.3%)
Radiation + Intraarterial chemotherapy	2	(6.7%)
Primary urothelial tumor site		
Bladder	9	(30.0%)
Renal pelvis ~ ureter	21	(70.0%)
Advanced disease at first visit	7	(23.3%)
Recurrence after surgery for primary tumor	23	(76.7%)
Site of metastasis or recurrence, or invasion from primary tumor		
Lung	6	(20.0%)
Lymph node	18	(60.0%)
Local recurrence	5	(16.7%)
Bone	2	(6.7%)

Table 2. Patient characteristics

our institution. All patients were evaluated for efficacy and for toxicity. The pretreatment characteristics of the patients are listed in Table 2. 23 patients (77%) had previously received combination chemotherapy of methotrexate / epirubicin / cisplatin (MEC).

3.2 Treatment plan

In the first cycle of the therapy, the creatinine clearance (Ccr) (ml / min) of each patient was measured prior to initiation of the therapy. In the patients with Ccr > 60, cisplatin was administered, while in those with Ccr < 60, carboplatin was administered as the platinum anti-cancer drug. Gemcitabine (1,000 mg / m^2) was given by intravenous infusion over 30 – 60 min on days 1, 8, and 15. Cisplatin (70 mg / m^2) was given by intravenous infusion over 30 – 60 min on day 2 in the cisplatin group, whereas carboplatin dosed to an AUC of 5 was given by intravenous infusion over 30 – 60 minutes on day 2 in the carboplatin group. Basically, each cycle consisted of 21 days. However, an extension of the days in each cycle was permitted based on the judgment of the physician in charge if any severe adverse events were noted. All toxicities were recorded according to the National Cancer Institute Common Toxicity Criteria (NCI-CTC) version 3.0. Dose adjustment during the treatment was based on hematological and non-hematological assessment of toxicities. In the hematological assessment of toxicities, leukocyte and platelet counts were generally measured weekly. For cases where leukocytes < 2,000 / mm^3 or platelets < 75,000 / mm^3, or where there was evidence of bleeding, gemcitabine was omitted. No new cycle was started unless leukocytes were > 2,000 / mm^3 and platelets were > 75,000 / mm^3. The platinum anti-cancer drug dose was reduced by 50% for grade 2 neurotoxicity, omitted for grade 3, and stopped for grade 4. For renal toxicity, the dose of platinum anti-cancer drug was reduced by 50% for Ccr 50 – 59, and omitted for Ccr < 50. For other grade 3 non-hematological toxicities (except nausea, vomiting, and alopecia), gemcitabine and platinum anti-cancer drug doses were reduced by 50% or omitted per the physician in charge. For grade 4 toxicities, doses were reduced by 50% or stopped (unless the patient was responding to the therapy).

3.3 Dose administration

The median number of consecutive cycles per patient was 3 (range: 1 – 7). 16 patients (53%) underwent more than 3 cycles of the therapy. Cisplatin was administered in 12 patients (40%), while carboplatin was administered in 18 patients (60%) as the platinum anti-cancer drug (Table 3).

3.4 Efficacy

All 30 patients were assessed with regard to clinical outcome and treatment efficacy according to RECIST criteria at the end of the study. With regard to clinical outcome (Table 3), we observed 2 (7%) cases of complete response (CR) and 7 (23%) cases of partial response (PR), with an overall response rate (ORR) of 30%. The visceral field of metastasis or relapse in patients of CR and PR was the lungs in 3 cases, lymph nodes in 5 cases, and local relapse (post-nephroureterectomy) in 1 case. There were no cases with responses in other visceral fields such as bone. Stable disease (SD) was identified in 10 patients (33%), and progressive disease (PD) in 9 patients (30%). 2 patients (7%) were not evaluated. The median time to follow-up was 11.7 months (range: 0.8 – 65.8 months). The median overall survival (OS) was 11.1 months. Kaplan-Meier curves for OS are shown in Fig. 1.

		No. of patients (%)
No. of chemotherapy cycles	1	6 (20.0)
	2	8 (26.7)
	3	10 (33.3)
	More than 4	6 (20.0)
Platinum drug	Cisplatin	12 (40.0)
	Carboplatin	18 (60.0)
Efficacy according to RECIST	CR	2 (6.7)
	PR	7 (23.3)
	SD	10 (33.3)
	PD	9 (30.0)
	NE	2 (6.7)
Outcome	NED	2 (6.7)
	Alive with cancer	8 (26.7)
	Dead due to cancer	20 (66.6)

Table 3. Treatment profile and efficacy

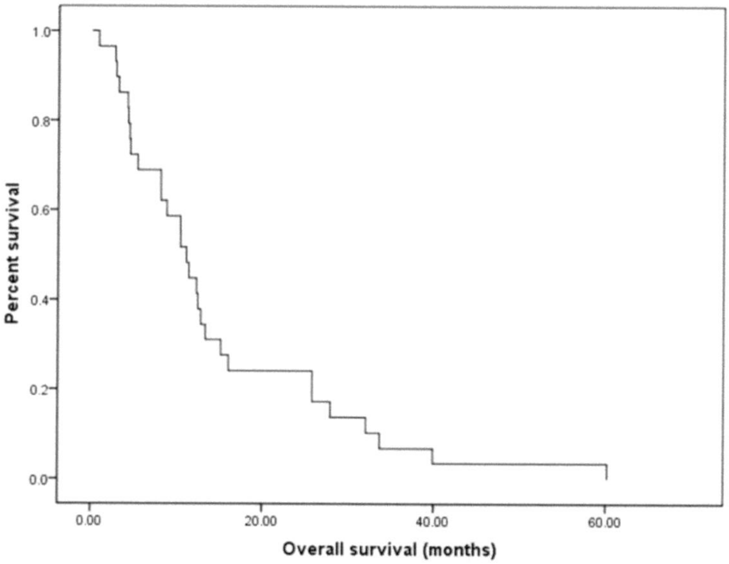

Fig. 1. Overall survival rate of all 30 patients with advance UC treated at Tottori University Hospital

3.5 Toxicity

Only 1 patient discontinued the therapy simply for reasons of toxicity; this patient showed a Grade 2 allergic reaction to gemcitabine, which was administered on day 15. Since this patient eventually received one whole cycle of the therapy, we assessed the efficacy of the treatment as such. Grade 3 / 4 neutropenia was the most frequent toxicity, occurring in 63% of the patients. Grade 3 / 4 thrombocytopenia was also a frequent toxicity, occurring in 57% of the patients. Grade 3 / 4 non-hematologic toxicities included nausea and vomiting in 1 patient (3%). Major toxicities according to NCI-CTC are summarized in Table 4. No other types of major toxicities such as nephrotoxicity or neurotoxicity were observed in any patients. In order to analyze the cumulative damage due to hematologic side effects, the nadir values of blood counts were analyzed. The nadir values of hemoglobin and the nadir counts of leukocytes and platelet cells in the first cycle were practically the same as those in the other progressive cycles. In other words, hematological toxicities were not enhanced by the progressive repetition of cycles (data not shown).

	No. of patients (%)			
	Grade 1	Grade 2	Grade 3	Grade 4
Neutropenia	4 (13.3)	6 (20.0)	16 (53.3)	3 (10.0)
Anemia	3 (10.0)	13 (43.3)	9 (30.0)	4 (13.3)
Thrombocytopenia	6 (20.0)	4 (13.3)	8 (26.7)	9 (30.0)
Vomiting	3 (10.0)	2 (6.7)	1 (3.3)	0 (0)
Allergy	0 (0)	1 (3.3)	0 (0)	0 (0)

Table 4. Mayor toxicities according to NCI-CTC

3.6 Conclusions

The efficacy of gemcitabine plus a platinum anti-cancer drug as a second-line chemotherapy for advanced UC was found to be modest. The toxicity of the therapy was tolerable despite damage from previous chemotherapy and repeated cycles. The present data, obtained as a result of particular limitations in the medical insurance industry in Japan, will be helpful when considering the best course of second-line chemotherapy for cases of advanced UC in the future.

4. Is there any effective combination chemotherapy except MVAC or GC for advanced UC?
— The combination therapy of methotrexate / epirubicin / cisplatin (MEC) —

The combination chemotherapy of methotrexate, epirubicin and cisplatin (MEC) was mainly developed in Japan for the purpose of establishing a regimen less toxic than MVAC but with equal efficacy. Several academic Japanese institutions including the Japanese Urothelial Cancer Research Group promoted a randomized trial comparing MEC and MVAC (Kuroda et al., 1998). Total of 89 patients were assigned to three groups receiving either standard MEC (S-MEC), dose-intensified MEC (I-MEC) or MVAC. The S-MEC regimen consisted of methotrexate (30 mg / m^2), epirubicin (50 mg / m^2) and cisplatin (100 mg / m^2), and that of the I-MEC regimen was methotrexate (36 mg / m^2), epirubicin (60 mg / m^2) and cisplatin (120 mg / m^2). In both groups, methotrexate was administered on day 1 and 15, epirubicin was administered on day 1, and cisplatin was administered on day 2. In the I-MEC group, G-CSF

(2μg / kg) was administered from day 3 until day 12 routinely. The response rates (CR + PR) were 52% with S-MEC, 76% with I-MEC and 47% with MVAC. All of the adverse events were rendered tolerable in the S-MEC and I-MEC groups through the use of G-CSF agents. We had been utilizing MEC as a first choice therapy until 2008 in our institution because it was less toxic than but as effective as MVAC. As a matter of fact, most of the patients in our study of second-line combination chemotherapy with gemcitabine and the platinum anti-cancer drugs described above had been receiving MEC as the first line chemotherapy at other institutions.

5. Prevention of micro metastasis and effort of tumor reduction by neoadjuvant chemotherapy at radical cystectomy

In T2-4 (invasive) bladder cancer, neoadjuvant chemotherapy with MVAC or cisplatin, methotrexate, and vinblastine has demonstrated significant progression-free survival (PFS) and OS benefit in several randomized trials. One representative trial is the Intergroup 8710 trials reported by Grossman et al. in which cystectomy alone was compared with neoadjuvant MVAC followed by radical cystectomy. The group receiving neoadjuvant chemotherapy had an increased likelihood of eliminating residual cancer in the cystectomy specimen (pT0) and had an associated improved survival. Moreover, neoadjuvant chemotherapy did not adversely affect the patient's chance of undergoing a cystectomy and did not increase the risk of postoperative complications (Grossman et al., 2003). In the combined analysis of 2 Nordic studies, neoadjuvant platinum-based combination chemotherapy was associated with an 8% increase in survival at 5 years (Sherif et al., 2004). A meta-analysis of randomized controlled trials demonstrated a survival benefit to receiving neoadjuvant chemotherapy (Winquist et al., 2004). Carboplatin-based regimens have been evaluated in the neoadjuvant setting only in phase 2 trials, and hence their use in the neoadjuvant or adjuvant setting cannot be recommended (Smith et al., 2008; deVele White et al., 2009). The studies of adjuvant chemotherapy have demonstrated conflicting results. They have had design flaws and small sample sizes and are therefore underpowered to give a conclusive answer regarding the benefits.

6. Other recent chemotherapeutic regimens including taxanes

The taxanes are diterpenes produced by the plants of the genus Taxus (yews), and include such compounds as docetaxel and paclitaxel, the latter of which was originally derived from the Pacific yew tree. The principal mechanism of action of the taxane class of drugs is the disruption of microtubule function. Microtubules are essential to cell division, and taxanes stabilize GDP-bound tubulin in the microtubule, thereby inhibiting the process of cell division. Thus, in essence, taxanes are mitotic inhibitors. Both paclitaxel and docetaxel have been studied as chemotherapeutic agents for metastatic bladder cancer. Paclitaxel-based regimens in combination with either cisplatin or carboplatin have been evaluated with response rates between 16% and 36% and median survival ranging from 6 to 10 months depending on the characteristics of the patients enrolled and whether they are ciplatin-sensitive or a refractory population (Vaishampayan et al., 2005; Uhm et al., 2007). A phase 3 study comparing docetaxel and cisplatin (DC) with G-CSF versus MVAC with G-CSF found MVAC to be more effective than DC for metastatic cancer; MVAC demonstrated both a superior median time to progression (9.4 vs 6.1 months; $P = 0.003$) and median survival time (14.2 vs 9.3 months; $P = 0.026$) (Bamias et al., 2004). Other recent representative reports of taxanes with cisplatin therapy are shown in Table 5. Antifolates such as trimetrexate and premetrexed have been better tolerated with promising response rates and should be promising for future evaluation (Witte et al. 1994; Sweeney et al., 2006). Oxaliplatin-based regimens have been evaluated and also shown to be of modest benefit (Carles et al., 2007).

Author	Previous therapy	Dose (mg / m²) Cisplatin	Taxane	No. of Cases	Efficacy (%) (CR + PR)	CR rate (%)	Median survival (M)
Dreicer	None	75	175 (P)	52	50	8	10.6
Burch	None	70	135 (P)	34	70	32	13
Sengelov	None	75	75 (D)	25	60	26	13.6
Dimopoulos	None	75	75 (D)	66	52	12	8

P, Paclitaxel; D, Docetaxel

Table 5. Recent representative reports of taxanes with cisplatin therapy for advanced urotherial cancer

7. Role of targeted therapies in bladder cancer

The actual clinical advent of targeted therapies has been slower in UC, as compared to other solid tumors due to large variations in histology worldwide, as well as the difficulty in accruing to clinical trials with this malignancy. Vaishampayan et al. evaluated and reported the frequency of overexpression of Her-2 in bladder cancer and correlated with the Her-2 expression in metastatic sites. Interestingly, the overexpression of her-2 by immunohistochemistry (IHC) (2+ or 3+) was 37% in primary bladder tumor tissue, the expression in metastatic sites such as lymph nodes was 63% and the expression in visceral metastases was 86% (Vaishampayan, 2009). 45% of Her-2/neu-negative primaries had Her-2/neu-positive lymph node metastases, while 92% of Her-2-positive primary tumors were associated with Her-2-positive metastasis. This finding suggested that Her-2 over-expression could be a useful therapeutic target for advanced UC. Hence, a phase 2 trial was conducted and reported evaluating the role of trastuzumab with chemotherapy in metastatic UC. An extremely promising 70% response rate and a favorable median survival of 14 months were noted despite 55% of the patients having visceral metastases (Hussain et al., 2007). Another novel approach using molecular targeted therapy for advanced UC patients is the combination therapy of bevacizumab and chemotherapeutic agents. A phase 2 study of bevacizumab in combination with cisplatin and gemcitabine in metastatic or locally advanced bladder cancer involving 36 patients showed a complete response in 6 (17%), and a partial response in 18 (50%); this combination is now being studied in a phase 3 trial (Dovedi & Davies, 2009; Hahn et al., 2011). Another study with anti-angiogenic therapy is the evaluation of sunitinib in a placebo-controlled double-blind trial with the goal of sustaining or prolonging response, after initial chemo-therapy in advanced bladder cancer (Bradley et al., 2007). Epithelial growth factor receptor has also been identified as an exciting target in UC. The over-expression of EGFR by IHC is noted in about 92% (35 of 38) of the bladder cancer cases at Wayne State University; however, its association with survival outcome has not been established (Bellmunt et al., 2003). Given the possibility of EGFR-targeted therapy, a phase 2 randomized trials of cisplatin and gemcitabine with or without cetuximab (a monoclonal antibody to EGFR) is ongoing as a frontline therapy for metastatic UC. Current and future additional trials of targeted therapy are listed in Table 6.

First line for metastatic disease	Therapy	Organization
(not renal insufficiency)		
Phase II	GC + BVZ	CALGB
Phase II	GC + Sorafenib	MSKCC, EORTC
Phase I	GC + Lapatinib	EORTC
First line metastatic disease		
(renal insufficiency)		
Phase II	GEM + CBDCA + BVZ	MSKCC
Phase II	Sunitinib	SOGUG
Second line		
(single agent)		
Phase II	Sunitinib	MSKCC
Phase II	Sunitinib randum	U. Michigan
Phase II	Sorafenib	PMH / SWOG

GC, gemcitabine + cisplatin; BVZ, bevacizumab; GEM, gemcitabine; CBDCA, carboplatin; CALGB, Cancer and Leukemia Group B; MSKCC, Memorial Sloan-Kettering Cancer Center; EORTC, European Organization for Research and Treatment of Cancer; SOGUG, Spanish Oncology Genitourinary Group; U. Michigan, University of Michigan; PMH, Princess Margaret Hospital; SWOG, Southwest Oncology Group

Table 6. Current and future trial with targeted therapy

8. Conclusions

Since the breakthrough progress of development MVAC chemotherapy by Sternberg for advanced UC patients, the survival of such patients has been prolonged compared with those of untreated patients. However, despite the development of anti-cancer drugs, metastatic bladder cancer is still not considered a curable disease. Numerous efforts to achieve improved curability are going, including investigations into molecular targeted therapy, which has just been developed as a breakthrough treatment for patients with advanced renal cell carcinoma in the same field of urologic oncology.

9. References

Bamias A, Aravantinos G, Deliveliotis C, Bafaloukos D, Kalofonos C, Xiros N, Zervas A, Mitropoulos D, Samantas E, Pectasides D, Papakostas P, Gika D, Kourousis C, Koutras A, Papadimitriou C, Bamias C, Kosmidis P, Dimopoulos MA; Hellenic Cooperative Oncology Group (2004): Docetaxel and cisplatin with granulocyte colony-stimulating factor (G-CSF) versus MVAC with G-CSF in advanced urothelial carcinoma: a multicenter, randomized, phase III study from the Hellenic Cooperative Oncology Group. *J Clin Oncol*: Jan 15;22(2):pp. 220-228. Epub 2003 Dec 9. Erratum in: *J Clin Oncol*: May 1;22(9): pp. 1771. PMID: 14665607

Bellmunt J, Hussain M, Dinney CP (2003): Novel approaches with targeted therapies in bladder cancer. Therapy of bladder cancer by blockade of the epidermal growth factor receptor family. *Crit Rev Oncol Hematol*: 46(Suppl): pp. 85-104. PMID: 12850530

Bradley DA, Dunn R, Nanus D, Stadler W, Dreicer R, Rosenberg J, Smith DC, Hussain M (2007): Randomized, double-blind, placebo-controlled phase II trial of maintenance sunitinib versus placebo after chemotherapy for patients with advanced urothelial carcinoma: scientific rationale and study design. *Clin Genitourin*: Dec;5(7): pp. 460-463. PMID: 18272031

Burch PA, Richardson RL, Cha SS, Sargent DJ, Pitot HC 4th, Kaur JS, Camoriano JK (2000): Phase II study of paclitaxel and cisplatin for advanced urothelial cancer. *J Urol*: Nov;164(5): pp. 1538-1542. PMID: 11025699

Carles J, Esteban E, Climent M, Font A, Gonzalez-Larriba JL, Berrocal A, Garcia-Ribas I, Marfa X, Fabregat X, Albanell J, Bellmunt J; Spanish Oncology Genito Urinary Group Study Group (2007): Gemcitabine and oxaliplatin combination: a multicenter phase II trial in unfit patients with locally advanced or metastatic urothelial cancer. *Ann Oncol*: Aug;18(8): pp. 1359-1362. PMID: 17693649

deVere White RW, Lara PN Jr, Goldman B, Tangen CM, Smith DC, Wood DP Jr, Hussain MH, Crawford ED (2009): A sequential treatment approach to myoinvasive urothelial cancer: a phase II Southwest Oncology Group Trial (S0219). *J Urol*: Jun;181(6): pp. 2476-2480; discussion 2480-2481. Epub 2009 Apr 16. PMID: 19371909

Dimopoulos MA, Bakoyannis C, Georgoulias V, Papadimitriou C, Moulopoulos LA, Deliveliotis C, Karayannis A, Varkarakis I, Aravantinos G, Zervas A, Pantazopoulos D, Fountzilas G, Bamias A, Kyriakakis Z, Anagnostopoulos A, Giannopoulos A, Kosmidis P (1999): Docetaxel and cisplatin combination chemotherapy in advanced carcinoma of the urothelium: a multicenter phase II study of the Hellenic Cooperative Oncology Group. *Ann Oncol*: Nov;10(11): pp. 1385-1388. PMID: 10631471

Dogliotti L, Cartenì G, Siena S, Bertetto O, Martoni A, Bono A, Amadori D, Onat H, Marini L (2007): Gemcitabine plus cisplatin versus gemcitabine plus carboplatin as first-line chemotherapy in advanced transitional cell carcinoma of the urothelium: results of a randomized phase 2 trial. *Eur Urol*: Jul;52(1): pp. 134-141. PMID: 17207911

Dovedi SJ, Davies BR (2009): Emerging targeted therapies for bladder cancer: a disease waiting for a drug. *Cancer Metastasis Rev*: Dec;28(3-4): pp. 355-367. PMID: 19997963

Dreicer R, Manola J, Roth BJ, Cohen MB, Hatfield AK, Wilding G (2000): Phase II study of cisplatin and paclitaxel in advanced carcinoma of the urothelium: an Eastern Cooperative Oncology Group Study. *J Clin Oncol*: Mar;18(5): pp. 1058-1561. PMID: 10694557

Gatzemeier U, Shepherd FA, Le Chevalier T, Weynants P, Cottier B, Groen HJ, Rosso R, Mattson K, Cortes-Funes H, Tonato M, Burkes RL, Gottfried M, Voi M (1996): Activity of gemcitabine in patients with non-small cell lung cancer: a multicentre, extended phase II study. *Eur J Cancer*: Feb;32A(2): pp. 243-248. PMID: 8664035

Grossman HB, Natale RB, Tangen CM, Speights VO, Vogelzang NJ, Trump DL, deVere White RW, Sarosdy MF, Wood DP Jr, Raghavan D, Crawford ED (2003): Neoadjuvant chemotherapy plus cystectomy compared with cystectomy alone for locally advanced bladder cancer. *N Engl J*: Aug 28;349(9): pp. 859-866. PMID: 12944571

Hahn NM, Stadler WM, Zon RT, Waterhouse D, Picus J, Nattam S, Johnson CS, Perkins SM, Waddell MJ, Sweeney CJ; Hoosier Oncology Group (2011): Phase II trial of cisplatin, gemcitabine, and bevacizumab as first-line therapy for metastatic urothelial carcinoma: Hoosier Oncology Group GU 04-75. *J Clin Oncol*: Apr 20;29(12): pp. 1525-1530. PMID: 21422406

Hussain MH, MacVicar GR, Petrylak DP, Dunn RL, Vaishampayan U, Lara PN Jr, Chatta GS, Nanus DM, Glode LM, Trump DL, Chen H, Smith DC; National Cancer Institute (2007): Trastuzumab, paclitaxel, carboplatin, and gemcitabine in advanced human epidermal growth factor receptor-2/neu-positive urothelial carcinoma: results of a multicenter phase II National Cancer Institute trial. *J Clin Oncol*: Jun 1;25(16): pp. 2218-2224. Erratum in: *J Clin Oncol*: 2008 Jul 1;26(19): pp. 3295. PMID: 17538166

Jemal A, Murray T, Samuels A, Ghafoor A, Ward E, Thun MJ (2003): Cancer statistics, 2003. *CA Cancer J Clin*: Jan-Feb;53(1):pp. 5-26. PMID: 12568441

Jemal A, Siegel R, Ward E, Hao Y, Xu J, Murray T, Thun MJ (2008): Cancer statistics, 2008. *CA Cancer J Clin*: Mar-Apr;58(2): pp. 71-96. PMID: 18287387

Kuroda M, Kotake T, Akaza H, Hinotsu S, Kakizoe T (1998):Efficacy of dose-intensified MEC (methotrexate, epirubicin and cisplatin) chemotherapy for advanced urothelial carcinoma: a prospective randomized trial comparing MEC and M-VAC (methotrexate, vinblastine, doxorubicin and cisplatin). Japanese Urothelial Cancer Research Group. *Jpn J Clin Oncol*: Aug;28(8): pp. 497-501. PMID: 9769784

Loehrer PJ Sr, Einhorn LH, Elson PJ, Crawford ED, Kuebler P, Tannock I, Raghavan D, Stuart-Harris R, Sarosdy MF, Lowe BA, et al (1992): A randomized comparison of cisplatin alone or in combination with methotrexate, vinblastine, and doxorubicin in patients with metastatic urothelial carcinoma: a cooperative group study. *J Clin Oncol*: Jul;10(7): pp. 1066-1073. Erratum in: *J Clin Oncol* 1993 Feb;11(2): pp. 384. PMID: 1607913

Moore M (1996): Activity of gemcitabine in patients with advanced pancreatic carcinoma. A review. *Cancer*: Aug 1;78(3 Suppl): pp. 633-638. Review. PMID: 8681302

Peters GJ, Bergman AM, Ruiz van Haperen VW, Veerman G, Kuiper CM, Braakhuis BJ (1995): Interaction between cisplatin and gemcitabine in vitro and in vivo. *Semin Oncol*: Aug;22(4 Suppl 11): pp. 72-79. PMID: 7481849

Saad A, Hanbury DC, McNicholas TA, Boustead GB, Morgan S, Woodman AC (2002): A study comparing various noninvasive methods of detecting bladder cancer in urine. *BJU Int*: Mar;89(4): pp. 369-373. PMID: 11872026

Saxman SB, Propert KJ, Einhorn LH, Crawford ED, Tannock I, Raghavan D, Loehrer PJ Sr, Trump D (1997): Long-term follow-up of a phase III intergroup study of cisplatin alone or in combination with methotrexate, vinblastine, and doxorubicin in patients with metastatic urothelial carcinoma: a cooperative group study. *J Clin Oncol*: Jul;15(7): pp. 2564-2569. PMID: 9215826

Sengeløv L, Kamby C, Lund B, Engelholm SA (1998): Docetaxel and cisplatin in metastatic urothelial cancer: a phase II study. *J Clin Oncol*: Oct;16(10): pp. 3392-3397. PMID: 9779718

Sherif A, Holmberg L, Rintala E, Mestad O, Nilsson J, Nilsson S, Malmström PU; Nordic Urothelial Cancer Group. (2004): Neoadjuvant cisplatinum based combination chemotherapy in patients with invasive bladder cancer: a combined analysis of two Nordic studies. *Eur Urol*: Mar;45(3): pp. 297-303. PMID: 15036674

Smith DC, Mackler NJ, Dunn RL, Hussain M, Wood D, Lee CT, Sanda M, Vaishampayan U, Petrylak DP, Quinn DI, Beekman K, Montie JE. (2008): Phase II trial of paclitaxel, carboplatin and gemcitabine in patients with locally advanced carcinoma of the bladder. *J Urol*: Dec;180(6): pp. 2384-2388; discussion pp. 2388. Epub 2008 Oct 18.

Soloway MS, Sofer M, Vaidya A (2002): Contemporary management of stage T1 transitional cell carcinoma of the bladder. *J Urol*: Apr;167(4): pp. 1573-1583. PMID: 18930256

Stadler WM, Kuzel T, Roth B, Raghavan D, Dorr FA (1997): Phase II study of single-agent gemcitabine in previously untreated patients with metastatic urothelial cancer. *J Clin Oncol*: Nov;15(11): pp. 3394-3398. PMID: 9363871

Sternberg CN, Yagoda A, Scher HI, Watson RC, Herr HW, Morse MJ, Sogani PC, Vaughan ED Jr, Bander N, Weiselberg LR, et al (1988): M-VAC (methotrexate, vinblastine, doxorubicin and cisplatin) for advanced transitional cell carcinoma of the urothelium. *J Urol*: Mar;139(3): pp. 461-469. PMID: 3343727

Sternberg CN, Yagoda A, Scher HI, Watson RC, Geller N, Herr HW, Morse MJ, Sogani PC, Vaughan ED, Bander N, et al (1989): Methotrexate, vinblastine, doxorubicin, and cisplatin for advanced transitional cell carcinoma of the urothelium. Efficacy and patterns of response and relapse. *Cancer*: Dec 15;64(12): pp. 2448-2258. PMID: 2819654

Sternberg CN (2000): Gemcitabine in bladder cancer. *Semin Oncol*: Feb;27(1 Suppl 2): pp. 31-39. Review. PMID: 10697034

Sweeney CJ, Roth BJ, Kabbinavar FF, Vaughn DJ, Arning M, Curiel RE, Obasaju CK, Wang Y, Nicol SJ, Kaufman DS (2006): Phase II study of pemetrexed for second-line treatment of transitional cell cancer of the bladder. *J Clin Oncol*: Jul 20;24(21): pp. 3451-3457. PMID: 16849761

Uhm JE, Lim HY, Kim WS (2007): Paclitaxel with cisplatin as salvage treatment for patients with previously treated advanced transitional cell carcinoma of the urothelial tract. *Neoplasia*: Jan;9(1): pp. 18-22. PMID: 17325740

Vaishampayan U (2009): Systemic therapy of advanced urothelial cancer. *Curr Treat Options Oncol*: Aug;10(3-4): pp. 256-266. Epub 2009 Apr 29. Review. PMID: 19408129

Vaishampayan UN, Faulkner JR, Small EJ, Redman BG, Keiser WL, Petrylak DP, Crawford ED (2005): Phase II trial of carboplatin and paclitaxel in cisplatin-pretreated advanced transitional cell carcinoma: a Southwest Oncology Group study. *Cancer*: Oct 15;104(8): pp. 1627-1632. PMID: 16138364

Van Echo DA, Egorin MJ, Aisner J (1989): The pharmacology of carboplatin. *Semin Oncol*: Apr;16(2 Suppl 5): pp. 1-6. Review. PMID: 2655093

von der Maase H, Hansen SW, Roberts JT, Dogliotti L, Oliver T, Moore MJ, Bodrogi I, Albers P, Knuth A, Lippert CM, Kerbrat P, Sanchez Rovira P, Wersall P, Cleall SP, Roychowdhury DF, Tomlin I, Visseren-Grul CM, Conte PF (2000): Gemcitabine and cisplatin versus methotrexate, vinblastine, doxorubicin, and cisplatin in advanced or metastatic bladder cancer: results of a large, randomized, multinational, multicenter, phase III study. *J Clin Oncol*: Sep;18(17): pp. 3068-3077. PMID: 11001674

Winquist E, Kirchner TS, Segal R, Chin J, Lukka H (2004): Neoadjuvant chemotherapy for transitional cell carcinoma of the bladder: a systematic review and meta-analysis. *J Urol*: Feb;171(2 Pt 1): pp. 561-569. PMID: 14713760

Witte RS, Elson P, Khandakar J, Trump DL. (1994): An Eastern Oncology Group phase II trial of trimetrexate in the treatment of advanced urothelial carcinoma. *Cancer*: Feb 1;73(3): pp. 688-691. PMID: 8299090

Xu N, Zhang XC, Xiong JP, Fang WJ, Yu LF, Qian J, Zhang L (2007): A phase II trial of gemcitabine plus carboplatin in advanced transitional cell carcinoma of the urothelium. *BMC Cancer*: Jun 9;7: pp. 98. PMID: 17559681

Part 7

Invasive Disease, Surgical Treatment and Robotic Approach

15

Robot-Assisted Radical Cystectomy as a Treatment Modality for Patients with Muscle-Invasive Bladder Cancer

Martin C. Schumacher[1,2]
[1]*Dept. of Urology, Karolinska University Hospital, Stockholm,*
[2]*Hirslanden Klinik Aarau,*
[1]*Sweden*
[2]*Switzerland*

1. Introduction

Over the last two decades open radical cystectomy and urinary diversion have become a widely accepted form of treatment in both men and women with transitional cell carcinoma of the bladder. In the mid-1980s orthotopic urinary diversion with anastomosis to the urethra became an oncologically and functionally acceptable option in appropriately selected male patients. With better understanding of the anatomy and of the continence mechanism, orthotopic urinary diversion was subsequently performed in the early 1990s in female patients[1].

Until today open radical cystectomy is still considered the gold standard treatment for patients with muscle-invasive transitional cell carcinoma of the bladder [2, 3]. This is based on the following observations: First, the best long-term survival rates and lowest local recurrence rates have been reported after radical cystectomy [4 5]. Second, the morbidity and mortality of radical cystectomy have significantly improved during the last decades, and good functional results in patients with orthotopic urinary diversions have been achieved [6 7]. Third, radical cystectomy and pelvic lymph node dissection provides the most accurate tumor staging, thus helps selecting patients for adjuvant treatment protocols [8 9].

Radical cystectomy performed through a laparoscopic approach was first described in 1992 [10]. Since then, laparoscopic radical cystectomy has been reported in over 500 patients and current results suggest that this approach may cause less blood loss, decreased postoperative pain and faster recovery compared to open surgery [11 12]. However, due to the technical difficulty (two-dimensional laparoscopic view, counterintuitive motion, poor ergonomics, and nonwristed instrumentation), the steep learning curve and the lack of long-term oncological results, this treatment has not been adopted by mainstream urology.

The introduction of robot assisted surgery for pelvic laparoscopy, especially in performing radical prostatectomy, has changed the possibilities of performing complicated operations in the small pelvis. Three-dimensional vision with ten-fold magnification and the dexterity provided by the endo-wrist (six degrees of freedom) allows the surgeon to operate the tips of the laparoscopic instruments like an open surgeon [13]. Thus, the surgeon will benefit from a faster learning curve as compared to conventional laparoscopy. Further, these advantages have allowed surgeons to translate standard open surgical procedures to a minimally invasive approach, especially its potential in operating in a narrow pelvis as well as for the reconstruction of the urinary tract.

With the beginning of robot-assisted pelvic surgery a decade ago, radical cystectomy and reconstruction of the urinary tract is currently possible. However, until today, results on robot-assisted radical cystectomy (RARC) are mainly reported from a few centers worldwide. Further, results on RARC with intracorporeal urinary diversion are sparse, as most surgeons perform the reconstructive part outside the abdomen due to technical difficulties and longer operative time.

2. Robot-assisted radical cystectomy

The history of robot-assisted radical cystectomy started with Beecken et al. who was the first to perform a RARC with intracorporeal formation of an ileal orthotopic bladder substitute in 2002 [14]. Operating time was 8.5 hours and blood loss 200ml. At five months post-operatively the oncological and functional result of the reservoir were considered excellent. Menon et al. reported the first series of RARC in 17 patients in 2003 [15]. In their series, an ileal conduit was performed in three patients, a W-pouch in ten, a double chimney in two, and a T-pouch in two cases. Mean operating time for radical cystectomy was 140 min and 120–168 min for the different urinary diversions, which were all performed extracorporeally. Mean blood loss was less than 150 mL, and surgical margins were negative in all cases.

Since then, several case series have been published, however, most RARC series comprise less than 100 cases per center [table 1]. Additionally, our current knowledge on RARC is mainly based on reports from less than twenty different surgical centers worldwide. In order to provide a better overview on the value of RARC, data from a mix of 15 academic and private centers from the USA and Europe are prospectively collected and the results reported by the International Robotic Cystectomy Consortium (IRCC) [16] [17] [18]. Despite increasing evidence that RARC seems as effective as open radical cystectomy, it is still too premature to draw any firm conclusions about the status of RARC.

3. Patient selection

Which patients are suitable for RARC using a minimal invasive approach? As patients planned for radical cystectomy are in general older and have a higher prevalence of smoking-related co-morbidities, pulmonary diseases may cause intraoperative problems. Some of these patients may even not be suitable for robot-assisted interventions because of the need for CO_2 insufflation and the steep Trendelenburg position. The cardiac and respiratory systems are especially vulnerable to the extreme and lengthy head-down position. However, in order to minimize these risks, a 25° Trendelenburg position during radical cystectomy and lymph node dissection is possible without affecting the surgical quality [19]. For the urinary diversion the Trendelenburg position can further be decreased to 15°, thus minimizing potential pulmonary complications.

A question mark regarding contra-indications in selecting patients for RARC remains. Presence of bulky disease, locally advanced disease, or enlarged lymph nodes have been considered relative contra-indications [20] [21]. Khan et al. reported specific surgery-related complications at RARC [22]. They found that patients with multiples intravesical therapies, such as mitomycin or BCG, are more likely to have adhesions between the bladder and the

Author (reference)	No. of pts.	Type of urinary diversion:	extracorporeal intracorporeal	Conversion to open surgery	Mean operative time (min)	Mean perioperative blood loss (ml)	Mean post op. hospital stay (days)	Positive margins (bladder)	No. of lymph nodes removed	Follow-up (months)
Beecken et al, 2003 [14]	1	Orthotopic neobladder	intracorporeal	no	510	200	n. a.	neg.	n. a.	n. a.
Menon et al, 2003 [15]	17	Cystectomy Ileal conduit (3) Orthotopic neobladder (14)	extracorporeal	1 pt	140 260 308	150	n. a.	neg.	x (4 – 27)	n. a.
Hemal et al, 2004 [	24	Ileal conduit (4) Orthotopic neobladder (20)	extracorporeal	no	228 - 348	100 - 300	4 - 5	neg.	3 - 27	n.a.
Galich et al, 2006 [33]	13	Ileal conduit (6) Orthotopic neobladder (5) Indiana pouch (2)	extracorporeal	no	697 (240 – 828)	500 (100 – 1000)	8 (4 – 23)	neg.	n. a.	n. a.
Rhee et al, 2006 [30]	7	Ileal conduit	extracorporeal	no	638 (592 – 684)	479	11 (6 – 16)	neg.	n. a.	n. a.
Abraham et al, 2007 [54]	14	Cystectomy Ileal conduit	extracorporeal	no	410 (340 – 545)	212 (50 – 500)	6 (4 – 7)	1 pt (pT4)	22.3 (13 – 42)	n. a.
Mottrie et al, 2007 [56]	27	Ileal conduit (19) Orthotopic neobladder (8)	extracorporeal	no	340 (150 – 450)	301 (50 – 550)	n. a.	neg.	23 (6 – 37)	10.2
Lowentritt et al, 2008 [38]	4/20#	Ileal conduit (4)	extracorporeal	no	350 (340 – 410)	300 (250 – 500)	5 (3 – 8)	neg.	12 (9 – 16)	n. a.
Murphy et al, 2008 [31]	23	Ileal conduit (19) Orthotopic neobladder (4)	extracorporeal	no	397 (314 – 480)	278 (49 – 507)	12 (8 – 15)	neg.	16 (7 – 25)	17 (4 – 40)
Wang et al, 2008 [32]	32	Ileal conduit (17) Orthotopic neobladder (12) Indiana pouch (3)	extracorporeal	no	390 (210 – 570)	400 (100 – 1200)	5 (4 – 18)	2 pts (pT3 N1)	17 (6 – 32)	n. a.
Woods et al, 2008 [34]	27	Ileal conduit (?) Orthotopic neobladder (?)	extracorporeal	no	400 (225 – 660)	277 (50 – 700)	n. a.	2 pts. (pT4)	12 (7 – 20)	n. a.
Hemal et al, 2008 [55]	6	Ileal conduit (5) Orthotopic neobladder (1)	extracorporeal	no	330	200 (150 – 1000)	9.2	no	12 (4 – 19)	n. a.

n. a. not available, # report on 4 female pts., ≠one case without urinary diversion, renal failure, ǂ results from pts. < 70years vs. ≥ 70 years)

Author (reference)	No. of pts.	Type of urinary diversion:	extracorporeal intracorporeal	Conversion to open surgery	Mean operative time (min)	Mean perioperative blood loss (ml)	Mean post op. hospital stay (days)	Positive margins (bladder)	No. of lymph nodes removed	Follow-up (months)
Yuh et al, 2008 [40]	54	n. a.	extracorporeal	2 pts.	n. a.	557	9.1	0 pts. (pT0- pT2) 7 pts. (pT3-pT4)	20 (SD 12) pT0 - pT2 15 (SD 7) pT3 - pT4	n. a.
Gamboa et al, 2009 [57]	41	Ileal conduit (24) Orthotopic neobladder (17)	intracorporeal	no	498 (320 – 805)	254 (50 – 700)	8 (5 -37).	2 pts. (pT4)	25 (4 – 68).	n. a.
Kauffman et al, 2009 [39]	79	Ileal conduit (46) Orthotopic neobladder (33)	extracorporeal	n. a.	378	460	5	6 pts.	18.4	n. a.
Schumacher et al, 2009 [63]	18	Ileal conduit (5) Orthotopic neobladder (13)	intracorporeal	3 pts.	501 (382 – 750)	525 (200 – 2200)	12 (6 – 79)	1 pt. (pT4)	20 (10 – 42)	25 (4 – 58)
Richards et al, 2010 [65]	35	Ileal conduit (30) Orthotopic neobladder (5)	extracorporeal	no	530 (458 – 593)	350 (250 – 600)	7 (6 – 9)	1 pt.	16 (11 – 24)	n.a.
Guru et al, 2010 [52]	26	Ileal conduit (13) Ileal conduit (13)	intracorporeal extracorporeal	no	391 387	315 454	8.8 (5 – 23) 8.5 (6 – 14)	1 pt. (pT4)	25 26	n. a.
Pruthi et al, 2010 [68]	100≠	Ileal conduit (61) Orthotopic neobladder (38)	extracorporeal (94) intracorporeal (5)	no	276	271	4.9	neg.	19 (8 - 40)	18.4 (5 - 44)
Lavery et al, 2010 [66]	15	n. a.		no	423 (300 – 506)	160 (50 – 500)	3.4 (3 – 7)	neg.	41.8 (18 – 67)	3
Coward et al, 2011‡[22]	99	Ileal conduit (60) Orthotopic neobladder (39)	extracorporeal	no	288 vs. 264	289 vs. 249	4.7 vs. 5.0	neg.	19.5 (8 – 40) 18.1 (10 – 37)	n. a.
Khan et al, 2011 [45]	50	Ileal conduit (45) Orthotopic neobladder (5)	extracorporeal	no	361 (240 – 600)	340 (100 1150)	10 (5 – 24)	1 pt. (pT4)	17 (11 – 28)	3
Manoharan et al, 2011 [67]	14	Orthotopic neobladder (14)	extracorporeal	no	310 (± 220)	360 (± 48)	8.5	neg.	12 (± 3)	n. a.
Cha et al, 2011 [72]	85	Ileal conduit Orthotopic neobladder	extracorporeal	no	n. a.	n. a.	n. a.	5.9%	19	18
Schumacher et al, 2011 [35]	45	Ileal conduit (9) Orthotopic neobladder (36)	intracorporeal	3 pts.	477 (325 – 760)	550 (200 – 2200)	9 (4 – 78)	1 pt. (pT4)	22.5 (10 – 52)	24 (3 – 77)

Table 1. Contemporary reports/series of robotic-assisted laparoscopic radical cystectomy (RARC) and urinary diversion for TCC of the bladder.

surrounding structures, especially the rectum, rendering dissection difficult. Thus, careful dissection is required in developing the rectovesical plane to avoid injury of the rectum. Prior abdominal surgery, radiotherapy or neoadjuvant chemotherapy may be relative-contraindications for RARC, as these factors can significantly increase the degree of technical difficulty [22 23].

Patient selection makes a direct comparison between open radical cystectomy series and smaller RARC series difficult. Results from open high-volume centers indicate that approximately two-thirds of patients at radical cystectomy have organ-confined disease, whereas one-third has non-organ-confined disease [24 25 26 27 28 29]. In general, the percentage of patients with non-organ-confined disease undergoing RARC is substantially lower than figures reported from major series from open radical cystectomy [table 2] [30 31 32 21, 33-40].

Recent multi-institutional results from the International Robotic Cystectomy Consortium (IRCC) of 527 patients treated with RARC show similar figures regarding the numbers of patients with organ-confined (65%) vs. non-organ-confined (35%) disease, as with open radical cystectomy series [18]. However, data on neoadjuvant chemotherapy were not reported in this series.

4. Surgery-related complications

Although the number of RARC cases reported in the literature is relatively small, the intraoperative complication rate seems comparable to open radical cystectomy series. Nix et al. found in a prospective randomized trial of robotic (n = 21) versus open (n = 20) radical cystectomy no difference in the absolute number of complications (p = 0.279) [41]. Less blood loss was observed in the robotic group (mean 258 mL) compared to the open group (mean 575 mL). Similarly, Wang et al. reported no difference regarding intraoperative complications in their prospective trial between robotic (n = 33) and open radical cystectomy (n = 21) [32]. Again, less blood loss was noted with RARC (mean 400 mL, range 100–1200 mL) compared to open radical cystectomy (mean 750 mL, range 250–2500 mL). Galich et al., in a comparative analysis of early postoperative outcomes following robotic (n = 13) and open (n = 24) radical cystectomy, found no difference between groups regarding surgery-related complications and blood loss [33]. Kauffman et al. collected data on 79 consecutive patients treated with RARC and extracorporeal urinary diversion [42]. In their series, high-grade complications (Clavien III–V) occurred in 16 patients (21%) during the first 3 months postoperatively. Urinary obstruction, intra-abdominal abscess, uro-enteric fistulas, and gastrointestinal bleeding were the most common high-grade complications. The high percentage of overall urinary obstruction (8%) despite extracorporeal urinary diversion without robotic assistance is of concern [42]. Khan et al. reported an 8% ureteric stricture rate, with 6% strictures occurring on the left side in their series of 50 RARC cases [22]. Results from open radical cystectomy series report an uretero-intestinal stricture rate of less than 3% [5]. Performing the anastomosis between the ureters and the urinary diversion outside the abdomen through a small abdominal incision may only be possible with relatively long ureters, thus increasing the risk for ischemic complications. Resection of the ureters at the level where they cross over the common iliac artery minimizes the risk of strictures at the uretero-intestinal anastomosis due to ischemia [43].

Different parameters may affect outcome and risk for surgery-related complications such as age, higher ASA score or previous surgery. Butt et al. did not find a significant association between age, BMI, ASA score and complication rate in their series of 66 RARC cases [44].

Author (reference)	No. of pts.	Age (years)	Organ-confined tumors ≤ pT2 (%)	Non-organ-confined tumors > pT2 (%)	Node positive disease (%)	Positive margins (%)	Follow-up (months)
Open radical cystectomy:							
Stein et al, 2001 [24]	1054	66 (range 22 - 93)	669 (64%)	385 (36%)	246 (23%)	1%	122 (range 0 - 336)*
Manoharan et al, 2009 [28]	432	69 (SD ± 9)	262 (60.5%)	170 (39.5%)	90 (21%)	5%	38 (range 1 - 172)
Dotan et al, 2007 [29]	1589	n. a.	858 (54%)	727 (46%)	288 (24%)	4.2%	up to 15 years
Hautmann et al, 2006 [26]	788	65 (SD ± 10)	528 (67%)	260 (33%)	143 (18%)	< 1%	54 (range 0.1 - 223)
Robot-assisted radical cystectomy:							
Galich et al, 2006 [33]	13	70 (range 38 - 88)	7 (54%)	6 (46%)	2 (15%)	0%	n. a.
Rhee et al, 2006 [30]	7	60 (SD ± 9)	6 (86%)	1(14%)	2 (28%)	0%	n. a.
Guru et al, 2008 [36]	58/ 67≠	67 (range 36 - 90)	29 (50%)	29 (50%)	17 (29%)	6 (10.3%)	n. a.
Wang et al, 2008 [32]	32	70 (range 41 - 84)	23 (72%)	9 (28%)	6 (19%)	2 (6%)	n. a.
Murphy et al, 2008 [31]	23	65 (SD ± 9.4)	17 (74%)	6 (26%)	2 (8.7%)	0%	17 (range 4 - 40)
Dasgupta et al, 2008 [37]	20	66 (range 36 - 77)	15 (75%)	5 (25%)	2 (10%)	0%	23 (range 7 - 44)
Lowentritt et al, 2008 [38]	4/ 20#	69.5 (SD ± 10.5)	1 (25%)	3 (75%)	1 (25%)	0%	n. a.
Woods et al, 2008 [34]	27	67 (range 49 - 80)	n. a.	n. a.	9 (33%)	2 (7.4%)	n. a.
Yuh et al, 2008 [40]	54	67	19 (35%)	35 (65%)	n. a.	7 (13%)	n. a.
Kauffman et al, 2009 [39]	79	71 (SD ± 11)	47 (59%)	32 (41%)	12 (15%)	6 (7.6%)	26.4
Pruthi et al, 2010 [68]	100	65.5 (range 33 - 86)	87 (87%)	13 (13%)	20 (20%)	0%	18.4 (range 5 - 44)
Schumacher et al, 2011 [35]	45	60.6 (range 37 – 79)	35 (77.8%)	10 (22.2%)	9 (20%)	1 (2.2%)	24 (range 3 – 77)

n. a. not available; * 91% of pts with FU > 3 years; # results on 4 female cases; ≠58 pats eligible for analysis

Table 2. Patient characteristic of contemporary robotic-assisted radical cystectomy (RARC) and open radical cystectomy series for TCC of the bladder.

Similar, Coward et al. did not find worse outcomes in terms of complications when comparing older patients (≥ 70 years) with higher ASA scores vs. younger patients (< 70 years) treated with RARC [45].

Schumacher et al. assessed the surgery-related complications at RARC with total intracorporeal urinary diversion during their learning curve [35]. A total of 45 patients were pooled in 3 consecutive groups of 15 cases each to evaluate the complications according to the Clavien classification [46]. Overall, fewer complications were observed between the groups over time, with a significant decrease in late versus early complications (P = 0.005 and P = 0.058). However, the early Clavien grade III complications remained significant (27%) and did not decline with time; thus indicating the complexity of the intracorporeal urinary diversion. Khan et al., assessed early surgery-related complications using also the Clavien Classification [22]. Early complications were observed in 34% of patients. Clavien grade IIIa/b complications were seen in 29% of their patients. Both series have somehow a lower complication rate compared to the 64% complication rate from a large series of 1142 open radical cystectomy patients from the Memorial-Sloan-Kettering Cancer Center (MSKCC) [47]. The higher percentage of non-organ-confined tumors in the open series from MSKCC may be one factor to explain this difference in favor of the robotic approach.

Hayn et al., from the IRCC assessed whether previous robotic surgical experience affects on the implementation and execution of robot-assisted radical cystectomy [17]. They found that previous robot-assisted radical prostatectomy (RARP) case volume might affect the operative time, blood loss, and lymph node yield at RARC. In addition, surgeons with increased RARP experience operated on patients with more advanced tumors. Previous RARP experience, however, did not appear to affect the surgical margin status.

5. Lymphadenectomy

Pelvic lymphadenectomy at radical cystectomy is the standard treatment for patients with muscle-invasive bladder cancer. Radical cystectomy series report that approximately 25% of patients initially staged T1–T4 N0 M0 who undergo lymphadenectomy have lymph node metastases; and the absolute number of positive nodes removed affects survival [9 48].

It has been stated that, as a guideline, removal of >20 nodes per patient should be the aim [48]. Others have reported an improved cancer-specific survival rate of 65% when ≥ 16 nodes were retrieved compared to 51% when < 16 nodes were retrieved [49]. Whereas some experts do recommend that at least 10 nodes should be removed at pelvic lymph node dissection [50 51]. While assessing the lymph node counts obtained after lymph node dissection at radical cystectomy from various institutional series, huge differences in node count are noted. Median node count has been reported to vary from 8 to 80, and is also affected by the extent of a pelvic lymphadenectomy [9 24 52 53 47 48 54 55 56 57 58]. Interindividual variances, sending separate or en-bloc nodal packages, and the pathologic work-up of the specimens may explain differences in reporting on the number of nodes removed/detected by the pathologist [58 59]. Other factors such as the commitment of the surgeon in performing a lymph node dissection or selecting patients for more or less extensive lymphadenectomy may explain differences in nodal count [60].

Controversy still persists regarding the boundaries and terminology used in lymph node dissection. Mills et al. describe a *standard* lymph node dissection that includes removal of nodal tissue up to and including the common iliac bifurcation, including the internal iliac vessels, presacral area, obturator fossa, external iliac vessels, and distal part of the common

iliac artery [61]. In order to avoid injury to the hypogastric nerves, nodes medial to the ureter (proximal half of the common iliac artery, aortic bifurcation) are not removed. In contrast, Stein et al. define an *extended* lymph node dissection as including all nodal tissue in the boundaries of: the aortic bifurcation and common iliac vessels (proximally); the genitofemoral nerve (laterally); the circumflex iliac vein and lymph node of Cloquet (distally); the hypogastric vessels (posteriorly), including the obturator fossa, pre-sciatic nodes bilaterally; and the presacral lymph nodes anterior to the sacral promontory [62].
Data on lymph node yield and oncological outcome in RARC series are still limited, however, node counts are similar to open radical cystectomy series [21 31 35 34 36 63]. Earlier reports from various RARC series describe mostly the boundaries of a *limited* (obturator fossa only) or *standard* template with less than a median of 20 nodes removed [63]. A recent report by Pruthi et al. performing an *extended* lymph node dissection, described a median node yield of 28 nodes (range 12–39) [64]. Schumacher et al. found similar node counts in their series of 45 patients with a mean of 22.5 nodes (range 10 - 52) removed [35]. Applying a template up to the aortic bifurcation resulted in a mean of 32 nodes removed. Richards et al. compared lymph node counts from 35 open radical cystectomy cases to their first 35 RARC cases [65]. Median total lymph node yield was similar between groups, with 15 nodes (range 11 - 22) in the open cystectomy group compared to 16 nodes (range 11 - 24) in the RARC group. Lavery et al, reported in their first 15 RARC cases undergoing an extended pelvic lymphadenectomy up to the aortic bifurcation a mean nodal yield of 41.8 nodes (range 18 - 67) [66]. Kauffmann et al. applying a similar template at RARC found a mean of 19.1 nodes (range 0 - 56) removed [42]. Evaluating the number of nodes removed from different institutions, the IRCC reported that at RARC 82.9% underwent a pelvic lymphadenectomy, which resulted in a mean of 17.8 nodes (range 0 - 68) removed [18]. According to these reports, it seems that robotic lymphadenectomy applying an *extended* lymph node dissection template, if indicated, up to the aortic bifurcation is technically feasible with intraoperative morbidity similar to open series [63].

6. Urinary diversion

The first case of RARC with intracorporeal urinary diversion was performed by Beecken et al. in 2002 [14]. Operative time was 8.5 hours, and therefore attention was turned towards extracorporeal urinary diversion in order to decrease operative times. Menon et al. were the first to describe their technique of extracorporeal diversion, using a 5–8 cm mid-line incision [15]. Until today, the majority of urinary diversions in conjunction with RARC are done extracorporeally [table 1] [67]. However, standardization of the intracorporeal procedure and decreasing operative times might turn the interest towards this approach [19 68]. We have previously reported our results in a series of 18 patients treated with RARC and totally intracorporeal urinary diversion, later, results in 45 patients were published [19 35]. Mean operative time was 476 min (range 325–760) and mean blood loss 669 mL (range 200–2200) [35]. Whether there is an advantage of performing the complete procedure intracorporeally or not is less clear. At least in female patients, the specimen can be removed through an incision via the vaginal wall, thus avoiding a mid-line incision. The technical difficulties in performing the urinary diversion totally intracorporeally have so far prevented its wide-spread adoption. Results reported by Schumacher and co-workers indicate at least at the beginning of their learning curve increased surgery-related complications using an intracorporeal urinary diversion approach [35]. Rehman et al. reported on 9 patients treated with RARC and totally intracorporeal confection of an ileal conduit [69]. One postoperative iatrogenous necrosis of the ileal conduit, probably caused by retraction of the organ bag occurred.

7. Oncologic outcome

To objectively assess oncological outcomes in patients treated either with open radical cystectomy or RARC for bladder cancer one needs to focus on: long-term cancer control, surgical quality (positive margins), tumor spillage, and port site metastasis.
Today, the highest long-term survival rates were reported for open radical cystectomy with an extended lymph node dissection. Stein et al. reported 5-year and 10-year recurrence-free survival rates of 68% and 60%, respectively, among 1,054 patients treated with radical cystectomy and extended lymph node dissection with curative intent [24]. For lymph node-negative, organ-confined disease, 5-year and 10-year recurrence-free survival rates were 85% and 82%. Similar results have been reported from other high-volume centers performing open radical cystectomy [25 26 27 28 29].
Whether the same cancer control rates equivalent to results from open radical cystectomy series can be achieved with RARC is still unknown; to date there are no long-term data available [70]. Median time to any recurrence after radical cystectomy is approximately 12 months, whereas 86% of recurrences occur within 3 years [24]. The mean follow-up in the current RARC series ranged from 3 to 77 months [tables 1 and 2]. However, in all of these RARC series median follow-up is short (<24 months), and reported survival data in which all patients have passed at least a 12 months follow-up do not exist.
The surgical quality at radical cystectomy independent of the surgical approach is essential for optimal local cancer control. Thus, negative margins must be achieved to avoid local tumor recurrence, which ultimately results in the death of the patient. Positive surgical margins have been reported to be 5% or less in high-volume open radical cystectomy series [25 26 27 28 29]. The incidence of positive margins at RARC ranged from 0% to 13% [21 30 31 32 34 36 37 38 39 40 71 72]. Guru et al, reported a 10.3% positive margin rate at RARC, whereas Yuh et al. found 13% positive margins in their patients [36 40]. Whether this high positive margin rate is attributable to the learning curve in these series is not clear. Data from the IRCC showed an overall 7% positive margin rate in their pooled 496 patients [17]. For patients with pathologic stage ≤ T3, 3.7% had a positive margin, whereas for patients with pathologic stage T3 or T4, 16% had a positive margin. The authors found with increasing surgical experience at RARC an improvement of their positive margin rate [17].
Port site metastasis in urological malignancies are of concern; they do occur, albeit infrequently. The etiology of port site metastasis is unknown. Port site metastasis has been reported after RARC and laparoscopic radical cystectomy for bladder cancer [73 74].

8. Post-operative recovery

Perioperative pathophysiology and care suggest that a multitude of factors contribute to postoperative morbidity, length of hospital stay, and convalescence in patients undergoing surgery [75]. Radical cystectomy is still associated with significant perioperative morbidity—this despite the implementation of accelerated postoperative recovery programs, or so-called "fast-track" surgery [76]. Comparison between historical cystectomy series and recent studies regarding post-operative recovery are difficult, as the concept of "fast-track" surgery has only been adopted by the urologic community during the last decade.

In order to reduce perioperative morbidity at cystectomy, Pruthi and co-workers have implemented and continuously improved the perioperative management in their 362 patients [77]. Reported findings from the last 100 (open and RARC) of these 362 cystectomy cases showed favorable return of bowel function (mean time to flatus 2.2 days, and mean time to bowel movements 2.9 days), the majority of patients being discharged after a mean of 5 days. Readmission was observed in 12% of patients, and the most common reasons for readmission were urinary tract infection (3%), gastrointestinal disorders (2%), and deep venous thrombosis (2%). The same group has published a randomized trial and assessed perioperative outcomes in patients treated with open versus robotic radical cystectomy [41]. Patients undergoing robotic cystectomy had longer operative times (4.2 versus 3.5 hours; $p < 0.001$) and less blood loss (258 versus 575 mL; $p < 0.001$) than did patients with open cystectomy. Further, patients in the robotic group demonstrated a faster return of bowel activity (median time to flatus 2.3 days versus 3.2 days, and time to bowel movement 3.2 days versus 4.3 days). Hospital stay did not differ between groups (robotic 5.1 days, open 6.0 days; $p = 0.239$). Patients in the robotic group required significantly less analgesia than did patients with the open approach ($p = 0.019$). Similar results have been reported by Ng et al., comparing 104 open cystectomy with 83 RARC cases [78]. The robotic group demonstrated decreased blood loss (460 mL versus 1172 mL; $p < 0.0001$) and shorter length of hospital stay (5.5 days versus 8 days; $p < 0.0001$) than did the open cystectomy group. Wang et al., comparing open radical cystectomy with RARC patients, reported reduced blood loss, faster return to regular diet, and shorter hospital stay in the robotic group [32]. One may argue that fewer non-organ-confined tumors (28%) in the RARC group may have influenced their results compared to 57% non-organ-confined tumors in the open group. A recent study by Coward et al. found similar results regarding time to flatus (median 2 days) and time to bowel movements (median 3 days) after RARC in their series [45].

Despite the presumed advantages of less postoperative pain, faster return of bowel movements, shorter hospital stay, and overall quicker recovery over open surgery, the exact role of laparoscopy in improving perioperative outcomes remains unclear.

9. Quality of life

Quality of life (QoL) and postoperative recovery after surgery are important factors with direct financial implications for the health care system. Karvinen et al. reported on the effect of exercise and QoL in survivors of bladder cancer [79]. Findings from their study indicate that exercise is positively associated with QoL and the ability to perform physical activity results in increased QoL. If patients are able to return more quickly to preoperative levels with minimally invasive surgery, i.e. robotic surgery, they might be able to initiate exercise sooner, which in turn improves their QoL.

Yuh et al. evaluated QoL in a small single-center study after RARC [20]. Despite some inheriting limitations of the study design, QoL appeared to return to base-line by 3 months after RARC, and improved further at 6 months. The authors postulated that short-term improvement in QoL might also have positive implications regarding initiating adjuvant treatment protocols in these patients. Further studies are required to assess the physical and psychological implications of robotic surgery on QoL in patients undergoing radical cystectomy.

Functional results have been reported after open nerve-sparing radical cystectomy and orthotopic bladder substitution, however, reports from RARC series assessing continence and potency rates are sparse [7 80].

10. Costs

The introduction of new and costly technologies into daily clinical practice has been criticized, especially during periods of economic uncertainty. With the introduction of expensive robotic technology cost-effectiveness has become more important. For robot-assisted radical prostatectomy some studies have shown volume-dependant cost advantages [81 82]. Less information on cost-analysis is available for RARCS.

Smith et al., from North Carolina, US, performed a cost analysis at their institution between robotic and open radical cystectomy [83]. The financial costs of robotic and open radical cystectomy were categorized into operating room and hospital components, and further divided into fixed and variable costs for each. Variable costs were related to several factors, such as length of hospital stay. For each procedure the means of 20 cases were used to perform a comparative cost analysis. Based on their results, robotic cystectomy is associated with an overall higher financial cost of $1,640.

Martin et al. performed a detailed cost-analysis for open radical cystectomy vs. RARC cases [84]. They found that the most critical parameters for increased costs were operative time and hospital stay, which favored the robotic approach at their institution. Further, they stated that the real cost advantages are mostly seen when indirect costs are considered, such as treatment of perioperative complications or readmission rates due to complications.

Costs are difficult to measure and comprise other factors than just the perioperative period. Thus, earlier return to normal activity and reduced sick-leave might be important factors justifying these additional costs offered by the robotic approach.

11. Conclusions

Based on the current literature RARC is evolving rapidly as an alternative technique to open surgery in patients requiring radical cystectomy and urinary diversion. Lymph node yield and perioperative outcomes are similar to open radical cystectomy series; however, long-term oncological results are unknown. Several small prospective or randomized single-center trials showed comparable results between RARC and open cystectomy. However, the surgical procedure is technically demanding, especially when performing the urinary diversion totally intracorporeal. It is advisable to concentrate this type of surgery to high-volume centers where robotic expertise and technology is available.

12. References

[1] Stein JP, Penson DF, Wu SD, Skinner DG. Pathological guidelines for orthotopic urinary diversion in women with bladder cancer: a review of the literature. J Urol 2007;178:756-60.

[2] Stein JP, Skinner DG. Radical cystectomy for invasive bladder cancer: long-term results of a standard procedure. World J Urol 2006;24:296-304.

[3] Stein JP. Improving outcomes with radical cystectomy for high-grade invasive bladder cancer. World J Urol 2006;24:509-16.
[4] Stein JP, Skinner DG. Results with radical cystectomy for treating bladder cancer: a 'reference standard' for high-grade, invasive bladder cancer. BJU Int 2003;92:12-7.
[5] Hautmann RE, Volkmer BG, Schumacher MC, Gschwend JE, Studer UE. Long-term results of standard procedures in urology: the ileal neobladder. World J Urol 2006;24:305-14.
[6] Leissner J. [Lymphadenectomy for bladder cancer. Diagnostic and prognostic significance as well as therapeutic benefit]. Urologe A 2005;44:638-44.
[7] Studer UE, Burkhard FC, Schumacher M, et al. Twenty years experience with an ileal orthotopic low pressure bladder substitute--lessons to be learned. J Urol 2006;176:161-6.
[8] Stein JP. The role of lymphadenectomy in patients undergoing radical cystectomy for bladder cancer. Curr Oncol Rep 2007;9:213-21.
[9] Dhar NB, Klein EA, Reuther AM, Thalmann GN, Madersbacher S, Studer UE. Outcome after radical cystectomy with limited or extended pelvic lymph node dissection. J Urol 2008;179:873-8; discussion 8.
[10] Parra RO, Andrus CH, Jones JP, Boullier JA. Laparoscopic cystectomy: initial report on a new treatment for the retained bladder. J Urol 1992;148:1140-4.
[11] Haber GP, Campbell SC, Colombo JR, Jr., et al. Perioperative outcomes with laparoscopic radical cystectomy: "pure laparoscopic" and "open-assisted laparoscopic" approaches. Urology 2007;70:910-5.
[12] Basillote JB, Abdelshehid C, Ahlering TE, Shanberg AM. Laparoscopic assisted radical cystectomy with ileal neobladder: a comparison with the open approach. J Urol 2004;172:489-93.
[13] Wiklund NP. Technology Insight: surgical robots--expensive toys or the future of urologic surgery? Nat Clin Pract Urol 2004;1:97-102.
[14] Beecken WD, Wolfram M, Engl T, et al. Robotic-assisted laparoscopic radical cystectomy and intra-abdominal formation of an orthotopic ileal neobladder. Eur Urol 2003;44:337-9.
[15] Menon M, Hemal AK, Tewari A, et al. Nerve-sparing robot-assisted radical cystoprostatectomy and urinary diversion. BJU Int 2003;92:232-6.
[16] Hellenthal NJ, Hussain A, Andrews PE, et al. Surgical margin status after robot assisted radical cystectomy: results from the International Robotic Cystectomy Consortium. J Urol 2010;184:87-91.
[17] Hayn MH, Hussain A, Mansour AM, et al. The learning curve of robot-assisted radical cystectomy: results from the International Robotic Cystectomy Consortium. Eur Urol 2010;58:197-202.
[18] Hellenthal NJ, Hussain A, Andrews PE, et al. Lymphadenectomy at the time of robot-assisted radical cystectomy: results from the International Robotic Cystectomy Consortium. BJU Int 2010;107:642-6.
[19] Schumacher MC, Jonsson MN, Wiklund NP. Robotic cystectomy. Scand J Surg 2009;98:89-95.
[20] Yuh B, Butt Z, Fazili A, et al. Short-term quality-of-life assessed after robot-assisted radical cystectomy: a prospective analysis. BJU Int 2009;103:800-4.

[21] Pruthi RS, Nielsen ME, Nix J, Smith A, Schultz H, Wallen EM. Robotic radical cystectomy for bladder cancer: surgical and pathological outcomes in 100 consecutive cases. J Urol 2010;183:510-4.

[22] Khan MS, Elhage O, Challacombe B, Rimington P, Murphy D, Dasgupta P. Analysis of early complications of robotic-assisted radical cystectomy using a standardized reporting system. Urology 2011;77:357-62.

[23] Haber GP, Crouzet S, Gill IS. Laparoscopic and robotic assisted radical cystectomy for bladder cancer: a critical analysis. Eur Urol 2008;54:54-62.

[24] Stein JP, Lieskovsky G, Cote R, et al. Radical cystectomy in the treatment of invasive bladder cancer: long-term results in 1,054 patients. J Clin Oncol 2001;19:666-75.

[25] Madersbacher S, Hochreiter W, Burkhard F, et al. Radical cystectomy for bladder cancer today--a homogeneous series without neoadjuvant therapy. J Clin Oncol 2003;21:690-6.

[26] Hautmann RE, Gschwend JE, de Petriconi RC, Kron M, Volkmer BG. Cystectomy for transitional cell carcinoma of the bladder: results of a surgery only series in the neobladder era. J Urol 2006;176:486-92; discussion 91-2.

[27] Yossepowitch O, Dalbagni G, Golijanin D, et al. Orthotopic urinary diversion after cystectomy for bladder cancer: implications for cancer control and patterns of disease recurrence. J Urol 2003;169:177-81.

[28] Manoharan M, Ayyathurai R, Soloway MS. Radical cystectomy for urothelial carcinoma of the bladder: an analysis of perioperative and survival outcome. BJU Int 2009;104:1227-32.

[29] Dotan ZA, Kavanagh K, Yossepowitch O, et al. Positive surgical margins in soft tissue following radical cystectomy for bladder cancer and cancer specific survival. J Urol 2007;178:2308-12; discussion 13.

[30] Rhee JJ, Lebeau S, Smolkin M, Theodorescu D. Radical cystectomy with ileal conduit diversion: early prospective evaluation of the impact of robotic assistance. BJU Int 2006;98:1059-63.

[31] Murphy DG, Challacombe BJ, Elhage O, et al. Robotic-assisted laparoscopic radical cystectomy with extracorporeal urinary diversion: initial experience. Eur Urol 2008;54:570-80.

[32] Wang GJ, Barocas DA, Raman JD, Scherr DS. Robotic vs open radical cystectomy: prospective comparison of perioperative outcomes and pathological measures of early oncological efficacy. BJU Int 2008;101:89-93.

[33] Galich A, Sterrett S, Nazemi T, Pohlman G, Smith L, Balaji KC. Comparative analysis of early perioperative outcomes following radical cystectomy by either the robotic or open method. JSLS 2006;10:145-50.

[34] Woods M, Thomas R, Davis R, et al. Robot-assisted extended pelvic lymphadenectomy. J Endourol 2008;22:1297-302.

[35] Schumacher MC, Jonsson MN, Hosseini A, et al. Surgery-related Complications of Robot-assisted Radical Cystectomy With Intracorporeal Urinary Diversion. Urology 2011;77:871-6.

[36] Guru KA, Sternberg K, Wilding GE, et al. The lymph node yield during robot-assisted radical cystectomy. BJU Int 2008;102:231-4; discussion 4.

[37] Dasgupta P, Rimington P, Murphy D, et al. Robotic assisted radical cystectomy: short to medium-term oncologic and functional outcomes. Int J Clin Pract 2008;62:1709-14.

[38] Lowentritt BH, Castle EP, Woods M, Davis R, Thomas R. Robot-assisted radical cystectomy in women: technique and initial experience. J Endourol 2008;22:709-12.
[39] Kauffman EC, Ng CK, Lee MM, et al. Critical analysis of complications after robotic-assisted radical cystectomy with identification of preoperative and operative risk factors. BJU Int 2009;105:520-7.
[40] Yuh B, Padalino J, Butt ZM, et al. Impact of tumour volume on surgical and pathological outcomes after robot-assisted radical cystectomy. BJU Int 2008;102:840-3.
[41] Nix J, Smith A, Kurpad R, Nielsen ME, Wallen EM, Pruthi RS. Prospective randomized controlled trial of robotic versus open radical cystectomy for bladder cancer: perioperative and pathologic results. Eur Urol 2010;57:196-201.
[42] Kauffman EC, Ng CK, Lee MM, et al. Critical analysis of complications after robotic-assisted radical cystectomy with identification of preoperative and operative risk factors. BJU Int 2010;105:520-7.
[43] Schumacher MC, Scholz M, Weise ES, Fleischmann A, Thalmann GN, Studer UE. Is there an indication for frozen section examination of the ureteral margins during cystectomy for transitional cell carcinoma of the bladder? J Urol 2006;176:2409-13; discussion 13.
[44] Butt ZM, Fazili A, Tan W, et al. Does the presence of significant risk factors affect perioperative outcomes after robot-assisted radical cystectomy? BJU Int 2009;104:986-90.
[45] Coward RM, Smith A, Raynor M, Nielsen M, Wallen EM, Pruthi RS. Feasibility and Outcomes of Robotic-assisted Laparoscopic Radical Cystectomy for Bladder Cancer in Older Patients. Urology 2011.
[46] Dindo D, Demartines N, Clavien PA. Classification of surgical complications: a new proposal with evaluation in a cohort of 6336 patients and results of a survey. Ann Surg 2004;240:205-13.
[47] Shabsigh A, Korets R, Vora KC, et al. Defining early morbidity of radical cystectomy for patients with bladder cancer using a standardized reporting methodology. Eur Urol 2009;55:164-74.
[48] Karl A, Carroll PR, Gschwend JE, et al. The impact of lymphadenectomy and lymph node metastasis on the outcomes of radical cystectomy for bladder cancer. Eur Urol 2009;55:826-35.
[49] Leissner J, Hohenfellner R, Thuroff JW, Wolf HK. Lymphadenectomy in patients with transitional cell carcinoma of the urinary bladder; significance for staging and prognosis. BJU Int 2000;85:817-23.
[50] Stein JP, Cai J, Groshen S, Skinner DG. Risk factors for patients with pelvic lymph node metastases following radical cystectomy with en bloc pelvic lymphadenectomy: concept of lymph node density. J Urol 2003;170:35-41.
[51] Herr H, Lee C, Chang S, Lerner S. Standardization of radical cystectomy and pelvic lymph node dissection for bladder cancer: a collaborative group report. J Urol 2004;171:1823-8; discussion 7-8.
[52] Guru K, Seixas-Mikelus SA, Hussain A, et al. Robot-assisted intracorporeal ileal conduit: Marionette technique and initial experience at Roswell Park Cancer Institute. Urology 2010;76:866-71.

[53] Hemal AK, Abol-Enein H, Tewari A, et al. Robotic radical cystectomy and urinary diversion in the management of bladder cancer. Urol Clin North Am 2004;31:719-29, viii.
[54] Abraham JB, Young JL, Box GN, Lee HJ, Deane LA, Ornstein DK. Comparative analysis of laparoscopic and robot-assisted radical cystectomy with ileal conduit urinary diversion. J Endourol 2007;21:1473-80.
[55] Hemal AK, Kolla SB, Wadhwa P. First case series of robotic radical cystoprostatectomy, bilateral pelvic lymphadenectomy, and urinary diversion with the da Vinci S system. J Robotic Surg 2008;2:35-40.
[56] Mottrie A, Caprpentier P, Schatteman P, et al. Robot-assisted laparoscopic radical cystectomy: initial experience on 27 consecutive patients. J Robotic Surg 2007;1:197-201.
[57] Gamboa AJ, Young JL, Dash A, Abraham JBA, Box GN, Ornstein DK. Pelvic lymph node dissection and outcomes of robot-assisted radical cystectomy for bladder carcinoma. J Robotic Surg 2009;3:7-12.
[58] Bochner BH, Cho D, Herr HW, Donat M, Kattan MW, Dalbagni G. Prospectively packaged lymph node dissections with radical cystectomy: evaluation of node count variability and node mapping. J Urol 2004;172:1286-90.
[59] Ather MH, Alam ZA, Jamshaid A, Siddiqui KM, Sulaiman MN. Separate submission of standard lymphadenectomy in 6 packets versus en bloc lymphadenectomy in bladder cancer. Urol J 2008;5:94-8.
[60] Kulkarni GS, Finelli A, Lockwood G, et al. Effect of healthcare provider characteristics on nodal yield at radical cystectomy. Urology 2008;72:128-32.
[61] Mills RD, Fleischmann A, Studer UE. Radical cystectomy with an extended pelvic lymphadenectomy: rationale and results. Surg Oncol Clin N Am 2007;16:233-45.
[62] Stein JP, Quek ML, Skinner DG. Lymphadenectomy for invasive bladder cancer. II. technical aspects and prognostic factors. BJU Int 2006;97:232-7.
[63] Schumacher MC, Jonsson MN, Wiklund NP. Does extended lymphadenectomy preclude laparoscopic or robot-assisted radical cystectomy in advanced bladder cancer? Curr Opin Urol 2009;19:527-32.
[64] Pruthi RS, Wallen EM. Robotic-assisted laparoscopic pelvic lymphadenectomy for bladder cancer: a surgical atlas. J Laparoendosc Adv Surg Tech A 2009;19:71-4.
[65] Richards KA, Hemal AK, Kader AK, Pettus JA. Robot assisted laparoscopic pelvic lymphadenectomy at the time of radical cystectomy rivals that of open surgery: single institution report. Urology 2010;76:1400-4.
[66] Lavery HJ, Martinez-Suarez HJ, Abaza R. Robotic extended pelvic lymphadenectomy for bladder cancer with increased nodal yield. BJU Int 2010.
[67] Manoharan M, Katkoori D, Kishore TA, Antebie E. Robotic-assisted radical cystectomy and orthotopic ileal neobladder using a modified Pfannenstiel incision. Urology 2011;77:491-3.
[68] Pruthi RS, Nix J, McRackan D, et al. Robotic-assisted laparoscopic intracorporeal urinary diversion. Eur Urol 2010;57:1013-21.
[69] Rehman J, Sangalli MN, Guru K, et al. Total intracorporeal robot-assisted laparoscopic ileal conduit (Bricker) urinary diversion: technique and outcomes. Can J Urol 2011;18:5548-56.

[70] Chade DC, Laudone VP, Bochner BH, Parra RO. Oncological outcomes after radical cystectomy for bladder cancer: open versus minimally invasive approaches. J Urol 2010;183:862-69.
[71] Guru KA, Kim HL, Piacente PM, Mohler JL. Robot-assisted radical cystectomy and pelvic lymph node dissection: initial experience at Roswell Park Cancer Institute. Urology 2007;69:469-74.
[72] Cha EK, Wiklund NP, Scherr DS. Recent advances in robot-assisted radical cystectomy. Curr Opin Urol 2011;21:65-70.
[73] El-Tabey NA, Shoma AM. Port site metastases after robot-assisted laparoscopic radical cystectomy. Urology 2005;66:1110.
[74] Stolla V, Rossi D, Bladou F, Rattier C, Ayuso D, Serment G. Subcutaneous metastases after coelioscopic lymphadenectomy for vesical urothelial carcinoma. Eur Urol 1994;26:342-3.
[75] Kehlet H, Dahl JB. Anaesthesia, surgery, and challenges in postoperative recovery. Lancet 2003;362:1921-8.
[76] Olbert PJ, Baumann L, Hegele A, Schrader AJ, Hofmann R. [Fast-track concepts in the perioperative management of patients undergoing radical cystectomy and urinary diversion: review of the literature and research results]. Urologe A 2009;48:137-42.
[77] Pruthi RS, Nielsen M, Smith A, Nix J, Schultz H, Wallen EM. Fast track program in patients undergoing radical cystectomy: results in 362 consecutive patients. J Am Coll Surg 2010;210:93-9.
[78] Ng CK, Kauffman EC, Lee MM, et al. A comparison of postoperative complications in open versus robotic cystectomy. Eur Urol 2009;57:274-81.
[79] Karvinen KH, Courneya KS, Venner P, North S. Exercise programming and counseling preferences in bladder cancer survivors: a population-based study. J Cancer Surviv 2007;1:27-34.
[80] Mottrie A, Schatteman P, Fonteyne E, Rotering J, Stockle M, Siemer S. [Robot-assisted laparoscopic radical cystectomy]. Urologe A 2008;47:414, 6-9.
[81] Lotan Y, Cadeddu JA, Gettman MT. The new economics of radical prostatectomy: cost comparison of open, laparoscopic and robot assisted techniques. J Urol 2004;172:1431-5.
[82] Scales CD, Jr., Jones PJ, Eisenstein EL, Preminger GM, Albala DM. Local cost structures and the economics of robot assisted radical prostatectomy. J Urol 2005;174:2323-9.
[83] Smith A, Kurpad R, Lal A, Nielsen M, Wallen EM, Pruthi RS. Cost analysis of robotic versus open radical cystectomy for bladder cancer. J Urol;183:505-9.
[84] Martin AD, Nunez RN, Castle EP. Robot-assisted Radical Cystectomy Versus Open Radical Cystectomy: A Complete Cost Analysis. Urology;77:621-5.

16

Robotic-Assisted Laparoscopic Radical Cystoprostatectomy and Intracorporeal Urinary Diversion (Studer Pouch or Ileal Conduit) for Bladder Cancer

Abdullah Erdem Canda, Ali Fuat Atmaca and Mevlana Derya Balbay
Ankara Atatürk Training and Research Hospital, 1st Urology Clinic, Ankara Turkey

1. Introduction

Bladder cancer is the fourth most common malignancy in American men and almost 25% is muscle invasive at the time of diagnosis (Cancer Facts and Figures, 2009; Nieder et al., 2008).

Currently, most effective local treatment of muscle invasive bladder cancer and non-invasive, high-grade bladder tumors that recur or progress despite intravesical therapies is open radical cystoprostatectomy with urinary diversion (Clinical Practice Guidelines in Oncology, 2010; Huang et al., 2007).

With the advancement of technology, minimally invasive surgical approaches including laparoscopic (Huang et al., 2010; Guazzoni et al., 2003) or robotic-assisted laparoscopic (Akbulut et al., 2011; Rehman et al., 2011; Kauffman et al., 2011; Hellenthal et al., 2010; Kasraeian et al., 2010; Pruthi et al., 2010; Schumacher et al., 2009) cystectomies are increasingly being performed.

This chapter summarizes the current state of the use of the surgical robot in performing radical cystoprostatectomy with urinary diversion in patients with bladder cancer.

2. Why to use a surgical robot?

Radical cystoprostatectomy with bilateral extended lymph node dissection and urinary diversion (Studer pouch reconstruction or ileal conduit formation) are complex and time consuming surgical procedures. Performing these complex procedures in an open surgical approach is well established. To perform these complex procedures pure laparoscopically is extremely difficult. However, the use of a surgical robot enables the operating surgeon to perform these procedures much more easily because it has the advantages of the 3-dimensional and magnified image capability, higher grades of wristed hand movements, decreased hand tremor leading to a shorter learning curve. Besides, having the 4th-robotic arm gives the advantage of additional assistance and tissue retraction and letting the console surgeon to operate in a comfortable sitting position rather than standing position for long hours. Menon et al suggested that robotic approach combines the oncological principles of

open surgery with technical advantages of the surgical robot which allows a precise, gentle, quick and safe surgery during performing radical cystectomy for bladder cancer (Menon et al., 2003).
Therefore, following the introduction of da Vinci-S 4-arm surgical robot (Intuitive Surgical, Sunnyvale, California) many centers have started to publish their experiences with the use of a surgical robot in performing these complex surgical procedures (Akbulut et al., 2011; Rehman et al., 2011; Kauffman et al., 2011; Hellenthal et al., 2010; Kasraeian et al., 2010; Pruthi et al., 2010; Schumacher et al., 2009).

3. Open versus robotic approach

3.1 Comparison of complications

A prospective study from Weill Cornell Medical College, Department of Urology, New York, NY, USA has recently evaluated prospective complications of open (n=104) versus robotic (n=83) cystectomy procedures (Ng et al., 2010). Complications were classified due to modified Clavien system. Significantly lower major complications were detected in the robotic group compared to the open surgical approach (17% versus 31%, p=0.03). Robotic cystectomy was found to be an independent predictor of fewer overall and major complications at 0-30 day (perioperative) and 31-90 day periods. Another well known study from The University of North Carolina at Chapel Hill, Division of Urologic Surgery, Chapel Hill, North Carolina, USA randomized 21 patients to robotic approach and 20 to the open technique. No significant difference in regard to overall complication rate or hospital stay was detected between the two groups of patients (Nix et al., 2010). In our initial experience of 12 cases whom we performed robot assisted laparoscopic nerve sparing radical cystoprostatectomy with bilateral extended lymph node dissection and intracorporeal Studer pouch construction, we had 6 minor complications (Grade 1 and 2) 2 major complications (Grade 3-5) in the perioperative period (0-30 day) and 3 minor and 2 major complications in the 31-90 day period due to modified Clavien system (Akbulut et al., 2011). Although the number of prospective and randomized studies comparing these two approaches is limited currently in the literature, robotic approach does not seem to add an additional complication risk when compared to open surgery.

3.2 Comparison of oncologic parameters

Lymph node yield, surgical margins, recurrence-free survival and overall survival are important parameters in evaluating surgical oncologic efficacy. The University of North Carolina study which randomized 21 patients to robotic approach and 20 to the open technique did not find any significant difference in the number of lymph nodes removed between two groups (19 versus 18, p>0.05). Likewise, surgical margins were negative in all patients in both approaches (Nix et al., 2010). The Weill Cornell Medical College study, having larger numbers of patients similarly did not find significant differences concerning these two parameters between the two approaches (Ng et al., 2010). Mean lymph node yield was 15.7 in the open surgical approach and was 17.9 in the robotic approach (p>0.05). Positive surgical margins were detected 8.7% of the patients in open approach and 7.2% of the patients in robotic approach (p>0.05). In our initial series of 12 patients, mean lymph node yield was 21.3±.8.8 (Akbulut et al., 2011).

A recent review from the Memorial Sloan-Kettering Cancer Center has recently evaluated the oncological outcomes after radical cystectomy for bladder cancer comparing open versus minimally invasive approaches (Chade et al., 2010). Although the follow-up is limited in robotic series compared to open surgical approach, robotic assisted studies reported recurrence-free survival rates of 86% to 91% at 1 to 2 years and 90% to 96% overall survival in 1 to 2 years of follow-up. On the other hand, large open surgery studies showed 62% to 68% recurrence-free survival at 5 years and 50% to 60% at 10 years, with overall survival of 59% to 66% at 5 years and 37% to 43% at 10 years.
With these limited current data, robotic approach seems to provide sufficient short-term surgical oncologic efficacy in patients with bladder cancer.

3.3 Comparison of cost

Controversial reports exist regarding the cost analysis of open versus robotic approaches. One study revealed that robotic assisted laparoscopic radical cystectomy is associated with a higher financial cost than the open approach in the perioperative setting (Smith et al., 2010). Whereas, another study suggested that although robotic approach is more expensive in terms of operative costs and robotic supplies, due to decreased hospital stay in robotic approach and higher complication rates with open surgical approach make total actual costs much higher than robotic approach (Martin et al., 2011).

4. Surgical oncologic safety of robotic approach (lymph node yield and surgical margins)

Regarding open radical cystectomy, lymph node yield and positive surgical margin rates are considered as the significant factors related to surgical quality (Herr et al., 2004; Skinner et al., 2007; Stein et al., 2003). Herr et al and Skinner et al suggested a lymph node yield of greater than 10 and a positive surgical margin rate of less than 10% in surgical oncologic adequacy (Herr et al., 2004; Skinner et al., 2007). Stein et al suggested a lymph node yield of greater than 15 obtained during open radical cystectomy in order to be oncologically acceptable and sufficient (Stein et al., 2003).
Guru et al evaluated whether robot assistance allows adequate pelvic lymph node dissection particularly during the initial experience (Guru et al., 2008). In a series of 67 patients, mean number of lymph nodes retrieved was 18 (6-43) (Guru et al., 2008). Mean lymph node yield was 41.8 (18-67) in another series of 15 consecutive patients who underwent robotic radical cystectomy for bladder cancer (Lavery et al., 2010). Recently, International Robotic Cystectomy Consortium (IRCC) evaluated 527 patients who underwent robotic cystectomy for bladder cancer and mean lymph node yield was 17.8 (range 0-68) (Hellenthal et al., 2011). Mean lymph node yield was 21.3 (range, 8-38) and 24.8±.9.2 in our initial series of 12 (Akbulut et al., 2011) and 27 cases (unpublihsed data), respectively.
Positive surgical margin rates were reported as 6.8%, 0%, 7.2% and 2% in 513, 83, 100 and 50 robotic cystectomy patients (Hellenthal et al., 2010; Pruthi et al., 2010; Ng et al., 2010; Shamim Khan et al., 2010). In our initial series of 12 patients, positive surgical margin rate was 0% (Akbulut et al., 2011). We had only one patient with positive surgical margin (3.7%) who had pT4b disease in the total of 27 patients underwent totally intracorporeal robotic cystectomy (unpublihsed data).

5. Learning curve of robotic approach

Robotic-assisted laparoscopic radical cystectomy with bilateral extended lymph node dissection and particularly intracorporeal urinary diversion (Studer or ileal conduit) are complex procedures. Therefore, a learning curve is required in order to perform these procedures successfully.

Regarding the completion of the learning curve of robotic cystectomy, some authors have suggested to perform a certain number of cases in the literature. International Robotic Cystectomy Consortium (IRCC) suggested that 21 cases were needed to be performed for operative time to reach 6.5 hours and 8, 20 and 30 patients were required to reach a lymph node yield of 12, 16 and 20, respectively (Hayn et al., 2010). On the other hand, others reported that after the first 20 cases of robotic cystectomy, no further significant improvement was detected in terms of intraoperative parameters, pathologic outcomes and complication rates (Pruthi et al., 2008). Following evaluation of 100 cases of robotic cystectomy, Guru et al stated that operative results and oncologic outcomes for robotic-assisted radical cystectomy constantly improve as the technique evolves (Guru et al., 2009).

We have started performing robotic urological procedures at our institution in February 2009, following initially performing more than 50 cases of robot assisted laparoscopic radical prostatectomy cases some of which also included pelvic lymph node dissection. We recommend to start performing robotic cystectomy cases after a certain experience gained particularly on robotic radical prostatectomy. Additionally, a good knowledge of the pelvic anatomy and adequate open surgical experience are essential.

6. Surgical technique

6.1 Patient position

Patient is placed in deep (30°) Trendelenburg position at the beginning of the procedure until the completion of robotic cystectomy, bilateral extended lymph node dissection and transposition of the left ureter under the mobilized sigmoid colon. During performing intracorporeal Studer pouch reconstruction or ileal conduit formation, patient position is adjusted to mild (5°) Trendelenburg position.

A Veress needle is introduced into the abdominal cavity about 2 cm above the umbilicus. Intra-abdominal pressure is set to 10-12 mmHg during performing bilateral extended lymph node dissection. Regarding rest of the surgery, intra-abdominal pressure is set to 16-18 mmHg.

6.2 Abdominal port locations

Overall, we use 6 trocars with the 4th-arm of the surgical robot placed on the patient's right which provides easy control to the right-handed console surgeon (Figure 1).

Camera port (12-mm) is placed 2 cm above the umblicus. Two robotic trocars (8-mm) are placed 8 cm apart from the camera port at the level of the umblicus. An 8-mm sized robotic trocar is placed 3 cm vertically above from the right iliac crest for the 4th-arm. We use 2 assistant trocars on the left abdomen for the assistant surgeon: A 15-mm trocar for introducing for tissue staplers for bowels and endobags for specimens is placed 3 cm vertically above from the left iliac crest and a 12-mm trocar is placed between the camera port and the 2nd-robotic arm.

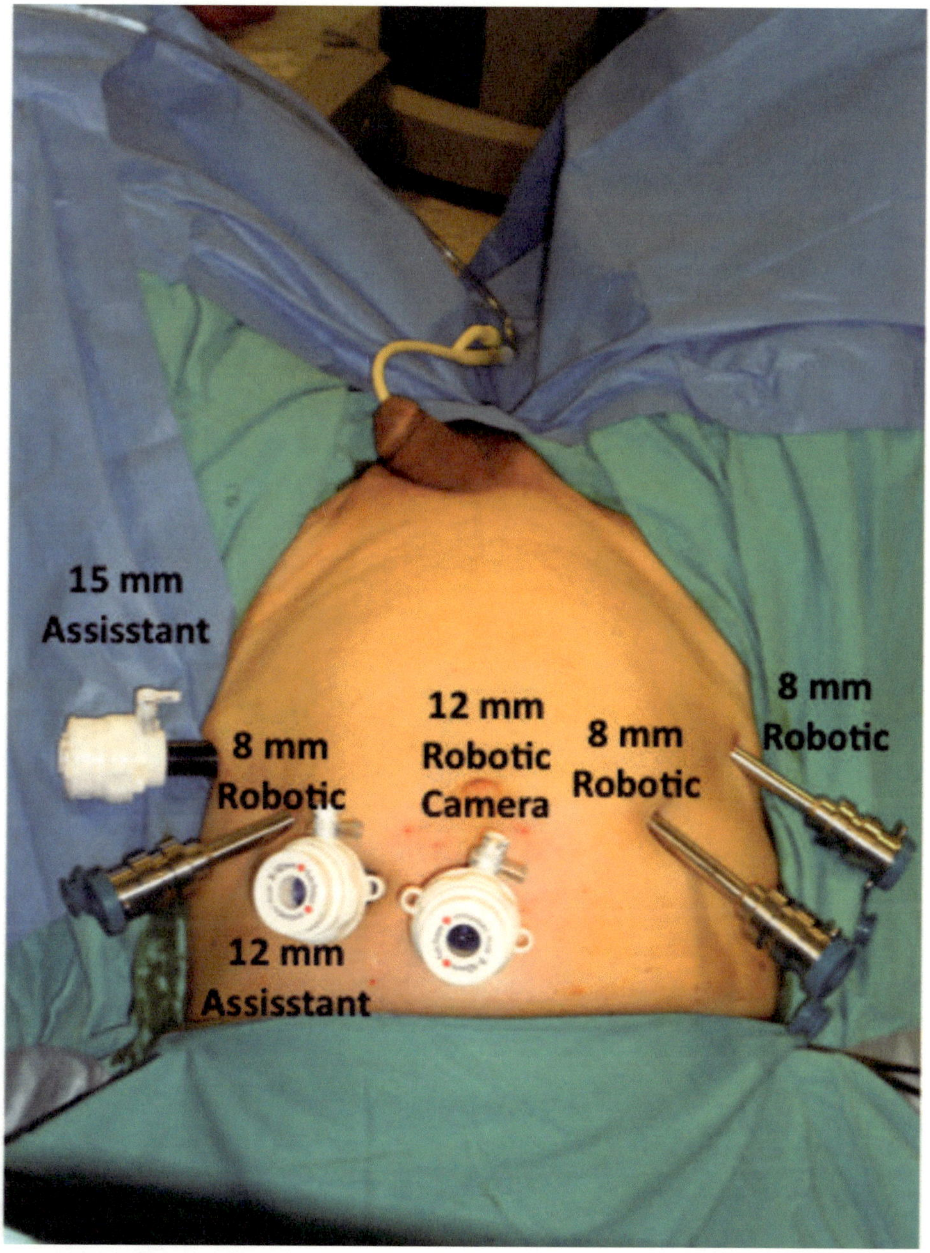

Fig. 1. Abdominal port locations (*Archive of Ankara Atatürk Training and Research Hospital, 1st Urology Clinic, Ankara, Turkey*)

6.3 Robotic-assisted laparoscopic bilateral neurovascular bundle sparing radical cystoprostatectomy in male patients (Akbulut et al., 2011; Canda et al., 2011; Canda et al., 2011; Akbulut et al., 2010)

Surgery starts with dissection of the ureters. They are double clipped and cut where they enter the bladder. Most distal parts are sent for frozen section analysis (Figure 2).

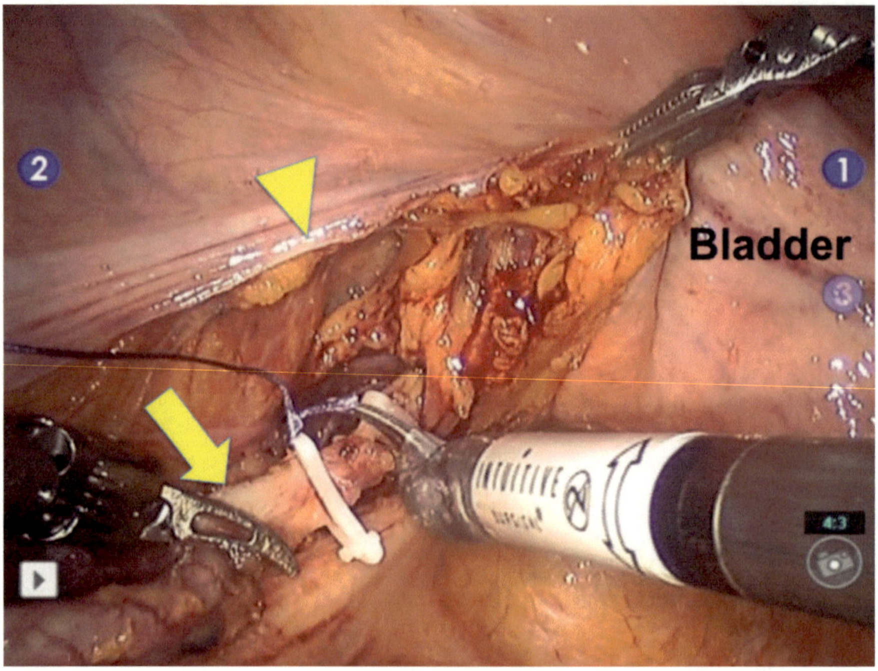

Fig. 2. Ureters are dissected, double clipped and cut where they enter the bladder (left side). Arrow: left ureter, arrowhead: incised and opened peritoneum on the left side. *(Archive of Ankara Atatürk Training and Research Hospital, 1st Urology Clinic, Ankara, Turkey)*

Peritoneum on the anterior wall of the Douglas' pouch is incised and posterior dissection of the prostate is carried out (Figure 3).

Following the identification of seminal vesicles, Denonvilliers' fascia is opened (Figure 4). Tissue lateral to the tip of the seminal vesicles corresponding to the mid point of the pararectal plexus is marked with Hem-o-lok® clips on both sides (Figure 5). Prostate is dissected off of the rectum. Lateral bladder pedicles are severed with vessel sealing system (Ligasure®) until the Hem-o-lok® clips placed at the tips of the seminal vesicles to mark pararectal plexus of which the neurovascular bundles originate (Figure 6). Then, endopelvic fascia is opened on both sides. Dorsal venous complex is ligated by 0/0 vicryl (40 mm ½ RB needle). High anterior release (intra-fascial) neurovascular bundle preservation is performed on both sides by dissecting the periprostatic fascia over the prostatic capsule alongside the prostate down until the dorsal venous complex suture and bilateral neurovascular bundle dissections are completed (Figure 7).

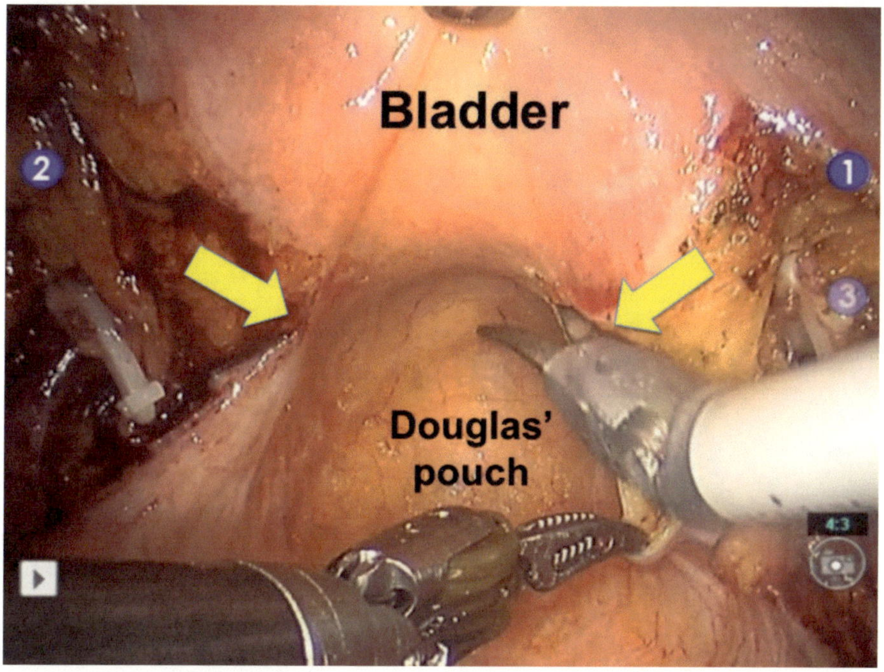

Fig. 3. Incision of the peritoneum on the anterior Douglas' pouch wall (arrows). (*Archive of Ankara Atatürk Training and Research Hospital, 1st Urology Clinic, Ankara, Turkey*)

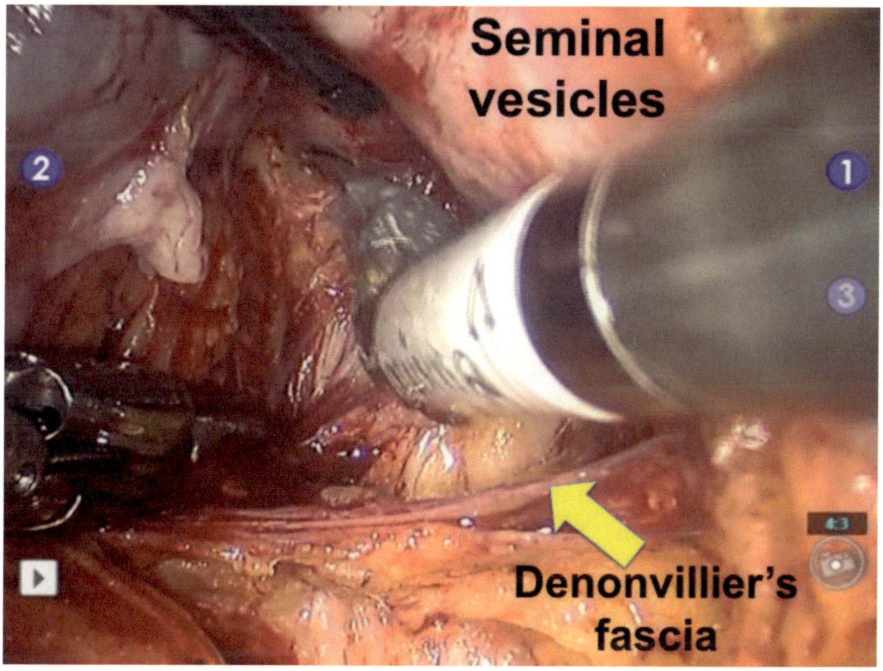

Fig. 4. Opening Denonvilliers' fascia (arrow). (*Archive of Ankara Atatürk Training and Research Hospital, 1st Urology Clinic, Ankara, Turkey*)

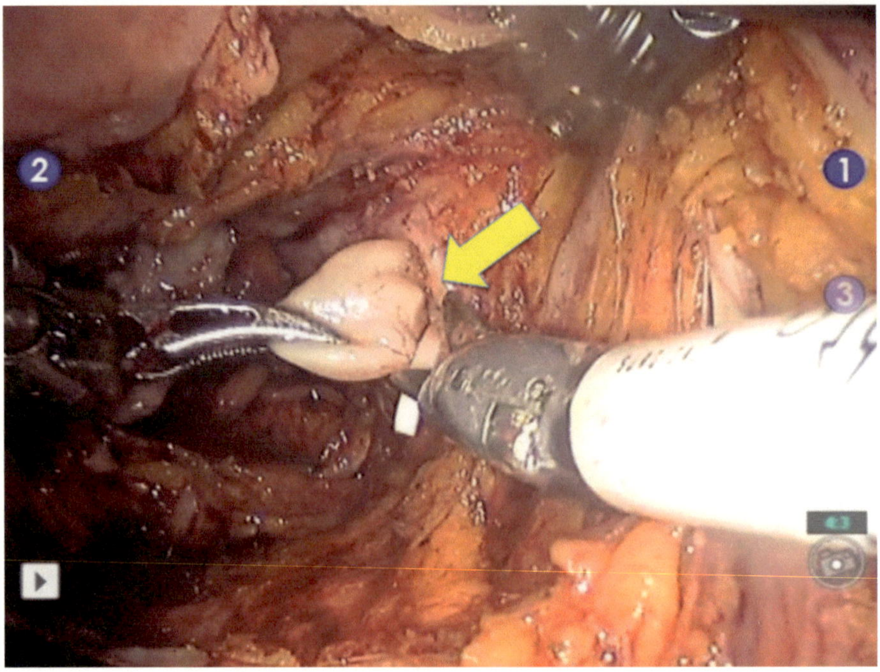

Fig. 5. Tip of the seminal vesicle is marked with a Hem-o-lok® clip and cut (arrow). (*Archive of Ankara Atatürk Training and Research Hospital, 1st Urology Clinic, Ankara, Turkey*)

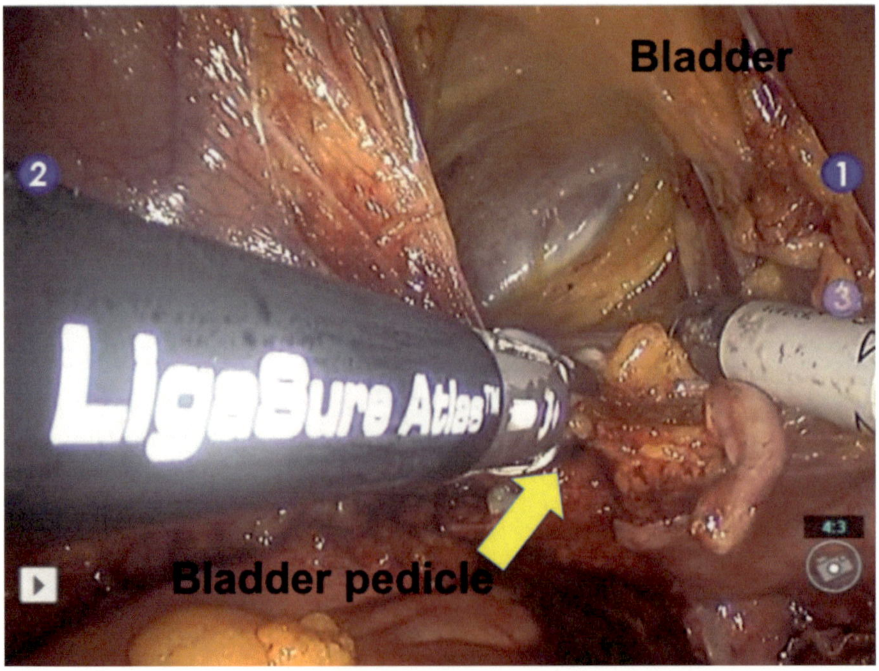

Fig. 6. Severence of lateral bladder pedicles with vessel sealing system (arrow). (*Archive of Ankara Atatürk Training and Research Hospital, 1st Urology Clinic, Ankara, Turkey*)

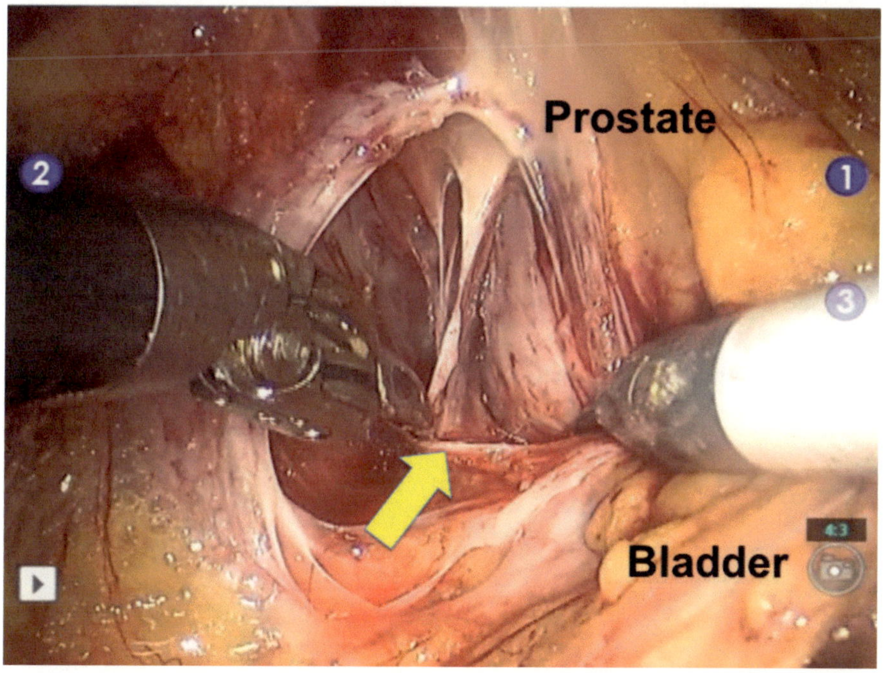

Fig. 7. High anterior release of the periprostatic fascia (arrow) over the prostatic capsule alongside the prostate in preserving neurovascular bundles on the left side. *(Archive of Ankara Atatürk Training and Research Hospital, 1st Urology Clinic, Ankara, Turkey)*

Starting from the umblical level, urachus is dissected by incising lateral to the medial umblical ligaments on the anterior abdominal wall. Puboprostatic ligaments are cut. Ligated dorsal venous complex (Figure 8) and ligated membraneous urethra (Figure 9) with 0/0 vicryl (40 mm ½ RB needle) to prevent tumor spillage are cut. Cystoprostatectomy is completed (Figure 10) and specimen is put into the endobag. Urethral stump is sampled for frozen section analysis.

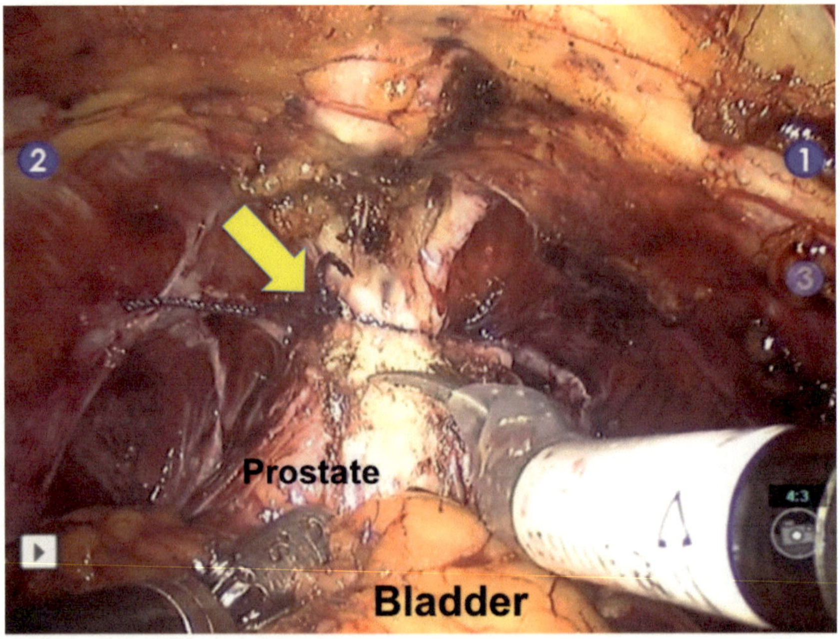

Fig. 8. Dorsal venous complex is ligated and cut (arrow). (Archive of Ankara Atatürk Training and Research Hospital, 1st Urology Clinic, Ankara, Turkey)

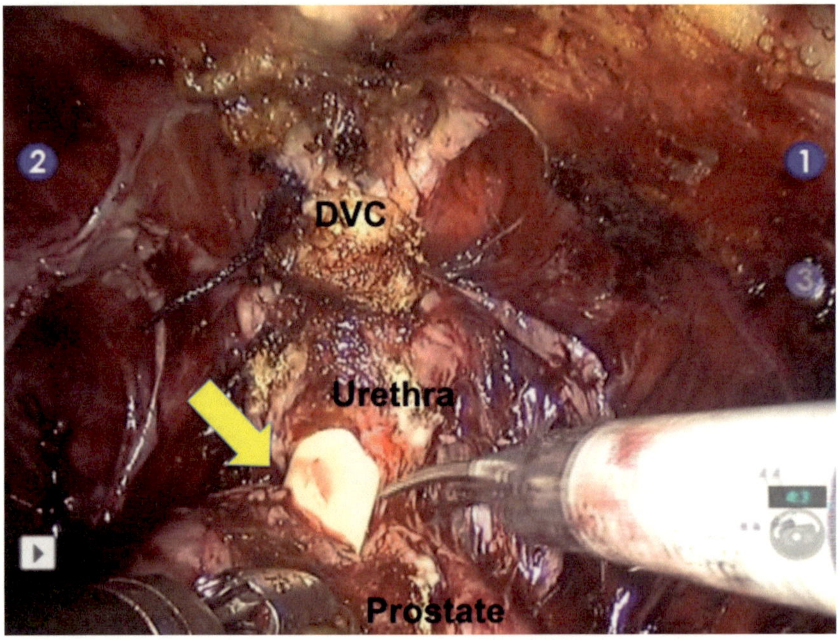

Fig. 9. Membraneous urethra is cut after being ligated and foley catheter is inserted back in until its tip reaches the specimen to show the anatomic details apparently. Arrow: appearance of the urethral catheter. DVC: dorsal venous complex (ligated and cut) *(Archive of Ankara Atatürk Training and Research Hospital, 1st Urology Clinic, Ankara, Turkey)*

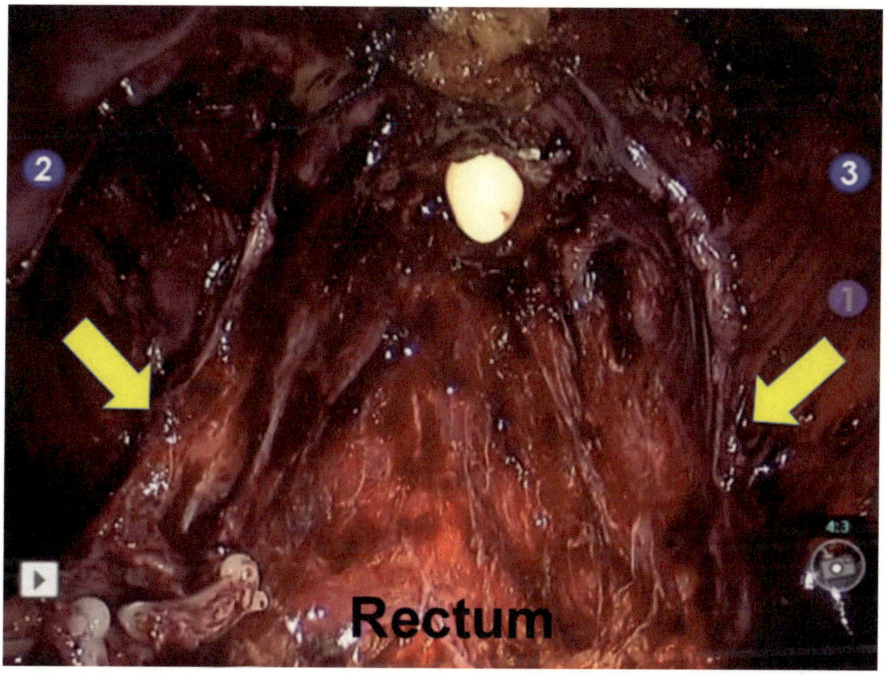

Fig. 10. Bilaterally preserved neurovascular bundles following the removal of the cystoprostatectomy specimen into the endobag (arrows). *(Archive of Ankara Atatürk Training and Research Hospital, 1st Urology Clinic, Ankara, Turkey)*

6.4 Robot assisted laparoscopic bilateral extended lymph node dissection (Canda et al., 2011; Akbulut et al., 2010; Akbulut et al., 2011)

We use the landmarks below during performing robot assisted laparoscopic bilateral extended lymph node dissection:

Superior border: inferior mesenteric artery and accompanying vena cava superior

Inferior border: node of Cloquet and circumflex iliac vein

Medial border: cut edge of the endopelvic fascia over the neurovascular bundles and internal iliac vessels

Lateral border: genitofemoral nerves, psoas muscles and ureters

Initially, starting from the genitofemoral nerve lymphatic tissue around external iliac artery & vein are removed until the obturator nerve is seen (Figure 11).

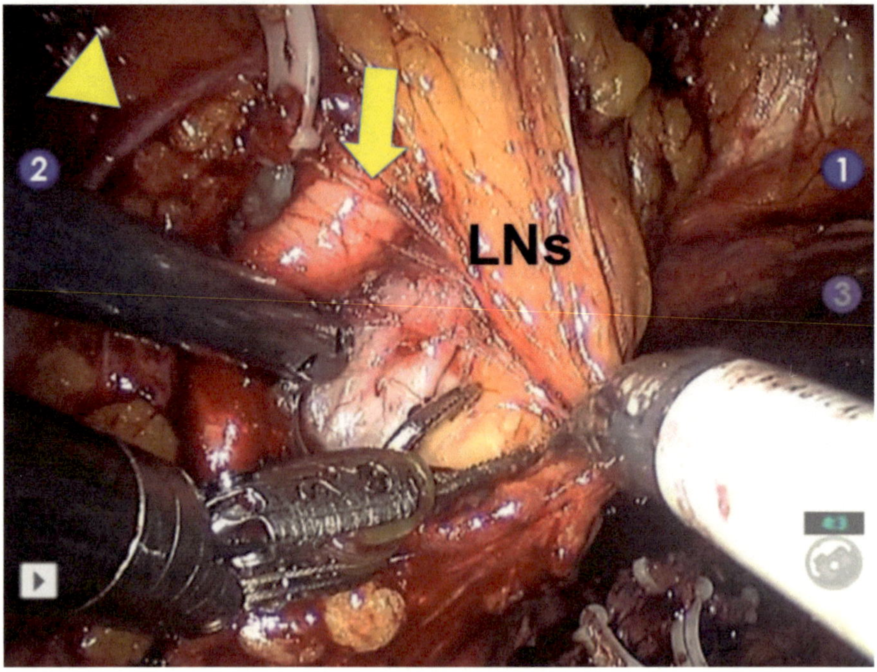

Fig. 11. Arrowhead: Genitofemoral nerve (left). Arrow: External iliac artery (left). LNs: Lymph node tissue. *(Archive of Ankara Atatürk Training and Research Hospital, 1st Urology Clinic, Ankara, Turkey)*

Then, bifurcation of common iliac artery are identified and lymphatic tissues located below the obturator nerve and surrounding the internal iliac artery are removed. Later, lymphatic tissues medial to the genitofemoral nerve and around the common iliac artery are dissected until the aortic bifurcation. Same lymphatic dissection is performed on the other side. Then, lymphatic tissues which are located distal to the aortic bifurcation, overlying and distally located to the vena caval bifurcation and common iliac arteries and veins are removed followed by presacral lymph nodes anterior to the sacrum. Lastly, preaortic and paracaval lymphatic dissections are performed. Inferior mesenteric artery on the aorta makes the most proximal end of the extended lymphatic dissection (Figure 12). Hem-o-lok® clips are used in order to tie off the most distal parts of the lymphatic vessels draining the limbs to prevent or reduce lymphatic leakage and lymphocele formation.

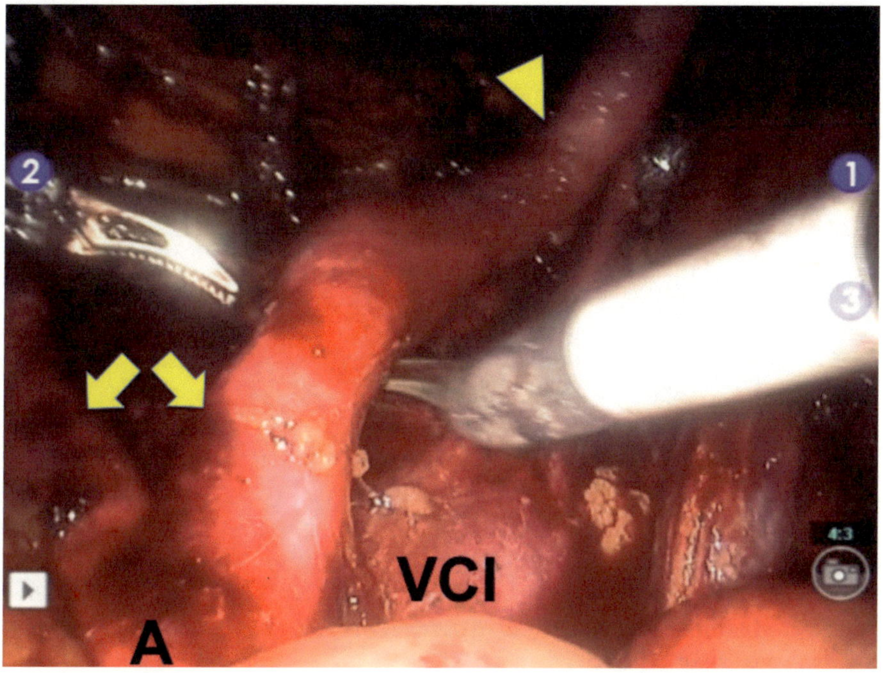

Fig. 12. Completed bilateral extended lymph node dissection and appearance of the major abdominal vasculature that are skeletonized. A: abdominal aorta, VCI: vena cava inferior, Arrows: right and left common iliac arteries, Arrowhead: right external iliac artery. *(Archive of Ankara Atatürk Training and Research Hospital, 1st Urology Clinic, Ankara, Turkey)*

Having completed the extended lymph node dissection, sigmoid colon is mobilized and left ureter is transposed to the right gutter underneath the sigmoid colon above the vasculature.

6.5 Robot assisted laparoscopic intracorporeal Studer pouch reconstruction (Canda et al., 2011; Akbulut et al., 2010; Akbulut et al., 2011)

Using a double armed 3/0 monocryl (17 mm ½c RB needle) urethral remnant is anostomosed to the assigned 1 cm opening on the antimesenteric wall of the most dependent part of the segregated ileum, initially (Figures 13,14). A 10 cm ileal segment on the right and a 40 cm ileal segment on the left side of urethroileal anastomosis are assigned for the pouch sparing the distal 20 cm ileal segment adjacent to the ceacum. Laparoscopic intestinal staplers are introduced through the 15 mm assistant port on the left side and placed perpendicular across the ileum and adjacent mesointestinum of approximately 2 cm (Figure 15). Side-to-side ileoileostomy is performed using two additional laparoscopic intestinal staplers between proximal and distal ends of the ileum (Figure 16).

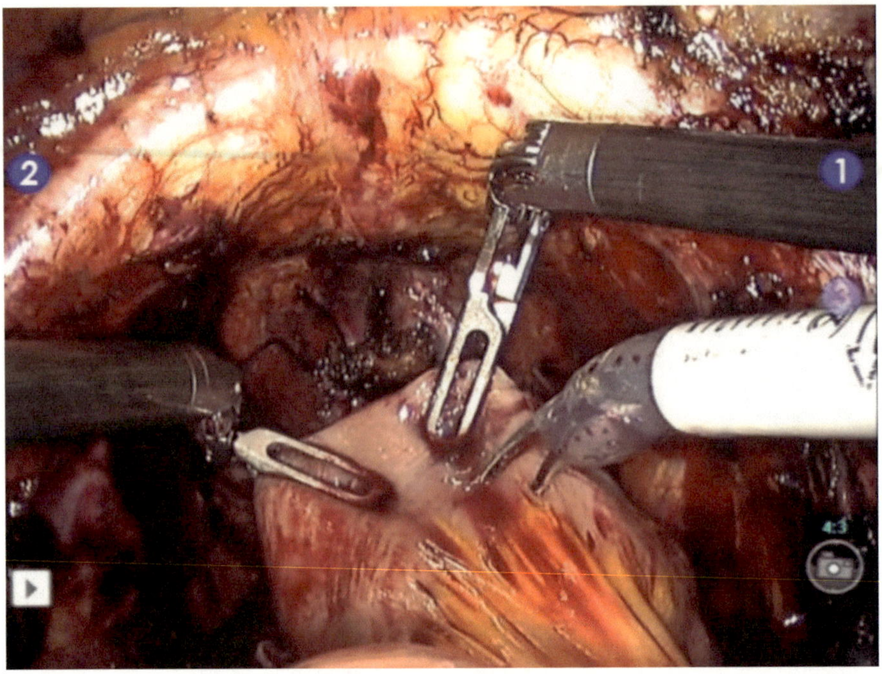

Fig. 13. Segregated antimesenteric ileal wall. (*Archive of Ankara Atatürk Training and Research Hospital, 1st Urology Clinic, Ankara, Turkey*)

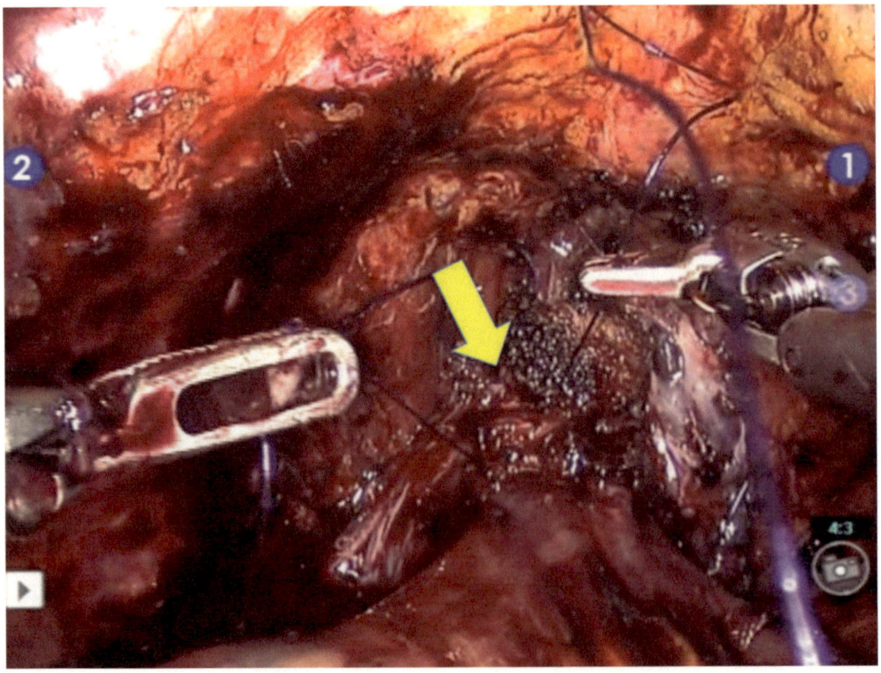

Fig. 14. Urethral remnant is sutured to the assigned antimesenteric ileal wall which is segregated. (*Archive of Ankara Atatürk Training and Research Hospital, 1st Urology Clinic, Ankara, Turkey*)

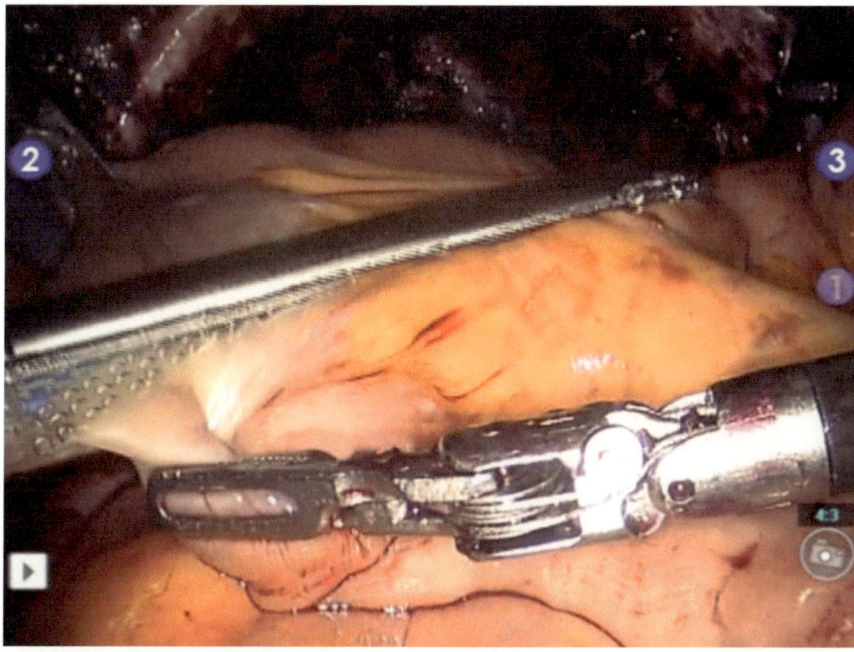

Fig. 15. Laparoscopic intestinal stapler introduced through the 15 mm assistant port on the left side and placed perpendicular across the ileum with adjacent 2 cm of mesointestinum included. *(Archive of Ankara Atatürk Training and Research Hospital, 1st Urology Clinic, Ankara, Turkey)*

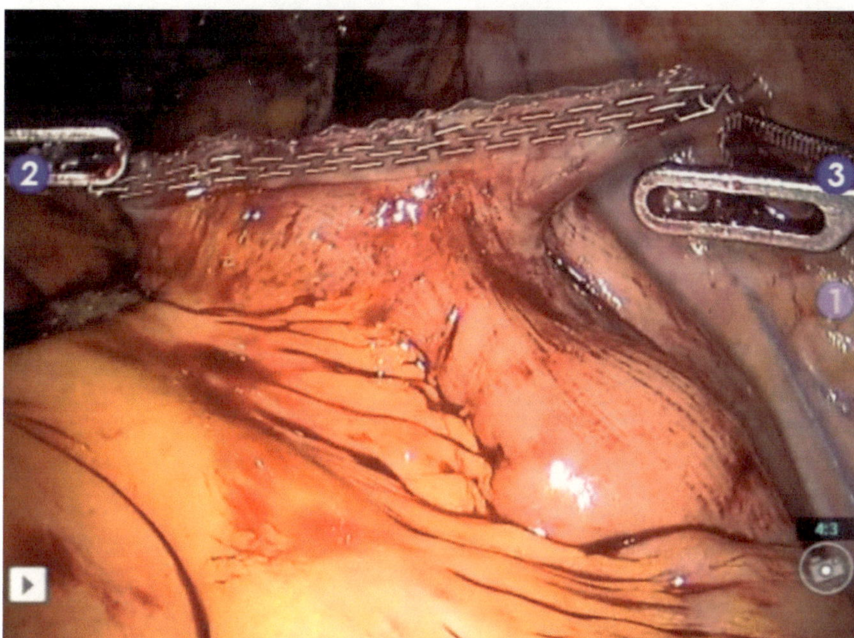

Fig. 16. Formation of side-to-side ileoileostomy by using laparoscopic intestinal staplers between proximal and distal ends of the ileum. *(Archive of Ankara Atatürk Training and Research Hospital, 1st Urology Clinic, Ankara, Turkey)*

Proximal 10 cm segment of the segregated ileum is spared as afferent loop. Then, a 60 cm feeding tube is inserted through the urethra and advanced within the lumen of the ileal segment until the proximal end of the afferent loop. Next, sparing the afferent loop, anti-mesenteric border of the remaining ileal segment is incised. Asymmetric closure of the posterior wall is accomplished with interrupted 2/0 vicryl (30 mm ½c RB needle) sutures followed by a running suture of 3/0 monocryl (26 mm ½c RB needle). Anterior wall anastomosis is accomplished using a running 3/0 monocryl (26 mm ½c RB needle) (Figure 17).

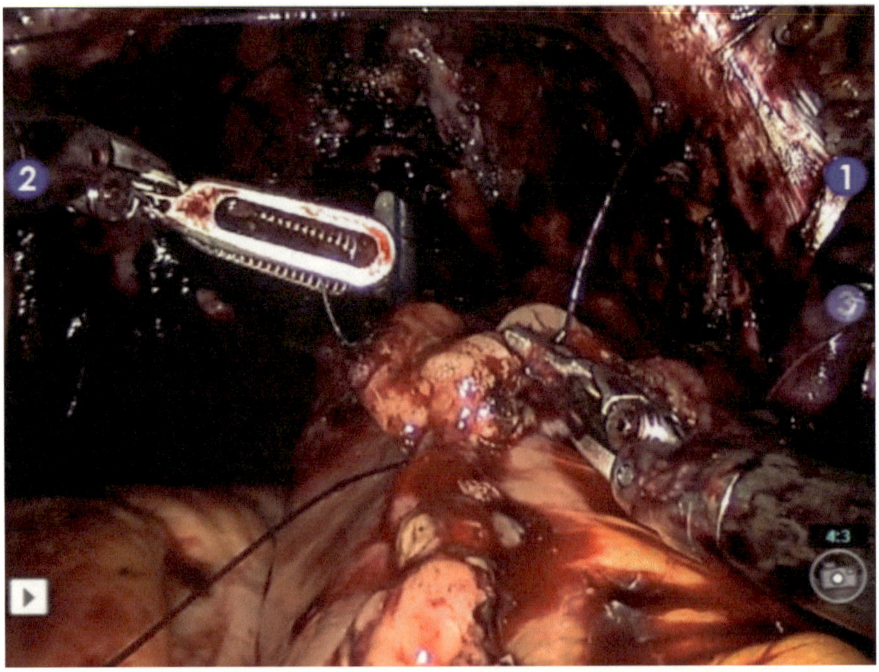

Fig. 17. Anterior wall closure. (*Archive of Ankara Atatürk Training and Research Hospital, 1st Urology Clinic, Ankara, Turkey*)

Distal ureteric ends are spatulated and anastomosed to each other at their medial edges in order to develop a common ureteral duct (Figure 18).

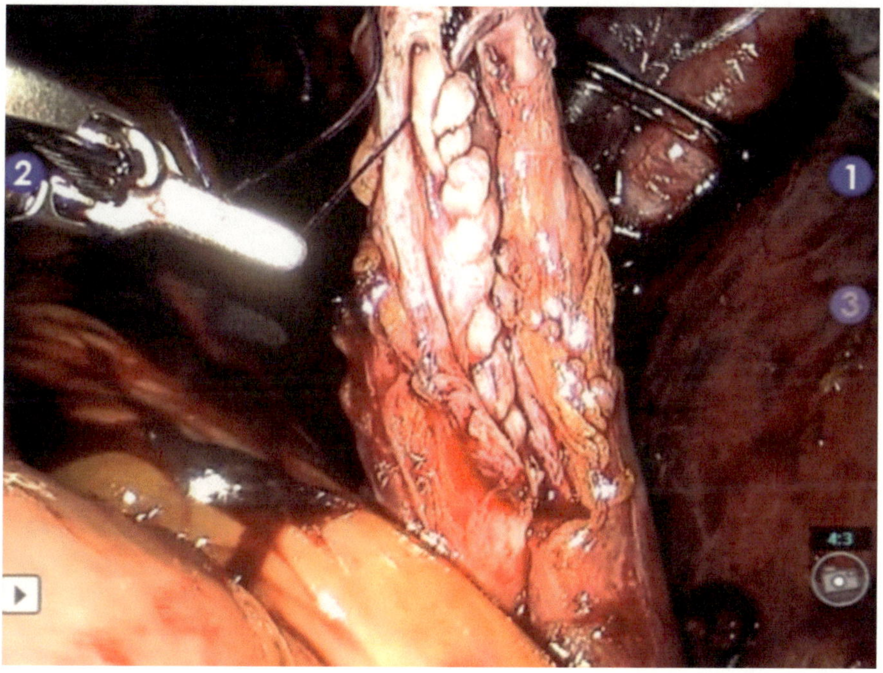

Fig. 18. Distal ureteric ends are spatulated and anastomosed to each other at their medial edges in order to develop a common ureteral duct before reconstruciton of a Wallace type uretero-ureteral and intestinal anastomosis. *(Archive of Ankara Atatürk Training and Research Hospital, 1st Urology Clinic, Ankara, Turkey)*

Double J stents with long strings at their distal ends are passed through inside the feeding tube over a guide wire to the uretero-intestinal anostomosis site and fed up to the ureters and renal pelves (Figure 19). Distal tips of the stents are tied to the tip of a 22F urethral catheter outside the body, which will then be passed through the urethra into the completed Studer pouch over a guide-wire.

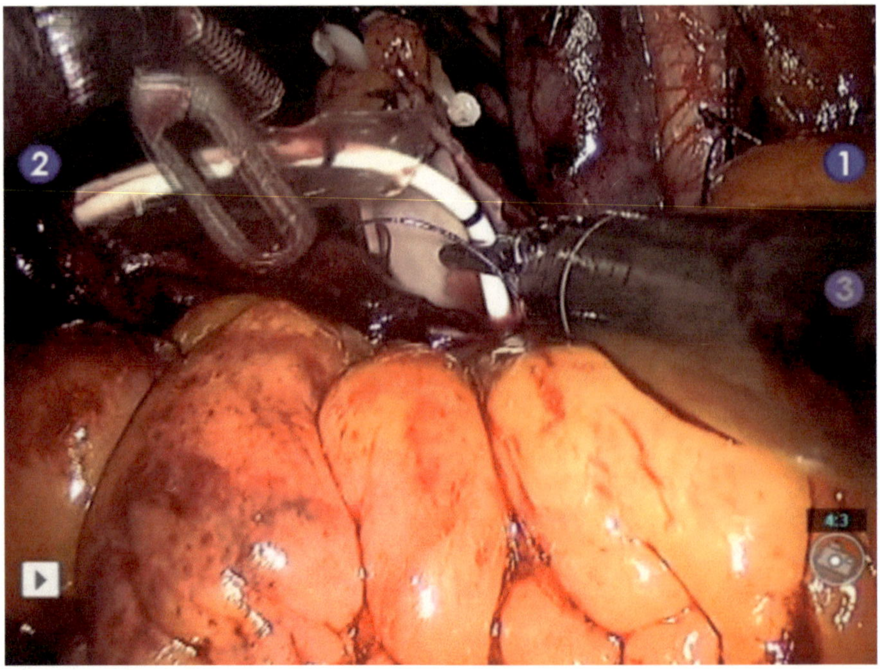

Fig. 19. Use of a feeding tube for inserting the double J catheters through the urethra, within the lumen of the ileum and into the ureters up to the renal pelves. *(Archive of Ankara Atatürk Training and Research Hospital, 1st Urology Clinic, Ankara, Turkey)*

A Wallace type uretero-intestinal anostomosis is performed between common ureteral duct and proximal end of the afferent loop. To do this anostomosis, medial edge of the ureteral duct is sutured to the medial edge of the ileal wall with a double armed 4/0 monocryl (22 mm ½c RB needle) running suture. After internalization of the double-J stents, rest of the ureteroileal anastomosis is completed (Figure 20). Ureteroileal anastomosis is retroperitonealized by using several interrupted sutures in the right gutter laterally.

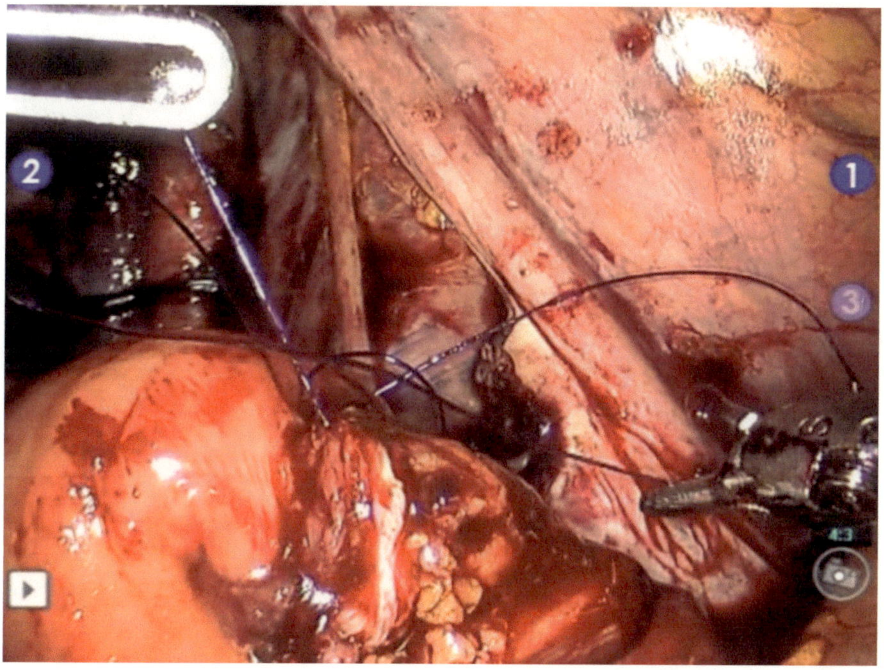

Fig. 20. Stapler line is excised at the proximal end of the afferent loop and posterior wall is anastomosed halfway between the ileal wall and medial edge of the uretero-ureteric anastomosis with a double armed 4/0 monocryl (22 mm ½c RB needle) running suture. *(Archive of Ankara Atatürk Training and Research Hospital, 1st Urology Clinic, Ankara, Turkey)*

Watertightness of the created Studer pouch is tested filling it with 150 cc of saline (Figure 21).

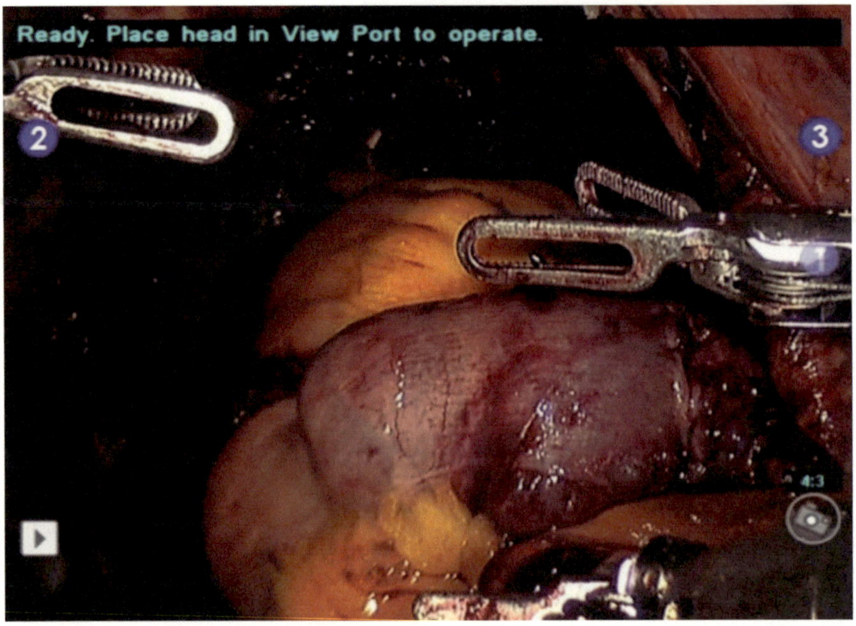

Fig. 21. Completed intracorporeal Studer pouch. (*Archive of Ankara Atatürk Training and Research Hospital, 1st Urology Clinic, Ankara, Turkey*)

Robotic-assisted laparoscopic radical cystoprostatectomy with intracorporeal Studer urinary diversion leads to better wound healing with excellent cosmetic result (Figure 22).

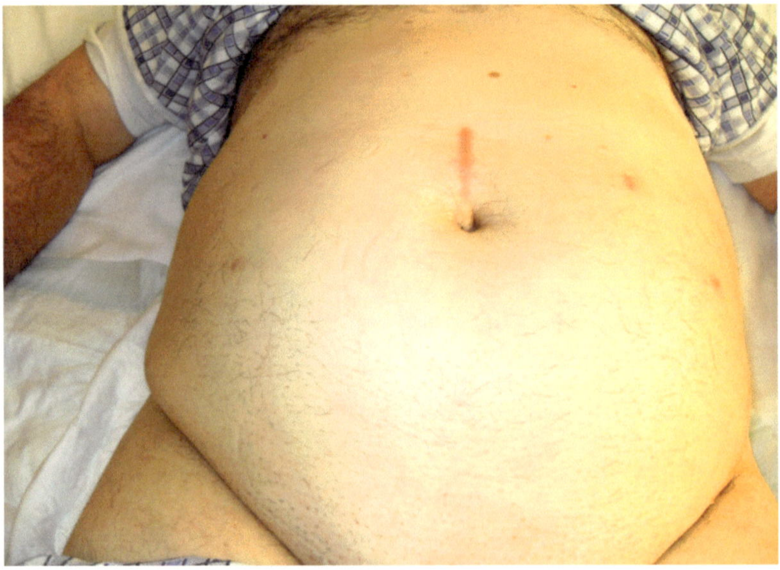

Fig. 22. Postoperative 6th-month abdominal appearance of a male patient who underwent robotic-assisted laparoscopic bilateral neurovascular bundle sparing radical cystoprostatectomy with bilateral extended lymph node dissection and intracorporeal Studer pouch formation for bladder cancer. *(Archive of Ankara Atatürk Training and Research Hospital, 1st Urology Clinic, Ankara, Turkey)*

Patients are discharged after tolerating an oral diet and sufficient ambulation following removal of the lodge drain. A cystography is done by filling the bladder with 200 cc of diluted contrast material on the postoperative 21st-day. When no leakage is seen, urethral catheter is removed. If leakage is detected, urethral catheter is kept for one more week and removed after another cystography.

6.6 Robotic-assisted laparoscopic intracorporeal ileal conduit formation (Canda et al., 2011)

Initially, sigmoid colon is mobilized and left ureter is transposed to the right gutter underneath the sigmoid colon above the vasculature. 20 cm ileal segment including the terminal ileum adjacent to the ceacum is spared and a 15-20 cm of ileal segment is segregated by using tissue staplers.

A Wallace type uretero-ureteric anastomosis is performed as explained above. For inserting the JJ stents into the renal pelves, a feeding tube is passed through the urethra and advanced within the lumen of the ileal segment. Its tip is held close to anastomozed ureteral lumens and JJ stents are passed over a guide wire up to the renal pelves. Then, uretero-ileal anostomosis is performed by using a double armed running 3/0 monocryl suture (Figure 23). Ureteroileal anastomosis is retroperitonealized by using several interrupted sutures in the right gutter laterally.

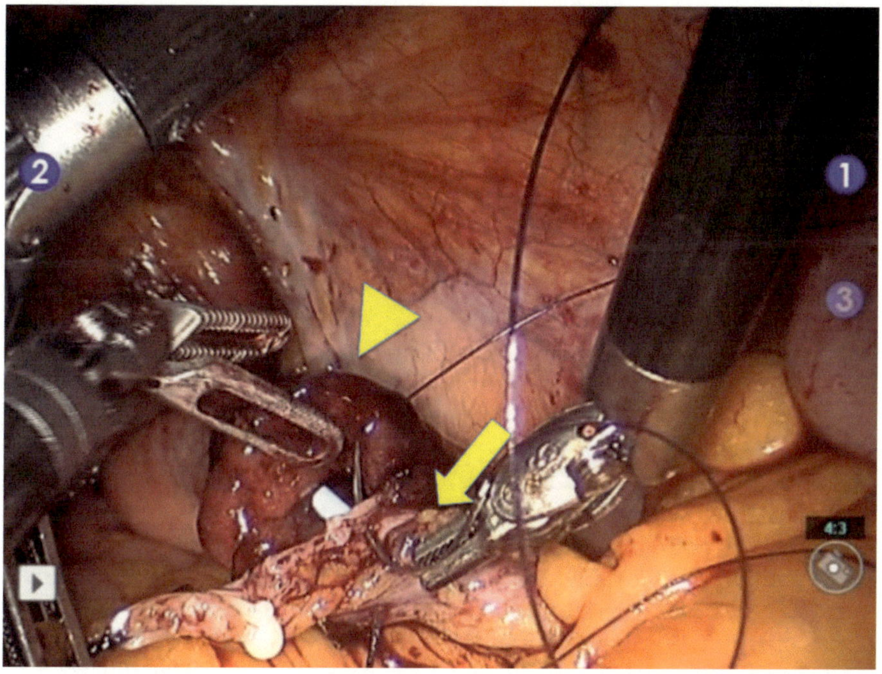

Fig. 23. Uretero-ileal anostomosis with JJ stents and intracorporeal ileal conduit. Arrowhead: ileal conduit, Arrow: Wallace type uretero-ureteric anastomosis. *(Archive of Ankara Atatürk Training and Research Hospital, 1st Urology Clinic, Ankara, Turkey)*

The 8-mm robotic trocar site opening located next to the supraumblical camera port on right is used for ileal conduit stoma following its enlargement. Interrupted 2/0 vicryl sutures are used in order to fix the ileal loop serosa to the anterior rectus sheet. Ileal opening is everted by interrupted 2/0 vicryl sutures to create a nipple type stoma.
Patients are discharged after tolerating an oral diet and sufficient ambulation following removal of the lodge drains.

7. References

Akbulut Z, Canda AE, Atmaca AF, Ozdemir AT, Asil E & Balbay MD. (2010) Robot assisted laparoscopic bilateral nerve-sparing radical cystoprostatectomy: Initial Ankara experience. *J Endourol* 24(Supplement 1):A360:VS8-14.

Akbulut Z, Canda AE, Atmaca AF, Ozdemir AT, Asil E & Balbay MD. (2010) Robot assisted laparoscopic extended pelvic lymph node dissection during radical cystoprostatectomy: Initial Ankara experience. *Eur Urol Suppl* 9(5):521.

Akbulut Z, Canda AE, Atmaca AF, Ozdemir AT, Asil E & Balbay MD. (2010) Robot assisted laparoscopic intracorporeal Studer pouch formation: Initial Ankara experience. *J Endourol* 24(Supplement 1):A359:VS8-12.

Akbulut Z, Canda AE, Ozcan MF, Atmaca AF, Ozdemir AT & Balbay MD. (2011) Robot assisted laparoscopic nerve sparing radical cystoprostatectomy with bilateral extended lymph node dissection and intracorporeal Studer pouch construction: Outcomes of first 12 cases. *J Endourol* In Press.

Canda AE, Atmaca AF, Altinova S, Akbulut Z, Balbay MD. (2011) Robot assisted nerve sparing radical cystectomy with bilateral extended lymph node dissection and intracorporeal urinary diversion for bladder cancer: Initial experience in 27 cases. *BJU Int* Accepted for publication.

Canda AE, Asil E & Balbay MD. (2011) An unexpected resident in the ileum detected during robot assisted laparoscopic radical cystoprostatectomy and intracorporeal Studer pouch formation: Taenia saginata parasite. *J Endourol* 25(2):1-3.

Canda AE, Dogan B, Atmaca AF, Akbulut Z & Balbay MD. (2011) Ureteric duplication is not a contrandication for robot assisted laparoscopic radical cystoprostatectomy and intracorporeal Studer pouch formation. *JSLS* In Press.

Cancer Facts and Figures 2009. Atlanta: American Cancer Society 2009.

Chade DC, Laudone VP, Bochner BH & Parra RO. (2010) Oncological outcomes after radical cystectomy for bladder cancer: open versus minimally invasive approaches. *J Urol* 183(3):862-69.

Clinical Practice Guidelines in Oncology, version 1.2010. Bladder Cancer. National Comprehensive Cancer Network. Available at http://www.nccn.org. Accessed March 15, 2010.

Guru KA, Perlmutter AE, Butt ZM, Piacente P, Wilding GE, Tan W, Kim HL & Mohler JL. (2009) The learning curve for robot-assisted radical cystectomy. *JSLS* 13(4):509-14.

Guru KA, Sternberg K, Wilding GE, Tan W, Butt ZM, Mohler JL, et al. (2008) The lymph node yield during robot-assisted radical cystectomy. *BJU Int.* 102(2):231-4.

Hayn MH, Hussain A, Mansour AM, Andrews PE, Carpentier P, Castle E, Dasgupta P, Rimington P, Thomas R, Khan S, Kibel A, Kim H, Manoharan M, Menon M, Mottrie A, Ornstein D, Peabody J, Pruthi R, Palou Redorta J, Richstone L, Schanne F,

Stricker H, Wiklund P, Chandrasekhar R, Wilding GE & Guru KA. (2010) The learning curve of robot-assisted radical cystectomy: results from the International Robotic Cystectomy Consortium. *Eur Urol.* 58(2):197-202.

Hellenthal NJ, Hussain A, Andrews PE, Carpentier P, Castle E, Dasgupta P, Kaouk J, Khan S, Kibel A, Kim H, Manoharan M, Menon M, Mottrie A, Ornstein D, Palou J, Peabody J, Pruthi R, Richstone L, Schanne F, Stricker H, Thomas R, Wiklund P, Wilding G & Guru KA. (2010) Surgical margin status after robot assisted radical cystectomy: results from the International Robotic Cystectomy Consortium. *J Urol.* 184(1):87-91.

Hellenthal NJ, Hussain A, Andrews PE, Carpentier P, Castle E, Dasgupta P, Kaouk J, Khan S, Kibel A, Kim H, Manoharan M, Menon M, Mottrie A, Ornstein D, Palou J, Peabody J, Pruthi R, Richstone L, Schanne F, Stricker H, Thomas R, Wiklund P, Wilding G & Guru KA. (2011) Lymphadenectomy at the time of robot-assisted radical cystectomy: results from the International Robotic Cystectomy Consortium. *BJU Int.* 107(4):642-6.

Herr H, Lee C, Chang S & Lerner S; Bladder Cancer Collaborative Group. (2004) Standardization of radical cystectomy and pelvic lymph node dissection for bladder cancer: a collaborative group report. *J Urol.* 171(5):1823-8.

Huang GJ & Stein JP. (2007) Open radical cystectomy with lymphadenectomy remains the treatment of choice for invasive bladder cancer. *Curr Opin Urol* 17:369-8.

Huang J, Lin T, Liu H, Xu K, Zhang C, Jiang C, Huang H, Yao Y, Guo Z & Xie W. (2010) Laparoscopic radical cystectomy with orthotopic ileal neobladder for bladder cancer: oncologic results of 171 cases with a median 3-year follow-up. *Eur Urol.* 58(3):442-9.

Kasraeian A, Barret E, Cathelineau X, Rozet F, Galiano M, Sanchez-Salas R & Vallancien G. (2010) Robot-assisted laparoscopic cystoprostatectomy with extended pelvic lymphadenectomy, extracorporeal enterocystoplasty, and intracorporeal enterourethral anastomosis: initial Montsouris experience. *J Endourol.* 24(3):409-13.

Kauffman EC, Ng CK, Lee MM, Otto BJ, Wang GJ & Scherr DS. (2011) Early oncological outcomes for bladder urothelial carcinoma patients treated with robotic-assisted radical cystectomy. *BJU Int.* 107(4):628-35.

Lavery HJ, Martinez-Suarez HJ & Abaza R. (2010) Robotic extended pelvic lymphadenectomy for bladder cancer with increased nodal yield. *BJU Int.* 11. doi: 10.1111/j.1464-410X.2010.09789.x. [Epub ahead of print]

Martin AD, Nunez RN, Castle EP. (2011) Robot-assisted Radical Cystectomy Versus Open Radical Cystectomy: A Complete Cost Analysis. *Urology.* 77(3):621-5.

Menon M, Hemal AK, Tewari A, Shrivastava A, Shoma AM, El-Tabey NA, Shaaban A, Abol-Enein H & Ghoneim MA. (2003) Nerve-sparing robot-assisted radical cystoprostatectomy and urinary diversion. *BJU Int.* 92(3):232-6.

Ng CK, Kauffman EC, Lee MM, Otto BJ, Portnoff A, Ehrlich JR, Schwartz MJ, Wang GJ & Scherr DS. (2010) A comparison of postoperative complications in open versus robotic cystectomy. *Eur Urol.* 57(2):274-81.

Nieder AM, Mackinnon JA, Huang Y, Fleming LE, Koniaris LG & Lee DJ. (2008) Florida bladder cancer trends 1981 to 2004: minimal progress in decreasing advanced disease. *J Urol.* 179(2):491-5

Nix J, Smith A, Kurpad R, Nielsen ME, Wallen EM & Pruthi RS. (2010) Prospective randomized controlled trial of robotic versus open radical cystectomy for bladder cancer: perioperative and pathologic results. *Eur Urol.* 57(2):196-201.

Pruthi RS, Smith A & Wallen EM. (2008) Evaluating the learning curve for robot-assisted laparoscopic radical cystectomy. *J Endourol.* 22(11):2469-74.

Pruthi RS, Nielsen ME, Nix J, Smith A, Schultz H & Wallen EM. (2010) Robotic radical cystectomy for bladder cancer: surgical and pathological outcomes in 100 consecutive cases. *J Urol.* 183(2):510-4.

Rehman J, Sangalli MN, Guru K, de Naeyer G, Schatteman P, Carpentier P & Mottrie A. (2011) Total intracorporeal robot-assisted laparoscopic ileal conduit (Bricker) urinary diversion: technique and outcomes. *Can J Urol.* 18(1):5548-56.

Schumacher MC, Jonsson MN & Wiklund NP. (2009) Robotic cystectomy. *Scand J Surg.* 98(2):89-95

Skinner EC, Stein JP & Skinner DG. (2007) Surgical benchmarks for the treatment of invasive bladder cancer. *Urol Oncol.* 25(1):66-71.

Shamim Khan M, Elhage O, Challacombe B et al: (2010) Analysis of early complications of robotic-assisted radical cystectomy using a standardized reporting system. *Urology.* Sep 7. [Epub ahead of print]

Smith A, Kurpad R, Lal A, Nielsen M, Wallen EM & Pruthi RS. (2010) Cost analysis of robotic versus open radical cystectomy for bladder cancer. *J Urol.* 183(2):505-9.

Stein JP, Cai J, Groshen S & Skinner DG. (2003) Risk factors for patients with pelvic lymph node metastases following radical cystectomy with en bloc pelvic lymphadenectomy: concept of lymph node density. *J Urol.* 170(1):35-41.

17

Current Trends in Urinary Diversion in Men

S. Siracusano, S. Ciciliato, F. Visalli, N. Lampropoulou and L. Toffoli
Department of Urology – Trieste University
Italy

1. Introduction

Prior to the introduction of the ileal conduit more than four decades ago, the options for urinary diversion after cystectomy were extremely limited. Direct cutaneous anastomoses of the collecting system (cutaneous pyelostomies, ureterostomies) offered patients a short-term diversion, but the benefits were outweighed by significant complications: recession or stenosis of the stoma. The first choice of diversion was the ureterosigmoidostomy with or without antireflux technique. Then it fell in popularity and was replaced with continent/non-continent uretero-ileo-cutaneous diversions. Only in the last years the continent orthotopic neobladder has been widely employed as first procedure choice. At present, patients can be offered a non-continent cutaneous diversion, a continent cutaneous diversion or an orthotopic neobladder urinary reconstruction (ONR).

2. Surgical indications

Urinary diversion is necessary in patients who undergo cystectomy.
The choice of a specific urinary diversion should be performed on the basis of the mental status of the patient, renal function and overall health (Table1).
The main surgical indications to perform a urinary diversion or a bladder replacement using transposed intestinal segments are bladder cancer, neurogenic bladder dysfunction, idiopathic detrusor overactivity and chronic inflammatory conditions (such as interstitial cystitis, tuberculosis, schistosomiasis and postradiation bladder contraction) [1].
If surgical cystectomy is indicated due to invasive bladder cancer the choice for replacing the lower urinary tract function rests between conduit diversion, bladder replacement or continent diversion [2].
In patients affected by neurogenic bladder dysfunction due to congenital or acquired disorders (e.g. Neural tube defect or spinal cord injured patients) the main indications for such surgery is represented by intractable incontinence, deteriorating renal function and high bladder pressures. The choices would include either bladder reconstruction, replacement or continent diversion [3].
Equally in subjects with severe idiopathic detrusor overactivity, if conservative measures fail the surgical therapy which may involve transposition of intestinal segments into the urinary tract (e.g. Clam enterocystoplasty) can provide effective treatment for some patients [4].

Finally in patients affected by idiopathic interstitial cystitis with a failure of all conservative treatments the surgical choices range from ileal conduit diversion to orthotopic neobladder reconstruction (ONR). In this context in case of bladder tuberculosis resulting in intolerable frequency, pain, urgency and haematuria with a small and incapable bladder the surgical therapy ranges from ileal conduit diversion to augmentation cystoplasty [5].

Choice of urinary diversion

At present urologists have a variety of urinary diversions using different types of bowel segments based on an individual patient's need and desire. In the past the ureterosigmoidostomy and the rectal neobladder as described by Mouclaire were the earliest forms of continent urinary diversion however, due to the rate of complications, these surgical solutions are at present abandoned. The ileal conduit remains the most common form of non-continent urinary diversion practiced worldwide today and it is the standard to which all other urinary diversions are compared [6]. Continent cutaneous diversions using detubularized colonic segments requiring timed intermittent self-catheterization. These diversions gained popularity in the 1980s and are still applied today in patients for whom an ONR is not indicated. In this way the ONR represents the most innovative surgical solution of the last thirty years because it seems to offer a satisfactory quality of life.

Urinary diversions used today in patients undergoing radical cystectomy can be categorized into three basic categories as follows : I) bowel conduits II) continent cutaneous stomal reservoirs using colonic segments III) orthotopic neobladder reconstruction (ONR) [7]. On the basis of the above reported classification we will restrict our focus on the ileal conduit, on the continent cutaneous diversions and the ONR by the use of ileal bowel.

The ileal conduit is the simplest and most commonly performed urinary diversion for which the longest follow-up is available and due to the short operative time it is often applied in patients with significant medical comorbidities in an attempt to minimize postoperative complications and the need for reoperation [8].

The continent urinary diversion involves the creation of a low pressure reservoir of good capacity using a detubularised intestinal segments as described by Kock [9]. In this setting several techniques can be used to maintain continence adopting the principle of the nipple valve and one of the most popular type is the flap valve by the use of the appendix implanted into the reservoir as described by Mitrofanoff [10]. In this surgical technique the distal end of the continence channel is brought out as a stoma through the abdominal wall for clean intermittent self-catheterisation, thus avoiding the use of a stoma bag but requiring the ability of the patient to catheterize the stoma.

In ONR the most used intestinal segment is the ileum due to its easy and ductile use while colonic segments although they had already been employed at the beginning of the "ONR era" they showed a higher number of late complications in comparison with ileum segments [11].

Patients selection criteria: Absolute and relative contraindications

The primary goals of urinary diversion are to provide the best local cancer control, to reduce the potential range of complications and to guarantee the best quality of life for the patient. The decision process is complex and involves consideration of issues related to cancer stage and location, medical comorbidities, technical surgical issues, treatment needs, and patient desires related to quality-of-life and lifestyle (Table 2). In this setting, patients should be aware that intraoperative pathological findings could modify the type of urinary diversion planned, as in the case of a short mesentery or cancer-related issues such as positive urethral margin, or gross extravesical disease precluding a negative surgical margin. For this reason, all patients planned for an ONR should have a stoma site marked preoperatively by an enterostomal therapist and at the same time have read and accepted the informed consent for an alternative urinary diversion [7,12,13].

In this way an absolute contraindication to continent diversion of any type is compromised renal function that results from long-standing obstruction or chronic renal failure, with serum creatinine levels above 150 to 200 mol/L.

In patients with borderline renal function, creatinine clearance should be evaluated because at least a creatinine clearance of 60 mL/min is recommended for continent diversions [14]. A severe hepatic dysfunction is also a contraindication for continent diversion [15] because the reabsorption and recirculation of urinary metabolites require normal liver function [16-17-20]. In fact the interposition of intestine in the urinary tract results in a marked increase in the absorption of urinary ammonia into the portal circulation resulting in a metabolic adaptation in a normal functioning liver without a hyperammonemia with a consequent altered mental status [19].

Regarding related contraindications, we know that these are steadily decreasing. However some, such as mental impairment, external sphincter dysfunction or recurrent urethral stricture, deserve serious consideration.

Notably, old age is not a contraindication for ONR. Older patients, as part of the informed consent, need to be aware that they have a greater incidence of enuresis or nocturnal incontinence than do younger men, but age by itself should not be a contraindication. In this context, physiologic rather than chronologic age must be taken into consideration [20]. Although urinary continence rates are somewhat lower in patients over 70 years of age, satisfactory continence rates and functional outcomes can be obtained. [21,22].

Obesity does not preclude orthotopic diversion and in some cases an orthotopic diversion may be advantageous because of the difficulty of constructing an optimal stoma for a urostomy appliance with conduits and the difficulty in negotiating a catheter through a thick abdominal wall for catheterization of a continent cutaneous pouch. In addition, large fluctuations in patient weight can change the angle of the originally constructed pouch making it difficult to catheterize [23].

Satisfactory functional outcomes with ONR after cystectomy have been reported in carefully selected patients who have received previous definitive, full dose pelvic irradiation [24,25]. However, these are technically complex and demanding procedures with a high risk for perioperative complications [26]. Common complications reported in post-radiation surgical series include ureteral stricture in up to 32% of patients, prolonged incontinence in up to 44%, stomal problems in up to 39%, and fistulas in up to 7%. Reoperations to address these complications occur in 8% to 69% of patients and the most common reasons for reoperation include stomal revisions, ureteral anastomotic revisions, and procedures to correct incontinence and repair of fistulas [24,27].

Patients with compromised intestinal function, particularly inflammatory bowel disease, may be better served by an incontinent bowel conduit. A thorough evaluation of the colon by a contrast enema, sigmoidoscopy, or colonoscopy is recommended when planning to use large bowel segments for the urinary diversions to rule out colonic pathology such as diverticulosis, inflammatory bowel disease, or occult colon cancer, which would prevent their use. A family or personal history of colon cancer or familial polyposis may predispose the patient to developing an adenocarcinoma in a colonic urinary reservoir segment and should be taken into consideration during the diversion selection process [28,29].

In conclusion the goal of patient counseling about urinary diversion should be to determine the method that is the safest for cancer control, that has the fewest complications over both the short and the long term and that provides the easiest adjustment for patients' lifestyle, thereby supporting the best quality of life [7]. The ileal conduit is still the best urinary diversion method in many patients who have bladder cancer with associated chronic medical disease or certain surgical factors that render other urinary diversion techniques difficult to carry out. Finally we believe that all patients are potentially candidates for an ONR although the main problem is to identify patients for whom an ONR may be not indicated.

Bowel Segment	Primary Indication
Gastric	Children requiring diversion (extrophy,pelvic radiation); Renal insufficiency
Jejunum	Pelvic radiation; Deficient ureteral length; Compromised viability of other small or large bowel
Ileum or ileal-colic reservoirs	Malignancies requiring removal of the bladder; Severe hemorrhagic cystitis; Incontinence
Colon (ureterosigmoidostomy)	Children requiring diversion (extrophy, pelvic radiation); No other bowel segment alternative
Transverse colon conduit	Malignancies requiring removal of the bladder; Small bowel not practical

Table 1. Indications for use of bowel segments in urinary diversion [1,6]

Absolute contraindications
Impaired renal function
Impaired hepatic function
Inadequate intellectual capacity
Positive apical urethral margin (for neobladder)
Unmotivated patient
Relative contraindications
Advanced age
Need for adjuvant chemotherapy
Prior pelvic radiation
Bowel disease (especially inflammatory bowel disease)
Urethral pathology
Local disease and high risk of local recurrence

Table 2. Absolute and Relative Contraindications for Continent Cutaneous/Orthotopic Neobladder Urinary Diversions [1,6]

3. Non continent cutaneous diversions: Surgical aspects and postoperarative complications

The ileal and the colon conduit represent the non-continent cutaneous urinary diversions. The ileal conduit has been the mainstay of urinary diversion over the past forty-five years and, in authors' opinion, it remains the first choice against all other compared urinary diversions. It consists of diverting urine to a short intestinal segment brought out through the anterior abdominal wall. The ileal resection can induce malabsorption of bile salts and vitamin B_{12}. The colon conduit was less employed because of resulted in electrolyte abnormalities and was more amenable to antireflux ureteral implantation techniques. The non-refluxing technique is employed for a better maintenance of upper urinary tract integrity.

Ileal conduit

Ureteroileal urinary diversion is the most common method of non-continent urinary diversion. The basic technique for creation of the ileal loop has not changed significantly since the original description by Seiffer 1935. The procedure was subsequently popularized by Bricker.

The patient is placed in supine position and a vertical midline or paramedian incision from the symphysis pubis to the umbilicus or beyond is required for good exposure [30].

The ureters are identified and transected approximately 3 or 4 cm above the bladder and then they are minimally mobilized taking care to preserve the surrounding adventitia and fat. The conduit is constructed using an ileal segment 15 to 20 cm long that is isolated approximately 20 cm proximal to the ileocecal valve [31,32,33].

Once the appropriate length of bowel is selected and isolated, the mesentery is divided proximally and distally and individual mesenteric blood vessels are ligated. The bowel is divided, thus isolating the segment selected for conduit construction. The continuity of the small intestine is reestablished, allowing for normal bowel function. The base of the conduit is closed and the ureters are reimplanted directly, creating an antirefluxing ureteroileal anastomosis.

Ureteral stents (small-diameter, multichannel, silicone catheters) are placed through the ureteral anastomosis, the conduit and into the pelvis to facilitate urinary drainage while the anastomosis is healing [33-34].The conduit is usually positioned in the right lower quadrant of the abdomen in an isoperistaltic direction [32].

To create the stoma, a small circle of skin is excised at the premarked site. And the underlying cylinder of fat is removed. The fascia is incised in a cruciate fashion. The end of the conduit is brought through the lateral aspect of the rectus abdominis muscle and anchored to the fascia, and the stoma is then formed [34]. The stoma should protrude, without tension approximately 2,5-3 cm above the skin surface. A Rutzen bag can be applied to the stoma on the fifth or sixth postoperative day with complete comfort for the patient [34].

Jejunal conduit

Jejunal conduit urinary diversion is used rarely, since many better alternatives are available. However, jejunal conduits have been used in cases in which there has been significant ileal and colonic disease caused by previous irradiation and inflammatory bowel disease or there has been loss of the middle and distal ureter [35].

As is discussed later, electrolyte disturbances can occur after incorporation of intestinal segments into the urinary tract; these are more common when the jejunum is used for conduit construction. In approximately 40% of patients with jejunal urinary conduits, hyponatremic, hyperkalemic, hypochloremic metabolic acidosis and azotemia develop [36]. The jejunum is unable to maintain large solute gradients, so large amounts of water and solute pass through the jejunal wall. Sodium and chloride are rapidly excreted into the conduit, and potassium is passively absorbed [36-37].

Aldosterone is produced, resulting in reabsorption of hydrogen and excretion of potassium into the distal tubule of the kidney and consequent acidosis and movement of potassium from the body's intracellular stores. As water is lost into the conduit, extracellular fluid volume is reduced, as is the glomerular filtration rate. The renin-angiotensin system is activated, which further stimulates aldosterone secretion. Urea may be absorbed from the jejunal lumen, which (with dehydration) contributes to azotemia [36]. As with other bowel segments incorporated into the urinary tract, the length of jejunum should be as short as possible to reduce metabolic abnormalities. The ureters are brought out from the retroperitoneum below the ligament of Treitz. An appropriate segment of jejunum is identified and isolated and it is important to preserve an adequate blood supply to the segment. In contrast to the ilal conduit, the isolated jejunum should lie above the reanastomosed jejunum. The proximal end of the conduit is directed towards the retroperitoneum and the conduit is oriented in an isoperistaltic direction. The ureters are anastomosed to the jejunum, with placement of stents to reduce early postoperative electrolyte abnormalities. The mesenteric window is closed using nonasorbable sutures. The stoma is created in the same way as described for an ileal conduit and is usually located in the right upper quadrant [38].

Colon conduit

There are several advantages to using the large bowel for the construction of urinary conduits: nonrefluxing ureterointestinal anastomoses are easily performed, possibly abrogating the deleterious effects of reflux on the upper urinary tracts [37-39].

In the colon conduit stomal stenosis is uncommon because of the wide diameter of the large bowel but limited absorption of electrolytes occurs; the blood supply to the transverse and sigmoid colon is abundant [39]. Either the transverse or the sigmoid colon can be used, allowing for placement of the conduit high or low in the abdomen, depending on the integrity and condition of the ureters. Use of the transverse colon for conduit construction is especially well suited for patients who have received extensive pelvic irradiation or when the middle and distal ureters are absent [37,39].

The blood supply of the transverse colon is based on the middle colic artery.

The greater omentum is separated from the superior surface of the transverse colon, and a segment of bowel, usually 15 cm in length, is selected for the conduit [39]. Short mesenteric incisions are made, and the colon is divided proximally and distally. Once the conduit is isolated, bowel continuity is reestablished. The proximal end of the conduit is closed and fixed in the midline posteriorly. The ureters are brought through small incisions in the posterior peritoneum and reimplanted into the base of the conduit [39]. The stoma may be positioned on either the patient's right or left side.

A sigmoid conduit is constructed in a similar manner. Great care should be taken to preserve the blood supply by carefully selecting a segment with a good blood supply and by

making short mesenteric incisions. The conduit is positioned lateral to the reapproximated sigmoid colon. Ureteral reimplantation and stoma construction are completed [39].
The ureters can be reimplanted into the large intestine either in a way that prevents reflux or by anastomosis directly into the bowel. Ureteral reflux is prevented by constructing a short tunnel (approximately 2-3 cm in length) of bowel mucosa, through which the distal ureter runs [37,39]. Frequently, this is accomplished by incising the tenia of the large bowel for a distance of 3-4 cm. The incision is carried through the muscular fibers of the bowel wall, sparing the mucosa. A small elliptic segment of mucosa is removed, and a mucosa-to-mucosa anastomosis is performed between the ureter and the mucosa of the bowel. The muscularis of the tenia is repositinated over the ureter to create the tunnel [39].

Cutaneous ureterostomy

This surgical technique is based on the simple bilateral ureterostomy or alternatively on the transureteroureterostomy. From a technical point of view the first surgical solution is easier and faster than the transureteroureterostomy. In particular, in order to carry out of a transureteroureterostomy with cutaneous ureterostomy the ureters are isolated with care to preserve the blood supply. A retroperitoneal course anterior to the great vessels for the least dilated is created [40,41]. If only a single ureter is obstructed, a simple stoma can be created by sewing the end of the ureter flush with the skin at the stoma site. Another option, when the ureter is narrow, is to create a V-flap stoma. If both ureters are dilated, a single stoma can be created by suturing the ureters together, everting them and anastomosing the ends to the skin. When a single ureter is dilated, transureterostomy with retroperitoneal passage of the smaller ureter to the controlatereral side is combined with the cutaneous ureterostomy [38].

Postoperative complications

Complications occurring after urinary diversion are generally a product of surgical technique, the underlying disease process and its treatment, the age of the patient, and the length of follow-up. Postoperative complications are divided into early and late.
Early complications (occurring in approximately 10% of patients) are wound infection, followed by ureteroileal leakage, intestinal obstruction, intestinal fistula and acute pyelonephritis [30].
Late complications (10-20% of patients) include metabolic disorders, stomal stenosis, cronic pyelonephritis, and calculi [30].

Metabolic and nutritional disorders

Fluid, electrolyte, nutrient, and waste product excretion or absorption normally occurs across the intestinal wall. The extent of absorption or excretion is dependent on the concentration of these substances in the lumen or blood and on which segment of bowel is in contact with them.
Metabolic abnormalities may occur when intestinal segments are interposed into the urinary tract [33].
The pathogenesis and nature of metabolic abnormalities occurring after incorporation of the ileum or colon into the urinary tract differ from those associated with jejunal conduits [35]; when such segments are used, sodium and chloride are absorbed across the bowel surface. Chloride is absorbed in slight excess of sodium, resulting in a net loss of bicarbonate into the bowel lumen. Preexisting renal failure contributes to the development and severity of the

disorder, as does a large bowel surface area and long contact time. Hyperchloremic acidosis is more common in patients who undergo ureterosigmoidostomy than in patients who undergo simple conduit construction using either the ileum or the colon, because of the larger surface area and longer contact time with urine associated with ureterosigmoidostomies [42].

Hyperchloremic metabolic acidosis may manifest clinically as weakness, anorexia, vomiting, Kussmaul breathing, and coma. One potential long-term complication of chronic acidosis may be decreased bone calcium content and osteomalacia [36].

Bile salts are important for fat digestion and uptake of vitamins A and D. Bile salt metabolism may be altered after ileal resection [43].

Resecton of small segments of the ileum may be associated with mild malabsorption and steatorrhea owing to increased concentrations of bile salts delivered to the colon.

The increased concentration of such salts leads to decreased colonic absorption of water and electrolytes [35].The distal ileum is important for reabsorption of bile acidis, the use of this part of intestine for uncontinent urinary diversion causes abnormal high concentrations of bile acids in the colon leading to diarrhea due to the altered sodium absorption [43].

Vitamin B12 deficiency may occur as a result of resecting the terminal ileum to resconstruct the lower urinary tract. The signs of vitamin B 12 deficiency include megaloblastic macrocytic anemia and neurologic injury, which become permanent if allowed to persist [33,35,42,44].

Stomal complications

Stoma related complications occurred in 15% of patients with the most frequent being parastomal hernia, stenosis and various skin irritations or fungal infections [32,33]. The majority of stoma related complications occurred within the first 5 years after surgery [32].

Stomal stenosis can lead to conduit elongation and upper-tract obstruction. This condition can be diagnosed relatively easily by catheterizing the stoma and measuring the residual urine volume. It is corrected by revision of the stoma [42].

Skin irritation or infections are most common in procedures in which an appliance is worn and there is prolonged contact of the skin with urine. Some patients' skin may be sensitive to adhesive agents [30].

Urinary tract infection and pyelonephritis

Pyelonephritis occurs in approximately 12% of patients who have undergone urinary diversion. The infectious complications occurred at a median of 1.8 years after surgery [45].

Treatment is based on a properly collected urine sample for culture. A urine sample should not be collected from the pouch; rather, the pouch should be removed, the stoma cleansed with an antiseptic, and a catheter advanced gently through the stoma.

If infection has occurred in a patient with a simple conduit, the volume of residual urine within the conduit should be recorded. Obstruction and stasis of urine within the reconstructed urinary tract are risk factors for the development of infection [32].

Although many patients with preexisting dilation of the upper urinary tract show improvement or resolution of the dilation after urinary diversion or bladder substitution, progressive renal deterioration as manifested by hydronephrosis or an increasing serum creatinine level (or both) occur in a certain percentage of patients who undergo these procedures [42]. The incidence of either complication increases after 10 years. Pyelographic

evidence of upper urinary tract deterioration has been noted in up to 50% of patients who have undergone urinary diversion at an early age.
Recurrent upper urinary tract infection and high-pressure ureteral reflux and obstruction, usually in combination, contribute to the likelihood of renal deterioration.

Calculi

Calculi occur in approximately 8% of patients who undergo urinary diversion, at a median of 2.5 years after surgery [33].
Such patients have several risk factors for the development of various calculi.
Nonabsorbable staples, mesh, or suture material used to construct conduits or reservoirs may act as a nidus for stone formation [33].
Colonization in either conduits or reservoirs is common, whereas symptomatic infection is much rarer.
Certain bacteria can contribute to stone formation; some bacteria commonly found in the urinary tract, including: Proteus, Klebsiella, and Pseudomonas species, produce urease, a urea-splitting enzyme that contributes to the formation of ammonia and carbon dioxide.
Hydrolysis of these products results in an alkaline urine supersaturated with magnesium ammonium phosphate, calcium phosphate, and carbonate apatite crystals.
Management of such infection-related stones requires stone removal, resolution of infection, and, often, use of adjunctive agents to complete stone dissolution [33].
The likelihood of stone formation is increased by the development of systemic acidosis, as described previously. Prolonged contact of the urine with the intestinal surface facilitates the exchange of chloride for bicarbonate [33].
Bicarbonate loss results in systemic acidosis and hypercalciuria. The combination of hypercalciuria and alkaline urine predisposes a patient to the development of calcium calculi. In addition, the terminal ileum is responsible for bile salt absorption; if this portion of the intestine is used for conduit or bladder reservoir construction, excess bile salts in the intestine may bind calcium and result in increased absorption of oxalate, which may lead to the development of oxalate-containing calculi [36].
Hypocitraturia may also be a risk factor for stone disease in patients undergoing bladder replacement [36].
Excess conduit length, urine stasis, and dehydration make the development of calculi more likely.

4. Orthotopic neobladder reconstruction (ONR): Surgical aspects and postoperative complications

In 1979, Camey and Le Duc published their clinical experience with ONR. This orthotopic bladder substitute has evolved into the most ideal form of urinary diversion available today and should be considered the gold standard with which other forms of diversion are compared. Before 1990, the orthotopic substitution was reserved for male patients with invasive bladder cancer while the same surgical approach was considered contraindicated in the female subjects because the urethra was removed during cystectomy to assure adequate oncological results. It was also believed that the female patient would be unable to maintain the continence mechanism if orthotopic diversion was performed after cystectomy. Actually, it has been shown that the urethra can be saved in the most women undergoing cystectomy for bladder cancer without compromising the oncological results [46].

Models of ONR

Radical cystectomy is the standard treatment for localized muscle-invasive bladder cancer. Different types of intestinal segments have been used for urinary diversion, including stomach, ileum, colon in humans and animals. However, the terminal ileum is most often used for bladder substitution. Therefore, the ideal diversion should be fully continent, cosmetically impeccable, allowing easy and complete emptying within socially acceptable intervals, and preserve renal function [47].

- In Camey II orthotopic substitution a total of 65 cm of ileum is isolated, with an area of the ileum identified to reach the region of the urethra in a tension-free manner. After the integrity of the bowel is restored, the mesenteric trap is closed, and the isolated portion of ileum is opened along the antimesenteric border for the entire length, except the area previously identified for urethral anastomosis. In this region, the ileal incision is directed toward the mesenteric border. The ileum is then placed in a transverse U orientation. The medial borders of the U are sutured together with a running absorbable suture. A fingertip opening is made in the preselected area for the ileourethral anastomosis, the entire ileal plate is brought down to the pelvis, and urethroenteric anastomosis is performed. The ureteroileal anastomosis is then performed by a Le Duc technique. The reservoir is completed by folding the ileal plate and suturing with a running absorbable suture. The ends of the U are anchored to the pelvic floor to reduce tension [48].
- The ileal neobladder developed by Hautmann was an ileal reservoir with a "W configuration" that wanted to guarantee a reduction of nighttime incontinence. A segment of terminal ileum of approximately 70 cm is selected. The bowel is reconstituted, and the mesenteric trap is closed. The ileal section that reaches the urethra most easily is identified and marked with a traction suture along the antimesenteric border. The isolated bowel segment is then arranged in either an M or W shape and is incised. The entire segment is opened along the antimesenteric border except for a 5-cm section along the traction suture, where the incision is directed toward the anterior mesenteric border to make a U-shaped flap. This facilitates anastomosis of the neobladder to the urethra. The four limbs of the M or W are then sutured to one another with a running absorbable suture. In the center of the previously developed flap, a segment of the ileal wall is excised. The ileourethral anastomosis is then performed with the sutures tied from "inside" the neobladder. Once the ileal neobladder is situated in the pelvis and the urethral sutures are tied, the ureters are implanted from inside the neobladder through a small incision in the ileum at a convenient site as reported by Abol-Enein (Fig.1) or in monolateral fashion as described by Siracusano [49]. The remaining portion of the anterior wall is then closed with a running absorbable suture.
- The Studer ileal bladder substitute uses a portion of terminal ileal segment: 54 to 60 cm is isolated approximately 25 cm proximal to the ileocecal valve. Bowel continuity is restored, and the ends of the isolated segment are closed with a running absorbable suture. The distal 40-cm segment of ileum is placed in a U shape and opened along the antimesenteric border. The ureters are split and anastomosed in an end-to-side fashion to the proximal afferent tubular portion of ileum. The two medial borders of the U-shaped ileum are then oversewn with a running absorbable suture. The bottom of the U is folded over between the two ends of the U. After the lower half of the anterior wall

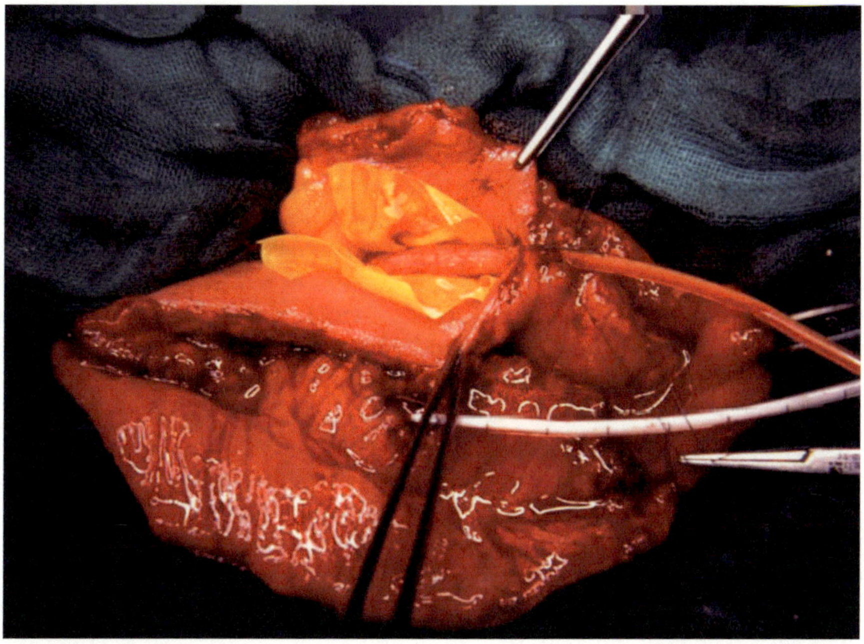

Fig. 1. Spatulated ureters are anastomosed to intestinal mucosa of the lateral wall of the trough. The ureters are anastomosed on 8 Fr anti-reflux double "J" stents (By Siracusano Eur Urol 38 : 313, 2000)

and part of the upper half are closed, a finger is introduced through the remaining reservoir opening to determine the most caudal part of the neobladder. A hole is cut out in this dependent portion of ileum, away from the suture line, which allows urethral anastomosis. The urethroenteric anastomosis is performed, and the remaining portion of the reservoir is then closed [50].

- The Kock ileal reservoir utilizes intussuscepted nipple valves for both the afferent and efferent limbs to prevent urinary reflux. A total of 61 cm of terminal ileum is isolated. 22-cm segments are placed in a U configuration and opened adjacent to the mesentery. The more proximal 17-cm segment of ileum will be used to make the afferent intussuscepted nipple valve. The posterior wall of the reservoir is then formed by joining the medial portions of the U with a continuous running suture. A 5- to 7-cm antireflux valve is made by intussusception of the afferent limb with the use of Allis forceps clamps. The afferent limb is fixed with two rows of staples placed within the leaves of the valve. The valve is fixed to the back wall from outside the reservoir. After completion of the afferent limb, the reservoir is completed by folding the ileum on itself and closing it (anterior wall). The most dependent portion of the reservoir becomes the neourethra. Ureteroileal anastomosis is performed first, and urethroenteric anastomosis is completed in a tension-free, mucosa-to-mucosa fashion [51].
- The "vescica ileale padovana" (VIP) is a modified form of Camey II with a more spherical reservoir. A portion of terminal ileum 40 cm long is isolated approximately 20 cm proximal to the ileocecal valve and opened along the antimesenteric border. The distal 10-cm segment is intended to constitute a tunnel for ileal-urethral anastomosis,

while the proximal 30-cm segment of ileum is folded in a jellyroll fashion to produce a posterior plate. The pouch is then closed anteriorly [52].

- The T pouch ileal neobladder is a variant of Koch ileal reservoir but with a new, safe and simple antireflux technique. The T pouch is constructed from a 44-cm segment of terminal ileum placed in a V formation with a more proximal 8- to 10-cm segment of ileum used to form the antireflux limb. The entire mesentery remains intact to provide excellent viability. Windows of Deaver are opened (with Penrose drains placed into each window) in the distal 3 to 4 cm of the isolated afferent limb. The blood supply remains intact to this afferent ileal segment. A series of interrupted silk sutures are used to approximate the serosa of the adjacent 22-cm limbs (cephalad portion), with the passage of sutures through the corresponding window of Deaver. After the silk suture is passed through the window of Deaver, it is placed at a corresponding site on the adjacent 22-cm segment and then brought back through the same window of Deaver and tied down. The anchored portion of afferent limb is tapered on the antimesenteric border. The ileal segments are opened adjacent to the mesentery beginning at the apex and carried upward to the ostium of the afferent limb. Once the incision reaches the ostium of the afferent limb, it is directed to the antimesenteric border and then carried upward. This provides excellent ileal flaps to cover the tapered afferent ileal segment that is anchored into the serous trough. The ostium of the afferent segment is sutured to the ileal flaps. The ileal flaps are then brought over and oversewn to cover the tapered afferent ileal segment. This completes the posterior wall of the reservoir and forms the antireflux flap-valve mechanism. The reservoir is folded and closed in the opposite direction from which it was opened. The ureteroileal anastomosis is performed to the proximal portion of the afferent ileal segment. The anterior suture line is stopped just short of the right side. Then the result will be anastomosed to the urethra [53].
- The surgeons of Turin University propose an operative technique of a new Y-shaped ileal neobladder reconstruction. The procedure is performed with the isolation of 40cm of ileum, 15-20cm before the ileocecal valve. The isolated segment is arranged in a Y-shape with two central segments of 14cm and two limbs of 6cm. The two central segments are brought together and detubularized, with a nonabsorbable mechanical stapler inserted through an opening made at the lowest point of the neobladder. The Y-neobladder is anastomosed to the urethra with five sutures in 2-0 polyglycolic acid, over a 22F silastic catheter. The ureters, resected above the crossing with the iliac vessels and spatulated anteriorly, are anastomosed to the dorsal aspect of the two limbs with 5.0 polyglycolic acid sutures, using the direct Nesbit technique. Ureteral stents, previously placed, are brought out through the distal portions of each chimney and then through the anterior abdominal wall. The two limbs are fixed to the psoas muscles [54].
- In relation to the use of colon for carrying out ONR we report Mansson's technique and the pouches described by the Mainz School and by Reddy respectively.

In particular Mansson proposes an orthotopic neobladder substitution using a right colon segment (Mansson pouch). The entire right colon and cecum are isolated, and a transverse ileocolonic anastomosis is performed to provide bowel continuity. The ileal stump at the ileocecal valve is closed with a running absorbable suture. The colonic segment is then opened along the anterior taenia, leaving the proximal 2 to 3 inches of cecum intact. An appendectomy is performed, and the ureters are implanted in an antireflux fashion within the reservoir. The colon is then folded in a Heineke-Mikulicz manner and closed with a running absorbable suture. The ureterocolonic anastomosis is then performed [55].

- The surgeons of Mainz Institute describe a surgical procedure with a segment of both ileum and right colon (Mainz pouch). A 10- to 15-cm segment of cecum, in continuity with a 20- to 30-cm segment of ileum, is isolated. An ascending ileocolostomy is performed. The entire segment of bowel is opened along the antimesenteric border, sacrificing the ileocecal valve. The bowel is placed in a W configuration, with the first limb of the W represented by cecum and the middle two limbs represented by ileum. The adjacent three limbs are sutured together with an absorbable suture, forming the posterior plate of the reservoir. At the cephalic portion of the cecum, tunneled ureterocolonic anastomosis is performed. A buttonhole incision is made in the cecum at the base of the reservoir, and a ureterocolonic anastomosis is performed. After this, the reservoir is closed side to side with absorbable suture [56].
- Reddy and Lange describe an orthotopic reconstruction with sigmoid segment (Reddy pouch). A 35-cm portion of descending colon and sigmoid is isolated and arranged in a U configuration. The medial taenia of the U is incised down to an area just short of the urethral anastomosis. The incised medial limbs of the U are then brought together with an absorbable suture. Ureteral implantation is performed in a tunnel antireflux fashion. A small button of colon is removed from the most dependent portion of the reservoir, and the urethroenteric anastomosis is performed. The reservoir is then closed side to side [57].

Complications

The patients may incur early and late complications as previously reported in non continent cutaneous diversions. The early post-operative complications may be identified as enterocolitis, acute pyelonephritis or lymphorrhoea. Therefore, chronic urinary retention, stricture of neobladder-urethra anastomosis, urosepsis secondary to bilateral hydronephrosis and neobladdder stones are the main late complications for this form of surgery [58]. Finally the utilization of small bowel for urinary diversion may interfere with the physiological renal acid and salt regulation while osteoporosis and osteomalacia might theoretically develop from a persistent hypokalemic, hyperchloremic acidosis.

5. Conclusions

For many years the ileal conduit and the ureterosigmoidostomy were considered the primary choice for urinary diversion following cystectomy. In the last twenty years the surgical procedures of urinary tract reconstruction after bladder removal have evolved from simply urinary diversions and protecting the upper tract to creating a socially and psychologically more acceptable quality of life. Nevertheless at present there is no optimal surgical urinary diversion for all patients but surgical solutions that must be applied to each type of patient.

6. References

[1] Ghulam Nabi, June D Cody, Norman Dublin, Samuel McClinton , James MO N'Dow, David E Neal, Robert Pickard, Sze M Yong. Urinary diversion and bladder reconstruction/replacement using intestinal segments for intractable incontinence or following cystectomy Cochrane Database of Systematic Reviews, 2009

[2] Manoharan M and AM Nieder: "surgical management: cystectomy and urinary diversion" pp348-360 in Urological Oncology, VH Nargund, D Raghavan, HM Sandler Ed, Springer-Verlag London ltd 2008.
[3] Stein R, Wiesner C, Beetz R, Schwarz M, Thüroff JW. Urinary diversion in children and adolescents with neurogenic bladder: the Mainz experience. Part I: Bladder augmentation and bladder substitution--therapeutic algorisms. Pediatr Nephrol. 2005;20(7):920-5
[4] Lewis DK, Morgan JR, Weston PM, Stephenson TP. The "clam": indications and complications. British Journal of Urology 1990;65:488–91.
[5] Benchekroun A, Lachkar A, Soumana A, Farih MH, Belahnech Z, Marzouk M, Faik M. Urogenital tuberculosis. 80 cases. Ann Urol, 1998;32(2):89-94.
[6] Bricker EM: Bladder substitution with isolated small intestine segments; a progress report. Am Surg 1952;18:654-664.
[7] Dipen J. Parekh and S. Machele Donat Urinary Diversion: Options,Patient Selection, and Outcomes Semin Oncol 2007;34:98-109,
[8] Turnbull RB Jr: Intestinal stomas. Surg Clin North Am 1958; 38:1361-1372,
[9] Kock NG, Nilson AE, Nilsson LO, Norlen LJ, Philipson BM. Urinary diversion via a continent ileal reservoir: clinical results in 12 patients. Journal of Urology 1982;128(3):469–75
[10] Sumfest JM, Burns MW, Mitchell ME. The Mitrofanoff principle in urinary reconstruction. J Urol. 1993;150, 1975-1878
[11] Hautmann RE: Urinary diversion: Ileal conduit to neobladder. J Urol 2003; 169:834-842,
[12] Henna as a durable preoperative skin marker. Henna as a durable preoperative skin marker. World J Surg. 2011;35(2):311-5
[13] Bass EM, Del Pino A, Tan A, Pearl RK, Orsay CP, Abcarian H. Does preoperative stoma marking and education by the enterostomal therapist affect outcome? Dis Colon Rectum. 1997;40(4):440-2
[14] Mills RD, Studer UE: Metabolic consequences of continent urinary diversion. J Urol 1999;161:1057-1066.
[15] Mills RD, Studer UE: Metabolic consequences of continent urinary diversion. J Urol 1999; 161:1057-1066.
[16] Koch MO, McDougal WS, Thompson CO: Mechanisms of solute transport following urinary diversion through intestinal segments: An experimental study with rats. J Urol 1991; 146:1390-1394.
[17] Koch MO, McDougal WS, Flora MD: Urease and the acidosis of urinary intestinal diversion. J Urol 1991;146:458-462.
[18] McDougal WS, Koch MO: Accurate determination of renal function in patients with intestinal urinary diversions. J Urol 1986; 135:1175-1178.
[19] Kaveggia FF, Thompson JS, Schafer EC, et al: Hyperammonemic encephalopathy in urinary diversion with urea-splitting urinary tract infection. Arch Intern Med 1990;150:2389-2392.
[20] Studer UE, Hautmann RE, Hohenfellner M, Mills RD, Okada Y, Rowland RG, et al. Indications for continent diversion after cystectomy and factors affecting long-term results. Urol Oncol 1998; 4:172-82

[21] Steven K, Poulsen AL: The orthotopic Kock ileal neobladder: Functional results, urodynamic features, complications and survival in 166 men. J Urol 2000;164:288-295.

[22] Elmajian DA, Stein JP, Esrig D, et al: The Kock ileal neobladder: Updated experience in 295 male patients. J Urol 1996; 156:920-925.

[23] Colwell JC, Fichera A: Care of the obese patient with an ostomy. J Wound Ostomy Continence Nurs 2005; 32:378-383.

[24] Gheiler EL, Wood DP Jr, Montie JE, et al: Orthotopic urinary diversion is a viable option in patients undergoing salvage cystoprostatectomy for recurrent prostate cancer after definitive radiation therapy. Urology 1997; 50:580-584.

[25] Bochner BH, Figueroa AJ, Skinner EC, et al: Salvage radical cystoprostatectomy and orthotopic urinary diversion following radiation failure. J Urol 1998; 160:29-33.

[26] Lebret T, Herve JM, Barre P, et al: Urethral recurrence of transitional cell carcinoma of the bladder. Predictive value of preoperative latero- montanal biopsies and urethral frozen sections during prostatocystectomy. Eur Urol 1998; 33:170-174.

[27] Chang SS, Alberts GL, Smith JA Jr, et al: Ileal conduit urinary diversion in patients with previous history of abdominal/pelvic irradiation. World J Urol 2004; 22:272-276.

[28] Albertini JJ, Sujka SK, Helal MA, et al: Adenocarcinoma in a continent colonic urinary reservoir. Urology 1998; 51:499-500.

[29] Pickard R: Tumour formation within intestinal segments transposed to the urinary tract. World J Urol 2004; 22:227-234.

[30] Oneeka W, Vereb M, Libertino J. Noncontinent urinary diversion. Urol Clin North Am. 1997; 24: 735-743

[31] Gburek B.M,Lieber M.M, Blute M.L. Comparison of studer ileal neobladder and ileal conduit urinary diversion with respect to perioperative outcome and late complications.J Urol. 1998; 160: 721-723

[32] Madersbacher S, Schmidt J, Eberle M.J, Thoeny H.C, Burkhard F, Hochreiter W, Studer E. Long-term outcome of ileal conduit diversion. J Urol. 2003; 169: 985-990.

[33] Shimko M, Tollefson M, Umbreit E, Farmer S, Blute M, Frank I. Long-Term Complications of Conduit Urinary Diversion. J Urol. 2011; 185: 562-567

[34] Bricker E. Bladder substitution after pelvic evisceration. J Urol. 2002; 167:1140-1145

[35] Hautmann R. Urinary diversion: ileal conduit to neobladder. J Urol. 2003; 169:834-842.

[36] Hall C, Koch M, McDouglas S. Metabolic Consequences of Urinary Diversion Through Intestinal Segment. Urol Clin North Am. 1991; 18: 725-735.

[37] Carroll P et all. Urinary Diversion & Bladder Substitution. Smith's General Urology 17th edition. Mc GrawHill.

[38] DownsT et all. Noncontinent and Continent Cutaneous Urinary Diversion. Urologic Oncology 2005. Elsevier.

[39] Richie J. Sigmoid Conduit Urinary Diversion. Urol Clin North Am. 1986; 13: 225-231.

[40] Beland G, laberge I. Cutaneous transureterostomy in children. J Urol. 1975; 114:588-590.

[41] Rainwater L, Leary F, Rife C. Transureteroureterostomy with cutaneous ureterostomy: a 25-year experience. J Urol. 1991; 146:13-15.

[42] Nieuwenhuijzen J, Vries R, Bex A, van der Poel H, Meinhardt W, Antonini N, Horenblas S. Urinary Diversion after Cystectomy: The Association of Clinical factors, Complications and Functional Results of Four Different Diversions. Eur Urol. 2008; 53:834-844.

[43] Olofsson G, Fjalling M, Kilander A, Ung k, Jonsson O. Bile acid malabsorption after continent urinary diversion with an ileal reservoir. J Urol. 1998; 160:724-727
[44] Terai A, Okada Y, Shichiri Y, Kakehi Y, Terachi T, Arai Y, Yoshida O. Vitamin B 12 Deficency in patients with Urinary Intestinal Diversion. Int J Urol. 1997; 4:21-25.
[45] Fitzgerald J, Malone M, Gaertner R, Zinman L. Stomal construction, complication, and reconstruction. Urol Clin North Am. 1997; 24: 729-733.
[46] Campbell-Walsh. *Urology.* (2007) Saunders IX Edition, Volume I
[47] Granberg CF et al. *Functional and oncological outcomes after orthotopic neobladder reconstruction in women.* BJU Int 2008; 102; 1551-1555
[48] Barre PH et al. *Update on the Camey II procedure.* World J Urol 1996; 14(1): 27-8
[49] Siracusano S. et Al. *Modified Ghoneim's technique using single serous-lined extramural orthotopic ileal W-bladder.* Eur Urol 2000; 38 : 313-5,
[50] Studer UE et al. *Orthotopic ileal neobladder.* BJU Int (2004) 93(1): 183-93
[51] Ghoneim MA et al. *An appliance-free, sphincter-controlled bladder substitute: the urethral Kock pouch.* J Urol 1987; 138(5): 1150-4
[52] Novara G et al. *Functional results following vescica ileale Padovana (VIP) neobladder: midterm follow-up analysis with validated questionnaires.* Eur Urol 2010; 57(6): 1045-51
[53] Stein JP et al. *The T pouch: an orthotopic ileal neobladder incorporating a serosal lined ileal antireflux technique.* J Urol 1998; 159(6): 1836-42
[54] Fontana D et al. *Y-neobladder: an easy, fast, and reliable procedure.* Urology. 2004; 63(4): 699-703
[55] Månsson W et al. *Continent urinary tract reconstruction - the Lund experience.* BJU Int. 2003; 92(3): 271-6
[56] Thuroff JW et al. *The Mainz pouch (mixed augmentation ileum 'n zecum) for bladder augmentation and continent urinary diversion. 1985.* Eur Urol 2006; 50(6): 1142-50
[57] Reddy PK. *The colonic neobladder.* Urol Clin North Am 1991; 18(4): 609-14
[58] Wyczolkowski M et al. *Studer orthotopic ileal bladder substitute construction – surgical techniqueand complication management: one center and 12-year experience.* Adv Med Sci 2010; 55(2); 146-15

Part 8

Future Treatments

The H19-IGF2 Role in Bladder Cancer Biology and DNA-Based Therapy

Imad Matouk[1,2,*] et al
[1]*Department of Biological Chemistry, Institute of Life Sciences, The Hebrew University of Jerusalem, Jerusalem*
[2]*Department of Biology, Science and Technology, Alquds Abu-Dis University, Jerusalem Israel*

1. Introduction

The H19-IGF2 locus within the imprinted cluster of the human chromosome 11, has been implicated in a variety of disorders and cancer pre-disposition including bladder cancer. BBN induced bladder cancer model in rats has identified both H19 and IGF2 among differentially expressed genes that are induced in response to carcinogen exposure.

In this chapter, the role of both H19 and IGF2 genes in cancer will be handled in general with special focus on bladder cancer. Although IGF2 role in human cancers is relatively well established, recent data from our laboratory and others have just revealed a critical role for H19 RNA in the process of tumorigenicity including that of the bladder. H19 functions as a stress modulator, being induced by hypoxia, and a survival factor that is involved in several fundamental processes of tumorigenesis. Furthermore, we uncovered a molecular mechanism that integrates H19, p53 and HIF1-α to hypoxic stress response. Placing the H19 gene product in this deadly circuit undoubtedly will have major impacts in its utility as a target for cancer gene therapy.

Regulatory sequences of both H19 and IGF2 have already been used to successfully target expression of a toxic protein, diphtheria toxin A (DT-A), in carcinoma cells in culture, in several xenograft, orthotopic animal models, and in chemically induced BBN model of bladder cancer. In case of H19, it is successfully used in patients with bladder carcinoma for a period of over 5 years and recently a clinical trial phase I/IIa using this therapeutic approach has been successfully completed. It is also successfully used in other types of human cancers but will not be handled in the current chapter.

We will discuss also novel approaches, to create a new family of plasmids. In one approach a cytotoxic gene is driven by two different regulatory sequences, selected from the cancer-specific promoters H19, IGF2-P3 and IGF2-P4 carried on a single construct. In a second

* Naveh Evantal[1], Doron Amit[1], Patricia Ohana[1], Ofer Gofrit[3], Vladimir Sorin[1], Tatiana Birman[1], Eitan Gershtain[1] and Abraham Hochberg[1]
[1]*Department of Biological Chemistry, Institute of Life Sciences, The Hebrew University of Jerusalem, Jerusalem, Israel*
[2]*Department of Biology, Science and Technology, Alquds Abu-Dis University, Jerusalem, Israel*
[3]*Department of Urology, Hadassah Hebrew University Medical Center, Jerusalem, Israel*

approach a single promoter is used to drive two cytotoxic genes having synergistic effect on a single construct. Both approaches show superior tumor growth inhibition activity, in preclinical studies of bladder cancer.
Bladder Cancer is the fourth most common cancer in men accounting for about 7% of all cancer cases and 3% of all cancer related mortality. Each year, more than 50,000 new patients are diagnosed with bladder cancer in the USA and about 10,000 die from this disease (Jemal et al., 2010). Carcinogens activity on a susceptible epithelium is believed to be the cause of bladder cancer. Many industrialized chemicals are causally related; benzidine, βnapthylamine, 4-aminobiphenyl, etc. However, the commonest cause of bladder cancer nowadays, is by far cigarette smoking accounting for about half of all bladder cancers (Burch et al., 1989). Whether bladder cancer arises from a single transformed cell (clonogenic theory) or from multiple transformed cells (field change theory), is still under debate.
Painless hematuria is the hallmark of bladder cancer. This dramatic symptom urgently brings the patient to see a doctor. Therefore, most bladder tumors are diagnosed during the lifetime of the patient. Bladder tumors can also present with irritative urinary symptoms (urinary urgency, frequency and dysuria). Bladder tumors can be diagnosed by ultrasonography, intravenous urography, or computerized tomography. The resolution of these radiologic techniques is low, and only a 5 to 10 mm lesion can be detected. Cystoscopy done by inserting an optical instrument into the bladder can diagnose bladder tumors as small as 1mm. Urinary cytology is an important adjunct to cystoscopy, especially for the diagnosis of the flat lesion carcinoma in-situ (CIS).
Most bladder tumors arise from the epithelial lining the urinary system-the transitional epithelium (urothelium), and are therefore, transitional cell carcinomas (or urothelial carcinomas). Bladder cancer is a heterogeneous disease with wide variations in molecular pathogenesis, morphology and prognosis. They are classified according to their depth of invasion into the bladder wall (stage) and according to the degree of histological anaplasia (grade).
As in most other types of cancer, it is believed that 4-6 DNA hits are required for malignant transformation (Duggan et al., 2004). These include deletions, mutations and loss of heterozygosity (LOH) of genetic material that carries tumor suppressor genes or proto-oncogenes, and epigenetic changes such as CpG methylations that modify gene expression. There are at least 2 major pathogenic pathways leading to 2 completely different bladder cancers. One pathway leads a low grade, papillary bladder cancer (about 75% of all bladder tumors). This type of tumor has a proliferative ability but no ability to invade the epithelial lamina propria and muscle of the bladder, to metastasize and to kill the patient. The second pathway leads to a high grade, solid tumor that has an invasive and metastatic potential (about 15% of the tumors). Possibly, there is a third pathway that leads to a high grade papillary tumor (about 10% of the tumors) (Goebell &Knowles, 2010). While low grade tumors tend to recur but almost never endanger the life of the patient, high grade tumors are often lethal.
It is believed that low grade tumors develop following this pathway: Urothelial hyperplasia→ urothelial atypia →low grade TCC. The most prominent molecular change in this group is mutation in FGFR3, found up to 88% of these tumors (van Rhijn et al., 2002). In most cases these are activation mutation that probably supports tumor proliferation by stimulating the RAS-MAPK pathway. The frequency of FGFR3 mutations in high grade tumors is much lower. Activation of the phosphatidylinositol 3-kinase (PI3K) pathway by a wide range of mechanisms is also typical to low grade tumors (Goebell &Knowles, 2010).

High grade bladder tumors develop following this pathway: Urothelial atypia →dysplasia → CIS →Invasive TCC→metastatic disease. The most prominent molecular changes in high grade tumors involve inactivation of the p53 and RB pathways. p53, whose activity is augmented in the presence of DNA damage, arrests cells at G1-S checkpoint by inducing the transcription of the CDK inhibitors-p21/Waf1, and GADD45. Then the cell may either correctly repair its DNA or undergo apoptosis. Deletions or mutations in the p53 pathway are found in about 70% of the high-grade tumors.

The Retinoblastoma gene codes for an 110kDa nuclear phosphoprotein acting as a tumor suppressor that also arrest cells at G1. It is often mutated by a truncating mutation of the carboxyl terminal. Mutations or deletions in Rb gene are found in 30% of the patients with advanced bladder cancers. They result in uncontrolled cellular proliferation even without mitogenic signals. Hypermethylation of the Rb promoter region can have the same effect. Similarly, loss of the cyclin dependent kinase inhibitor p16 either by mutation, deletion, or by promoter hypermethylation, as documented in 20-45% of the bladder cancers prevents Rb activation by hyper-phosphorylation, or leads to uncontrolled cell cycle progression (Schultz, 1998).

Epithelial to mesenchymal transition (EMT) is an important process typical to high grade tumors. It is characterized by down regulation of the adhesion molecule E-cadherin and of proteins associated with cell polarity along with up regulation of fibronectin, vimentin and matrix metalloproteases (MMPS). EMT is induced by cytokines like the TGFβ and is associated with increased invasion, migration and angiogenesis.

Alterations in chromosome 9 are the most common cytogenetic findings in bladder cancer. Of these, the most common are deletions and LOH in the short arm, home of the tumor suppressor genes and cell-cycle regulators CDKN2A (encoding for p16 and $p14^{ARF}$) and CDKN2B (encoding for p15). In a rather consistent manner high grade tumors demonstrate LOH of 3p, 8p, 13q, and 17p, while low grade tumors demonstrate LOH of chromosome 9 only (Knowles et al., 2001).

Animal models are critical in the understanding of bladder cancer pathogenesis and in the quest for new treatments. Most animal models in bladder cancer are in rodents. Although various models exist, we'll focus on carcinogen induced bladder cancer model.

1.1 Carcinogen induced bladder cancer in mice and rats

In this model, the rodent is given a carcinogen, most commonly in the drinking water. BBN (N -butyl-N- (4-hydroxybutyl) nitrosamine) is a carcinogen given to the rodents in a concentration of 0.05% in the drinking water. It induces bladder tumors in 95% of the rodents after 25 weeks of administration (Okada et al., 1975). The tumors produced by the carcinogen resemble human bladder cancer in histology, etiology, and in kinetics (25 rat weeks equal 10 human years- the believed incubation period of human bladder cancer). Molecular events occurring during chemical carcinogenesis can be followed (Ariel et al., 2004). Tumor development and the response to novel treatments can be assessed non-invasively, without scarifying the animal using ultrasonography (Gofrit et al., 2006). The main disadvantages of this model are necessity to handle a carcinogen and the long period required for tumor production.

In our lab we used this model to "fish up" genes involved in bladder tumorigenesis using microarray analyses. We identified both H19 and IGF2 among differentially expressed genes that are induced in response to carcinogen exposure (Elkin et al., 1998, Ariel et al., 2004)

In the following sections we will present the role of both H19 and IGF2 genes in tumorigenicity. Then we will discuss pre-clinical and clinical data for the successful treatment of bladder cancer by DNA-based drug developed in our laboratory based on both the H19 and IGF2 regulatory sequences to drive the expression of a toxic protein, diphtheria toxin A (DT-A). This approach also proved to be successful in other cancer types; ovarian (Mizrahi et al., 2010), prostate (submitted) in human patients, and pre-clinically under development in glioblastoma (under preparation), lung (Hasenpusch et al., 2011), and colorectal liver metastasis (Ohana et al., 2005). This chapter will focus only on bladder cancer. Pre-clinical data using novel approaches for the treatment of bladder cancer with improved cytotoxic effect will be presented as well.

2. The H19-IGF2 locus and tumorigenesis

The IGF2 and H19 genes are both located on the short arm of chromosome 11 and are reciprocally imprinted. Genomic imprinting of the IGF2 and H19 genes has been shown to play a role in the regulation of the IGF2 and H19 expressions during embryonic development and in cancer. The role of genomic imprinting in tumor development is not well understood and it is beyond the scope of this chapter. Over-expressions of H19 and IGF2 genes in many tumors may or may not be associated with loss of imprinting.

2.1 The pivotal role of H19 RNA in tumorigenesis

H19 is an oncofetal gene that expresses only RNA and not protein, being expressed in the embryo, repressed in the adult, and re-expressed in a variety of human tumors, for review (Matouk et al., 2005). *H19* is emerging as one of the key players in cancer biology. We and others have demonstrated an essential role of H19 RNA in tumor development, and the association and contribution of H19 RNA with various aspects of tumorigenic process. This contradicts the initial proposal that H19 gene product has a tumor suppressive activity (Hao et al., 1993).

Our strategy to delineate the role of H19 RNA in tumor development is based on determining if tumor development is dependent on H19 expression through both over-expression and knockdown approaches in different tumor models including bladder cancer. To shed light into its mechanism of action our strategy is based on identifying upstream effectors and also downstream targets by applying the global gene expression profiling to identify genes modulated by both H19 over-expression and knockdown. Here again bladder cancer model is included.

Our results, supported by results from others, reveal that H19 RNA harbors oncogenic properties, enhancing the development of carcinogenesis. In this section we'll present major findings that support this issue and highlight its relevance to bladder cancer where possible.

2.1.1 H19 RNA is essential for human tumor growth

Although H19 over-expression sometimes associated with loss of imprinting have been reported in a large arrays of human cancers, direct evidence of its tumorigenic role was lacking. Using two cell line models including bladder carcinoma, we provided evidences, that H19 is critical for tumor development. Our in vivo results show that bladder carcinoma formed from UMUC3 cells in which the H19 RNA have been knocked down , induce a very significant retardation of tumor growth. Similar results were reproduced using other carcinoma model (Matouk et al., 2007).

Moreover we showed that ectopic H19 expression enhances the tumorigenic potential of bladder carcinoma cells in vivo. Tumors induced from T24P bladder carcinoma cell line ectopically over-expressing H19 RNA, differ significantly in their growth properties and growth kinetics in vivo relative to the control, and are well vascularized with evidences of tumor hemorrhage (Matouk et al., 2007). H19 RNA also enhances entry to S-phase of the cell cycle of bladder cancer cells under serum starved condition, but not under normal cell culture condition (Ayesh et al., 2002). Further supports for the tumorigenic properties have been reported in other cancer models. H19 over-expression of ectopic origin confers a proliferative advantage for breast epithelial cells in a soft agar assay and in several combined immunodeficient mice (Lottin et al., 2002). c-Myc induces the expression of the H19 RNA. c-Myc binds to the E-boxes near the imprinting control region to facilitate histone acetylation and transcriptional initiation of the H19 gene, to potentiate tumorigenesis (Barsyte-Lovejoy et al., 2006). The H19 is reported to be a target gene for the hepatocyte growth factor (HGF), further signifying the potential role of H19 RNA in hepatocellular carcinoma development (Adriaenssens et al, 2002). Furthermore, H19 RNA is important for entry into S-phase after serum starvation recovery by E2F binding to its promoter (Berteaux et al, 2005). Recently, it was reported that the Retinoblastoma tumor suppressor gene is a target gene for miR-675 which is produced from exon-1 of the H19 gene (Tsang et al., 2010).

2.1.2 H19 is induced by hypoxia – the P53 brakes and the HIF-1α engine

It is well established that every solid tumor encounters hypoxic regions beyond certain diameters. Hypoxia is a major trigger for tumor angiogenesis, metastasis, chemo-resistance and also associated with poor prognosis at least in some types of human cancers. All of these conditions as discussed below are associated with an increase of H19 RNA expression.
Over-expression of *H19* RNA, is accompanied with up-regulation of a 95 kDa membrane glycoprotein (p95) observed in a variant of breast and lung carcinomas that are multi- drug resistance (Doyle et al., 1996). Moreover, results show that the level of H19 RNA is elevated in the multidrug resistance variant of HCC cell lines. Here doxorubicin resistance phenotype is related to H19 over-expression (Tsang et al., 2007).
H19 provides a novel and clinically useful diagnostic marker for prognosticating human bladder carcinoma. More striking is the predictive value of H19 for tumor recurrence. We have found that in transitional cell carcinoma of the bladder with tumors that express H19 in most cells have shorter median disease-free survivals (Ariel et al., 2000).
We have identified downstream targets modulated by H19 over-expression in the T24P bladder carcinoma cell line (Ayesh et al., 2002); comparing the m-RNA levels of many genes between cells containing high levels of H19 RNA (from H19 expressing plasmid) to that of the same cells lacking H19 RNA, showed a clear preference towards genes promoting cellular migration, angiogenesis and metastasis.
All of these observations prompted us to explore the effect of hypoxia on H19 expression and to delineate the mechanism of action involved. Indeed, under hypoxic conditions, we have reported that in bladder carcinoma cell lines T24P and UMUC3, and hepatocellular carcinoma cell line Hep3B the H19 RNA is significantly elevated (Matouk et al., 2007).
Following these initial studies we screened about thirty different carcinomas cell lines of different lineages and origins for their ability to induce H19 RNA in hypoxic stress (Matouk et al., 2010). We observed very different patterns of response to hypoxia. To gain insight into

the possible mechanism associated with the H19 response to hypoxia, we searched for a common denominator among these cell lines.

It is well established today that the tumor suppressor signaling pathway of p53 can be activated by stress signals such as hypoxic stress and can either trans-activate or trans-repress its target genes to influence the cellular response. The key processes regulated by p53 pathway include cell cycle arrest, apoptosis, DNA repair, senescence, metastasis and angiogenesis, depending on cell types, nature of the inducer, cell intrinsic environment, and the activities of other signal transduction pathways. These observations suggests a possible association between the status of p53 (wild type or mutant) and H19 responsiveness to hypoxic stress. Moreover the involvement of the wild type tumor suppressor gene p53 in the down regulation of the H19 promoter activity which lacks a p53 consensus site and a TATA box was previously shown by (Dugimont et al., 1998). Taking all of these observations into account and the availability of IARC TP53 mutation database, we explored the possible involvement of p53 in determining H19's behavior in hypoxic response.

We recently demonstrated a tight correlation between *H19* RNA elevation by hypoxia and the status of the p53 tumor suppressor. In cells harboring wild type p53 ($p53^{wt}$) *H19* RNA is not induced upon hypoxia, whereas in cells carrying a mutated p53 ($p53^{mt}$) the *H19* message is significantly induced most strongly in p53-null cells. Furthermore through both over-expression and knockdown approaches we identified HIF1-α as the factor that is responsible for H19 elevation under hypoxic stress (Matouk et al., 2010).

H19 functions, consequently, as a stress modulator and a survival factor and is involved in several fundamental processes, including epithelial-mesenchymal transition (EMT), malignant transformation, cell-cycle transition, metastasis and neo-angiogenesis. EMT is an important process on the way to the malignant phenotype; notably- H19 up-regulation occurs in the stroma as well as in the epithelium. In the metastatic tumor stage, which bears a striking similarity to the embryonic stage, H19 involvement appears to be essential: adherent and cohesive cells lose their anchorage, migrate under stressful conditions to remote sites and replicate with neovascular support. Thus, H19 is a central figure in the cancer embryonic shift (Matouk et al., 2008).

In the light of our study, a molecular mechanism that integrates H19, p53 and HIF1-α to hypoxic stress response is uncovered. As hypoxia readily occurs in the majority of solid tumors driving critical steps in tumor development and metastasis and resistance to therapeutic modalities, placing the H19 gene product in this deadly circuit undoubtedly will have major impacts in its utility as a target for cancer gene therapy. Indeed a DNA-based drug depending on H19 regulatory sequence and diphtheria toxin is now in clinical trial with promising results (Ohana et al., 2004, Sidi et al., 2008, Mizrahi et al., 2010). We'll concentrate on bladder cancer.

2.1.3 Targetted therapy for bladder cancer mediated by a plasmid expressing DTA under the control of H19 regulatory sequences – clinical data

During the past few years we have developed a DNA based therapy strategies for treating tumors expressing H19 RNA. The successful development of anti-tumor gene therapy depends on the use of a combinatorial approach aimed at targeted delivery and specific expression of effective anti-tumor agents. We exploit the unique H19 transcriptional regulatory sequences for directing tumor-selective expression of toxins. For this purpose we use non-viral vectors due to their potential to circumvent the main disadvantage of adenoviral vectors, caused by immune responses directed against adenovirus proteins which limit their ability to be administered iteratively. As a toxic gene, we used the diphtheria toxin A chain (DT-A), which has suitable properties for achieving efficacious cancer cell killing. DT-A peptide catalyzes ADP-ribosylation at the dipthamide residue of the cellular translation elongation factor 2 (eEF-2), inhibiting protein synthesis and causing cell death. While a very low level of DT-A expression suffices for cell killing, DT-A released from the lysed cells is not able to enter the neighboring cells in the absence of the DT-B chain.

All preclinical studies needed to set up the stage for using this approach to treat bladder cancer patients will not be handled in this chapter, and are reviewed elsewhere (Matouk et al., 2005).

Clinical studies

The goals of treatment are to reduce tumor recurrence, decrease the risk of disease progression, avoid cystectomy (bladder sparing treatment), and improve survival. Preventing progression to muscle invasive disease is of key importance because even with aggressive treatment, including radical cystectomy, as few as 50% of patients with muscle invasive disease will survive 5 years (Dalbagni et al., 2001).

The primary factors that influence risk of disease progression include: 1. the number of tumors at primary diagnosis; 2. recurrence rate in a previous period or an early recurrence at 3 months after the first resection; 3. size of the tumor (tumors larger than 3 cm are more likely to recur than smaller tumors); and stage and grade of the tumor.

The initial clinical development plan for DTA-H19/PEI for bladder cancer is in the intermediate-risk patient population who has failed prophylactic therapy with either BCG or chemotherapy. In the Phase 1/2a study, the safety and preliminary efficacy was examined in this population. Having determined that the highest dose tested in this trial, the 20 mg dose of DTA-H19, was well tolerated and elicited complete responses in 2 of 5 evaluable patients, the Phase 2b clinical protocol will assess the safety of this regimen in a larger patient population as well as the efficacy in a marker tumor clinical trial design.

Compassionate Use in Bladder Cancer. Two patients had recurrent superficial TCC of the bladder and had failed multiple courses of Bacille Calmette-Guérin (BCG) and chemotherapy, and two additional patients that underwent nephrourectomy due to a diagnosis of recurrent superficial TCC that showed BCG intolerance.

The investigations in the first two bladder cancer patients demonstrated that intravesical instillation of DTA-H19/PEI is safe up to a dose of 5 mg in a single administration or a cumulative dose of 70 mg intravesically. No local or systemic adverse effects considered attributable to DTA-H19 treatment were observed throughout treatment. In addition, DTA-H19 DNA was not detectable in the circulation by PCR analysis of blood samples taken after the first and second week of treatment, and 2 hours after plasmid administration. DTA-H19 DNA was detectable in a tumor biopsy taken 18 hours after intravesical administration and in voided urine for 1 week after treatment. Tumor regression (75% reduction in marker tumor size) was observed in marker tumors of both patients. One of the 2 compassionate patients was treated over a nearly 5 year period with 22 intravesical administrations of either a 2 mg or 4 mg dose of DTA-H19/PEI for a cumulative dose of 70 mg of plasmid DNA. Treatments were well tolerated, and although the marker tumor persisted, it did not increase in size, stage or grade during the 14-month period before it was finally resected along with one other new low grade papillary tumor. No increase in stage or grade of TCC was observed.

The patient that had a nephroureterectomy due to a diagnosis of high-grade TCC in the renal pelvis was treated with 6 weekly 10 mg injections of DTA-H19/PEI via the left nephrostome at a total volume of 15 ml each. After completion of the 6 plasmid infusions the patient underwent nephroscopy that revealed the following: renal pelvis with no presence of tumors and several papillary tumors on the left bladder wall in the trigon. Findings were biopsied, analyzed, and diagnosed as low grade TCC. Four months later, the patient underwent nephrography during which no tumors were observed. Urine cytology confirmed the absence of tumor cells.

There were no significant events or side effects throughout the patient's treatments. Overall, this was a good tumor response in a patient with only one kidney who was considered to be anephric and with dialysis during the last year. The treatment was well-tolerated by the patient, and there was no evidence of any negative systemic or urinary tract effect. During the treatments, the patient was fully functional, continued to work, and did not suffer any effect to his quality of life (QOL). The second patient that had nephroureteterectomy had multiple recurrences with the appearance of multi-focal lesions in the bladder. The patient underwent additional resection of a number of lesions that were localized inside and on the walls of the bladder. Since the patient was not a candidate to receive BCG treatment due to his compromised immune system, and after being refractory to Mitomycin C or Synergo, and refusal to undergo cystectomy, he was offered treatment with DTA-H19/PEI. He was treated with 20 mg of DTA-H19/PEI twice a week for the period of 4 weeks and once a week for another 2 weeks. Cytoscopy conducted at the end of the treatment showed an improvement in the number of lesions and in the general appearance of the bladder. The histological diagnosis of the biopsy showed low grade Ta.

Phase 1/2a Clinical Trial in Conventional Treatment Refractory Bladder Cancer Patients. A Phase 1/2a clinical trial was designed to determine the maximum tolerated dose (MTD) and assess the safety and preliminary efficacy of 5 different doses (2 mg, 4 mg, 6 mg, 12 mg, and 20 mg of DTA-H19) of DTA-H19/PEI given as 6 intravesical infusions into the bladder of patients with superficial bladder cancer (stages Ta and carcinoma *in situ* (CIS)) who had failed intravesical therapy with BCG. Patients had a diagnosis of superficial Stage Ta or CIS, grade 1 or 2 superficial bladder cancer that was confirmed by histopathology and that expressed H19 which was shown by *in situ* hybridization (ISH). Treatments were given weekly for 3 weeks followed 1 week later by safety and disease assessments, then another 3 weekly instillations were performed. Each dose cohort received the same dose for all treatments. Doses were escalated if none of the first 3 patients in the preceding dose cohort experienced a dose-limiting toxicity (DLT) after the first 3 weekly intravesical treatments. A DLT was defined as any grade 3 or greater toxicity by the National Cancer Institute Common Terminology Criteria for Adverse Events (NCI-CTCAE) that was considered to be related to the investigational product during the first 3 weekly intravesical treatments. Prior to initiating treatment, papillary tumors were resected leaving a single marker tumor. Videocystoscopy was performed 4, 8, and 12 weeks after the start of treatment for a safety evaluation of the bladder and also to record the presence or absence of the marker tumor and any other lesions suspicious for TCC of the bladder. If the marker tumor was still present at the Week 12 assessment, it was to be resected. If any new lesions were observed at Week 12, they were also to be resected. Patients whose disease had not progressed (i.e., no new tumors, increase in the size of the marker tumor by at least 50%, or increase in stage or any grade 3) were offered continued once monthly treatments and follow-up for up to 1 year.

A total of 18 patients were enrolled in this study. No DLTs were observed in this study. As the highest dose of product tested was the 20 mg dose of DTA-H19/PEI, this dose was considered the MTD for this study. The most frequently reported adverse events (AEs) considered at least possibly related to investigational products for any dose cohort were mild to moderate in severity and were most commonly renal and urinary disorders.

Of the 18 patients evaluable for tumor response at Week 12, a total of 4 patients had a complete response (CR) [complete disappearance of the marker tumor and no recurrence) including 2 of the 3 patients in the 2 mg dose cohort, and 2 of 6 patients in the 20 mg dose cohort. In addition, 2 patients (one in each of the 2 mg and 12 mg dose groups) had an incomplete partial response [IPR - complete disappearance of the marker tumor but with new tumor(s) occurring] suggesting that DTA-H19/PEI did have an effect on these marker tumors as well. Other responses included 1 partial response (PR - reduction in size of marker tumor by 50% and no new tumors present) (12 mg dose cohort) and 5 patients with SD (marker tumor still present but has not increased in size by more than 50% and no new tumors) (3 patients in the 4 mg dose cohort, 1 patient in the 12 mg dose cohort, and 1 patient in the 20 mg dose cohort). Thus, in this small study, there was evidence of tumor ablation over the dose range from 2 to 20 mg of DTA-H19/PEI. The 20 mg dose of DTA-H19/PEI was selected for evaluation in the Phase 2b clinical trial because this dose had an acceptable safety profile, showed objective tumor responses, and as the mechanism of action of DTA-H19/PEI is tumor-specific cytotoxicity, theoretically the highest safe dose has the greatest likelihood of an efficacious outcome.

2.2 Insulin-like growth factor 2 (IGF2) and tumorigenesis

IGF2 expression is driven by four different promoters (P1-P4) that produce 4 different transcripts all of which give rise to the same mature protein, a 67-amino acid polypeptide. The four promoters are activated in a development-dependent and tissue-specific manner. In fetal liver, promoters P2–P4 are active, of which P3 is the most active promoter, and promoter P1 is inactive. However, in liver tissue, shortly after birth, the IGF2 promoter P1 is exclusively active. The imprinting of the human IGF2 gene is promoter-specific. The P2, P3 and P4 promoters display monoallelic activity in embryonic, neonatal and postnatal liver specimens, whereas in adult, P1 is transcribed from both alleles.

The IGF2 peptide is a member of the insulin-like growth-factor family and is known to play an important role in the growth and differentiation of various tissues (Rechler 1990). This family also includes IGF1, insulin and relaxin. IGF2 is released to the extracellular fluid where it interacts with different cell membrane receptors and binding proteins. IGF2 binds three different types of receptors: IGF type 1 (IGF-1R), insulin receptor (IR) and IGF-2/mannose 6-phospate receptors (IGF-2R/M6P). The receptors, however, differ completely in structure and function (Yu and Rohan 2000). Ligand binding to IGF-1R and IR mediates mitogenic and anti-apoptotic effects. IGF-2R/M6P has tumor suppressor function and it mediates IGF2 degradation (Morison and Reeve 1998, Randhawa and Cohen 2005).

IGF2 can promote different functions depending on the cell type in which it is acting, and is a strong mitogen for a wide variety of cancer cell lines. It acts on the cell division cycle (DNA replication and mitosis) and on the cell growth (cellular enlargement), possibly by interfering with control cell checkpoint proteins. Moreover, IGF2 functions as an anti-

apoptotic agent. For example, it blocks c-Myc and SV40 T-antigen induced apoptosis in Raf-1 fibroblast cells (Ishii et al., 1993, Morali et al., 2000).
The mitogenic and metabolic actions of IGF2 in embryonic development and tumorigenesis are mediated by the IGF-1R and/or IR-A and are tightly regulated at different levels. These levels include the IGF-receptors availability, IGF2 interaction with its receptors and binding proteins (IGFBPs) and its degradation following internalization of the IGF2 after binding to its receptor, especially IGF-2R. Moreover, the IGF2 mRNA and protein levels are regulated by different ways. Any abnormality at one or more of these levels can be correlated to tumorigenesis. Over-expression of growth factors, or their receptors is a common event in malignancy and provides the underlying mechanisms for one of the hallmarks of cancer, namely uncontrolled proliferation (Hanahan and Weinberg 2000).
Transgenic mice, over-expressing the IGF2 gene, developed spontaneous tumors at a high frequency (Bates et al., 1995, Moorehead et al., 2003, Rogler et al., 1994), suggesting that over-expressed IGF2 may be involved not only in the progression of tumors but also in the initiation of neoplasia. IGF2 over-expression is significantly correlated to the increased tumor progression and proliferative activity as well as to decreased patient survival (Kawamoto et al., 1998, Rogler et al., 1994, Takanami et al., 1996)
Several mechanisms can potentially result in IGF2 over-expression in cancer, including, loss of imprinting (LOI) of the maternal allele, loss of heterozygosity (LOH) with paternal duplication, amplification of the IGF2 gene and abnormally activated signaling pathway leading to transcriptional up-regulation of the active alleles reviewed by (Hahn et al., 2000). IGF2 imprinting is relaxed in many different types of tumors, including bladder cancer (Byun et al., 2007).
The link between IGF2 and metastasis may be the basis for the identification of IGF2 and IGF-IR as predictors of poor outcome in many types of cancer.
In the rat model of bladder cancer induced by BBN, we observed over-expression of igf2 in the tumor, relative to the low level of expression in the normal tissue (Ariel et al., 2004).
Moreover we detected high levels of IGF2 mRNA expression from P3, P4 or both promoters in TCC samples. Whereas normal bladder samples showed no expression from either promoter. The human IGF2-P3 and IGF2-P4 promoters are highly active in bladder carcinoma. We showed that these constructs were able to selectively kill tumor cell lines and inhibit tumor growth in-vitro and in-vivo in accordance to the transcriptional activity of the above-mentioned regulatory sequences, when they are used to drive the expression of DTA (Ayesh et al., 2003, Amit et al., 2011).

3. Double promoter vectors: Novel approaches for the treatment of bladder cancer with improved cytotoxic effect

3.1 Double promoter DTA-expressing vectors

We have shown that IGF2 or H19 are significantly expressed in 50-84% of human bladder carcinoma respectively (Elkin et al, 1995) but not in normal bladder. Whereas combined expression (e.g. H19 and IGF2-P3/P4) was detected at high levels in nearly 100% of human bladder cancer samples. By that proving that the double promoter vectors are suitable for treating all bladder cancer patients. P3 and P4 were able to express the DTA in tumor cells in vitro, and inhibited tumor growth of mice heterotopic model, proving that both promoters could be used successively, in addition to H19 promoter, as part of the double promoter constructs (Ayesh et al., 2003, Amit et al., 2010, Amit et al., 2011).

Double promoter expressing vectors were created, carrying on a single construct two separate DNA sequences expressing the diphtheria toxin A-fragment (DTA), from two different regulatory sequences, selected from cancer-specific promoters H19, IGF2-P3 and IGF2-P4. This novel approach, create a new family of plasmids regulated by two regulatory sequences, which in their natural genome position are both proximately located and are reciprocally imprinted.

These vectors were then used to transfect and to eradicate tumor cells in culture or to inhibit tumor growth (*in vivo*), in heterotopic and orthotopic CD1 nude mice, bladder tumor models.

The activity of the double promoter vectors was tested and compared to the activity of the single promoter vectors. The double promoter vectors exhibited superior activity compared to the single promoter vectors. Furthermore, an augmented-than-additive activity was exhibited, compared to combination activity of the single promoter vectors, in cell lines and in heterotopic bladder cancer mice (Amit et al., 2010, Amit et al., 2011).

3.2 A single promoter driving two cytotoxic genes with synergistic effect

Because it is unlikely that gene transfer reaches every cell of a cancer, DNA based therapy approaches are thought to require the induction of a 'bystander' effect. An interesting approach for this purpose is cytokine DNA based therapy. TNF-α is a multifunctional and immuno-regulatory cytokine that exhibits direct tumor cell cytotoxicity, possesses anti-angiogenic properties, and enhances antitumor immunity by activating immune cells such as dendritic cells and T cells. Systemic delivery of the TNF-α protein has had limited success clinically because of severe dose limiting toxic effects. This limitation can be overcome by the use of a gene delivery approach, combined with a tumor specific promoter to express TNF-α in the tumor tissue.

In this approach, an enhanced cytotoxic effect could be achieved that could also overcome the resistance developed by tumor cells to either one of the toxin. It was reported that several cell lines - none are bladder cancer- are resistant to Diphtheria toxin and therefore would not be affected by the pH19-DTA vector. Adding TNF-α to the existing system was in agreement with supporting evidence of some publications showing a synergistic effect in cell cytotoxicity mediated by TNF-α and diphtheria toxin. This was shown on ovarian cancer cell lines- sensitive or resistant to both diphtheria toxin and TNF-α and on renal cell carcinoma cell lines (Morimoto et al., 1991, Mizutani et al., 1994). Using a construct in which both TNF-α and DTA expressions are driven by H19 tumor specific promoter, would overcome the dose limiting toxic effects of the systemic delivery of TNF-α protein.

So, we investigated a plasmid carrying, in addition to DTA, the gene for human hTNF-α. The pH19-TNF-IRES-DTA plasmid was built while the construct carries a viral IRES sequence (from the ECMV virus) 3' of the TNF. This IRES construct is 619 pb long and responsible the synthesis of DTA from the m-RNA transcript.

3.2.1 Synergistic effect in the killing activity of DTA and TNF in vitro using different cell line models

In vitro the cytotoxic effect in cells treated with the pH19-TNF-IRES-DTA plasmid was determined by luciferase assay (Ohana et al., 2004). To test for potency of this construct, cells

were also treated with a plasmid carrying either the DTA or TNF under the control of the H19 promoter. Cells from human, mouse and rat origin expressing H19 RNA were co-transfected with 2 µg/well of LucSV40 and the indicated concentrations of pH19-DTA, pH19-TNF or pH19-TNF-IRES-DTA plasmids. Luciferase activity was determined and compared to that of cells transfected with LucSV40 alone (**Figure 1**). In order to rule out the possibility of a false positive result due to the combined plasmid's structure effect, we reversed the TNF sequence in the pH19-TNF-IRES-DTA plasmid to eliminate the expression of TNF (pH19-TNFrev-IRES-DTA). The killing potency of the pH19-TNF-IRES-DTA plasmid was significantly higher compared to the pH19-DTA plasmid alone, even at very low concentrations. As the concentrations got higher the difference was diminished (**Figure 1**).
It should be noted that the use of the pH19-DTA plasmid alone was sufficient to cause a substantial decrease in luciferase activity, leading to 80-90% decrease in high concentrations, whereas the use of pH19-TNF alone showed little decrease, if any, and in some cases even an increase. When expressed in conjunction with the DTA domain, it clearly enhances cell death.

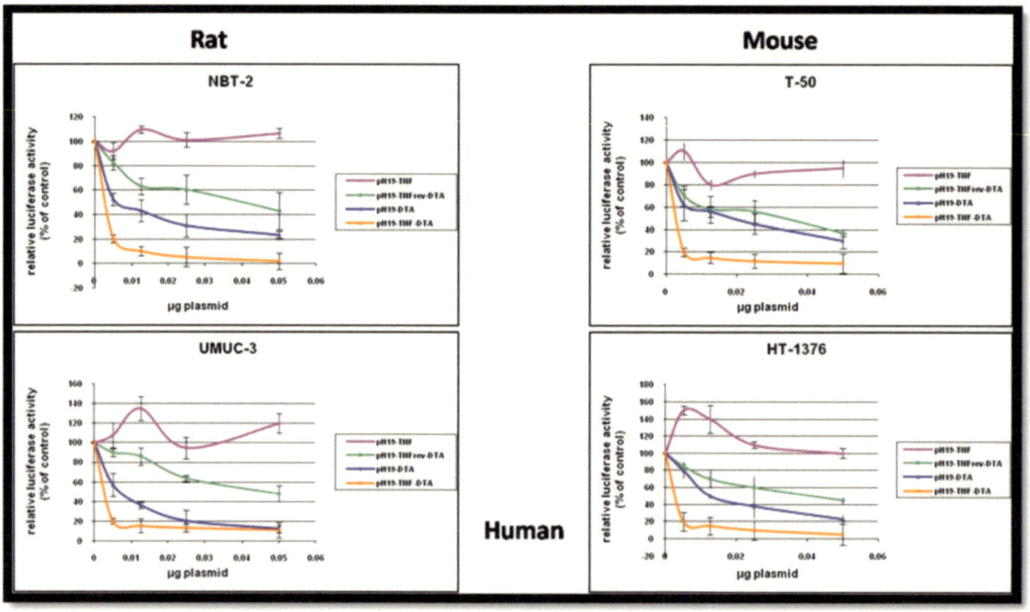

Fig. 1. Enhanced killing activity of pH19-TNF-IRES-DTA vector in different bladder carcinoma cell lines.

The killing potential of the pH19-DTA (blue), pH19-TNF (pink) or pH19-TNF-IRES-DTA(orange) vectors in human UMUC-3 and HT-1376, mouse T-50 and rat NBT-II was measured as a reduction of luciferase activity induced by LucSV40. Cells were co-transfected with 2 µg/well of LucSV40 and the indicated concentrations of pH19-DTA, or pH19-TNFa, or pH19-TNF-IRES-DTA. The pH19-TNFrev-IRES-DTA(green) served as a control.

3.2.2 In-vivo tumor growth inhibition by the pH19-DTA, pH19-TNF or pH19-TNF-IRES-DTA vectors in a carcinogen rat bladder cancer model

In vivo we utilize the carcinogen (BBN) induced rat bladder cancer model. Rats were treated with the above mentioned plasmids used in the in-vitro studies. An additional control

plasmid carrying the gene of Luciferase under the regulation of the H19 promoter (pH19-Luc) was included.
The therapeutic plasmid was given at two different times in order to investigate the correlation of the treatment efficiency to the severity and invasiveness of the disease. In the first, the plasmid treatments started after the rats received BBN for 20 weeks. By this time, the rats had developed visible tumors is their bladders. In the second, the plasmid treatment started only 16 weeks after the beginning of BBN administration in which tumors were visible only by histopathological examination.

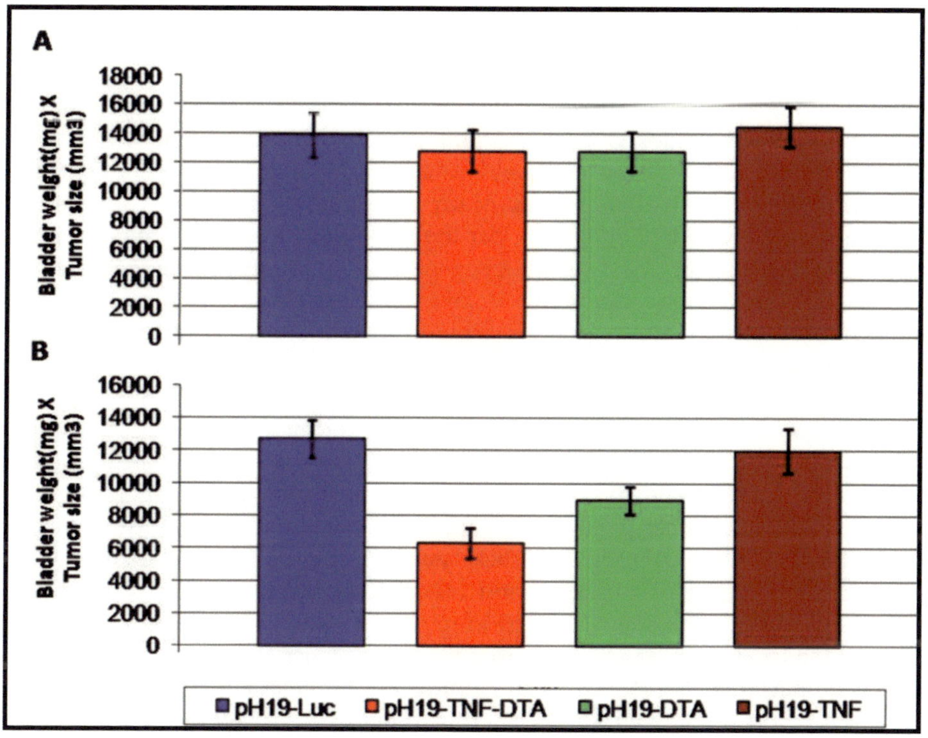

Fig. 2. Enhanced killing activity of pH19-TNF-IRES-DTA vector in the BBN rat bladder cancer model depending on time schedule of the treatments.

Tumor index (volume X weight) of rat's bladders as measured after treatment with three injections of pH19-DTA(green), pH19-TNF(brown) or pH19-TNF-IRES-DTA(red), and pH19-Luc(blue). A. Results of tumor index of rat's bladders which started treatments after 20 weeks. B. Results of tumor index of rat's bladders which started treatments after 16 weeks.

Each rat, in both experiments and in each group, received intravesical injection of 50 µg of the plasmid administered 3 times with an interval of 3 days between treatments. Four days after the last treatment, all rats were sacrificed and bladders were removed, weighed, photographed, excised and taken either for histological analysis or for DNA/RNA preparation. Tumor index was derived as mentioned. **Figure 2** shows the results of the in vivo experiments, where rats were treated from these two time points and onward.
We decided to try and estimate the tumor's volume by picturing each tumor at several angles, allowing us to use image analysis software in order to receive a reasonable

estimation. This was multiplied by the bladder's weight in order to give us a new, more comprehensive index of the tumor's status. It can be seen in the results that when starting the treatments after 20 weeks of BBN administration, virtually no effect is achieved in any of the plasmids. On the other hand, starting the treatments after 16 weeks showed a remarkable inhibition of tumor progression compared to the control. When administrated with pH19-DTA the tumor was delayed by approximately 30%, while when using the pH19-TNF-IRES-DTA vector about 50% inhibition was measured. No effect was seen when pH19-TNF was used. These results suggest that when treatment begins in an early stage it can be a highly potent one.

4. Concluding remarks and future perspectives

Our ability to understand the biology of bladder cancer at the molecular level utilizing the ever growing biotechnologies is an important step for understanding a wide range of signaling events in both healthy cells and in the context of carcinogenesis. Substantial progress has been made in this avenue. Many new genes that are involved in bladder carcinogenesis have been identified. It is clear the H19-IGF2 locus is playing a central role in this aspect. As the role of IGF2 in embryogenesis and tumorigenesis is relatively well understood, H19 as a stress modulator is recently emerging to be involved in several fundamental processes of tumorigenesis including that of the bladder. Yet the exact molecular mechanisms that integrate H19 to such diverse events and circuits that are malfunctioning in cancer need further investigations.

In our lab, different regulatory sequences, selected from cancer-specific promoters of H19, IGF2-P3 and IGF2-P4 linked to the potent toxin (DTA), have been successfully used to drive cytotoxicity to cancer cells in vitro, in vivo, in different tumor models, and more importantly in bladder cancer patients, at least in the case of H19, with promising results. Similar approaches are also used in other types of human cancers including ovarian, hepatocellular, and pancreatic cancers and are clinically encouraging. Preclinically, this approach also shows promising results in lung cancer, glioblastoma and colorectal cancer metastasis to the liver. We are working on novel approaches to increase the cytotoxicity of the therapeutic plasmids, and to increase the numbers of patients that can benefit from this therapy. Furthermore, and given the central role of hypoxia and also p53 in the resistance of conventional therapeutic options and the involvement of the IGF2-H19 locus, we are developing sequential treatments of the therapeutic plasmids with conventional chemotherapeutic drugs with encouraging results. Moreover, the preclinical utility of short interfering RNA to knockdown both H19 and IGF2 is under development.

5. Acknowledgement

We thank BioCancell Therapeutic for financial support. Additional support was provided through the grant from Phillip Morris.

6. References

Adriaenssens, E. Lottin, S. Berteaux, N. Hornez, L. Fauquette, W. et al. (2002) Cross-talk between mesenchyme and epithelium increases H19 gene expression during scattering and morphogenesis of epithelial cells. *Exp Cell Res* 275:215-229.

Amit, D. & Hochberg, A. (2010) Development of targeted therapy for bladder cancer mediated by a double promoter plasmid expressing diphtheria toxin under the control of H19 and IGF2-P4 regulatory sequences. *J Transl Med.* 8:134-152.

Amit, D. Tamir, S. Birman, T. Gofrit, ON. & Hochberg, A. (2011) Development of targeted therapy for bladder cancer mediated by a double promoter plasmid expressing diphtheria toxin under the control of IGF2-P3 and IGF2-P4 regulatory sequences. *Int J Clin Exp Med.* 4:91-102.

Ariel, I. Sughayer, M. Fellig, Y. Pizo, G. Ayesh, S. et al. (2000) The imprinted H19 gene is a marker of early recurrence in human bladder carcinoma. *Mol Pathol* 53: 320-323.

Ariel, I. Ayesh, S. Gofrit, O. Ayesh, B. Abdul-Ghani, R. et al. (2004) Gene expression in the bladder carcinoma rat model. *Mol Carcinog* 41: 69-76.

Ayesh, B. Matouk, I. Ohana, P. Sughayer, MA. Birman, T. et al. (2003) Inhibition of tumor growth by DT-A expressed under the control of IGF2 P3 and P4 promoter sequences. *Mol Ther.* 2003 7:535-41.

Ayesh, S. Matouk, I. Schneider, T. Ohana, P. Laster, M. et al. (2002) Possible physiological role of H19 RNA. *Mol Carcinog* 35: 63-74.

Barsyte-Lovejoy, D. Lau, SK. Boutros, PC. Khosravi, F. Jurisica, I. et al. (2006) The c-Myc oncogene directly induces the H19 noncoding RNA by allele-specific binding to potentiate tumorigenesis. *Cancer Res* 66: 5330-5337.

Bates, P. Fisher, R. Ward, A. Richardson, L. Hill, DJ. Et al. (1995) Mammary cancer in transgenic mice expressing insulin-like growth factor II (IGF-II). *Br J Cancer* 72: 1189-1193.

Berteaux, N. Lottin, S. Monte, D. Pinte, S. Quatannens, B. et al. (2005) H19 mRNA-like noncoding RNA promotes breast cancer cell proliferation through positive control by E2F1. *J Biol Chem* 280: 29625-26636.

Burch, JD. Rohan, TE. Howe, GR. Risch, HA. Hill, GB. et al. (1989) Risk of bladder cancer by source and type of tobacco exposure: a case-control study. *Int J Cancer* 44: 622-628.

Byun, HM. Wong, HL. Birnstein, EA. Wolff, EM. Liang, G. et al. (2007) Examination of IGF2 and H19 loss of imprinting in bladder cancer. *Cancer Res* 67: 10753-10758.

Clemmons, DR. Busby, WH. Arai, T. Nam, TJ. Clarke, JB. et al. (1995) Role of insulin-like growth factor binding proteins in the control of IGF actions. *Prog Growth Factor Res* 6: 357-366.

Dalbagni, G. et al. (2001) Cystectomy for bladder cancer: a contemporary series. *J Urol* 165: 1111-1116.

Doyle, LA. Yang, W. Rishi, AK. Gao, Y. & Ross, DD. (1996) H19 gene overexpression in atypical multidrug-resistant cells associated with expression of a 95-kilodalton membrane glycoprotein. *Cancer Res* 56: 2904-2907.

Duggan, BJ. Gray, SB. McKnight, JJ. Watson, CJ. Johnston, SR. et al. (2004) Oligoclonality in bladder cancer: the implication for molecular therapies. *J Urol* 171: 419-25.

Dugimont, T. Montpellier, C. Adriaenssens, E. Lottin, S. Dumont, L. et al. (1998) The H19 TATA-less promoter is efficiently repressed by the wild- type tumor suppressor gene product p53. *Oncogene* 16: 2395-2401.

Elkin, M. Shevelev, A. Schulze, E. Tyckocinsky, M. Cooper, M. et al. (1995) The expression of the H19 and IGF-2 genes in human bladder carcinoma. *FEBS Lett* 374: 57-61.

Elkin, M. Ayesh, S. Schneider, T. de Groot, N. Hochberg, A. et al. (1998) The dynamics of the imprinted H19 gene expression in the mouse model of bladder carcinoma induced by N-Butyl-N-(4-hydroxybutyl)nitrosamine.*Carcinogenesis*19:2095-99

Goebell, PJ. & Knowles, MA. (2010) Bladder cancer or bladder cancers? Genetically distinct malignant conditions of the urothelium. *Urol Oncol* 28: 409-28.

Gofrit, ON. Birman, T. Dinaburg, A. Ayesh, S. Ohana, P. et al. (2006) Chemically induced bladder cancer--a sonographic and morphologic description. *Urology* 68: 231-235.

Hahn, H. et al. (2000) Patched target Igf2 is indispensable for the formation of medulloblastoma and rhabdomyosarcoma. *J Biol Chem* 275: 28341-28344.

Hanahan,D. & Weinberg, RA. (2000) The hallmarks of cancer. *Cell* 100: 57-70.

Hao, Y. Crenshaw, T. Moulton, T. Newcomb, E. & Tycko, B. (1993) Tumor-suppressor activity of H19 RNA. *Nature* 365: 764-767.

Hasenpusch, G. Pfeifer, C. Aneja, MK. Wagner, K. Reinhardt, D. et al. (2011) Aerosolized BC-819 Inhibits Primary but Not Secondary Lung Cancer Growth. *PLoS One* 6: e20760.

Ishii, DN. Glazner, GW. & Whalen LR. (1993) Regulation of peripheral nerve regeneration by insulin-like growth factors. *Ann N Y Acad Sci* 692: 172-182.

Jemal, A. Siegel, R. Xu, J. & Ward, E. (2010) Cancer statistics, 2010. CA Cancer J Clin. 60: 277-300.

Kawamoto, K. Onodera, H. Kan, S. Kondo, S. & Imamura, M. (1999) Possible paracrine mechanism of insulin-like growth factor-2 in the development of liver metastases from colorectal carcinoma. *Cancer* 85: 18-25.

Liu, Y. Lehar, S. Corvi, C. Payne, G. & O'Connor, R. (1998) Expression of the insulin-like growth factor I receptor C terminus as a myristylated protein leads to induction of apoptosis in tumor cells. *Cancer Res* 58: 570-576.

Lottin, S. Adriaenssens, E. Dupressoir, T. Berteaux, N. Montpellier, C. et al. (2002) Overexpression of an ectopic H19 gene enhances the tumorigenic properties of breast cancer cells. *Carcinogenesis* 23:1885-95.

Matouk, I. Ohana, P. Ayesh, S. et al. (2005) The oncofetal H19 RNA in human cancer, from the bench to the patient. *Cancer Therapy* 3: 249-266.

Matouk, IJ. deGroot, N. Mezan, S. Ayesh, S. Abu-Lail, R. et al. (2007) The H19 non-coding RNA is essential for human tumor growth PloS ONE 2 : e845.

Matouk, IJ. Ohana, P. Galun, E. & Hochberg, A. (2008) The pivotal role of the oncofetal H19 RNA in human cancer, A new hope. Gene therapy and cancer research focus. Nova publisher. 241-260.

Matouk, IJ. Mezan, S. Mizrahi, A. Ohana, P. Abu-Lail, R. et al. (2010) The oncofetal H19 RNA connection: hypoxia, p53 and cancer. *Biochim Biophys Acta.* 1803:443-51.

Mizrahi, A. Czerniak, A. Ohana, P. Amiur, S. Gallula, J. et al. (2010) Treatment of ovarian cancer ascites by intra-peritoneal injection of diphtheria toxin A chain-H19 vector: a case report. *J Med Case Reports*. 4:228.

Mizutani, Y. Bonavida, B. & Yoshida, O. (1994) Cytotoxic effect of diphtheria toxin used alone or in combination with other agents on human renal cell carcinoma cell lines. *Urol Res.* 22:261-6.

Moorehead, RA. Sanchez, OH. Baldwin, RM. & Khokha, R. (2003) Transgenic overexpression of IGF-II induces spontaneous lung tumors: a model for human lung adenocarcinoma. *Oncogene* 22: 853-857.

Morali, OG. Jouneau, A. McLaughlin, KJ. Thiery, JP. & Larue, L. (2000) IGF-II promotes mesoderm formation. *Dev Biol* 227:133-45:

Morimoto, H. Safrit, JT. & Bonavida, B. (1991) Synergistic effect of tumor necrosis factor-alpha- and diphtheria toxin-mediated cytotoxicity in sensitive and resistant human ovarian tumor cell lines. *J Immunol* 147:2609-16.

Morison, IM. & Reeve, AE. (1998) Insulin-like growth factor 2 and overgrowth: molecular biology and clinical implications. *Mol Med Today* 4: 110-115.

Ohana, P. Schachter, P. Ayesh, B. Mizrahi, A. Birman, T. et al. Regulatory sequences of H19 and IGF2 genes in DNA-based therapy of colorectal rat liver metastases. *J Gene Med.* 3:366-74.

Ohana, P. Gofrit, O. Ayesh, S. Al-Sharef, W. Mizrahi, A. et al. (2004) Regulatory sequences of the H19 gene in DNA based therapy of bladder cancer. *Gene Therapy Molecular Biology* 8: 181-192.

Okada, M. Suzuki, E. & Hashimoto, Y. (1976) Carcinogenicity of N-nitrosamines related to N-butyl-N-(4-hydroxybutyl) nitrosamine and N,N,-dibutylnitrosamine in ACI/N rats. *Gann* 67: 825-34.

Randhawa, R. & Cohen, P. (2005) The role of the insulin-like growth factor system in prenatal growth. *Mol Genet Metab* 86: 84-90.

Rogler, CE. Yang, D. Rossetti, L. Donohoe, J. Alt, E. et al. (1994) Altered body composition and increased frequency of diverse malignancies in insulin-like growth factor-II transgenic mice. *J Biol Chem* 269: 13779-13784.

Schulz, WA. (1998) DNA methylation in urological malignancies. *Int J Oncol* 13: 151-67.

Shapiro, A. Kelley, DR. Oakley, DM. Catalona, WJ. & Ratliff, TL. (1984) Technical factors affecting the reproducibility of intravesical mouse bladder tumor implantation during therapy with Bacillus Calmette-Guerin. *Cancer Res* 44: 3051-4.

Sidi, AA. Ohana, P. Benjamin, S. Shalev, M. Ransom, JH. et al. (2008) Phase I/II marker lesion study of intravesical BC-819 DNA plasmid in H19 over expressing superficial bladder cancer refractory to bacillus Calmette-Guerin. *J Urol.*180:2379-83.

Takanami, I. Imamuma, T. Hashizume, T. Kikuchi, K. Yamamoto, Y. et al. (1996) Insulin-like growth factor-II as a prognostic factor in pulmonary adenocarcinoma. *J Surg Oncol* 61: 205-208.

Tsang, WP. & and Kwok, TT. (2007) Riboregulator H19 induction of MDR1-associated drug resistance in human hepatocellular carcinoma cells. *Oncogene* 26: 4877-4881.

Tsang, WP. Ng, EK. Ng, SS. Jin, H. Yu, J. et al. (2010) Oncofetal H19-derived miR-675 regulates tumor suppressor RB in human colorectal cancer. *Carcinogenesis.* 31:350-8.

van Rhijn, BW. Montironi, R. Zwarthoff, EC. Jöbsis, A. & van der Kwast, TH. (2002) Frequent FGFR3 mutations in urothelial papilloma. *J Pathol.* 198:245-51.

Yu, H. & Rohan, T. (2000) Role of the insulin-like growth factor family in cancer development and progression. *J Natl Cancer Inst* 92: 1472-1489.

Part 9

Basic Science Research and Bladder Cancer

19

Animal Models for Basic and Preclinical Research in Bladder Cancer

Ana María Eiján[1,2], Catalina Lodillinsky[2] and Eduardo Omar Sandes[1]
[1]*Research Area of the Institute of Oncology Angel H. Roffo, University of Buenos Aires,*
[2]*Consejo Nacional de Investigaciones Científicas y Técnicas (CONICET)*
Argentina

1. Introduction

Bladder cancer is one of the most common cancers in the world. In 2006, there were about 61,240 diagnosed cases of bladder cancer and approximately 13,060 deaths attributable to this disease, being the prevalence estimated worldwide more than 1,000,000 patients (Jemal *et al.*, 2006; Lerner, 2005). Taking into account that its incidence seems to be increasing, bladder cancer is clearly a significant public health issue around the world. Thus, it is necessary to intensify research on this topic.

Urinary bladder cancer originates mainly from epithelial cells of the urothelium (Lopez-Beltran *et al.*, 2004; Montironi *et al.*, 2005). When initially diagnosed, most bladder cancers (about 70%) do not present muscle invasion, and are thus known as non-muscle invasive bladder cancer (pTa and pT1). In these cases, a simple transurethral resection is sufficient to remove the tumor. However, some patients experience recurrence or even tumor progression. The progression of the tumor involves invasion of tumor cells, which penetrate deeper layers of the bladder such as the detrusor muscle (pT2), perivesical tissue (pT3) and extravesical organs (pT4) (Figure 1). Since this progression threatens the patient's life, more aggressive therapies are necessary (Sobin *et al.*, 1997).

Intensive research in bladder cancer, as well as that in most tumors, is being carried out to elucidate the reason for the appearance of tumors, and to find out which factors are involved in their development and which are related to the tumor progression process. These investigations, which provide insights into the biology of the tumor, are essential for the implementation of new therapeutic and/or preventive modalities (Bhattacharya *et al.*, 2010; Zhang *et al.*, 2011).

Research on basic science is focused on the mechanisms that lead cells towards transformation and development of cancer, using simple experimental models where it is easier to interpret the results. Cell culture techniques are widely used to study different oncological processes. The cell culture is the growth of any cell type, usually tumor cells, in with nutrient-containing solutions. The cells grow attached to the plastic surface, forming a monolayer, usually in a two-dimensional way. This technique allows studying processes such as mutagenesis, invasion, migration, and production of proteolytic enzymes. Although cell culture is a very important tool, it has certain limitations. Many biological processes depend on the three-dimensional architecture. In addition, monolayer culture is usually restricted to a single or at most two cell types. In contrast, tumors are complex and consist of tumor cells and other cell types such as stroma and immune cells that interact to either promote or inhibit tumor growth. To overcome these limitations, it is necessary to use three-dimensional models, such as tissue or organ cultures (Varley *et al.*, 2011).

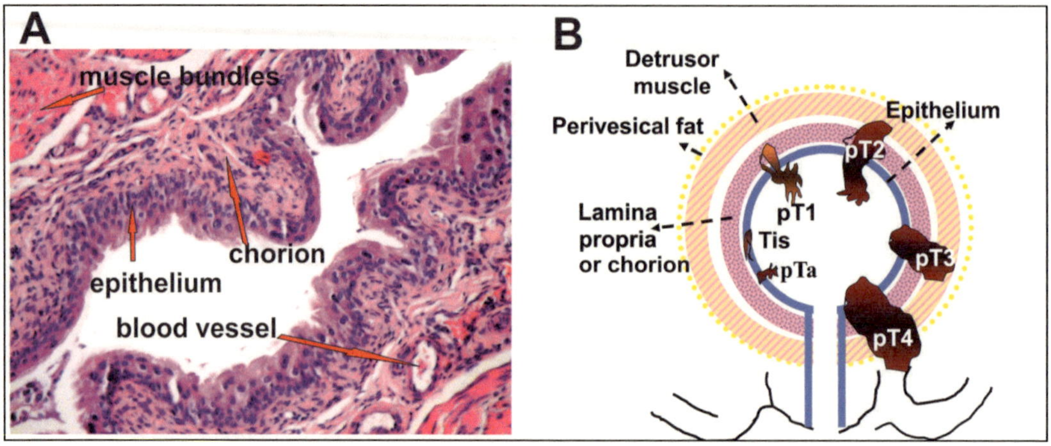

Fig. 1. A: Histology of a normal bladder from a C57BL/6J mouse (Hematoxylin- eosin).
B: Scheme of the invasion status of bladder tumors. Non-muscle invasive tumors pTa when are confined to epithelium, and pT1 when penetrating into the chorion. Invasive tumors when penetrate deeper layers of the bladder such as the detrusor muscle (pT2), perivesical tissue (T3) and extravesical organs (pT4).

To corroborate in vitro results, the next step in the investigation is the assay in a living organism. Animal models are important tools which allow studying the mechanisms of carcinogenesis as well as carrying out preclinical studies of new therapeutic modalities. It is important to design a model as similar to human disease as possible, so that observations can be readily transferred to clinical studies.

2. General characteristics of animal models

Animal models constitute the essential link between cell-based experiments and the translation of novel agents into human patients with cancer. They are used to study the development and progression of diseases and to test new treatments before they are provided to humans. Therefore, models should be as close to human pathology as possible.
In evolutionary biological terms, large animals have more similarity to humans. However, the most widely used animal models are rodents, in particular mice and rats. Although imperfect in their translatability into clinical efficacy, these animals have the advantage that they reproduce easily in short time, are easy to maintain with low cost, and can be manipulated genetically, thus remaining a critical tool in bladder cancer research.
Models allow researchers to study different characteristics of the tumor biology such as tumor growth, latency, growth rate, invasion and metastasis. Studies of carcinogenic substances or prevention of carcinogenesis may be carried out in animal models. Also, analysis of the response to cytotoxicity and immunotherapy treatments can be performed (Bhattacharya *et al.*, 2010; Takeuchi *et al.*, 2011; Zhang *et al.*, 2011).

According to the site of tumor inoculation, models are classified as heterotopic or orthotopic (see points 2.1.4 and 2.1.5.). In addition, depending on the species in which the tumor cell lines are inoculated, models may be xenogeneic or syngeneic models (see below).

2.1 Mouse models in bladder cancer

2.1.1 Xenogeneic models

Animals with transplanted human cancers are called xenogeneic or xenograft models. Nude mice are commonly used to inoculate human tumor fragments or bladder cancer cells. These mice have a spontaneous mutation in chromosome 11 named *nude* (*nu*), which gives certain phenotypic and functional changes. Homozygous nude mice show absence of hair, the feature that gave the name to the mutation. However, a few years after the appearance of the mutation, it was found that nude mice do not have a functional thymus. As a consequence, these animals have a low number of mature T lymphocytes, which allows them to accept xenograft transplantation. This feature of nude mice has contributed to the development of research in cancer, making these animal models useful to study the in vivo growth of human tumors and human cancer cell lines in which the efficacy of therapeutic agents such as monoclonal antibodies, cytotoxic drugs and radiotherapy can be tested. Below are a few examples of the relevant experiments in bladder cancer therapy using xenograft models.

One of the main features of tumors is their capacity to grow uncontrollably, invading the surrounding tissue, inducing neoformation of blood (angiogenesis) and lymphatic vessels and spreading in the body, forming secondary tumors or metastasis. In most cases, the death of patients with bladder cancer is due to the generation of metastasis. Angiogenesis, which is intricately involved in growth and metastasis and is in fact a prerequisite for these processes (Fidler, 1990; Folkman, 1986), is regulated by a fine balance between stimulatory and inhibitory factors produced by the tumor and the surrounding stroma (Liotta *et al.*, 1991). Bladder tumors produce high levels of several stimulatory factors, being the vascular endothelial growth factor (VEGF) overexpressed in bladder cancer (Crew *et al.*, 1997; O'Brien *et al.*, 1995). The action of this factor is mediated by its membrane receptor (VEGFR). Both VEGF and VEGFR are considered as important therapeutic targets. Some papers have studied the effects of a neutralizing monoclonal antibody targeted at murine VEGFR by using a xenograft model. In combination with cytotoxic compounds, such as paclitaxel, this monoclonal antibody impairs tumor growth and angiogenesis and. thus prevents metastatic spread and prolongs mouse survival (Davis *et al.*, 2004; Inoue *et al.*, 2000).

Xenograft models have also been used in radiopharmaceutical studies (Pfost *et al.*, 2009). Pfost et al. coupled monoclonal antibodies that recognize epidermal growth factor receptors on bladder cancer cells with ^{213}Bi, a radioactive alpha particle emitter, and found that therapy with 0.37 MBq of radiation after tumor cell inoculation in the bladder of nude mice results in higher survival of mice when compared with conventional treatment with Mitomycin C. These authors were also able to show that Mitomycin C produces nephrotoxicity, whereas ^{213}Bi-anti-EGFR-mAb treatment showed no signs of nephrotoxicity. These results suggest that radioimmunotherapy using intravesically instilled ^{213}Bi-anti-EGFR-mAb is a promising option for the treatment of bladder cancer in patients.

Xenogeneic models have also been used for the detection of growth and metastasis spread by bioluminescence techniques (Hadaschik *et al.*, 2007). To monitor tumor growth and therapeutic efficacy, noninvasive imaging concepts are preferable. For that purpose, tumor

cells are stably transfected with genes coding for fluorescent proteins (Tanaka *et al.*, 2003) or enzymes catalyzing bioluminescence (Hadaschik *et al.*, 2007), allowing for the continuous visualization of tumor development after intravesical instillation of tumor cells.
Although, as described above, xenograft models are important tools to study the behavior of human tumors in vivo, they also have an important limitation: they are immunodeficient. This makes this animal model not suitable to study interactions between the host immune system and the tumor. Furthermore, xenograft models are useless for research on the biological mechanisms related to carcinogenesis or on the possible compounds able to prevent carcinogenesis. In contrast, syngeneic animal models are more appropriate to approach these issues.

2.1.2 Syngeneic models

Syngeneic models include the appearance of spontaneous tumors, induction of tumors by chemical carcinogens, and inoculation of tumor cells in mice genetically identical to those in which tumors were developed. All of them are useful for studies in which the host-tumor interaction must be taken into account.

Immunotherapy

In patients, non-muscle invasive bladder cancers are usually managed with transurethral resection followed by the intravesical administration of Bacillus Calmette-Guerin (BCG). This immune therapy has been used without modification since 1976 (Morales *et al.*, 1976). In addition to the direct anti-tumor effect (Sandes *et al.*, 2007), it is widely recognized that intravesical BCG therapy is more potent in preventing tumor recurrence than any other intravesical chemotherapy (Sylvester, 2009). However, about 20% of patients either fail to respond initially or relapse within the first five years of treatment (Smaldone *et al.*, 2009). The exact mechanisms of BCG action have not been completely elucidated yet. However, it is known that BCG generates a local immunological reaction with activation of immune cells as well as secretion of cytokines involving Th1 cell cytotoxicity (Riemensberger *et al.*, 2002). To investigate the immune mechanisms by which BCG prevents bladder tumor recurrence and progression as well as the mechanisms of immune suppression to explain the lack of effectiveness of BCG observed in some patients, animal models with a competent immune system are needed. Syngeneic mouse bladder cancer models have thus been used for this purpose.
Animal models using subcutaneous or orthotopic inoculation of bladder cancer cell lines are being designed to study potential therapies to reverse these immune suppressive mechanisms. Mangsbo et al. have studied a syngeneic model by inoculating MB49 bladder cancer cell lines in the subcutis of C57BL/6J mice. This experimental model closely mimicks human bladder cancer, because MB49 cells express negative regulatory proteins of the immune response (Inman *et al.*, 2007; Nakanishi *et al.*, 2007). Among others, the programmed death ligand 1 (PD-L1) and the cytotoxicity T lymphocyte antigen-4 (CTLA-4) render T regulatory cells (Tregs) that can oppose to BCG immunotherapy. Antibodies able to block PD-L1 and CTLA-4 administered intratumorally improves long-term survival and leads to increased levels of tumor-reactive T cells and decreased numbers of Tregs at the tumor site. Therefore, this experimental model has allowed an approach to the understanding of immune suppression during immune therapy with BCG and represents a new therapeutic option in the treatment of bladder cancer (Mangsbo *et al.*, 2010).

It is known that BCG is neither free of mild or intermediate side effects such as fever and granulomatous prostatitis nor of severe side effects such as pneumonitis, hepatitis and BCG sepsis (DeHaven *et al.*, 1992). To avoid such unfavorable events, it is necessary to develop a more active and less toxic immunotherapeutic agent. A mouse syngeneic model using subcutaneous inoculation of MBT2 bladder cancer cell lines has been used to evaluate the effectiveness of liposomes containing walls from BCG bacteria as immune therapy. With this experimental design, Joraku et al. have demonstrated inhibition of tumor growth with increased immunity. Thus, this non-live bacterial agent may contribute to providing a more active and less toxic tool as a substitute for live BCG in immunotherapy (Joraku *et al.*, 2009).

Besides the study of the immune mechanism, other studies involving the tumor-host interaction have used syngeneic models. For example, in our laboratory, we have evaluated the mechanism of action of BCG using animals inoculated subcutaneously with MB49 bladder cancer cells, and found that macrophages from tumor-bearing mice treated with BCG intratumorally were able to produce soluble factors including fibroblast growth factor-2 (FGF-2), which induces fibroblast proliferation. We also found that in vivo BCG therapy reduces tumor growth with a concomitant increase in collagen deposition and expression of alpha-smooth muscle actin and FGF-2. These results suggest that tissue repair mechanisms similar to healing are involved in BCG immunotherapy of bladder cancer (Lodillinsky *et al.*, 2010).

Carcinogenesis and chemo-prevention

Bladder cancer is a candidate for chemo-prevention intervention for several reasons. In the first place, bladder cancer patients present successive recurrences that must be prevented. Also, in addition to genetic susceptibility, this cancer is closely related to exposure to environmental contaminants, including cigarette smoking, which implies the constant contact of carcinogenetic substances with the urothelium.

Animal models are widely used to select chemical synthesis products, purified natural products or even mixtures of natural products with potential to prevent tumor development, which can then be used in clinical trials. The idea is to use organ-specific animal models to determine which agents are likely to be helpful in preventing specific forms of cancer. These animal models can be obtained by chemical induction, spontaneous occurrence or use of transgenic animals.

To be useful, animal models must meet several characteristics. The model should be of clinical relevance, not only in terms of organ specificity but also in terms of the histology and the genetic abnormalities. Furthermore, premalignant lesions should be developed with genetic and histological features as similar as possible to those observed in the development of human cancer. In addition, the model must be consistent in generating tumors in a significant number of animals in a reasonable period. Finally, the model must be predictive in terms of clinical efficacy, i.e. that the positive or negative results obtained in the animal model should later correlate with positive and negative results in human trials (Steele *et al.*, 2010).

One of most useful models is the induction of bladder cancer in mice and rats with hydroxybutyl(butyl)nitrosamine (OH-BBN). This carcinogen compound induces premalignant lesions that progress to transitional bladder tumors, and in little proportion of squamous tumors (Grubbs *et al.*, 2000). Recent studies by Lu et al. have compared bladder tumors in rats and mice induced by OH-BBN with human bladder tumors, using a global gene expression approach cross-species analysis, and shown the similarity between this

animal model and bladder cancer in humans. These genes are likely to have conserved functions contributing to bladder carcinogenesis. To strengthen this analysis, these authors studied the molecular pathway commonly activated in both human and rodent bladder cancer and found a number of pathways that affect the cell cycle, HIF-1 and MYC expression, and regulation of apoptosis in both rodent and human bladder cancer. Also, they compared expression changes at mRNA and protein levels in the rat model and identified several genes/proteins exhibiting concordant changes in human bladder tumors. They concluded that rodent models (in OH-BBN-treated B6D2F1 mice and Fischer-344 rats) of bladder cancer accurately represent the clinical situation to an extent that will allow successful miming of target genes, showing that these models are powerful tools for chemoprevention research (Lu *et al.*, 2010). Using this experimental model, it has been demonstrated that NSAIDs (such as indomethacin, naproxen, NO-naproxen, and celecoxib), various EGFR inhibitors, and purified natural compounds (such as tea polyphenols and sulforaphane) have striking efficacy to prevent bladder tumor development (Ding *et al.*, 2010; Grubbs *et al.*, 2000; Lubet *et al.*, 2005; Steele *et al.*, 2009; Yao *et al.*, 2004).
Two disadvantages inherent in these models are the long experimental times (usually periods between 8 to 12 months) and the occupational exposure of workers. To avoid the use of carcinogens, knockout or transgenic mouse models can be used. These models are used in chemoprevention trials as well as in studies on the relevance of each gene in tumor development.

2.1.3 Transgenic models

Activation of oncogenes or inactivation of tumor suppressors in the urothelium is considered critical for the development of urothelial cancer. Transgenic mice have proven to be powerful tools to unravel the mechanisms of carcinogenesis and to understand the molecular basis of the disease. Transgenic mice are a particular case of syngeneic models, which are genetically modified to study the importance of a particular gene in cancer development and progression. Knockout mice, which are genetically modified mice, can be used to study the effect on the deficiency of a particular gene.
Alterations in the suppressor genes RB1 and p53 as well as the activation of oncogenes such as Ha-ras are commonly found in human urothelial tumors. Transgenic mice with alterations in these genes have been designed. By way of example, we will next describe some of the models developed and the conclusions that have been reached.
Mouse embryos lacking the retinoblastoma (Rb) gene die 14 days into gestation and mice lacking the p53 gene succumb to thymic lymphomas at seven months of age. So, the role of these genes in the analysis of tumorigenesis was delayed until conditional transgenic mice were developed. These models achieve the loss of gene function only in a particular tissue. The specific urothelium knockout system was developed using the Cre/loxP strategy. Transgenic mouse lines in which a 3.6-kb mouse uroplakin II promoter is used to drive the expression of Cre recombinase (Cre) have been generated (Mo *et al.*, 2005). The use of this model has allowed understanding the role of antitumor genes such as RB, p53 and PTEN in bladder carcinogenesis (Ahmad *et al.*, 2011; Ayala de la Pena *et al.*, 2011; He *et al.*, 2009). Conditional inactivation of both RB1 alleles in the mouse urothelium instead of accelerate urothelial proliferation, profoundly activated the p53 pathway, leading to extensive apoptosis in urothelial cells. Thus, pRb loss triggers fail-safe mechanisms whereby urothelial cells can evade tumorigenesis. Additional loss of p53 in pRb-deficient urothelial cells can

remove these p53-dependent tumor barriers, resulting in hyperplasia or umbrella cell nuclear atypia. Also, superficial papillary bladder tumors of low-grade (rare occurrence) but not invasive carcinomas have been detected. Furthermore, mice deficient in both pRb and p53 are highly susceptible to carcinogen exposure, developing invasive carcinomas that resemble human bladder cancer (He *et al.,* 2009). Another transgenic mouse with inactivation of the tumor suppressor p53 has been obtained by expression of SV40 large T antigen, directed to the urothelium with the specific promoter uroplakin-II. In the same way as in the transgenic mice described above, this construction has allowed demonstrating that the elimination of p53 alone is not sufficient for the generation of bladder tumor (Ayala de la Pena *et al.,* 2011). The function of proto-oncogene activation has been assessed by using Ha-ras trangenic mice (Zhang *et al.,* 2001).

Transgenic mice with compromised immune systems have also been developed. Mice knockout to IFN gamma (IFNɣ -/-), interleukins 17, 12 and 23 (IL-17 -/-; IL-12-/- and IL-23 -/-), among others, are being used to understand how different components of the immune system either promote or inhibit the development of bladder tumors (Kortylewski et al., 2009; Langowski et al., 2006; Wang *et al.,* 2009).

In both syngeneic and xenogeneic models, tumors can grow in heterotopic or orthotopic sites. Below we describe the advantages and disadvantages of both modalities.

2.1.4 Heterotopic tumor growth

This site of inoculation refers to the growth of a tumor in a site different from its target organs, generally using subcutaneous inoculation. This approach is advantageous in cases where the orthotopic inoculation (see below) is complex such as in bladder, kidney, and bowels. Tumor inoculation is simple and can be carried out by an operator with minimum training. Furthermore, the tumor can be easily detected and the tumor evolution can be easily assessed by using palpation of the skin and measurement with a caliper, respectively. To assess tumor growth, at least two perpendicular diameters, the larger diameter (D) and the smaller diameter (d), must be measured. Some researchers also measure depth (Figure 2). However, the latter is difficult to determine and generally produces large errors. Tumor size can be calculated from these data, using various formulas such as geometric mean ($\mathbf{(Dxd)^{1/2}}$ expressed in millimeters), arithmetic average (**Dxd/2** expressed in mm^2), or volume of the ellipsoid ($\mathbf{4/3\ \pi\ Dxd^2}$, expressed mm^3). Not all tumors grow in the same way; some of them are more compact, whereas others develop necrosis. Therefore, to choose the most appropriate formula for each tumor, it is first necessary to validate the formula that best fits, when compared with tumor weight.

The main disadvantage of the heterotopic model is the fact that an anatomic site other than an orthotopic site can differentially develop tumor growth. The tumorigenesis and metastatic potential of tumors depend not only on the characteristics of the tumor cells, but also on the tumor environment and therefore on the site of injection. Human tumors can be formed by different cell subpopulations with varying ability to metastasize and susceptibility to treatment, depending on the site of inoculation (Fidler, 1986). It has been observed that subcutaneous inoculation of murine MB49 bladder cancer cell lines induces lung metastases, and that inoculation of these cells in the bladder does not (Lodillinsky *et al.,* 2009). Similar observations have been made for human tumors using 253J B-V cells (Black *et al.,* 2007). After 28 days of tumor growth either in the bladder or in the subcutis, Black et al. were able to determine that the tumor size was similar in both sites, but that only tumors growing orthotopically in the bladder developed metastasis to lymph nodes and lungs. The orthotopic tumors, as compared to the subcutaneous tumors, have an increased microvessel density, increase in growth factors expression and proteolytic enzyme activity. Therefore, models of orthotopic growth are more appropriate for studies related to metastasis dissemination or response to any treatment.

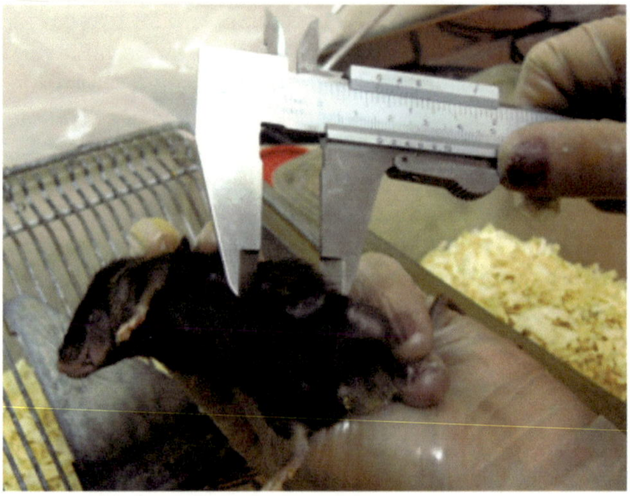

Fig. 2. Heterotopic tumor growth: MB49 bladder cancer cells growing in the subcutis of C57BL/6J mice.

There are some heterotopic models such as inoculation into the tail vein or the left ventricle of the heart which have been widely used to evaluate the process of extravasations and colonization in the lung or bone, respectively (Growcott, 2009; Wu *et al.*, 2010). Although very used, these models consider only a limited aspect of the metastatic process (Figure 3).

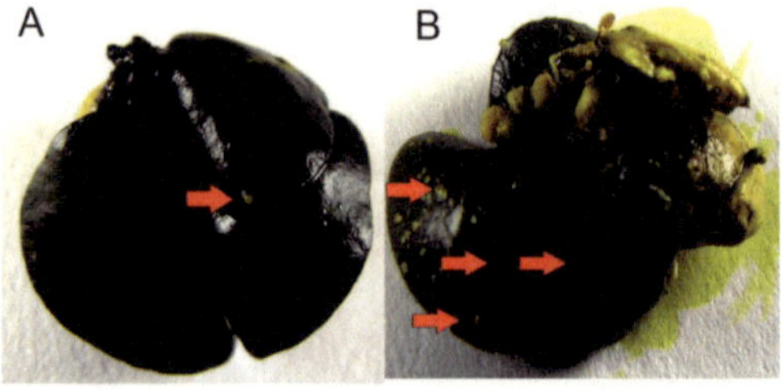

Fig. 3. Lung metastases: inoculation of MB49 (panel A) or MB49-I (panel B) bladder cancer cell lines into the tail vein induces lung metastasis. The lungs are colored in black by intratracheal inoculation of Indian ink. Metastases are seen in yellow by the stain and Bouin's fixative solution.

2.1.5 Orthotopic tumor growth

Growth in the target organ allows for better analysis of the interaction between the host and the tumor. When tumors are chemically induced, the carcinogen is chosen such that the tumor develops in the desired organ. Thus, tumor growth occurs in the orthotopic site. However, in the case that the tumor is generated by inoculation of a tumor fragment or tumor cell lines, the orthotopic inoculation is not always easy to perform. However, this difficulty must be overcome since the results obtained with heterotopic models are not always easy translated into clinical trials.

As previously mentioned, there are examples showing that different results are observed when the tumor is inoculated subcutaneously or orthotopically in the bladder. In studies of chemoprevention, inhibition of bladder cancer development by allyl isothiocyanate was detected for tumors growing orthotopically but not in the subcutis (Bhattacharya *et al.*, 2010). Furthermore, as described in the previous section, considerable variation has been detected between the two models in assays of immunotherapy, angiogenesis, invasion and metastatic spread, among others. Taking these limitations into account, to achieve a correct interpretation of results and a translatable preclinical model, it is necessary to inoculate the tumor in the bladder.

Inoculation into the bladder requires a qualified technician. Mice must first be anesthetized and subsequently, a 24-gauge Teflon i.v. catheter must be inserted through the urethra into the bladder using an inert lubricant to avoid discomfort in mice. For successful implantation of the bladder tumor cells, the urothelium must first be damaged. There are different techniques to induce such damage in the bladder. One of them involves the use of hydrochloric acid (0.1 ml 0.1 M HCl for 15 minutes) and subsequent neutralization with alkali and extensive washing with saline (Zhang *et al.*, 2011). Another technique involves instillation of a solution of silver nitrate (NO_3Ag) (Chade *et al.*, 2008). Both forms of injury allow the generation of tumors uniformly distributed in the bladder. The inoculation of MB49 tumor cells ($1x10^5$ to $5x10^5$) in syngeneic mice generates superficial tumors in about 7 to 15 days. Other techniques, using polylysine instillation, intramurally inoculation via laparotomy, or electro cauterization of the urothelium, are also used (Black *et al.*, 2010).

Cauterization of the bladder mimics transurethral resection of bladder tumor and therefore should facilitate adherence of instilled tumor cells to the bladder wall. The method was designed by Gunther et al. for the inoculation of MB49 cells in syngeneic mice (Gunther *et al.*, 1999). However, it is also used for inoculation of cells from human bladder tumors in nude mice (Pfost *et al.*, 2009). The technique involves the insertion of a guiding wire into the bladder of a mouse positioned dorsally on the ground plate of the cautery unit via the teflon catheter. When it is verified that the wire touches the bladder wall, the wire is attached to the cautery unit, and a monopolar coagulation mode is applied for 2 seconds at the lowest level (7 W). Then, via the same catheter, an appropriate number of tumor cells are inoculated and should remain in the bladder for at least 30 minutes (Figure 4A).

Another difficulty to be overcome is the determination of the evolution of bladder tumor growth. Unlike what happens in the case of a subcutaneous tumor growth, where its size can be easily determine at different times of evolution, the growth evolution in the bladder is more uncertain. However, hematuria is the hallmark of tumor presence (Figure 4B). Mice with $1x10^4$ or $1x10^5$ MB49 cell lines, inoculated by electrocautery, present hematuria about 15 or 9 days post-inoculation, respectively (Lodillinsky *et al.*, 2009). Inoculation of $5x10^3$ cells in the bladder previously treated with NO_3Ag generates hematuria in all mice about 7 days after tumor implantation (Chade *et al.*, 2008). Palpation of the bladder may give an idea of the extent of the tumor, but it is difficult to carry out because the bladder is retropubic. Also, in some cases, palpation could be given a wrong interpretation. When there is an obstruction of the urethra by blood clots, the bladder is greatly enlarged as a product of the accumulation of urine, and may thus lead to a wrong estimate of the extension of the tumor

(Figure 4C and D). Therefore, in these cases, the true evaluation of tumor size can be obtained at the end of the experiment, either by measuring the bladder with a caliper or by determining its weight (Figure 4E and F). Experiments of this type, also called end-point, have the disadvantage that they focus only on one measure of tumor size and not on its evolution throughout the experiment. This problem will soon be overcome by the design of non-invasive diagnostic equipment for small animals, similar to those used in medical practice in humans, such as ultrasound-doppler, infrared (IR) or bioluminescence imaging. By way of example, ultrasound-Doppler sagittal images have been used to evaluate angiogenesis in a mouse bladder cancer model (Sugano *et al.*, 2011). Also, bladder cancer cells that have been engineered to express certain proteins that emit fluorescence are being used in bioluminescence detection of tumor development (Black *et al.*, 2010).

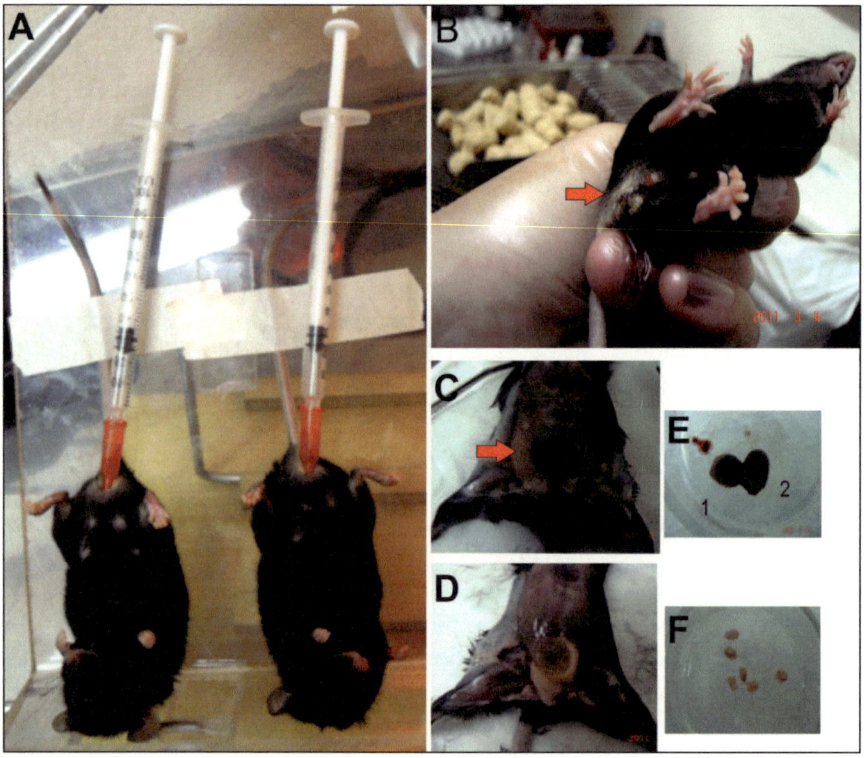

Fig. 4. Bladder tumor growth: A) orthotopic inoculation: after cauterization and inoculation of the appropriate number of tumor cells, mice should remain upside-down for at least 30 minutes so that cells can adhere to the bladder epithelium. B) Hematuria is the hallmark of tumor presence. C) Mouse with bladder tumor. D) Mouse with bladder containing urine but without tumor. E) Two bladders with tumor. F) Bladders from normal mice.

2.2 Mouse bladder cancer model for study of invasion and metastasis

2.2.1 Invasion and metastasis

The process of tumor invasion and metastasis is the most devastating stage of neoplastic disease and worsens prognosis of cancer patients. Adverse effects of systemic anti-tumor therapy and organ failure invaded with metastatic tissue are the leading causes of death in these patients (Steeg *et al.*, 2006). It is currently accepted that tumors have a clonal origin, which means that they are derived from a single cell. The high proliferative capacity, coupled with the genetic instability of tumor cells, generates new mutations, and thus the generation of other cell populations conferring tumor heterogeneity. This is considered part of an evolutionary process of genetic and epigenetic changes that allow some of the primary tumor cells acquire an adaptive advantage to migrate and colonize new environments. However, new findings have shown the possibility of a parallel development of cells capable of early metastatic spread. This parallel progression model urges to review the current diagnostic and treatment (Klein *et al.* 2009).

The local invasion process that gives rise to metastatic spread is a multi-step event called metastatic cascade. This is a phenomenon with low efficiency, indicating that only a few of the cells that emerge from the primary tumor are able to generate metastases.

Initially, tumor cells release proteolytic enzymes, such as MMPs and cathepsins, which degrade the extracellular components of basement membrane, thereby creating gaps that allow the invasion of the underlying connective tissue. The tumor cells migrate through the extracellular matrix and some may penetrate the lymphatic and blood capillaries, a phenomenon knows as intravasation. Once in the bloodstream, cells that manage to survive must leave the vessel (extravasation) into different organs (Figure 5). When the microenvironment of the target organ is appropriate, colonizing tumor cells can form metastases.

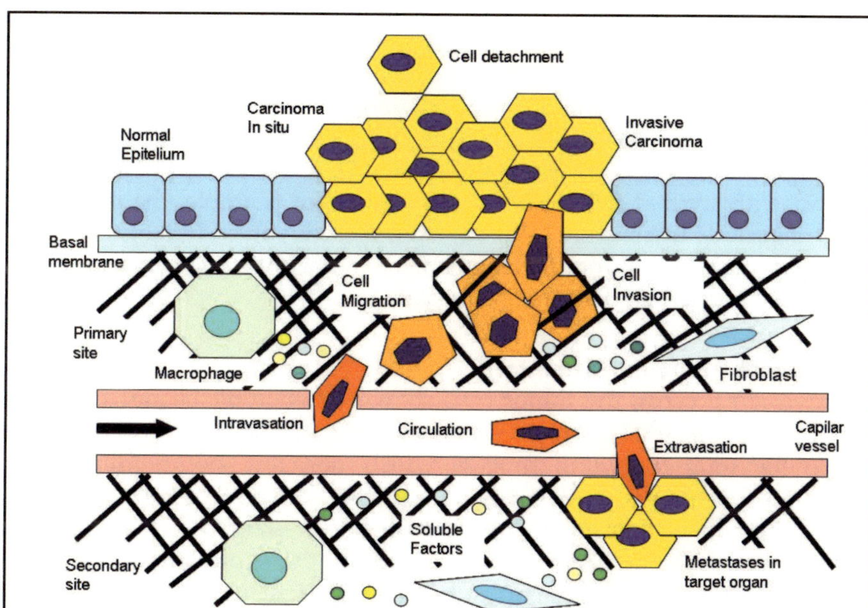

Fig. 5. During the metastatic cascade, tumor cells undergo genotypic and phenotypic changes that increase their capacity for invasion and migration. Some tumor cells are capable of degrading the basal membrane and migrating through connective tissue. Cells from connective tissue, such as macrophages and fibroblasts, through the release of growth factors, cytokines and proteolytic enzymes, can enhance the invasive behavior of tumor cells.

2.2.2 Metastogenes

The study of gene expression in primary tumor cells and metastatic cells has begun to lift the veil that prevented the understanding of the complex process of metastasis. These studies have identified a set of genes involved in the development of metastasis, called "metastogenic genes". Although there may be some overlap, these genes have been classified into three categories: a) initiation genes, b) progression genes and c) virulence genes (Nguyen *et al.*, 2007).

Initiation genes are associated with the processes of invasion, angiogenesis and epithelial-mesenchymal transition (EMT). Since during invasion the migration of cells is an important step, genes encoding for GTPases involved in cytoskeleton remodeling such as RhoC have been included in this category. Among those involved in angiogenesis are those encoding the vascular endothelium growth factor, and matrix metalloproteinase 9 (MMP9). EMT allows changes that give advantages in terms of migration and invasion. Certain genes that encode for transcription factors associated with this transition such as TWIST1 are also included in this group.

Progression genes are linked to the negative regulation of the immune response, vascular remodeling and extravasations. Examples are the gene coding for cyclooxygenase 2 (COX-2), matrix metalloproteinase 1 (MMP-1) and angiopoietin-like 4 (ANGPTL4), among others.

Finally, virulence genes are those which give the tumor cell an adaptive advantage to survive within an organ-specific microenvironment (Chiang *et al.*, 2008). Among them are intercellular signaling molecules such as cytokines and interleukins (CXCR4 and IL-11), molecules of the family of tumor necrosis factor (TNF) that are associated with bone metabolism (RANKL) and mediators of the angiogenic process such as the Endothelin-1.

Recent findings have identified the expression pattern characteristic of primary tumor gene, which is similar to a genetic signature that predicts the metastatic potential of the tumor (Bertucci *et al.*, 2007, Van't Veer *et al.*, 2002). This implies that the genetic profile expressed in metastases in specific organs is not always the same. Different groups of genes allow tumor cells to interact with stromal cells of the target organ. For example, the genes involved in breast cancer metastasis to bone are different from those involved in metastasis to the lung. This knowledge would allow the development of therapeutic strategies specific for each gene expression pattern or "signature " of a metastasis.

2.2.3 Epithelial-mesenchymal transition

During the invasion process, the tumor cells show a phenotypic change called epithelial-mesenchymal transition (EMT), which is characterized by a morphological change that is due to a genetic reprogramming process which normally occurs during embryonic development and tissue repair such as scarring (Peinado *et al.*, 2007). This reprogramming involves the expression of a group of transcriptional repressors (Zeb-1 and 2, Twist, Snail and Slug) that recruit histone deacetylases, controlling the expression of genes associated with the epithelial phenotype. An example of this is the decreased expression of E-cadherin, which leads to a loss of homotypic adhesion. Certain cytokines of the family of transforming growth factor beta (TGFbeta) and bone morphogenetic protein (BMP) are responsible for increasing the expression of these repressors (McConkey *et al.*, 2009).

Simultaneously with an underexpression of proteins of the epithelial phenotype, an overexpression of molecules associated with the mesenchymal phenotype has been detected. The expression of vimentin and loss of apical-basal polarization is a characteristic change of cells undergoing EMT (Peinado *et al.*, 2007).

2.2.4 Proteolytic enzymes in bladder cancer invasion

Proteolytic activity is of fundamental importance for the development, growth and maintenance of homeostasis of all the tissues in any organism. In each particular tissue, the activity of proteolytic enzymes is regulated at different levels, both at gene expression, transcriptional regulation and by specific endogenous inhibitors (Durkan *et al.*, 2003; Kumar *et al.*, 2010). In addition, these enzymes can activate each other through a mechanism cascade that also regulates their activity. The genetic instability of tumor cells leads to alterations in the genes encoding proteolytic enzymes and/or their inhibitors, which lead to an increased proteolytic activity in the tumor. It is well documented that proteolytic enzymes are involved in the process of invasion and metastasis. Matrix metalloproteinases (MMPs),cathepsins (B, L) and urokinase-type plasminogen activator (uPA) are the three main groups of enzymes described in the process of tumor invasion.

MMPs, of which several isoforms are known, have a major role in matrix destruction and are involved in metastasis by mediating basement membrane destruction and angiogenesis (Kim *et al.*, 2004). Of all known isoforms, MMP-2 and MMP-9 are strongly associated with invasion in bladder cancer (Eissa *et al.*, 2007; Papathoma *et al.*, 2000).

Cathepsins have also been involved in cancer invasion. Cathepsin B (CB) is one of the most abundant lysosomal cysteine proteinase in mammalian tissue. It is synthesized as a glycosylated zymogen named pro-CB and subsequently converted to an active form of 33 kDa or 27-29 kDa. CB has an important role in the lysosomal degradation of proteins and is also involved in the degradation of the extracellular matrix in neoplastic and inflammatory diseases. Particularly, results from our laboratory have shown that the high expression of the active form of CB in transitional bladder tumors is associated with worse prognosis factors such as invasiveness and high histological grade (Eiján *et al.*, 2003).

The proteolytic activity of uPA is a system regulated by urokinase, its specific receptor uPAR and the specific plasminogen activator inhibitor 1 (PAI-1). This system plays a major role in tumorigenesis, tumor progression, tumor invasion and metastasis formation. It is generally assumed that the pro-malignant effect of the uPA-uPAR system is mediated by increased local proteolysis, thus favoring tumor invasion, as well as by the pro-angiogenic effect (Binder *et al.*, 2008). Consistent with this activity it has been shown, in a rat orthotopic model, that intravesical administration of PAI-1, which inhibits uPA activity in tumors, reduces the growth and progression of bladder cancer (Chen *et al.*, 2009).

2.2.5 Orthotopic mouse bladder cancer invasion model

Certain fundamental properties of metastatic cells such as migration and invasion can be studied in the laboratory using tumor cell cultures. Using various tools of genetic engineering, genes that encode molecules that emit fluorescence (green fluorescent protein), bioluminescent molecules (luciferase) or molecules with color (beta galactosidase) can be introduced into the cell. This technique is known as reporter gene and has allowed the analysis of molecular processes at the level of cell groups or isolated cells (Ghajar *et al.*, 2008; Menon *et al.*, 2009). In vitro experiments have also been useful to shed light on genes that might be involved in certain steps of the metastatic cascade. So, the use of genetic and pharmacological methods has shown that the expression of certain genes facilitate the assembly of new tumor blood vessels, tumor cells out of circulation and the passage of circulating tumor cells through the pulmonary capillaries to grow lung metastases (Gupta *et al.*, 2007; Valastyan *et al.*, 2009). However, in vitro models allow a simple analysis and do not always allow evaluating interactions with the tumor microenvironment. It is therefore important to develop animal models to analyze the factors associated with tumor progression (Bos *et al.*, 2010). To this end, we have added the advances in multiphoton intravital microscopy, which allows observing the in vivo behavior of tumor cells labeled with green fluorescent protein in the process of invasion and metastasis (Condeelis *et al.*, 2003).

There are only few useful animal models to study the processes of invasion and metastasis. Dinney et al. have designed an orthotopic murine model with different degrees of invasion. To this end, they seeded human 253J cells into the bladder wall of immunodeficient mice (nude) and then selected subpopulations of the parental line by in vivo reimplantation in the bladder. After five serial passages, tumors were more tumorigenic and showed metastatic capacity (Dinney *et al.*, 1995). These authors observed that these variants had a tumoral abnormal karyotype, increased expression of molecules such as epidermal growth factor receptor (EGFR), interleukin 8 (IL-8) and MMP-9, and also observed an increased anchorage-independent growth and increased capacity to migrate in Matrigel ® (trade name of a protein mixture secreted by mouse sarcoma cells Engelbreth-Holm-Swarm), commonly used in the study of invasive and migratory behavior of tumor cells in contact with extracellular matrix components.

This is a xenogeneic model in which it is possible to study the changes experienced by the tumor cells to acquire their invasive and metastatic phenotype. While this is an ingenious and very useful model, the fact that it is an immunodeficient mouse slightly restricts the applicability of the model.

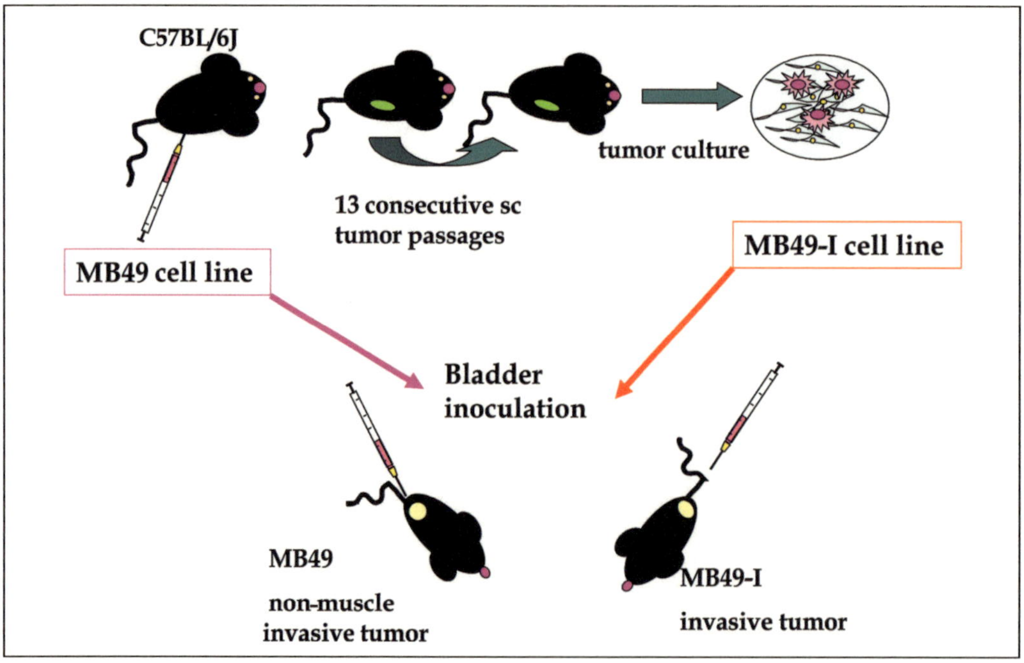

Fig. 6. MB49-I cell line obtained by successive in vivo passages of primary tumor obtained by inoculation of the MB49 bladder tumor cell line. The orthotopic inoculation in bladder of MB49 or MB49-I generates non-muscle invasive or muscle invasive tumors respectively.

In our laboratory, following the methodology of Dinney, but with subcutaneous inoculation, we developed a syngeneic murine model that reproduces the human pathology in terms of invasion status. A single cell suspension of the MB49 cell line was inoculated subcutaneously in the flank of syngeneic C57BL/6J mice. After 24 days, tumors were surgically removed and 2-mm tumor pieces were transplanted by trocar into the left flank of mice. This process was repeated 13 consecutive times. We found that the growth rate was increased in transplants #6 to #10 and then became stable. Therefore, primary culture from transplant #13 was carried out and the cell line originated was named MB49-I. The orthotopic inoculation of MB49 or MB49-I in the bladder generates non-muscle invasive or muscle invasive tumors respectively (Figure 6).

This new line has more aggressive characteristics. The MB49-I cell line has higher activity of the MMP-9, uPA and CB as well as increased in vitro invasion of Matrigel ®. Given the association of these enzymes with bladder cancer progression, our model has close similarities to human disease. The histopathological study in vivo showed results consistent with in vivo tests. Intravesical inoculation of MB49 cells was able to develop tumors without muscle invasion. By contrast, inoculation of the MB49-I cell line generated carcinoma with a disorganized structure and larger tumors with cellular atypia, muscle layer invasion and lung metastasis (Figure 7).

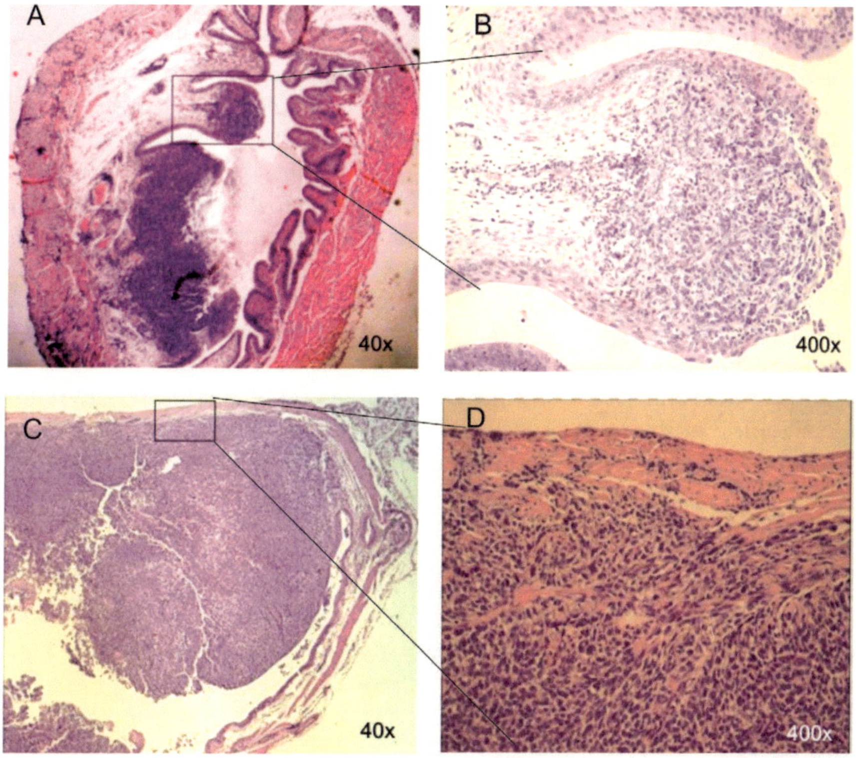

Fig. 7. Haematoxylin-eosin staining for bladder tumors. A: It can see two formations of a tumor of bladder MB49: one sessile and one pedunculated, which do not invade the muscle wall. B: MB49 the polypoid formation is magnified 400X. C: image of a tumor MB49-I, we observe a large tumor invading the muscular layer. D: MB49-I bladder tumor with higher magnification, where the tumor cells are intermingled with the muscle fibers.

Cellular plasticity is a fundamental process during tumor progression. It is now accepted that epithelial-mesenchymal transition is associated with tumor progression. A mark of this transition is the loss of cytokeratin and an increase in vimentin. MB49-I has not only morphological diversity, but also decreased cytokeratin and increased vimentin expression in vitro and in vivo.

Since both the xenogeneic and syngeneic models described here resemble human bladder cancer, they could be useful to study tumor progression, tissue remodeling, and invasive and metastatic processes, and to assay anti-invasive and metastatic agents.

3. Conclusions

Since animal models can reproduce the tumor-host interactions, performing studies using these models is a mandatory step to translate from basic research to the clinic. Taking into account that animal experiments are performed to obtain an improvement for human-health, but must generate a reduced impact on the animals, these experiments should be made according to international rules of bioethics. To accomplish the maximum welfare of the animal, every protocol, indicating the justification of each experiment and the methodology to be used, must be approved by the institutional ethics committee for the use of laboratory animals.

The ideal animal model should meet all the characteristics of the human pathology, such as growth parameters, histology, evolution and metastatic dissemination. However, in the practice, the ideal model does not always have a complete similarity. The researcher must thus decide which model best fits the question to be answered. Alternatively, the researcher can design his/her own model that most closely approaches the point of interest.

The generation of transgenic animals is one of the most developed branches in animal models. Technical refinements have allowed generating genetically modified mice either stable or conditional, making them a valuable tool.

Animal models that mimic human bladder cancer in terms of invasion have also been developed. The use of successive transplants of tumors derived from a cancer cell line can generate invasive bladder tumors. Both the syngeneic and xenogenic invasive models of tumor are useful in the study of tumor progression. Finally, it is important to note that for a better understanding of the tumor mechanism and the relationship with the host, the best models are those, like MB49-I, in which the tumor is inoculated in an orthotopic site.

4. Acknowledgments

This publication was supported by grants from the Consejo Nacional de Investigaciones Científicas y Técnicas (CONICET: www.conicet.gov.ar), and Universidad de Buenos Aires - UBACYT M017 (www.uba.ar). We thank M. Krasnapolsky and D. Belgorosky for their help in preparing the manuscript.

5. References

Ahmad, I.; Morton, J.P.; Singh, L.B.; Radulescu, S.M.; Ridgway, R.A.; Patel, S.; Woodgett, J.; Winton, D.J.; Taketo, M.M.; Wu, X.R.; Leung, H.Y. & Sansom, O.J. (2011). beta-Catenin activation synergizes with PTEN loss to cause bladder cancer formation. *Oncogene,* 30,2, (Jan 13, 2011), 178-89, 1476-5594 (Electronic) 0950-9232 (Linking).

Ayala De La Pena, F.; Kanasaki, K.; Kanasaki, M.; Tangirala, N.; Maeda, G. & Kalluri, R. (2011). Loss of p53 and acquisition of angiogenic microRNA profile is insufficient to facilitate progression of bladder urothelial carcinoma in situ to invasive carcinoma. *J Biol Chem*, (Mar 9, 2011), 1083-351X (Electronic) 0021-9258 (Linking).

Bertucci, F.; Cervera, N. & Birnbaum, D. (2007). A gene signature in breast cancer. *N Engl J Med*, 356,18, (May 3, 2007), 1887-8; author reply 1887-8, 1533-4406 (Electronic) 0028-4793 (Linking).

Bhattacharya, A.; Tang, L.; Li, Y.; Geng, F.; Paonessa, J.D.; Chen, S.C.; Wong, M.K. & Zhang, Y. (2010). Inhibition of bladder cancer development by allyl isothiocyanate. *Carcinogenesis*, 31,2, (Feb, 2010), 281-6, 1460-2180 (Electronic) 0143-3334 (Linking).

Binder, B.R. & Mihaly, J. (2008). The plasminogen activator inhibitor "paradox" in cancer. *Immunol Lett*, 118,2, (Jun 30, 2008), 116-24, 0165-2478 (Print) 0165-2478 (Linking).

Black, P.C. & Dinney, C.P. (2007). Bladder cancer angiogenesis and metastasis--translation from murine model to clinical trial. *Cancer Metastasis Rev*, 26,3-4, (Dec, 2007), 623-34, 0167-7659 (Print) 0167-7659 (Linking).

Black, P.C.; Shetty, A.; Brown, G.A.; Esparza-Coss, E.; Metwalli, A.R.; Agarwal, P.K.; Mcconkey, D.J.; Hazle, J.D. & Dinney, C.P. (2010). Validating bladder cancer xenograft bioluminescence with magnetic resonance imaging: the significance of hypoxia and necrosis. *BJU Int*, 106,11, (Dec, 2010), 1799-804, 1464-410X (Electronic) 1464-4096 (Linking).

Bos, P.D.; Nguyen, D.X. & Massague, J. (2010). Modeling metastasis in the mouse. *Curr Opin Pharmacol*, 10,5, (Oct, 2010), 571-7, 1471-4973 (Electronic) 1471-4892 (Linking).

Chade, D.C.; Andrade, P.M.; Borra, R.C.; Leite, K.R.; Andrade, E.; Villanova, F.E. & Srougi, M. (2008). Histopathological characterization of a syngeneic orthotopic murine bladder cancer model. *Int Braz J Urol*, 34,2, (Mar-Apr, 2008), 220-6; discussion 226-9, 1677-5538 (Print) 1677-5538 (Linking).

Chen, S.C.; Henry, D.O.; Hicks, D.G.; Reczek, P.R. & Wong, M.K. (2009). Intravesical administration of plasminogen activator inhibitor type-1 inhibits in vivo bladder tumor invasion and progression. *J Urol*, 181,1, (Jan, 2009), 336-42, 1527-3792 (Electronic) 0022-5347 (Linking).

Chiang, A.C. & Massague, J. (2008). Molecular basis of metastasis. *N Engl J Med*, 359,26, (Dec 25, 2008), 2814-23, 1533-4406 (Electronic) 0028-4793 (Linking).

Condeelis, J. & Segall, J.E. (2003). Intravital imaging of cell movement in tumours. *Nat Rev Cancer*, 3,12, (Dec, 2003), 921-30, 1474-175X (Print) 1474-175X (Linking).

Crew, J.P.; O'brien, T.; Bradburn, M.; Fuggle, S.; Bicknell, R.; Cranston, D. & Harris, A.L. (1997). Vascular endothelial growth factor is a predictor of relapse and stage progression in superficial bladder cancer. *Cancer Res*, 57,23, (Dec 1, 1997), 5281-5, 0008-5472 (Print) 0008-5472 (Linking).

Davis, D.W.; Inoue, K.; Dinney, C.P.; Hicklin, D.J.; Abbruzzese, J.L. & Mcconkey, D.J. (2004). Regional effects of an antivascular endothelial growth factor receptor monoclonal antibody on receptor phosphorylation and apoptosis in human 253J B-V bladder cancer xenografts. *Cancer Res*, 64,13, (Jul 1, 2004), 4601-10, 0008-5472 (Print) 0008-5472 (Linking).

DeHaven, J.I.; Traynellis, C.; Riggs, D.R.; Ting, E. & Lamm, D.L. (1992). Antibiotic and steroid therapy of massive systemic bacillus Calmette-Guerin toxicity. *J Urol*, 147,3, (Mar, 1992), 738-42, 0022-5347 (Print) 0022-5347 (Linking).

Ding, Y.; Paonessa, J.D.; Randall, K.L.; Argoti, D.; Chen, L.; Vouros, P. & Zhang, Y. (2010). Sulforaphane inhibits 4-aminobiphenyl-induced DNA damage in bladder cells and tissues. *Carcinogenesis,* 31,11, (Nov, 2010), 1999-2003, 1460-2180 (Electronic) 0143-3334 (Linking).

Dinney, C.P.; Fishbeck, R.; Singh, R.K.; Eve, B.; Pathak, S.; Brown, N.; Xie, B.; Fan, D.; Bucana, C.D.; Fidler, I.J. & Et Al. (1995). Isolation and characterization of metastatic variants from human transitional cell carcinoma passaged by orthotopic implantation in athymic nude mice. *J Urol,* 154,4, (Oct, 1995), 1532-8, 0022-5347 (Print) 0022-5347 (Linking).

Durkan, G.C.; Nutt, J.E.; Marsh, C.; Rajjayabun, P.H.; Robinson, M.C.; Neal, D.E.; Lunec, J. & Mellon, J.K. (2003). Alteration in urinary matrix metalloproteinase-9 to tissue inhibitor of metalloproteinase-1 ratio predicts recurrence in nonmuscle-invasive bladder cancer. *Clin Cancer Res,* 9,7, (Jul, 2003), 2576-82, 1078-0432 (Print) 1078-0432 (Linking).

Eijan, A.M.; Sandes, E.O.; Riveros, M.D.; Thompson, S.; Pasik, L.; Mallagrino, H.; Celeste, F. & Casabe, A.R. (2003). High expression of cathepsin B in transitional bladder carcinoma correlates with tumor invasion. *Cancer,* 98,2, (Jul 15, 2003), 262-8, 0008-543X (Print) 0008-543X (Linking).

Eissa, S.; Ali-Labib, R.; Swellam, M.; Bassiony, M.; Tash, F. & El-Zayat, T.M. (2007). Noninvasive diagnosis of bladder cancer by detection of matrix metalloproteinases (MMP-2 and MMP-9) and their inhibitor (TIMP-2) in urine. *Eur Urol,* 52,5, (Nov, 2007), 1388-96, 0302-2838 (Print) 0302-2838 (Linking).

Fidler, I.J. (1986). Rationale and methods for the use of nude mice to study the biology and therapy of human cancer metastasis. *Cancer Metastasis Rev,* 5,1, (1986), 29-49, 0167-7659 (Print) 0167-7659 (Linking).

Fidler, I.J. (1990). Critical factors in the biology of human cancer metastasis: twenty-eighth G.H.A. Clowes memorial award lecture. *Cancer Res,* 50,19, (Oct 1, 1990), 6130-8, 0008-5472 (Print) 0008-5472 (Linking).

Folkman, J. (1986). How is blood vessel growth regulated in normal and neoplastic tissue? G.H.A. Clowes memorial Award lecture. *Cancer Res,* 46,2, (Feb, 1986), 467-73, 0008-5472 (Print) 0008-5472 (Linking).

Ghajar, C.M. & Bissell, M.J. (2008). Extracellular matrix control of mammary gland morphogenesis and tumorigenesis: insights from imaging. *Histochem Cell Biol,* 130,6, (Dec, 2008), 1105-18, 0948-6143 (Print) 0948-6143 (Linking).

Growcott, J.W. (2009). Preclinical anticancer activity of the specific endothelin A receptor antagonist ZD4054. *Anticancer Drugs,* 20,2, (Feb, 2009), 83-8, 1473-5741 (Electronic) 0959-4973 (Linking).

Grubbs, C.J.; Lubet, R.A.; Koki, A.T.; Leahy, K.M.; Masferrer, J.L.; Steele, V.E.; Kelloff, G.J.; Hill, D.L. & Seibert, K. (2000). Celecoxib inhibits N-butyl-N-(4-hydroxybutyl)-nitrosamine-induced urinary bladder cancers in male B6D2F1 mice and female Fischer-344 rats. *Cancer Res,* 60,20, (Oct 15, 2000), 5599-602, 0008-5472 (Print) 0008-5472 (Linking).

Gunther, J.H.; Jurczok, A.; Wulf, T.; Brandau, S.; Deinert, I.; Jocham, D. & Bohle, A. (1999). Optimizing syngeneic orthotopic murine bladder cancer (MB49). *Cancer Res,* 59,12, (Jun 15, 1999), 2834-7, 0008-5472 (Print) 0008-5472 (Linking).

Gupta, G.P.; Nguyen, D.X.; Chiang, A.C.; Bos, P.D.; Kim, J.Y.; Nadal, C.; Gomis, R.R.; Manova-Todorova, K. & Massague, J. (2007). Mediators of vascular remodelling co-opted for sequential steps in lung metastasis. *Nature,* 446,7137, (Apr 12, 2007), 765-70, 1476-4687 (Electronic) 0028-0836 (Linking).

Hadaschik, B.A.; Black, P.C.; Sea, J.C.; Metwalli, A.R.; Fazli, L.; Dinney, C.P.; Gleave, M.E. & So, A.I. (2007). A validated mouse model for orthotopic bladder cancer using transurethral tumour inoculation and bioluminescence imaging. *BJU Int,* 100,6, (Dec, 2007), 1377-84, 1464-410X (Electronic) 1464-4096 (Linking).

He, F.; Mo, L.; Zheng, X.Y.; Hu, C.; Lepor, H.; Lee, E.Y.; Sun, T.T. & Wu, X.R. (2009). Deficiency of pRb family proteins and p53 in invasive urothelial tumorigenesis. *Cancer Res,* 69,24, (Dec 15, 2009), 9413-21, 1538-7445 (Electronic) 0008-5472 (Linking).

Inman, B.A.; Sebo, T.J.; Frigola, X.; Dong, H.; Bergstralh, E.J.; Frank, I.; Fradet, Y.; Lacombe, L. & Kwon, E.D. (2007). PD-L1 (B7-H1) expression by urothelial carcinoma of the bladder and BCG-induced granulomata: associations with localized stage progression. *Cancer,* 109,8, (Apr 15, 2007), 1499-505, 0008-543X (Print) 0008-543X (Linking).

Inoue, K.; Slaton, J.W.; Davis, D.W.; Hicklin, D.J.; Mcconkey, D.J.; Karashima, T.; Radinsky, R. & Dinney, C.P. (2000). Treatment of human metastatic transitional cell carcinoma of the bladder in a murine model with the anti-vascular endothelial growth factor receptor monoclonal antibody DC101 and paclitaxel. *Clin Cancer Res,* 6,7, (Jul, 2000), 2635-43, 1078-0432 (Print) 1078-0432 (Linking).

Jemal, A.; Siegel, R.; Ward, E.; Murray, T.; Xu, J.; Smigal, C. & Thun, M.J. (2006). Cancer statistics, 2006. *CA Cancer J Clin,* 56,2, (Mar-Apr, 2006), 106-30, 0007-9235 (Print) 0007-9235 (Linking).

Joraku, A.; Homhuan, A.; Kawai, K.; Yamamoto, T.; Miyazaki, J.; Kogure, K.; Yano, I.; Harashima, H. & Akaza, H. (2009). Immunoprotection against murine bladder carcinoma by octaarginine-modified liposomes incorporating cell wall of Mycobacterium bovis bacillus Calmette-Guerin. *BJU Int,* 103,5, (Mar, 2009), 686-93, 1464-410X (Electronic) 1464-4096 (Linking).

Kim, S.; Park, H.S.; Son, H.J. & Moon, W.S. (2004). [The role of angiostatin, vascular endothelial growth factor, matrix metalloproteinase 9 and 12 in the angiogenesis of hepatocellular carcinoma]. *Korean J Hepatol,* 10,1, (Mar, 2004), 62-72, 1738-222X (Print) 1738-222X (Linking).

Klein, C.A. (2009). Parallel progression of primary tumours and metastases. *Nat Rev Cancer,* 9,4, (Apr, 2009), 302-12, 1474-1768 (Electronic) 1474-175X (Linking).

Kortylewski, M.; Xin, H.; Kujawski, M.; Lee, H.; Liu, Y.; Harris, T.; Drake, C.; Pardoll, D. & Yu, H. (2009). Regulation of the IL-23 and IL-12 balance by Stat3 signaling in the tumor microenvironment. *Cancer Cell,* 15,2, (Feb 3, 2009), 114-23, 1878-3686 (Electronic) 1535-6108 (Linking).

Kumar, B.; Koul, S.; Petersen, J.; Khandrika, L.; Hwa, J.S.; Meacham, R.B.; Wilson, S. & Koul, H.K. (2010). p38 mitogen-activated protein kinase-driven MAPKAPK2 regulates invasion of bladder cancer by modulation of MMP-2 and MMP-9 activity. *Cancer Res,* 70,2, (Jan 15, 2010), 832-41, 1538-7445 (Electronic) 0008-5472 (Linking).

Langowski, J.L.; Zhang, X.; Wu, L.; Mattson, J.D.; Chen, T.; Smith, K.; Basham, B.; Mcclanahan, T.; Kastelein, R.A. & Oft, M. (2006). IL-23 promotes tumour incidence and growth. *Nature,* 442,7101, (Jul 27, 2006), 461-5, 1476-4687 (Electronic) 0028-0836 (Linking).

Lerner, S.P. (2005). Bladder cancer clinical trials. *Urol Oncol,* 23,4, (Jul-Aug, 2005), 275-9, 1078-1439 (Print) 1078-1439 (Linking).

Liotta, L.A.; Steeg, P.S. & Stetler-Stevenson, W.G. (1991). Cancer metastasis and angiogenesis: an imbalance of positive and negative regulation. *Cell,* 64,2, (Jan 25, 1991), 327-36, 0092-8674 (Print) 0092-8674 (Linking).

Lodillinsky, C.; Langle, Y.; Guionet, A.; Gongora, A.; Baldi, A.; Sandes, E.O.; Casabe, A. & Eijan, A.M. (2010). Bacillus Calmette Guerin induces fibroblast activation both directly and through macrophages in a mouse bladder cancer model. *PLoS One,* 5,10, 2010), e13571, 1932-6203 (Electronic) 1932-6203 (Linking).

Lodillinsky, C.; Rodriguez, V.; Vauthay, L.; Sandes, E.; Casabe, A. & Eijan, A.M. (2009). Novel invasive orthotopic bladder cancer model with high cathepsin B activity resembling human bladder cancer. *J Urol,* 182,2, (Aug, 2009), 749-55, 1527-3792 (Electronic) 0022-5347 (Linking).

Lopez-Beltran, A. & Montironi, R. (2004). Non-invasive urothelial neoplasms: according to the most recent WHO classification. *Eur Urol,* 46,2, (Aug, 2004), 170-6, 0302-2838 (Print) 0302-2838 (Linking).

Lu, Y.; Liu, P.; Wen, W.; Grubbs, C.J.; Townsend, R.R.; Malone, J.P.; Lubet, R.A. & You, M. (2010). Cross-species comparison of orthologous gene expression in human bladder cancer and carcinogen-induced rodent models. *Am J Transl Res,* 3,1, (2010), 8-27, 1943-8141 (Electronic)

Lubet, R.A.; Huebner, K.; Fong, L.Y.; Altieri, D.C.; Steele, V.E.; Kopelovich, L.; Kavanaugh, C.; Juliana, M.M.; Soong, S.J. & Grubbs, C.J. (2005). 4-Hydroxybutyl(butyl)nitrosamine-induced urinary bladder cancers in mice: characterization of FHIT and survivin expression and chemopreventive effects of indomethacin. *Carcinogenesis,* 26,3, (Mar, 2005), 571-8, 0143-3334 (Print) 0143-3334 (Linking).

Mangsbo, S.M.; Sandin, L.C.; Anger, K.; Korman, A.J.; Loskog, A. & Totterman, T.H. (2010). Enhanced tumor eradication by combining CTLA-4 or PD-1 blockade with CpG therapy. *J Immunother,* 33,3, (Apr, 2010), 225-35, 1537-4513 (Electronic) 1524-9557 (Linking).

McConkey, D.J.; Choi, W.; Marquis, L.; Martin, F.; Williams, M.B.; Shah, J.; Svatek, R.; Das, A.; Adam, L.; Kamat, A.; Siefker-Radtke, A. & Dinney, C. (2009). Role of epithelial-to-mesenchymal transition (EMT) in drug sensitivity and metastasis in bladder cancer. *Cancer Metastasis Rev,* 28,3-4, (Dec, 2009), 335-44, 1573-7233 (Electronic) 0167-7659 (Linking).

Menon, M.B.; Ronkina, N.; Schwermann, J.; Kotlyarov, A. & Gaestel, M. (2009). Fluorescence-based quantitative scratch wound healing assay demonstrating the role of MAPKAPK-2/3 in fibroblast migration. *Cell Motil Cytoskeleton,* 66,12, (Dec, 2009), 1041-7, 1097-0169 (Electronic) 0886-1544 (Linking).

Mo, L.; Cheng, J.; Lee, E.Y.; Sun, T.T. & Wu, X.R. (2005). Gene deletion in urothelium by specific expression of Cre recombinase. *Am J Physiol Renal Physiol,* 289,3, (Sep, 2005), F562-8, 1931-857X (Print)

Montironi, R. & Lopez-Beltran, A. (2005). The 2004 WHO classification of bladder tumors: a summary and commentary. *Int J Surg Pathol,* 13,2, (Apr, 2005), 143-53, 1066-8969 (Print) 1066-8969 (Linking).

Morales, A.; Eidinger, D. & Bruce, A.W. (1976). Intracavitary Bacillus Calmette-Guerin in the treatment of superficial bladder tumors. *J Urol,* 116,2, (Aug, 1976), 180-3, 0022-5347 (Print) 0022-5347 (Linking).

Nakanishi, J.; Wada, Y.; Matsumoto, K.; Azuma, M.; Kikuchi, K. & Ueda, S. (2007). Overexpression of B7-H1 (PD-L1) significantly associates with tumor grade and postoperative prognosis in human urothelial cancers. *Cancer Immunol Immunother,* 56,8, (Aug, 2007), 1173-82, 0340-7004 (Print) 0340-7004 (Linking).

Nguyen, D.X. & Massague, J. (2007). Genetic determinants of cancer metastasis. *Nat Rev Genet,* 8,5, (May, 2007), 341-52, 1471-0056 (Print) 1471-0056 (Linking).

O'Brien, T.; Cranston, D.; Fuggle, S.; Bicknell, R. & Harris, A.L. (1995). Different angiogenic pathways characterize superficial and invasive bladder cancer. *Cancer Res,* 55,3, (Feb 1, 1995), 510-3, 0008-5472 (Print) 0008-5472 (Linking).

Papathoma, A.S.; Petraki, C.; Grigorakis, A.; Papakonstantinou, H.; Karavana, V.; Stefanakis, S.; Sotsiou, F. & Pintzas, A. (2000). Prognostic significance of matrix metalloproteinases 2 and 9 in bladder cancer. *Anticancer Res,* 20,3B, (May-Jun, 2000), 2009-13, 0250-7005 (Print) 0250-7005 (Linking).

Peinado, H.; Olmeda, D. & Cano, A. (2007). Snail, Zeb and bHLH factors in tumour progression: an alliance against the epithelial phenotype? *Nat Rev Cancer,* 7,6, (Jun, 2007), 415-28, 1474-175X (Print) 1474-175X (Linking).

Pfost, B.; Seidl, C.; Autenrieth, M.; Saur, D.; Bruchertseifer, F.; Morgenstern, A.; Schwaiger, M. & Senekowitsch-Schmidtke, R. (2009). Intravesical alpha-radioimmunotherapy with ^{213}Bi-anti-EGFR-mAb defeats human bladder carcinoma in xenografted nude mice. *J Nucl Med,* 50,10, (Oct, 2009), 1700-8, 1535-5667 (Electronic) 0161-5505 (Linking).

Riemensberger, J.; Bohle, A. & Brandau, S. (2002). IFN-gamma and IL-12 but not IL-10 are required for local tumour surveillance in a syngeneic model of orthotopic bladder cancer. *Clin Exp Immunol,* 127,1, (Jan, 2002), 20-6, 0009-9104 (Print) 0009-9104 (Linking).

Sandes, E.; Lodillinsky, C.; Cwirenbaum, R.; Arguelles, C.; Casabe, A. & Eijan, A.M. (2007). Cathepsin B is involved in the apoptosis intrinsic pathway induced by Bacillus Calmette-Guerin in transitional cancer cell lines. *Int J Mol Med,* 20,6, (Dec, 2007), 823-8, 1107-3756 (Print) 1107-3756 (Linking).

Smaldone, M.C.; Gayed, B.A.; Tomaszewski, J.J. & Gingrich, J.R. (2009). Strategies to enhance the efficacy of intravescical therapy for non-muscle invasive bladder cancer. *Minerva Urol Nefrol,* 61,2, (Jun, 2009), 71-89, 0393-2249 (Print) 0393-2249 (Linking).

Sobin, L.H. & Fleming, I.D. (1997). TNM Classification of Malignant Tumors, fifth edition (1997). Union Internationale Contre le Cancer and the American Joint Committee on Cancer. *Cancer,* 80,9, (Nov 1, 1997), 1803-4, 0008-543X (Print) 0008-543X (Linking).

Steeg, P.S. (2006). Tumor metastasis: mechanistic insights and clinical challenges. *Nat Med,* 12,8, (Aug, 2006), 895-904, 1078-8956 (Print) 1078-8956 (Linking).

Steele, V.E. & Lubet, R.A. (2010). The use of animal models for cancer chemoprevention drug development. *Semin Oncol,* 37,4, (Aug, 2010), 327-38, 1532-8708 (Electronic) 0093-7754 (Linking).

Steele, V.E.; Rao, C.V.; Zhang, Y.; Patlolla, J.; Boring, D.; Kopelovich, L.; Juliana, M.M.; Grubbs, C.J. & Lubet, R.A. (2009). Chemopreventive efficacy of naproxen and nitric oxide-naproxen in rodent models of colon, urinary bladder, and mammary cancers. *Cancer Prev Res (Phila),* 2,11, (Nov, 2009), 951-6, 1940-6215 (Electronic) 1940-6215 (Linking).

Sugano, G.; Bernard-Pierrot, I.; Lae, M.; Battail, C.; Allory, Y.; Stransky, N.; Krumeich, S.; Lepage, M.L.; Maille, P.; Donnadieu, M.H.; Abbou, C.C.; Benhamou, S.; Lebret, T.; Sastre-Garau, X.; Amigorena, S.; Radvanyi, F. & Thery, C. (2011). Milk fat globule--epidermal growth factor--factor VIII (MFGE8)/lactadherin promotes bladder tumor development. *Oncogene,* 30,6, (Feb 10, 2011), 642-53, 1476-5594 (Electronic) 0950-9232 (Linking).

Sylvester, R.J. (2009). Bacillus Calmette-Guerin versus mitomycin C for the treatment of intermediate-risk non-muscle-invasive bladder cancer: the debate continues. *Eur Urol,* 56,2, (Aug, 2009), 266-8; discussion 268-9, 1873-7560 (Electronic) 0302-2838 (Linking).

Takeuchi, A.; Dejima, T.; Yamada, H.; Shibata, K.; Nakamura, R.; Eto, M.; Nakatani, T.; Naito, S. & Yoshikai, Y. (2011). IL-17 production by gammadelta T cells is important for the antitumor effect of Mycobacterium bovis bacillus Calmette-Guerin treatment against bladder cancer. *Eur J Immunol,* 41,1, (Jan, 2011), 246-51, 1521-4141 (Electronic) 0014-2980 (Linking).

Tanaka, M.; Gee, J.R.; De La Cerda, J.; Rosser, C.J.; Zhou, J.H.; Benedict, W.F. & Grossman, H.B. (2003). Noninvasive detection of bladder cancer in an orthotopic murine model with green fluorescence protein cytology. *J Urol,* 170,3, (Sep, 2003), 975-8, 0022-5347 (Print) 0022-5347 (Linking).

Valastyan, S.; Reinhardt, F.; Benaich, N.; Calogrias, D.; Szasz, A.M.; Wang, Z.C.; Brock, J.E.; Richardson, A.L. & Weinberg, R.A. (2009). A pleiotropically acting microRNA, miR-31, inhibits breast cancer metastasis. *Cell,* 137,6, (Jun 12, 2009), 1032-46, 1097-4172 (Electronic) 0092-8674 (Linking).

Van 'T Veer, L.J.; Dai, H.; Van De Vijver, M.J.; He, Y.D.; Hart, A.A.; Mao, M.; Peterse, H.L.; Van Der Kooy, K.; Marton, M.J.; Witteveen, A.T.; Schreiber, G.J.; Kerkhoven, R.M.; Roberts, C.; Linsley, P.S.; Bernards, R. & Friend, S.H. (2002). Gene expression profiling predicts clinical outcome of breast cancer. *Nature,* 415,6871, (Jan 31, 2002), 530-6, 0028-0836 (Print) 0028-0836 (Linking).

Varley, C.L. & Southgate, J. (2011). Organotypic and 3D reconstructed cultures of the human bladder and urinary tract. *Methods Mol Biol,* 695, (2011), 197-211, 1940-6029 (Electronic) 1064-3745 (Linking).

Wang, L.; Yi, T.; Kortylewski, M.; Pardoll, D.M.; Zeng, D. & Yu, H. (2009). IL-17 can promote tumor growth through an IL-6-Stat3 signaling pathway. *J Exp Med,* 206,7, (Jul 6, 2009), 1457-64, 1540-9538 (Electronic) 0022-1007 (Linking).

Wu, Z.; Owens, C.; Chandra, N.; Popovic, K.; Conaway, M. & Theodorescu, D. (2010). RalBP1 is necessary for metastasis of human cancer cell lines. *Neoplasia,* 12,12, (Dec, 2010), 1003-12, 1476-5586 (Electronic) 1476-5586 (Linking).

Yao, R.; Lemon, W.J.; Wang, Y.; Grubbs, C.J.; Lubet, R.A. & You, M. (2004). Altered gene expression profile in mouse bladder cancers induced by hydroxybutyl (butyl) nitrosamine. *Neoplasia,* 6,5, (Sep-Oct, 2004), 569-77, 1522-8002 (Print) 1476-5586 (Linking).

Zhang, Z.; Xu, X.; Zhang, X.; Chen, X.; Chen, Q.; Dong, L.; Hu, Z.; Li, J. & Gao, J. (2011). The therapeutic potential of SA-sCD40L in the orthotopic model of superficial bladder cancer. *Acta Oncol,* (Jan 19, 2011), 1651-226X (Electronic) 0284-186X (Linking).

Zhang, Z.T.; Pak, J.; Huang, H.Y.; Shapiro, E.; Sun, T.T.; Pellicer, A. & Wu, X.R. (2001). Role of Ha-ras activation in superficial papillary pathway of urothelial tumor formation. *Oncogene,* 20,16, (Apr 12, 2001), 1973-80, 0950-9232 (Print) 0950-9232 (Linking).

20

Intracellular Arsenic Speciation and Quantification in Human Urothelial and Hepatic Cells

Ricarda Zdrenka, Joerg Hippler, Georg Johnen, Alfred V. Hirner and Elke Dopp
University of Duisburg-Essen, Ruhr-University Bochum, University Hospital Essen Germany

1. Introduction

Arsenic can be found in nearly every part of the geosphere. It is viewed as the most harmful toxin in drinking water worldwide. At many places on earth the drinking water contains concentrations above 10 µg/l, which significantly exceed the tolerable value recommended by the WHO (World health organization [WHO], 2001). This is considered as a health threat for millions of people, especially in Bangladesh, Vietnam, and Latin America, where the geogenic origin has already been proved (Ng et al., 2003). The sources of this considerable arsenic occurrence (Fig. 1) are geogenic (erosion), mining activities, and geothermal waters (Smedly & Kinniburgh, 2002).

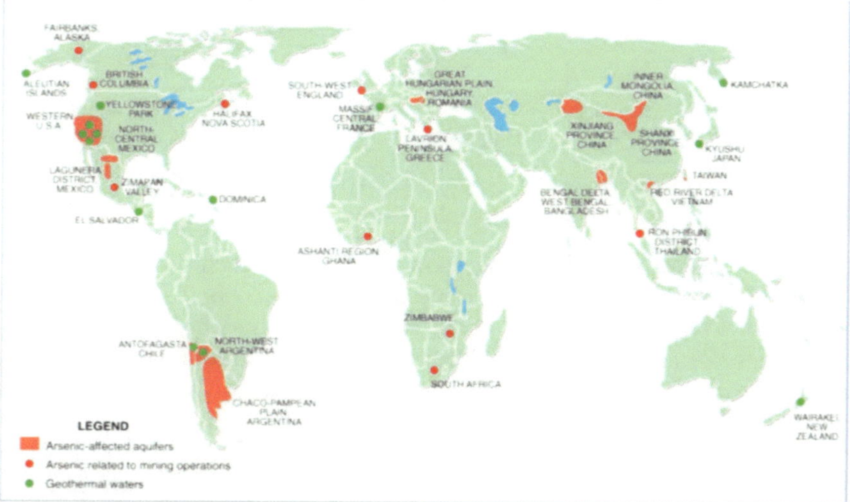

Fig. 1. Map of arsenic affected aquifers (Smedly & Kinniburgh, 2002)

The main arsenic species detected in drinking water are arsenite and arsenate. But the geothermal waters (Hot Spots) in the Yellowstone Nationalpark, USA, predominantly contain several mg/l of methylated thioarsenicals such as mono-, di-, tri-, and tetrathioarsenate, as well as methylated arsenoxy- and -thioanions (Planer-Friedrich et al., 2007). In the surrounding atmosphere 0.5 – 200 mg/m^3 of volatile arsenic species can be detected, which have been identified, among others, as $(CH_3)_2AsCl$, $(CH_3)_3As$, $(CH_3)_2AsSCH_3$, and CH_3AsCl_2 (Planer-Friedrich et al., 2006).

A second important source of arsenic is the air, whereas only one third of the occurring arsenic is of natural origin. Further anthropogenic sources are ore mining, smelteries, and the combustion of fossil fuels [Lozna & Biernat, 2008].

Among polluted air and contaminated drinking water also the human diet is of importance. For example, high doses of arsenic can be detected in fish, seafood, and algae, so that in 2004 the Food Agency of the UK warned against the consumption of Hijiki (hijikia fusiforme, black sea weed) (Food Standards Agency of the UK, 2004) as it contains inorganic arsenic up to 100 mg/kg. High arsenic concentrations can be found in the urine of the consumers (Nakjima et al., 2006). Francesconi published in 2010 the detection of up to 50 different arsenic compounds in fish and seafood, whereas their toxicity still is widely unknown (Francesconi, 2010).

Especially rice and rice products exhibit considerable noxious effects as they contain high doses of toxic inorganic arsenic (Meharg et al., 2008; Signes-Pastor et al., 2009; Sun et al., 2009) and form the nutrition base especially of the Asian people. But not only the rice from Asia but also the rice from the middle of the USA is contaminated with arsenic, the latter sustaining its contaminant not basically from natural sources but from pesticides anciently used on the cotton plantations. Finally DDT was introduced replaced arsenic in biocides (Hirner & Hippler, 2011). Fig. 2 summarises the several pathways of the human exposure to arsenic.

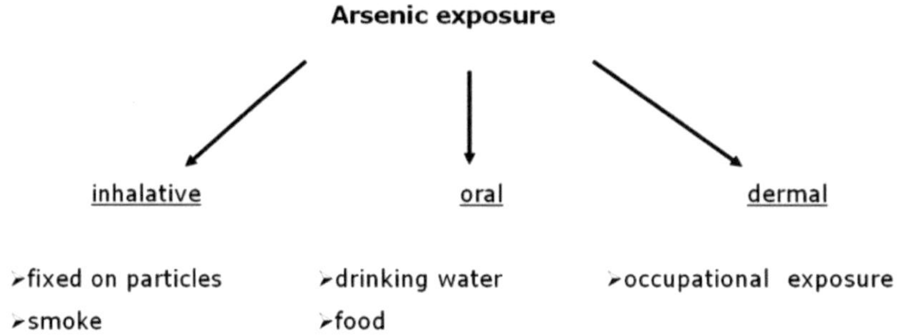

Fig. 2. Pathways of human exposure to arsenic (Dopp, 2007)

Chronic low-dose exposure may cause various diseases including bladder and other cancers. After ingestion arsenic is distributed to several organs, where it undergoes biotransformation. In 2005 Hayakawa et al. suggested a metabolic pathway (Fig. 3) for arsenic in rat liver tissue homogenate. Hereby arsenic-glutathione complexes are formed, which are then methylated by arsenic methyltransferase (Cyt19) and S-adenosyl-L-methionine (SAM) (Hayakawa et al., 2005).

This biotransformation of arsenic is generally regarded as a detoxifying process. Nevertheless, the trivalent arsenic intermediates and metabolites such as MMA(III) (monomethylarsonous acid) and DMA(III) (dimethylarsinous acid) are considered the most cyto- and genotoxic species (Dopp et al., 2010a). The liver is the main site of arsenic metabolism, and the renal route is the most important excretion pathway. A number of human studies have revealed that predominantly monomethylarsonic acid (MMA(V)) and dimethylarsinic acid (DMA(V)) can be detected in urine samples of arsenic-exposed individuals. Furthermore, Aposhian et al.

detected concentrations of about 50 nM MMA(III) in the urine of an arsenic-exposed human population in Romania (Aposhian et al., 2000). Studies in rats have shown that ingestion of DMA(V) causes bladder cancer (Wei et al., 1999) after chronic exposure. Subsequent experiments indicated that a large number of secondary arsenic metabolites are formed and renally excreted. For example, thiolated arsenicals such as dimethylmonothioarsonic acid (DMMTA(V)) were detected in the urine of DMA(V)-exposed rats (Yoshida et al., 1998). It is still unknown, however, which of the various arsenic metabolites is responsible for the development of bladder cancer. The metabolism of arsenic is of great importance for toxicological studies. As summarised by Dopp et al. (2010b) and Hirner & Rettenmeier (2010), the cyto- and genotoxic effects are highly dependent on the particular arsenic species, its cellular uptake, and its intracellular metabolism. For example, the toxicity of MMA(III) is 20 times greater than that of As(III) (Styblo et al., 2002; Bredfeldt et al., 2006).

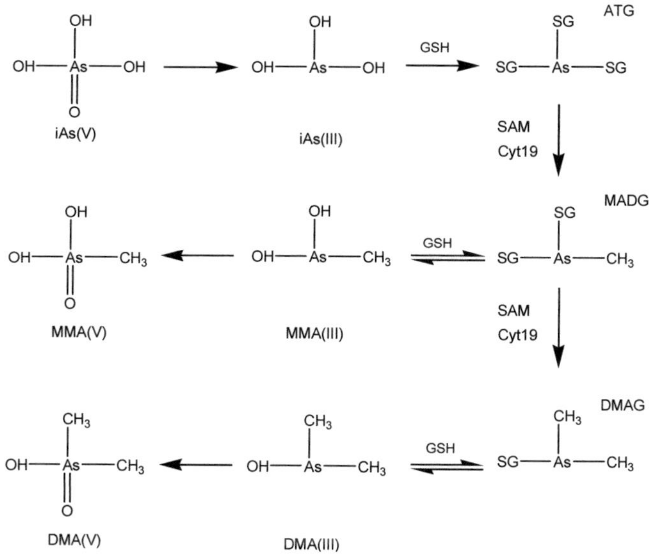

Fig. 3. Mechanism of arsenic biomethylation according to Hayakawa (Hayakawa et al., 2005)

Acute arsenic toxicity causes abdominal pain, nausea and faintness, vomiting, diarrhoea, and seizures (Gorby & Albuquerque, 1988). In contrast, chronic arsenic toxicity is less conspicuous. Characteristic symptoms are Mees' lines and hyperkeratosis predominantly at palms and soles of the feet. Furthermore, vascular diseases and peripheral neuropathy, and diabetes mellitus may occur (Smith et al., 2000). Until now, more than 60 million people in Bangladesh and India are still at risk of arsenic induced diseases due to arsenic concentrations of 10 - 50 µg/l or even higher (Chakraborti et al., 2004).

Moreover, chronic arsenic exposure is also associated with an increased risk of cancer. Especially arsenic induced lung cancer, as well as skin, kidney, and bladder cancer were reported (Chiou et al, 1995; Chen et al., 2010; Tseng, 2007).

The mechanisms of arsenic toxicity are only poorly understood. The structural likeness of arsenate and phosphate (Fig. 4), which is called molecular mimicry, results for example in the use of the same cellular transporters. Furthermore, there are plenty of biomolecules known, in which arsenate replaces phosphate, such as arsenosugars, arsenolipids and arsenobetaine (Rosen et al., 2011).

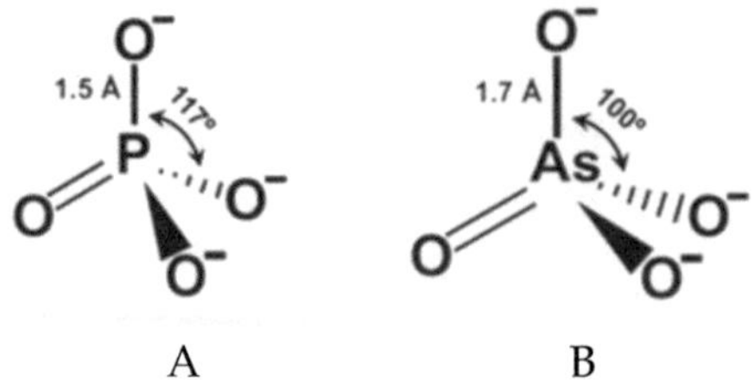

Fig. 4. Molecular mimicry of phosphate (A) and arsenate (B) (Rosen et al., 2011, modified)

The relevance of this molecular mimicry is pointed out in the study of Wolfe-Simon et al. (2011), reporting that phosphate can be substituted by arsenate in macromolecules of a bacterium, strain GFAJ-1 of the Halomonadaceae, isolated from Mono Lake, CA. However, these data are currently controversially discussed in the literature. Hereby few points have to be considered, first the rapid hydrolysis of arsenate esters, and second the notably altered three dimensional structure of macromolecules like DNA (Rosen et al., 2011).

One generally accepted mechanism for arsenic toxicity is the generation of reactive oxygen species (ROS). While ROS physiologically occur during cellular respiration or aerobic metabolism they also can result from exposure to oxidants. Already low levels of As(III) and MMA(III) are reported to generate ROS and therefore cause oxidative stress (Eblin et al., 2008; Wnek et al., 2009). These highly reactive radicals are discussed to exhibit their toxicity via induction of DNA damage, formation of DNA adducts, or alteration of DNA methylation and histone modifications (Wnek et al., 2009), and finally leading to carcinogenesis (Kitchin & Ahmad, 2003; Huang et al., 2004). In addition, arsenic is known to interfere with nucleotide and base excision repair at very low, non-cytotoxic concentrations and was observed for both trivalent and pentavalent metabolites. Hereby, MMA(III) and DMA(III) were reported to exhibit the strongest effects (Hartwig et al., 2003). One key mechanism is the inactivation of poly (ADP-ribose) polymerase (PARP) already at extremely low, environmentally relevant concentrations (Hartwig et al., 2002; Hartwig et al., 2003). Wnek et al. (2009) reported that the relative PARP activity was significantly reduced during chronic exposure of immortalised human urothelial cells (UROtsa) to 50 nM MMA(III). After removal of MMA(III) PARP activity increased again. Trivalent arsenic species are known to attach to zinc-binding structures generally found in DNA repair enzymes leading to alteration or inhibition of those proteins and finally the loss of genomic integrity (Kitchin & Wallace, 2008). In contrast, former studies report the insensitivity of isolated and purified DNA repair enzymes against inhibition by arsenic (Hu et al., 1998). This leads to the assumption that there are different modes of action for arsenic inhibited DNA repair, on the one hand by directly targeting DNA repair proteins, and on the other hand by altered signal transduction or gene expression.

Another mechanism of arsenic induced carcinogenesis is the altered cytoplasmic and nuclear signal transduction, modifying proteins involved in cell proliferation, differentiation, and apoptosis (Wnek et al., 2009). Hereby ROS were detected to be one key mechanism for the influence of As(III) and MMA(III) on the mitogen-activated protein kinase (MAPK) signaling pathway leading to consistent changes in cellular signalling (Eblin et al., 2008). The persistence of MMA(III)-induced altered cellular functions even after the removal of arsenic exposure point to lasting genomic or epigenetic changes and thus the highly carcinogenic potential of arsenic and its metabolites.

Furthermore, not only the molecular changes in the genome of arsenic exposed tissue and the altered signal transduction are of interest, but also the resulting phenotypical alterations. For the medical treatment of cancer it is of great interest whether the tumour has metastatic potential. Therefore, the tumour requires invasive growth into the surrounding tissue and the blood vessels. For example, the decrease of E-cadherin expression on the cellular surface is necessary for the detachment from the original tumour, and the increased expression of integrins is an important requirement for the attachment in the surrounding tissues like cells or extracellular matrix.

To better understand the underlying mechanisms of arsenic toxicity and carcinogenicity, further studies have to be carried out to correlate genotypic and metabolic effects with phenotypical alterations, especially under chronic exposure conditions. Therefore, it is important to detect and analyse intracellular arsenic species and their metabolic products. In own studies we have investigated the cellular uptake of arsenic species in non-methylating human urothelial (UROtsa) and methylating human hepatic cells (HepG2) and have speciated and quantified the intracellularly detected arsenic. Induced genotoxic effects in UROtsa cells were measured with the Alkaline Comet Assay and the malignant transformation after chronic arsenic treatment was assayed by using the Colony Formation Assay and the Migration and Invasion Assay. Our latest results are presented here.

2. Experimental

2.1 Cell culture

Studies were carried out using the human immortalized urothelial cell line UROtsa (generous gift from Prof. M. Styblo, University of North Dakota, USA). The UROtsa cells were maintained in Earle's minimal essential medium (MEM) (CC-PRO, Oberdorla, Germany) enriched with 10 % FBS (fetal bovine serum; GIBCO, Darmstadt, Germany), 0.5 % Gentamycin (CC-Pro GmbH, Oberdorla, Germany) and 1 % L-glutamine (CC-Pro GmbH, Oberdorla, Germany).

For comparison of a methylating and non-methylating cell line, HepG2 cells (human liver cells, methylating cells) were used as a second cell line. HepG2 cells were obtained from ATCC (HB 8065; ATCC, Manassas, VA, USA) and cultured in Earle's minimal essential medium (MEM) (CC-PRO, Oberdorla, Germany) enriched with 10 % FBS (GIBCO, Darmstadt, Germany), 0.5 % Gentamycin (CC-Pro GmbH, Oberdorla, Germany), 1 % L - glutamine (CC-Pro GmbH, Oberdorla, Germany), 1 % non essential amino acids (CC-Pro GmbH, Oberdorla, Germany) and 1 % sodium pyruvate (CC-Pro GmbH, Oberdorla, Germany).

All cells were grown under typical cell culture conditions (37 °C, 5 % CO_2, humidified incubator) and medium was replaced every 2 – 3 days. Cells were grown to 75 - 80 % confluence. For subculture the cells were washed with PBS (Phosphate buffered saline; GIBCO, Darmstadt, Germany) and UROtsa and HepG2 cells were detached using 0.25 % trypsine containing 0.1 % EDTA (2-[2-[bis(carboxymethyl]amino]ethyl-(carboymethyl) amino]acetic acid (CC-Pro GmbH, Oberdorla, Germany)) and finally split into ¼ and transferred into new flasks.

For chronic treatment 300,000 UROtsa cells were seeded into 75 cm^2 flasks and fed with 25 ml medium containing 50 nM, 75 nM, or 100 nM MMA(III), respectively. UROtsa cells fed with medium without any arsenic compound served as negative control. Once a week the cells were subcultured and fed with fresh exposure medium and 4 days later the exposure medium was replaced again. For cell detachment 0.25 % trypsin without EDTA (CC-Pro GmbH, Oberdorla, Germany) was used to prevent the complexation of arsenic.

2.2 Intracellular arsenic speciation and quantification

The following methodology (Hippler et al., 2011) was used for intracellular arsenic speciation and quantification: Cells were seeded into 150 cm² flasks and grown to confluence before experiments were performed. Both cell lines (UROtsa and HepG2) were incubated for five minutes to 24 hours in fresh growth medium containing 5 µM MMA(III) (exposure medium). The negative control consisted of cells incubated in fresh medium without any arsenic compound and subsequently they were handled the same way as the exposed cells. Additionally, a second negative control was trypsinised for cell counting.
After incubation the exposure medium was withdrawn and stored at -80°C. Cells were washed with 10 ml PBS and 10 ml Ampuwa (sterile deionised water). For the next washing step 10 ml 0.1 mM DMPS (2,3-bis(sulfanyl)propane-1-sulfonic acid) were used to remove traces of extracellular uncombined arsenic ions. The last washing step with 10 ml PBS was carried out to remove the residues of DMPS before lysis (Fig. 5.). All washing solutions were retained and stored at -80 °C until arsenic speciation analysis.

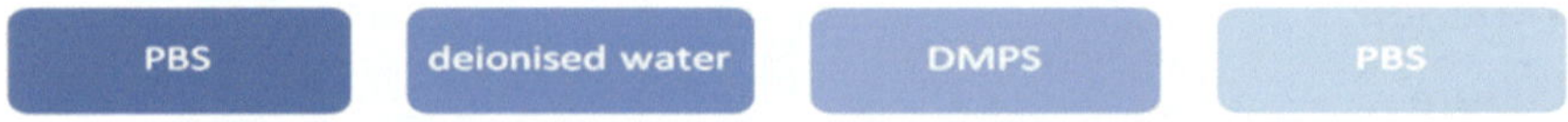

Fig. 5. Washing process prior the intracellular arsenic speciation and quantification: Exhaustive cell washing ensures the removal of all extracellular arsenic residues after the exposure (Hippler et al., 2011, modified).

The cell lysis was performed using the Precellys®24 tissue homogeniser (Peqlab Biotechnologie GmbH, Erlangen, Germany) as a tool for mechanical lysis. Therefore the cells were first detached from the culture flasks using a cell scraper and transferred to 0.5 ml tubes containing ceramic beads with a diameter of 1.4 mm (Peqlab Biotechnologie GmbH, Erlangen, Germany). Exhaustive homogenisation was obtained within three intervals of 20 seconds and 6500 rpm. Final centrifugation using a MiniSpin plus centrifuge at 14.000 x g (Eppendorf AG, Hamburg, Germany) assured a complete separation of the cell lysates from membranes and other solid, insoluble cellular structures. This non-soluble fraction of each sample was then digested using Proteinase K until the pellet was dissolved. Further oxidation with hydrogen peroxide (30 %) assured the release of arsenic from peptides and other cellular molecules.
After exposure, lysis and centrifugation all solutions and samples were stored at -80 °C. The cell lysates were thawed immediately before HPLC-ICP/MS analysis. Depending on the arsenic content of the samples, 1 to 25 µl were injected onto the HPLC-column.
For quantification a multi-As species standard containing 2 pg to 200 pg As(III), MMA(III), DMA(V), MMA(V), DMA(III), and As(V) was injected. Peak areas were obtained by monitoring transient signals for As at m/z 75 in non-collision cell mode at dwell times of 100 ms. The linearity of the external calibration resulted in an excellent calibration (e.g. MMA(V): r^2 = 0.9999; DMA(V): r^2 = 0.999). Limits of detection were approximately 3 pg As, varying slightly depending on the arsenic species. Table 1

presents the conditions for the high performance liquid chromatography (HPLC) and inductive coupled plasma mass spectrometry (ICP/MS). For reproduction the whole experiment was performed twice.

HPLC conditions		ICP/MS conditions	
HPLC Column	Phenomenex Luna 3µ C18(2) 100 Å	Forward power (RF)	1580 W
Column temperature	30 °C	Plasma gas rate (cool gas flow)	15 L Argon min^{-1}
Eluent flow rate	0.5 ml min^{-1}	Carrier gas flow rate	~ 0.8 L min^{-1}
Injection volume	1 - 25µl	Make-up gas flow rate	~ 0.25 L min^{-1}
		Sample depth	5.7 mm
Eluent:		Spray chamber	Quarz, cooled, 2 °C
Malonic acid	2 mM		
Tetrabutylammonium hydroxide (TBAH)	6 mM	Isotopes monitored	^{75}As, ^{35}Cl, $^{77}(^{40}Ar^{37}Cl)^{34}S$, ^{71}Ga, ^{73}Ge, ^{115}In, ^{103}Rh
Methanol	5 v/v%		
Water	95 v/v%		
pH	6.0		

Table 1. Conditions for the high performance liquid chromatography (HPLC) and inductive coupled plasma mass spectrometry (ICP/MS) (Hippler et al., 2011, modified)

2.3 Alkaline Comet Assay

For detection of genotoxic effects caused by arsenic exposure, the Alkaline Comet Assay was used. This assay detects single and double strand breaks of the DNA by single cell gel electrophoresis. Therefore UROtsa cells were seeded with a density of 100,000 cells / 2 ml medium into each well of a 24-well-plate and incubated over night. For exposure cell culture medium was removed and 2 ml of the exposure medium containing the arsenic compounds As(III) (arsenite), As(V) (arsenate), MMA(III) (monomethylarsonous acid), MMA(V) (monomethylarsonic acid), DMA(V) (dimethylarsinous acid) and TMAO (trimethylarsine oxide) in different concentrations were added. The negative control consisted of untreated cells; the positive control was exposed to 1 mg/ml N-ethyl-nitrosourea. For exposure to the volatile species DMA(III) (dimethylarsinous acid) 1,000,000 cells/10 ml medium were seeded into 25 cm^2 cell culture flasks with vent caps.

After incubation for 30 min exposure media were removed and the cells were trypsinised as described above. The cells were resuspended in PBS and 5,000 cells were seeded into each agarose gel consisting of 0.79 % low melting point agarose in PBS. The gels were solidified on ice and the cells were lysed over night.

For electrophoresis the gels were washed with Ampuwa and incubated in 4 °C cold electrophoresis solution at pH 13 for 15 min. After electrophoresis for 30 min the gels were washed with Ampuwa and neutralised to pH 7.5. Finally the gels were washed with deionised water again and incubated in ethanol p.a. to remove the water residues. The gels were now dried over night at 4 °C.

Image analysis was performed with Comet Assay IV Software (Perceptive Instruments Ltd., Haverhill, UK) using a fluorescence microscope (Leica Microsystems GmbH, Wetzlar, Germany) and a digital camera (Leica Microsystems GmbH, Wetzlar, Germany). Therefore the cells were stained with SYBR GREEN (Sigma-Aldrich, Saint Louis, Missouri, USA) and 50 cells / gel were evaluated.

2.4 Colony formation assay

When a normal cell is transformed to a cancer cell it loses its ability to grow in monolayers. After cell transformation (a step towards malignancy) the cells grow in colonies. With help of the colony formation assay (Bredfeldt et al., 2006) the development of an anchorage independent growth after chronic exposure of cells to arsenic can be determined. The colony formation assay was prepared in a 24-well plate. First 500 µL of a base agar containing 0.6 % low melting point agarose in cell culture medium were added to each well, solidified at room temperature and sterilised under UV light over night.

UROtsa cells were seeded with a density of 10,000 cells / 500 µL into each well. Additional wells were prepared without cells containing only base and top agar for background detection. The cells were fed with 250 µL of fresh cell culture medium every 3 – 4 days.

Image analysis was performed after 2 weeks of incubation using an inverted microscope (Leica Microsystems GmbH, Wetzlar, Germany) combined with a Leica digital camera (Leica Microsystems GmbH, Wetzlar, Germany).

2.5 Cellular migration and invasion

Typical features of transformed and cancer cells are increased proliferation, migration and invasion. For the detection of invasion the xCELLigence DP system (Roche Applied Science, Mannheim, Germany) was conducted. Therefore CIM-Plates (Roche Applied Science, Mannheim, Germany) were coated with 50 µl of 0.02 % collagen (SERVA Electrophoresis GmbH, Heidelberg, Germany) on each side of the microporous membrane for 1 h. After removing the collagen residues the CIM-Plates were dried for approximately 1 h at room temperature under the laminar flow. In between UROtsa cells originated from the chronic exposure were trypsinised as described above and brought to a concentration of 1.5 Mio cells / ml. For the detection of migration uncoated CIM-Plates were conducted.

160 µl of the pre-warmed cell culture medium were added to each well of the lower chamber and 100 µl were added to each well of the upper chamber. The CIM-Plates were then placed into the xCELLigence devices and the background was measured. Now 100 µl of the prepared cell suspensions were added (duplicate wells) and the CIM-Plates were placed into the xCELLigence again. The measurement was performed for 24 h with intervals of 15 min.

2.6 Statistics

All experiments were performed in triplicate unless stated otherwise. The statistical evaluation for the Alkaline Comet Assay was performed using GraphPad Prism (GraphPad Software, San Diego, USA). The mean values of the detected Olive Tail Moments are presented in bar graphs with the standard error of mean. For statistical analysis the non-parametric Mann-Whitney-Test was applied, which approximates the Gaussian distribution for more than 20 random samples and compares each test group to the untreated control group. The results are given in significance levels p for the confidence interval of 95 %. Then one has $p > 0.05$: non-significant, $p \leq 0.05$: *, $p \leq 0.01$: **, $p \leq 0.001$: ***.

3. Results

3.1 Intracellular arsenic speciation and quantification

To study the intracellular arsenic biotransformation of MMA(III) we incubated UROtsa and HepG2 cells with 5 µM MMA(III) for 5 min up to 24 hours, followed by a newly developed sample preparation process (Hippler et al., 2011). Using HPLC-ICP/MS analysis we were able to detect more than 99.99% of the total arsenic in the non-soluble fraction of both cell lines and only 0.003% in the soluble fraction of UROtsa cells and 0.01% of HepG2 cells, respectively. While in the non-soluble fraction of UROtsa cells the arsenic content consisted only of a monomethylated species, in HepG2 cells a time dependent occurrence of a dimethylated arsenic species additionally to monomethylated arsenic was observed (Fig. 6.). The differentiation between trivalent and pentavalent arsenic metabolites was impossible due to their oxidative release from the cellular structures.

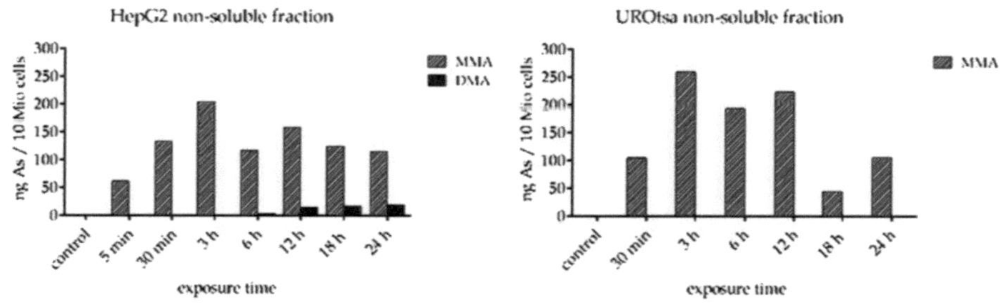

Fig. 6. Quantification of the metabolites in the non-soluble fraction after exposure of HepG2 and UROtsa cells to 5 µM MMA(III). The analysis was performed using HPLC-ICP/MS technique.

In the soluble fractions of both HepG2 and UROtsa cells only pentavalent arsenic species were detected (Fig 7.). In HepG2 cells a time dependent increase and decrease of MMA(V) was observed. Additionally we analysed the increase of DMA(V) by time. In contrast, in UROtsa cells only MMA(V) but no DMA(V) was detected. The occurrence of MMA(III) after 18 and 24 hours of exposure is believed to be the result of cytotoxic effects and can be correlated with membrane damage (data not shown).

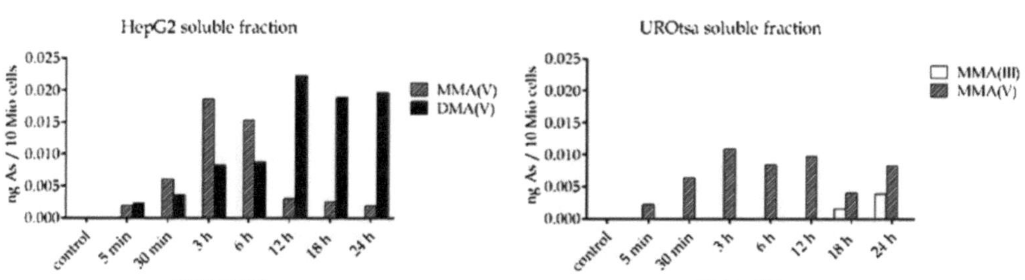

Fig. 7. Quantification of the metabolites in the soluble fraction after exposure of HepG2 and UROtsa cells to 5 µM MMA(III). The analysis was performed using HPLC-ICP/MS technique.

3.2 Alkaline Comet Assay

The Alkaline Comet Assay was conducted to examine the genotoxic effects of different arsenic metabolites. Testing the trivalent species we observed significant single and double strand breaks in UROtsa cells already after 30 min of exposure (Fig. 8.). Although the biotransformation initially was discussed to serve as a detoxification process, MMA(III) still is highly genotoxic and DMA(III) even exhibits the most genotoxic effects. In contrast, pentavalent arsenic species did not show any genotoxic effect except for As(V) at very high concentrations (Fig. 9).

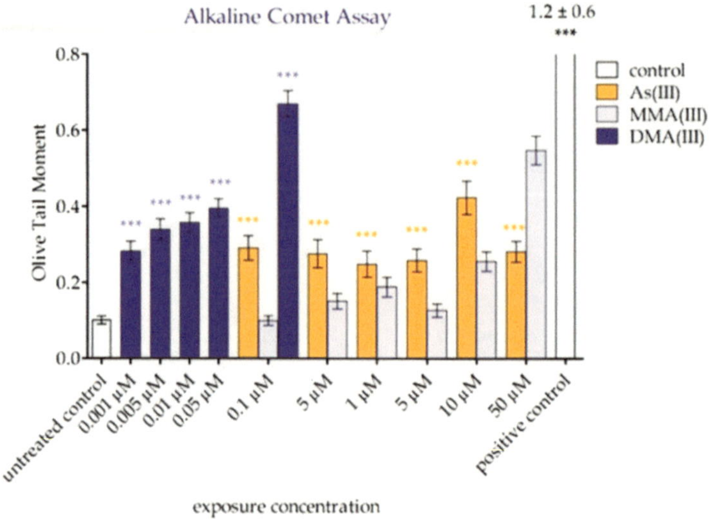

(mean ± SEM with $p > 0.05$: non-significant, $p \leq 0.05$: *, $p \leq 0.01$: **, $p \leq 0.001$: ***)

Fig. 8. The Alkaline Comet Assay was conducted to assay single and double strand breaks of the DNA after 30 min of exposure to the trivalent arsenic species As(III), MMA(III) and DMA(III). The DNA damage is given in the Olive Tail Moment.

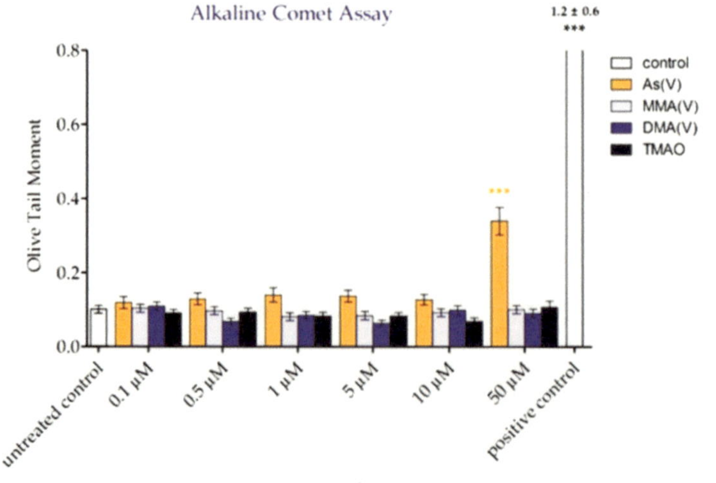

(mean ± SEM with $p > 0.05$: non-significant, $p \leq 0.05$: *, $p \leq 0.01$: **, $p \leq 0.001$: ***)

Fig. 9. The Alkaline Comet Assay was conducted to assay single and double strand breaks of the DNA after 30 min of exposure to the pentavalent arsenic species As(V), MMA(V), DMA(V) and TMAO. The DNA damage is given in the Olive Tail Moment.

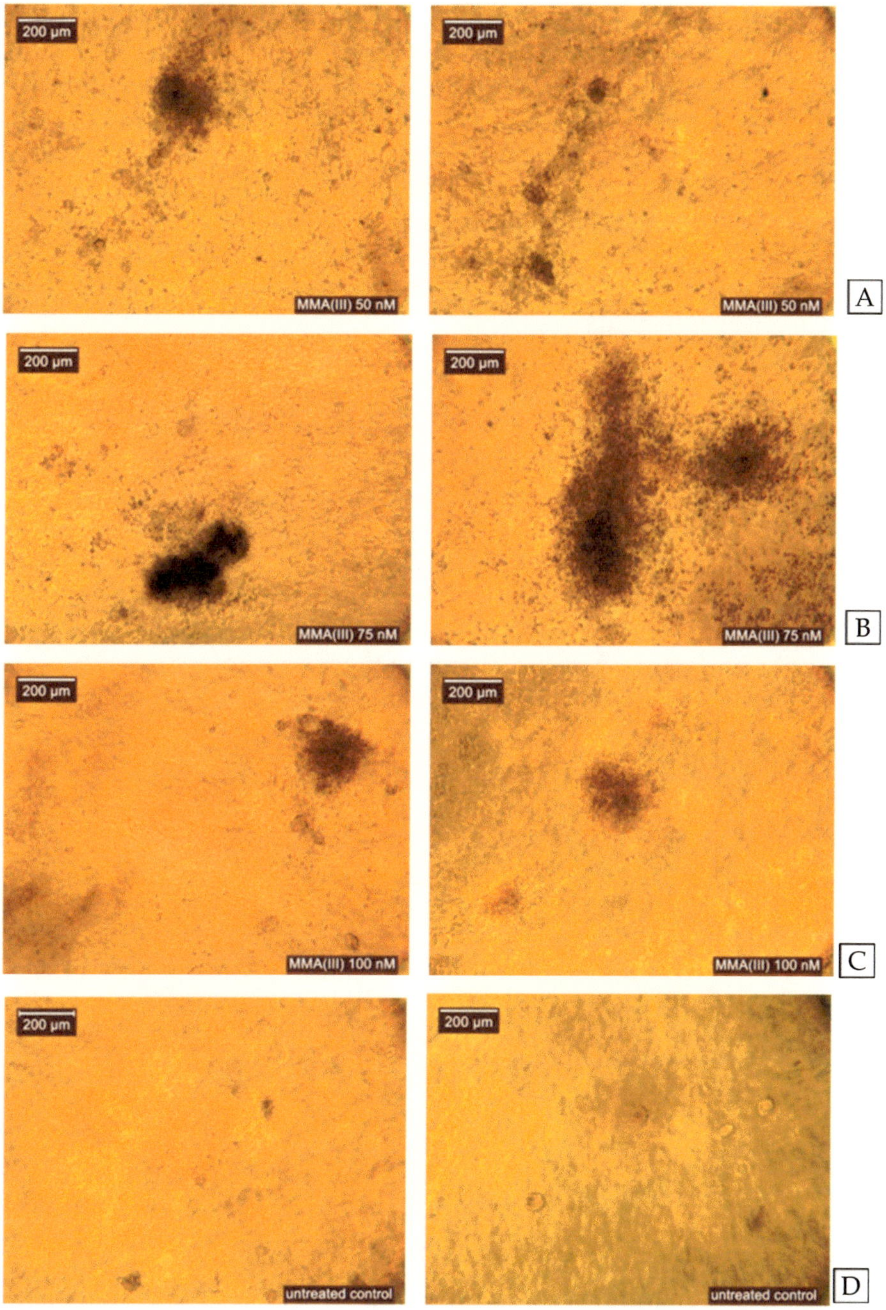

Fig. 10. The Colony formation assay was conducted for the analysis of an anchorage independent growth after chronic treatment of UROtsa cells with 50 nM (**A**), 75 nM (**B**), or 100 nM (**C**) MMA(III), respectively, for 93 weeks. The negative control (**D**) consisted of untreated UROtsa cells of the same passage. Given are two pictures of parallel treated samples.

3.3 Colony formation assay

To analyse the carcinogenic potential of one of the most important arsenic metabolites, MMA(III), UROtsa cells were cultured for 93 weeks and treated twice a week with fresh exposure medium containing 50 nM, 75 nM, and 100 nM MMA(III), respectively. Untreated UROtsa cells of the same passage served as negative control. The colony formation assay was determined to assay the loss of an anchorage dependent growth. As proven by the negative control, UROtsa cells are adherent cells and hence they cannot be cultured in soft agar (Bredfeldt et al., 2006). In contrast, after chronic exposure to MMA(III) UROtsa cells exhibit an anchorage independent growth and form notable colonies after two weeks of incubation in soft agar (Fig. 10.).

3.4 Cellular migration and invasion

To estimate the malignant potential of chronically exposed human urothelial cells to arsenic, their altered motility and invasiveness were examined. The xCELLigence system was conducted to assay the migration and invasion ability of UROtsa cells after 92 weeks of exposure to MMA(III). Hereby the cells moved through a microporous membrane and attached at the opposite side on the electrodes. For the analysis of the invasiveness the membranes and electrodes were coated with collagen, a typical extracellular matrix. The results show that after exposure to 75 nM and 100 nM MMA(III) for 92 weeks the motility of UROtsa cells was increased in comparison to the untreated control of the same passage. Only the exposure to 50 nM MMA(III) did not lead to an increase of migrated cells (Fig. 11.).

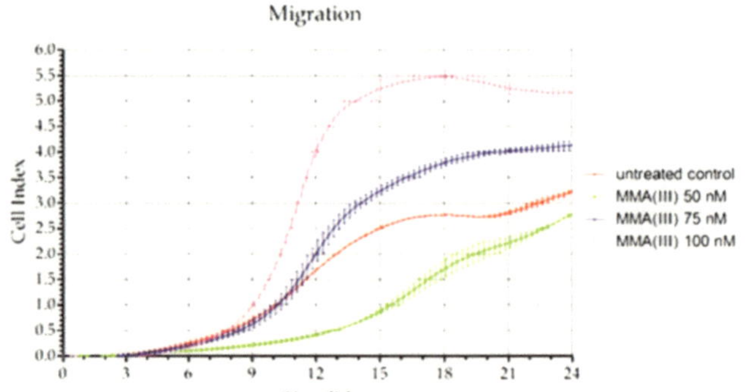

Fig. 11. The xCELLigence system was conducted for the analysis of the ability of migration after chronic treatment of UROtsa cells with 50 nM, 75 nM, or 100 nM MMA(III), respectively, for 92 weeks.

The examination of the invasion led to similar results. After coating the plate surface with collagen all samples exhibited an increased invasion property compared to the untreated control (Fig. 12.). In both migration and invasion assays the cells treated with 100 nM MMA(III) exhibited the strongest effects, leading to the assumption of an dose-dependent manner.

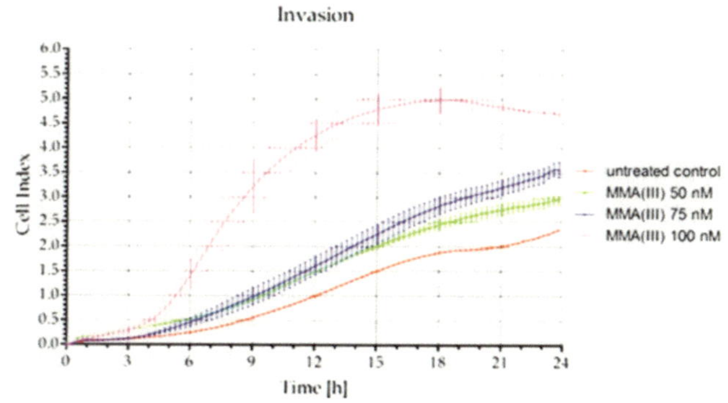

Fig. 12. The xCELLigence system was conducted for the analysis of the ability of invasion after chronic treatment of UROtsa cells with 50 nM, 75 nM, or 100 nM MMA(III), respectively, for 92 weeks. CIM-Plates were coated with collagen to simulate a biological matrix.

4. Discussion and conclusion

Arsenic is one of the most harmful toxins in drinking water worldwide and at many places on earth millions of people are at risk of arsenic induced diseases including cancer. In our study we have investigated the cellular uptake and biotransformation of arsenic species in non-methylating human urothelial (UROtsa) and methylating human hepatic cells (HepG2) using HPLC-ICP/MS technique. The induced genotoxic effects of several arsenic species in UROtsa cells were measured with the Alkaline Comet Assay and the malignant transformation after chronic arsenic treatment was assayed by using the Colony Formation Assay and the Migration and Invasion Assay.

The data presented here demonstrate that MMA(III) is rapidly taken up by human urothelial cells (UROtsa) and human hepatoma cells (HepG2). MMA(III) is known to be an important arsenic metabolite due to its high toxicity. Many studies report monomethylated and dimethylated arsenic species as the main metabolites in the urine (Aposhian et al., 2000; Fillol et al., 2010). Using an improved isolation method and HPLC-ICP/MS technique we were able to analyse not only the fast association of MMA(III) to large membrane structures, high-molecular-weight proteins, and other insoluble cell components, but also the presence of unbound pentavalent arsenic metabolites in the soluble fractions which only amount to 0.003% of the total intracellular arsenic in UROtsa cells and 0.01% in HepG2 cells, respectively. Furthermore we were able to differentiate between the various methylated metabolites and also their oxidation state in this complex cellular matrices.

The data demonstrate for both cell lines a fast cellular uptake of MMA(III) and the subsequent oxidation to MMA(V) already within 5 min of exposure and further increasing with time. Additionally, in HepG2 cells we observed a time dependent methylation to DMA(V). These findings appear to be in contrast to the reductive intracellular milieu (Du et al., 2009) due to glutathione concentrations up to millimolar ranges (Anderson, 1998). However, taking different cell compartments and specific metabolic effects of arsenic into account could provide a possible explanation. It is largely known from the literature that in contrast to their pentavalent analogues trivalent arsenicals bind to proteins (Styblo & Thomas, 1997; Yan et al., 2009). This leads to the assumption that MMA(III) rapidly binds to proteins after uptake, which is in compliance with the detection of more than 99.99 % of the total arsenic in the non-soluble fraction in both cell lines. We suggest that there is a fast subsequent degradation of at least part of the arsenic-conjugated or arsenic-inhibited proteins. Protein degradation is predominantly mediated by the proteasomes but can also take place in lysosomes, especially during turnover of membrane proteins (Clague & Urbé, 2010). An increased turnover of arsenic-bound proteins is in agreement with the evidence of the catabolism of arsenic-induced improperly folded or damaged proteins via the ubiquitin-dependent protein degradation pathway in zebrafish liver (Lam et al., 2006). Several studies report that protein ubiquitination not only targets protein degradation using the proteasome pathway but also the lysosomal pathway (Marques et al., 2004; Barriere et al.; 2007, Shenoy et al, 2008; Arancibia-Cárcamo et al, 2009). The lysosome is known to exhibit cellular oxidative activities (Chen, 2002) and during oxidative stress large amounts of hydrogen peroxide enter the lysosome, leading to the formation of hydroxyl radicals and lysosomal destabilisation (Terman et al., 2006). In addition, the lysosome is an important organelle in autophagy, helping the cells to remove toxic aggregation-prone proteins and even damaged organelles that are incompatible with the unfolding mechanism of the proteasome (Yang et al., 2008; Clague & Urbé, 2010; Mehrpour et al., 2010). The increase of protein catabolism, the elimination of excess or damaged organelles by autophagy, and the sequestering of toxicants is ubiquitous and believed to be a kind of "first-response reaction" to delay apoptosis (Kundu & Thompson, 2008; Yang et al., 2008). In the early stage of cell death autophagy is activated in HL60 cells soon after exposure to As_2O_3 to maintain cell survival under stress conditions (Yang et al., 2008).

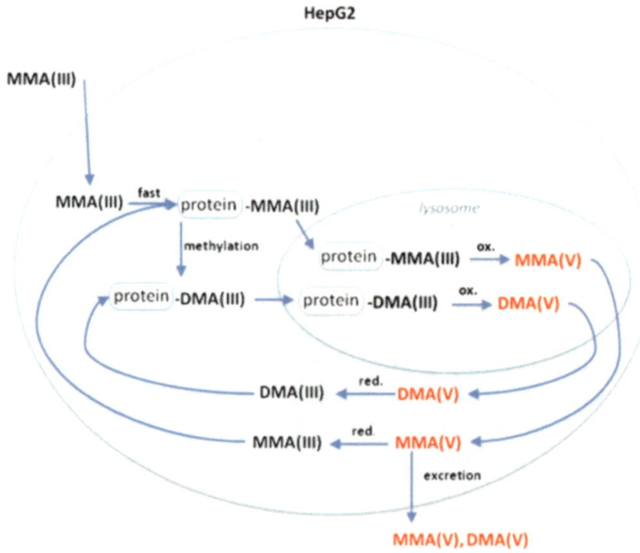

Fig. 13. Proposed arsenic cycle in HepG2 cells after exposure to MMA(III) (Hippler et al. 2011, modified)

Summarising all these data we conclude from our results that MMA(III) is immediately taken up and rapidly bound to proteins and other cellular structures, followed by, first, the generally accepted methylation to dimethylarsinic in HepG2 cells only, and second, the degradation of affected proteins and cellular structures in the lysosome in both HepG2 and UROtsa cells (Fig. 13. and 14.). During oxidative degradation in the lysosome arsenic is released as MMA(V) and DMA(V), which are either excreted from the cell or reduced by antioxidants in the cytosol. The reduced species MMA(III) and DMA(III) can then re-associate with proteins and cellular structures. In HepG2 cells most of the incorporated MMA(III) is methylated and oxidised to DMA(V) after passing this cycle; in UROtsa cells the cycle is limited to oxidation and reduction, and finally excretion, due to the fact that urothelial cells are non methylating (Hippler et al., 2011).

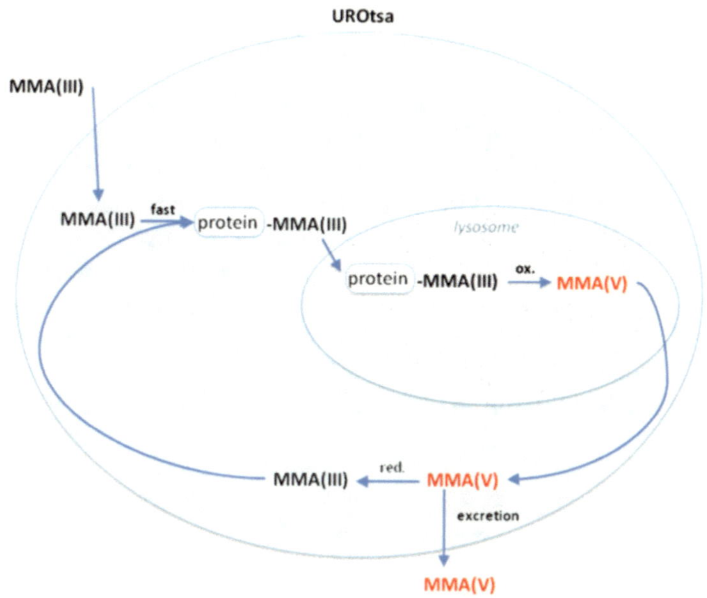

Fig. 14. Proposed arsenic cycle in UROtsa cells after exposure to MMA(III).

Especially the trivalent arsenicals are known to exhibit strong genotoxic effects (Dopp et al., 2010a). These effects can either be detected as DNA damage using the micronucleus test or the comet assay (Dopp et al., 2008), as oxidative damage by assaying the amount of 8-oxo-dG (8-Oxo-2'-deoxyguanosine) or in form of chromosomal aberrations (Dopp et al., 2004). In our study we determined the Alkaline Comet Assay to analyse single and double strand breaks of the DNA. We detected significant genotoxic effects of all tested trivalent arsenic compounds (As(III), MMA(III), and DMA(III)) and the pentavalent arsenate already after 30 min of exposure. These results are in compliance with the findings of previous studies using several mammalian cell types (Schwertdtle et al., 2003; Raisuddin & Jha, 2004; Dopp et al., 2005). This emphasises how urgently the knowledge of the tissue-dependent arsenic biotransformation (Fig. 13. and 14.) is needed, as the genotoxic effect of arsenic metabolites is not only dependent on its oxidative state but also on the state of methylation (Hirner & Rettenmeier, 2010; Dopp et al., 2010b). Wnek et al. (2009) reported that in UROtsa cells DNA damage caused by MMA(III) is not only a phenomenon of acute treatment but also an important effect in chronic, low-level exposure for 12 - 52 weeks.

The occurrence of single- and double-strand breaks is significantly decreased after the removal of MMA(III) for 2 weeks, but still significantly increased compared to the untreated control. The relative poly (ADP-ribose) polymerase (PARP) activity was significantly reduced during this chronic exposure and increased again after removal of MMA(III). Trivalent arsenic species are known to attach to zinc binding structures generally found in DNA repair enzymes and transcription factors, leading to alteration or inhibition of those proteins (Kitchin & Wallace, 2008). Together with the findings of Hu et al. (1998) it is likely that DNA repair is inhibited by both direct protein interaction and altered signal transduction or gene expression. Taken together, this leads to the fact that not only direct DNA damage plays a pivotal role in arsenic induced carcinogenesis. Inorganic arsenic and its metabolites are also known to be potent epigenetic modulators leading to (tissue specific) altered cellular functions, malignant transformation and tumorigenesis. Many studies report arsenic induced aberrant DNA methylation patterns (Sutherland & Costa, 2003; Smeester et al., 2011; Ren et al.; 2011), resulting in changes in the promoter activity that lead to altered gene expression (Jensen et al., 2009). Aberrant DNA methylation patterns might be the result of arsenic-induced altered global histone modification finally leading to, among others, the silencing of tumour suppressor genes (Zhou et al., 2008). Altered global DNA methylation levels have also been correlated with the arsenic metabolism as both systems use the same methyl donor SAM (S-adenosyl-methionine). Sam is known to transfer methyl groups to DNA methyltransferases on the one hand, and to AS3MT (arsenic (+3 oxidation state) methyltransferase) to the other hand (Ren et al., 2011). Jensen et al. (2009) correlated the occurrence of aberrant DNA methylation patterns after chronic low-dose exposure to MMA(III) with the development of a malignant phenotype of UROtsa cells (Table 2.).

Cell Line	Treatment	Exposure	Duration	Hyperproliferation	AIG	Tumors in mice
UROtsa	None	None	None	NA	No	No
URO-MSC12	MMA (III)	50 nM	12 weeks	Yes	No	No
URO-MSC24	MMA (III)	50 nM	24 weeks	Yes	Yes	No
URO-MSC36	MMA (III)	50 nM	36 weeks	Yes	Yes	ND
URO-MSC52	MMA (III)	50 nM	52 weeks	Yes	Yes	Yes
URO-MSC24 + 3mo	MMA (III)	50 nM	24 weeks	ND	Yes	ND
URO-MSC24 + 6mo	MMA (III)	50 nM	24 weeks	ND	Yes	ND
URO-MSC52 + 3mo	MMA (III)	50 nM	52 weeks	ND	Yes	Yes
URO-MSC52 + 6mo	MMA (III)	50 nM	52 weeks	ND	Yes	Yes
URO-ASSC	As (III)	1 µM	52 weeks	Yes	Yes	Yes
URO-CDSC	Cd (II)	1 µM	52 weeks	Yes	Yes	Yes

NA=not applicable; ND=not determined. (Jensen et al., 2009, modified)

Table 2. Cell line name, the treatment metal, concentration (exposure), and duration of treatment for each cell line are shown. In addition, the phenotypic properties of each cell line including increased growth rate relative to UROtsa (hyperproliferation), anchorage independent growth (AIG), and ability of each cell line to form tumours when injected subcutaneously into immunocompromised mice are described. The reference cites previous publications describing part or all of the information presented for a given cell line.

In our study we analysed the development of the malignant phenotype of UROtsa cells by assaying the ability of an anchorage independent growth as well as the ability of migration and invasion. Both characteristics are negative in untreated UROtsa cells, but occurred after chronic low-dose treatment to MMA(III) (50 nM, 75 nM, and 100 nM, respectively) for more than 90 weeks. The results of the soft agar assay do not provide evidence for a dose-dependent development of anchorage independent growth. In contrast, the data of the migration and invasion assays indicate that the motility of UROtsa cells is dose-dependently increased after chronic exposure to MMA(III). Both, the loss of anchorage independent growth and the increased motility / invasive potential, provide evidence for the formation of a malignant phenotype in UROtsa cells after chronic low-dose exposure to MMA(III). These *in vitro* results point to a possible model system to study the mechanisms of metastasis in arsenic-induced bladder cancer. Further studies have to be conducted analysing established molecular markers to support our presented data and proposals. For example, the analysis of cell-cell adhesion concerning the protein E-cadherin (encoded by the *CDH1* gene) and its regulation by the ZEB2 protein and *CDH1* promoter methylation would be of great interest for the investigation of the epithelial-mesenchymal transition (EMT), a basic mechanism required for the acquisition of an invasive and subsequently metastatic phenotype in epithelial tumours (Vandewalle et al., 2005). Furthermore, TWIST overexpression is known to increase migration and decrease the sensitivity to arsenic induced cell death in gastric cancer cells (Feng et al., 2009) and could serve as another interesting marker to study EMT and metastasis in arsenic-induced bladder cancer.

Fig. 15 summarises the molecular mechanisms of MMA(III)-induced toxicity and malignancy in UROtsa cells *in vitro* after chronic low-dose exposure. In this extended model we propose that after uptake and parallel to the fast conjugation to proteins and other cellular structures that is followed by lysosomal degradation and autophagy MMA(III) also induces DNA damage and epigenetic changes. This might lead to the observed alteration of signal transduction and cellular functions as well as the accumulation of (epi)genetic aberrations that are supposed to be the basis of transformation into a malignant phenotype.

Because this hypothetic model is based on *in vitro* research, there is an urgent need for further *in vivo* studies. While *in vitro* assays give important data for the investigation of molecular mechanisms, there is a lack of information concerning the defence of a whole organism against cancer including, e. g., the immune response.

In summary, we were able to present the tissue-dependent metabolism of MMA(III) in methylating HepG2 and non-methylating UROtsa cells. We analysed genotoxic effects of arsenic species in UROtsa cells and illustrated the dependence of genotoxicity on the methylation and oxidation state. This reveals how important the knowledge of the arsenic metabolism is, as each metabolite has its unique mechanisms of toxicity. MMA(III) is known as one of the most important metabolites due to its high toxicity. We analysed the malignant transformation of UROtsa cells after chronic low-dose exposure to MMA(III) and illustrated the loss of anchorage dependent growth and the development of increased migration and invasion properties. Both are serious phenotypical characteristics in the development of cancer. With our *in vitro* study we were able to give further evidence to arsenic-induced bladder cancer.

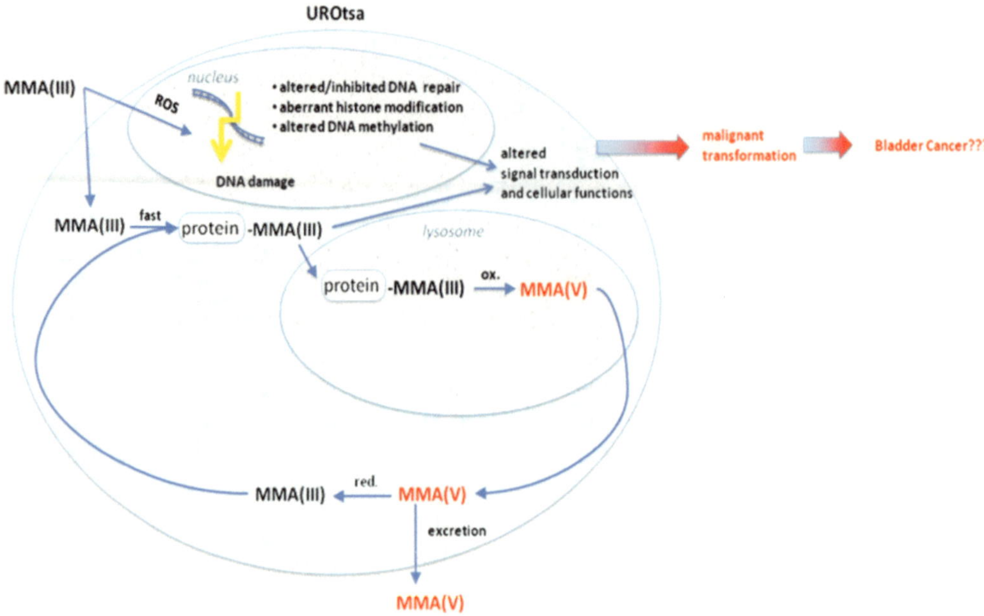

Fig. 15. Proposed molecular mechanisms of MMA(III) induced toxicity and malignancy in UROtsa cells after chronic low-dose exposure.

5. Acknowledgment

The authors would like to thank G. Zimmer, M. Gerhards and U. Zimmermann for their assistance of cell culturing. This work was kindly founded by the German research Foundation (DFG) Grant No: DO 332/8-1, JO 753/2-1 and HI 276/16-1.

6. References

Anderson, M. E. (1998). Glutathione: an overview of biosynthesis and modulation. *Chem Biol Interact,* Vol. 112, (April 1998), pp. 1-14, ISSN 0009-2797

Aposhian, H. V., Gurzau, E. S., Le, X. C., Gurzau, A., Healy, S. M., Lu, X. F., Ma, M. S., Yip, L., Zakharyan, R. A., Maiorino, R. M., Dart, R. C., Tircus, M. G., Gonzales-Ramirez, D., Morgan, D. L., Avram, D. & Aposhian, M. M. (2000). Occurrence of Monomethylarsonous acid in urine of humans exposed to inorganic arsenic. *Chem. Res. Toxicol.*, Vol. 13, No. 8, (August 2000), pp. 693-967, ISSN 0893-228X

Arancibia-Cárcamo I. L., Youen E. Y., Muir J., Lumb M. J., Michels G., Saliba R. S., Smart T. G., Yan Z., Kittler J. T. & Moss S. J. (2009). Ubiquitin-dependent lysosomal targeting of GABA(A) receptors regulates neuronal inhibition *PNAS,* Vol. 106, No. 41, (October 2009), pp. 17552-17557, ISSN 0027-8424

Barriere H., Nemes C., Du K. & Lukacs G. L. (2007). Plasticity of polyubiquitin recognition as lysosomal targeting signals by the endosomal sorting machinery. *MBoC,* Vol. 18, No. 10, (October 2007), pp. 3952-3965, ISSN 1059-1524

Bredfeldt, T. G., Jagadish, B., Eblin, K. E., Mash, E. A. & Gandolfi, A. J. (2006). Monomethylarsonous acid induces transformation of human bladder cells. *Toxicol. Appl. Pharmacol.*, Vol. 216, No. 1, (October 2006), pp. 69-79, ISSN 0041-008X

Chakraborti D., Sengupta M. K., Rahman M. M., Ahamed S., Chowdhury U. K., Hossain M. A., Mukherjee S. C., Pati S., Saha K. C., Dutta R. N. & Quamruzzaman Q. (2004). Groundwater arsenic contamination and its health effects in the Ganga-Meghna-Brahmaputra plain. *Journal of Environmental Monitoring,* Vol. 6, No. 6, (May 2004), pp. 74N-83N, ISSN 1464-0325

Chen C. L., Chiou H. Y., Hsu L. I., Hsueh Y. M., Wu M. M., Wang Y. H. & Chen C. J. (2010). Arsenic in Drinking Water and Risk of Urinary Tract Cancer: A Follow-up Study from Northeastern Taiwan. *Cancer Eepidemiology Biomarkers & Prevention,* Vol. 19, No. 1, (January 2010), pp. 101-110, ISSN 1055 9965

Chen C.-S. (2002). Phorbol ester induces elevated oxidative activity and alkalization in a subset of lysosomes. *BMC Cell Biology,* Vol. 3, (August 2002), pp. 21, doi:10.1186/1471-2121-3-21

Chiou H. Y., Hsueh Y. M., Liaw K. F., Horng S. F., Chiang M. H., Pu Y. S., Lin J. S. N., Huang C. H. & Chen C. J. (1995). Incidence of internal cancers and ingested Inorganic Arsenic - a 7- year follow-up-study in Taiwan. *Cancer Research,* Vol. 55, No. 6, (March 1995), pp. 1296-1300, ISSN 0008-5472

Clague M. J. & Urbé S. (2010). Ubiquitin: Same Molecule, Different Degradation Pathways. *Cell,* Vol. 143, No. 5, (November 2010), pp. 682-685, ISSN 0092-8674

Dopp E., Hartmann L. M., Florea A.-M., von Recklinghausen U., Pieper R., Shokouhi B., Rettenmeier A. W., Hirner A. V. & Obe G. (2004). Uptake of inorganic and organic derivates of arsenic associated with induced cytotoxic and genotoxic effects in Chinese hamster ovary (CHO) cells. *Toxicol Appl Pharmacol,* Vol. 201, No. 2, (December 2004), pp. 156-165, ISSN 0041-008X

Dopp E., Hartmann L. M., von Recklinghausen U., Florea A. M., Rabieh S., Zimmermann U., Shokouhi B., Yadav S., Hirner A. V. & Rettenmeier A. W. (2005). Forced Uptake of Trivalent and Pentavalent Methylated and Inorganic Arsenic and Its Cyto-/Genotoxicity in Fibroblasts and Hepatoma Cells. *Toxicol. Sciences,* Vol. 87, No. 1, (September 2005), pp. 46-56, ISSN 1096-6080

Dopp E. (2007) Neue Aspekte zur Arsen-induzierten Kanzerogenese. *ErgoMed.* Vol. 4, (n. d. 2007), pp. 100-1009

Dopp E., von Recklinghausen U., Hartmann L. M., Stueckradt I., Pollok I., Rabieh S., Hao L., Nussler A., Kartier C., Hirner A. V. & Retenmeier A. W. (2008). Subcellular Distributioan of Inorganic and Methylated Arsenic Compounds in Human Urothelial Cells and Human Hepatocytes. *Drug Metabolism and Disposition,* Vol. 36, No. 5, (May 2008), pp. 971-979, ISSN 0090-9556

Dopp E., von Recklinghausen U., Diaz-Bone R. A., Hirner A. V. & Rettenmeier A. W. (2010a). Cellular uptake, subcellular distribution and toxicity of arsenic compounds in methylating and non-methylating cells. *Environmental Research,* Vol. 110, No. 5, (July 2010), pp. 435-442, ISSN 0013-9351

Dopp E., Kligermann A. D. & Diaz-Bone R. A. (2010b). Organoarsenicals, Uptake, Metabolism, and Toxicity, In: *Metal Ions in Life Sciences,* Sigel A., Sigel H. & Sigel R.K.O. (Eds.), 231-265, RSC Publishing, ISSN 1559-0836, Cambridge, England

Du, Z.-X., Zhang, H.-Y., Meng, X., Guan, Y. & Wang, H.-Q. (2009). Role of oxidative stress and intracellular glutathione in the sensitivity to apoptosis induced by proteasome inhibitor in thyroid cancer cells. *BMC Cancer,* Vol. 9, No. 1, 56, DOI: 10.1186/1471-2407-9-56

Eblin, K. E., Hau, A. M., Jensen, T. J., Futscher, B.W. & Gandolfi, A. J. (2008). The role of arsenite and monomethylarsonous acid-induced signal transduction in human bladder cells: Acute studies. *Toxicology,* Vol. 250, No. 1, (August 2008), pp. 47-54, ISSN 0300-483X

Feng M.-Y., Wang K., Song H.-T., Yu H.W., Qin Y., Shi Q.-T. & Geng J.-S. (2009). Metastasis-induction and apoptosis-protection by TWIST in gastric cancer cells. *Clin Exp Metastasis,* Vol. 26, No. 8, (December 2008), pp. 1013-1023, ISSN 0262-0898

Fillol C., Dor F., Labat L., Boltz P., Le Bouard J., Mantey K., Mannschott C., Puskarczyk E., Viller F., Momas I. & Seta N. (2010). Urinary arsenic concentrations and speciation in residents living in an area with naturally contaminated soils. Science *of the Total Environment,* Vol. 408, No. 5, (February 2010), pp. 1190-1194, ISSN 0048-9697

Food Standards Agency of the UK, (2004). Seaweed warning. *Food Survey Information Sheet* (R938 - 28).

Francesconi K. A. (2010). Arsenic species in seafood: Origin and human health implications. *Pure and Applied Chemistry,* Vol. 82, No. 2, (February 2010), pp. 373-381, ISSN 0033-4545

Gorby M. S. & Albuquerque M. D., (1988). Arsenic Poisoning. *The Western Journal of Medicine,* Vol. 149, No. 3, (September 1988), pp. 308-315, ISSN 0093-0415

Hartwig A., Asmuss M., Ehleben I., Herzer U., Kostelac D., Pelzer A., Schwerdtle T. & Burkle A. (2002). Interference by toxic metal ions with DNA repair processes and cell cycle control: Molecular mechanisms. *Environmental Health Perspectives,* Vol. 110, Suppl. 5, (October 2002), pp. 797-799, ISSN 0091-6765

Hartwig A., Blessing H., Schwerdtle T. & Walter I. (2003), Modulation of DNA repair processes by arsenic and selenium compounds. *Toxicology,* Vol. 193, No. 1-2, (November 2003), pp. 161-169, ISSN 0300-483X

Hayakawa T., Kobayashi Y., Cui X. & Hirano S. (2005). A new metabolic pathway of arsenite: arsenic-glutathione complexes are substrates for human arsenic methyltransferase Cyt19. *Archives of Toxicology,* Vol. 79, No. 4, (April 2005), pp. 183-191, ISSN 0340-5761

Hippler J., Zdrenka R., Reichel R. A. D., Weber D. G., Rozynek P., Johnen G., Dopp E. & Hirner A. V. (2011). Intracellular, time resolved speciation and quantification of arsenic compound in human urothelial and hepatoma cells. *J. Anal. At. Spectrom.,* DOI:10.1039/C1JA10150A.

Hirner A. V. & Rettenmeier A. W. (2010). Methylated Metal(loid) Species in Humans, In: *Metal Ions in Life Sciences,* Sigel A., Sigel H. & Sigel R. K. O. (Eds.), pp. 465-512, RSC Publishing, ISSN 1559-0836, Cambridge, England

Hirner A. V. & Hippler J. (2011). Trace Metal(loids) (As, Cd, Cu, Hg, Pb, PGE, Sb, and Zn) and Their Species, In: *Treatise on water science,* Vol. 3, Wilderer P. (Ed.), pp. 31-57, Oxford: Academic Press, ISBN 0444531939

Hu, Y. Su, L. & Snow, E. T. (1998). Arsenic toxicity is enzyme specific and its affects on ligation are not caused by the direct inhibition of DNA repair enzymes. *Mutaion Research,* Vol. 408, No. 3, (September 1998), pp. 203-218, ISSN 0921-8777

Huang, C., Ke, Q., Costa, M. & Shi, x. (2004). Molecular Mechanisms of arsenic carcinogenesis. *Mol. Cell. Biochem.* Vol. 255, No. 1-2, (January 2004), pp. 57-66, ISSN 0300-8177

Jensen T. J., Novak P., Wnek S. M., Gandolfi A. J. & Futscher B. W. (2009). Arsenicals produce stable progressive changes in DNA methylation patterns that are linked to malignant transformation of immortalized urothelial cells. *Toxicol Appl Pharmacol,* Vol. 241, No. 2, (December 2009), pp. 221-229, ISSN 0041-008X

Kitchen, K. T. & Ahmad, S. (2003). Oxidative stress as a possible mode of action for arsenic carcinogenesis. *Toxicol. Lett.,* Vol. 137, No. 1-2, (January 2003), pp. 3-13, ISSN 0378-4274

Kitchen, K. T. & Wallace, K. (2008). The role of protein binding of trivalent arsenicals in arsenic carcinogenesis and toxicity. *J. Inorg. Biochem.,* Vol. 102, No. 3, (March 2008), pp. 532-539, ISSN 0162-0134

Kundu M. & Thompson C. B. (2008). Autophagy: Basic principles and relevance to disease. *Annu. Rev. Pathol. Mech. Dis.,* Vol. 3, (October 2008), pp. 427-455, ISSN 1553-4006

Lam S. H., Winata C. L., Tong Y., Korzh S., Lim W. S., Korzh V., Spitsbergen J., Mathavan S., Miller L. D., Liu E. T. & Gong Z. (2006). Transcriptome kinetics of arsenic-induced adaptive response in zebrafish liver. *Physiol. Genomics,* Vol. 27, No. 3, (November 2006), pp. 351-361, ISSN 1094-8341

Lozna, K. & Biernat, J. (2008). The occurrence of arsenc in the environment and food. *Rocz Panstw Zakl Hig,* Vol. 59, No. 1, (October 2008), pp. 19-31, ISSN 0035-7715

Marques C., Pereira P., Taylor A., Liang J. N., Reddy V. N., Szweda L. I. & Shang F.(2004). Ubiquitin-dependent lysosomal degradation of the HNE-modified proteins in lens epithelial cells. *The FASEB Journal,* Vol. 18, No. 10, (July 2004), pp. 1424-1426, ISSN 0892-6638

Meharg A. A., Ceacon C., Campbell R. C. J., Carey A. M., Williams P. N., Feldmann J. & Raab A. (2008). Inorganic arsenic levels in rice milk exceed EU and US drinking water standards. *Journal of Environmental Monitoring,* Vol. 10, No. 4, (March 2008), pp. 428-431, ISSN 1464-0325

Mehrpour M., Esclatine A., Beau I. & Codogno P. (2010). Overview of macroautophagy regulation in mammalian cells. *Cell Research,* Vol. 20, No. 7, (July 2010), pp. 748-762, ISSN 1001-0602

Nakajima Y., Endo Y., Inoue Y., Yamanaka K., Kato K., Wanibuchi H. & Endo G. (2006). Ingestion of Hijiki seaweed and risk of arsenic poisoning. *Applied Organometallic Chemistry,* Vol. 20, No. 9, (September 2006), pp. 557-564, ISSN 0268-2605

Naranmandura H., Suzuki N. & Suzuki K. T. (2006). Trivalent Arsenicals are bound to Proteins during reductive Methylation. *Chemical Research in Toxicology,* Vol. 19, No. 8, (August 2006), pp. 1010-1018, ISSN 0893-228X

Ng J. C., Wang J. & Shraim A. (2003). A global health problem caused by arsenic from natural sources. *Chemosphere*, Vol. 52, No. 9, (September 2003), pp. 1353-1359, ISSN 0045-6535

Planer-Friedrich B., Lehr C., Matschullat J., Merkel B. J., Nordstrom D. K. & Sandstrom M. W. (2006). Speciation of volatile arsenic at geothermal features in Yellowstone National Park. *Geochimica et Cosmochimica Acta,* Vol. 70, No. 10, (May 2006), pp. 2480-2491, ISSN 0016-7037

Planer-Friedrich B., London J., McCleskey R. B., Nordstrom D. K. & Wallschlaeger D. (2007). Thioarsenates in Geothermal Watersof Yellowstone National Park: Determination, Preservation, and Geochemical Importance. *Environmental Science & Technology,* Vol. 41, No. 15, (August 2007), pp. 5245-5251, ISSN 0013-936X

Raisuddin S. & Jha A. N. (2004). Relative Sensitivity of Fish and Mammalian Cells to Sodium Arsenate and Arsenite as Determined by Alkaline Single-Cell Gel Electrophoresis and Cytokinesis-Block Micronucleus Assay. *Environmental and Molecular Mutagenesis*, Vol. 44, No.1 , (June 2004), pp. 83-89, ISSN 0893-6692

Ren X., McHale C. M., Skibola C.F., Smith A. H., Smith M. T. & Zhang L. (2011). An Emerging Role for Epigenetic Dysregulation in Arsenic Toxicity and Carcinogenesis. *Environmental Health Perspectives,* Vol. 119, No. 1 (January 2011), pp. 11-19, ISSN 0091-6765

Rosen B. P., Ajees A. A. & McDermott T. R. (2011). Life and dead with arsenic, *Bioessays*, Vol. 33, No. 5, (May 2011), pp. 350-357, ISSN 0265-9247

Schwerdtle T., Walter I., Mackiw I. & Hartwig A. (2003). Induction of oxidative DNA damage by arsenite and its trivalent and pentavalent methylated metabolites in cultured human cells and isolated DNA. *Carcinogenesis*, Vol: 24, No. 5, (May 2003), pp. 967-974, ISSN 0143-3334

Shenoy S. K., Xiao K., Venkataramanan V., Snyder P. M., Freedmann N. J. & Weissmann A. M. (2008). Nedd4 mediates agonist-dependent ubiquitination, lysosomal targeting, and degradation of the beta(2)-adrenergic receptor. *J. Biol. Chem.*, Vol. 283, No. 32, (August 2008), pp. 22166-22176, ISSN 0021-9258

Signes-Pastor A. J., Deacon C., Jenkins R. O., Haris P. I., Carbonell-Barrachina A. A. & Meharg A. A. (2009). Arsenic speciation in Japanese rice drinks and condiments. *Journal of Environmental Monitoring*, Vol. 11, No. 11, (October 2009), pp. 1930-1934, ISSN 1464-0325

Smedley P. L. & Kinniburgh D. G. (2002). A review of the source, behaviour and distribution of arsenic in natural waters. *Applied Geochemistry,* Vol. 17, No. 5, (May 2002), pp. 517-568, ISSN 0883-2927

Smeester L. Rager J. E., Bailey K. A., Guan X., Smith N., Garcia-Vargas G., Del Razo L.-M., Drobná Z., Kelkar H., Stýblo M. & Fry R. C. (2011). Epigenetic Changes in Individuals with Arsenicosis. *Chem Res Toxicol,* Vol. 24, No. 2, (February 2011), pp. 165-167, ISSN 0893-228X

Smith A. H., Lingas E. O. & Rahman M. (2000). Contamination of drinking-water by arsenic in Bangladesh: a public health emergency. *Bulletin of the World Health Organization,* Vol. 78, No. 9, (n. d. 2000), pp. 1093-1103, ISSN 00429686

Styblo, M., Drobna, Z., Jaspers, I., Lin S. & Thomas, D. J. (2002). The role of biomethylation in toxicity and carcinogenicity of arsenic: a research update. *Environ. Health. Perspect.,* Vol. 110, Suppl. 5, (October 2002), pp. 767-771, ISSN 0091-6765

Styblo, M. & Thomas, D. J. (1997). Binding of arsenicals to proteins in an in vitro methylation system. *Toxicol Appl Pharmacol,* Vol. 147, No. 1, (November 1997), pp. 1-8, ISSN 0041-008X

Sun G. X., Williams P. N., Zhu Y. G., Deacon C., Carey A. M., Raab A., Feldmann J. & Meharg A. A. (2009). Survey of arsenic and its speciation in rice products such as breakfast cereals, rice crackers and Japanese rice condiments. *Environmental International,* Vol. 35, No. 3, (April 2009), pp. 473-475, ISSN 0160-4120

Sutherland J. E. & Costa M. (2003). Epigenetics and the Environment, In: *Ann. N.Y. Acad. Sci.,* Vol. 983, Verma M., Dunn B. K. & Umar A. (Ed.), pp. 151-160, NEW YORK ACAD SCIENCES, ISBN 1-57331-430-7

Terman A., Kurz T., Gustafsson B. & Brunk U. T. (2006). Lysosomal labilization. *IUBMB Life,* Vol. 58, No. 9, (September 2006), pp. 531-539, ISSN 1521-6543

Tseng C. H. (2007). Arsenic methylation, urinary arsenic metabolites and human diseases: Current perspective. *Journal of Environmental Science and Health, Part C Environmental Carcinogenesis and Ecotoxicology Reviews,* Vol. 25, No. 1, (2007), pp. 1-22, ISSN 1059-0501

Vandewalle C., Comijn J., De Craene B., Vermassen P., Bruyneel E., Andersen H., Tulchinsky E., Van Roy F. & Berx G. (2005). SIP1/ZEB2 induces EMT by repressing genes of different epithelial cell-cell junctions. *Nucleic Acids Research,* Vol. 33, No. 20, (November 2005), pp. 6566-6578, ISSN 0305-1048

Wei M., Wanibuchi H., Yamamoto S., Li W. & Fukushima S. (1999). Urinary bladder carcinogenicity of dimethylarsinic acid in male F344 rats. *Carcinogenesis,* Vol. 20, No. 9, (September 1999), pp. 1873–1876, ISSN 0143-3334

WHO (2001). *Arsenic compounds, Environmental health criteria 224, 2nd ed..* Geneva: World health organization

Wnek, S. M., Medeiros, M. K., Eblin, K. E. & Gandolfi A. J. (2009). Persistence of DNA damage following exposure of human bladder cells to chronic monomethylarsonous acid. *Toxicol. Appl. Pharmacol.,* Vol. 241, No. 2, (December 2009), pp. 202-209, ISSN 0041-008X

Wolfe-Simon F., Switzer Blum J., Kulp T. R., Gordon G. W., Hoeft S. E., Pett-Ridge J., Stolz J. F., Webb S. M., Weber P. K., Davies P. C. W., Anbar A. D. & Oremland R. S. (2010). A Bacterium That Can Grow by Using Arsenic Instead of Phosphorus. *Science,* Vol. 332, No. 6034, (June 2011) pp. 1163-1166, ISSN 0036-8075

Yan H. Wang N., Weinfeld M., Cullen W. R. &. Le X. C. (2009). Identification of Arsenic-Binding Proteins in Human Cells by Affinity Chromatography and Mass Spectrometry. *Anal. Chem.,* Vol. 81, No. 10, (May 2009), pp. 4144-4152, ISSN 0003-2700

Yang Y., Liang Z., Gao BJia., Y. & Qin Z. (2008). Dynamic effects of autophagy on arsenic trioxide-induced death of human leukemia cell line HL60 cells. *Acta Pharmacol Sin,* Vol. 29, No. 1, (January 2008), pp. 123-134, ISSN 1671-4083

Yoshida K., Inoue Y., Kuroda K., Chen H., Wanibuchi H., Fukushima S. & Endo G. (1998). Urinary excretion of arsenic metabolites after long-term oral administration of various arsenic compounds to rats. *J. Toxicol. Environ.Health,* Vol. 54, No. A, (June 1998), pp. 179-192, ISSN 0098-4108

Zhou X., Sun H., Ellen T. P., Chen H. & Costa M. (2008). Arsenite alters global histone H3 methylation. *Carcinogenesis,* Vol. 29, No. 9, (September 2008), pp. 1831-1836, ISSN 0143-3334

Part 10

Chemoprevention

21

Chemoprevention and Novel Treatments of Non-Muscle Invasive Bladder Cancer

Adam Luchey, Morris Jessop, Claire Oliver, Dale Riggs,
Barbara Jackson, Stanley Kandzari and Stanley Zaslau
Division of Urology
West Virginia University
Morgantown, WV,
USA

1. Introduction

The Cancer Journal for Clinicians reports there will be 69,250 newly diagnosed cases of bladder cancer in 2011, with 52,020 being men and 17,230 being women with an increase by 50% of annual cases since 1985. Approximately 1 in 5 of those who develop bladder cancer will die due to the disease (relative mortality 20.8%, [Siegel et al., 2011, Golijanin et al., 2006]). Bladder cancer has become the second most prevalent cancer after cancer of the prostate in middle-aged to elderly male individuals. Many patients do not die from their disease, but typically have multiple recurrences (Pelucchi et al., 2006). This lends to a five-year cost to Medicare attributed to bladder cancer of over one billion dollars (Yabroff et al., 2008). Tobacco use and exposure to aromatic amines are well established etiologic contributors to bladder cancer and by eliminating or reducing contact with these substances has been shown to reduce such risk.

BCG (bacillus Calmette-Guerin) has become the standard of care in the treatment of carcinoma in situ as well as high grade T1 (invasion into the lamina propria) and when not appropriate, Mitomycin-C, has been proven to be an acceptable, albeit, less effective alternate. The goal of this chapter will be to describe novel agents that may show promise in the treatment of bladder cancer. This will include descriptions of the agents, their respective mechanism of action (e.g. molecular/biochemical pathways, cell cycle interaction, necrosis), clinical data, combinations of combinations of regimens and mode of delivery. and mode of delivery. A second goal of this chapter will be to consider whether any of these novel agents may have a role in the prevention of bladder cancer.

2. Chemoprevention

Kamat in his review of superficial bladder cancer stated that chemoprevention is needed for a multitude of reasons: high recurrence rates, increased morbidity from repeat resections, a tedious course of disease to see treatment outcomes, ability of agents to be concentrated in the urine, and the ability to monitor recurrence with cytology/cystoscopy (Kamat, 2003). Table 1 lists potential agents that may be considered for chemoprevention of bladder cancer.

POTENTIAL CHEMOPREVENTION AGENTS
• Vitamin A
• Vitamin E
• Vitamin C
• Selenium
• Cactus Pear
• Isoflavones
• Garlic
• Green Tea
• Difluoromethlyornithine (DFMO)
• Non-Steroidal Anti-Inflammatory Drugs
• Statins

Table 1. Potential Chemoprevention agents for Bladder Cancer

2.1 Vitamin A

Vitamin A is necessary for light absorption in the retina and is also known to have a role in epithelial growth. Additionally, vitamin A has been researched as a chemotherapeutic and chemopreventive agent for a variety of malignancies. Currently, it is utilized to treat acute promyelocytic leukemia (Zusi et al., 2002). The mechanism of vitamin A's inhibition of tumor growth is thought to work through modulation of gene expression in cell growth, differentiation, and apoptosis (Zanardi et al., 2006). Evidence suggests that it does this through a variety of molecular pathways including binding to nuclear retinoic acid receptors (RAR) and ligand activating transcription factors such as retinoid X receptors (RXR) (Simeone & Tari, 2004). Additionally, vitamin A's anti-tumor activity may involve, among others, interactions with growth factors and cytokines, neoplastic stem cell pathways such as WNT, cAMP pathways, mitogen activated protein kinases (MAPKs), PI3K/AKT, cyclin-dependent kinases (CDKs), protein kinase C, and epigenetic modulation of gene expression (Garattini et al., 2007). Other studies indicate that some synthetic retinoids may even reduce VEGF expression, which is an important angiogenic factor in bladder cancer growth (Hameed & el-Metwally, 2008).

Several studies have examined vitamin A and its derivatives for chemoprevention of bladder cancer. The first clinical trial was performed in 1978 (Gunby, 1978) and was followed by several other prospective and controlled trials. Results for these trials were mixed, with some showing significant preventative effects (Alfthan et al., 1983; Studer et al., 1995; Yoshida et al., 1986) and others showing less promising results (Decensi et al., 2000; Prout & Barton, 1992). Mild to severe toxicities were also noted in many of these studies and may potentially limit vitamin A's use as a chemopreventive agent (Hameed & el-Metwally, 2008). More recently, to enable lower doses of retinoic acids and decrease unwanted side effects, combinations of retinoic acid and inhibitors of the CYP26A enzyme (involved in degradation of vitamin A) have been explored with some success (Hameed & el-Metwally, 2008). Although a recent cohort study showed no significant association of several vitamins including retinoids with urothelial carcinoma risk (Hotaling et al., 2011), other past studies provide some compelling evidence for vitamin A's efficacy. Thus further research into vitamin A's use in preventing bladder cancer is warranted.

2.2 Vitamin E

Vitamin E is a lipid soluble anti-oxidant and is known to be important in a variety of biological processes. It is also thought to possibly lower the risk of many malignancies through free radical scavenging, inhibition of N-nitroso compound formation (Mirvish, 1995), immunological stimulation (Beisel et al., 1981), and potent induction of apoptosis (Kline et al., 2004; Sigounas et al., 1997).

The clinical evidence for vitamin E in bladder cancer prevention has mixed results. A large Cohort study with Vitamin E and C and risk of bladder cancer mortality showed a reduced risk of mortality with regular intake of vitamin E (Jacobs et al., 2002). A phase III clinical trial using megadoses of several vitamins including E, when compared to patients who just received the recommended daily allowance (RDA) of the same vitamins, had a 40% reduction in bladder tumor recurrence after the first 10 months of the study (Lamm et al., 1994). However, in this same study, patients also received BCG therapy, which is known to promote immune response to tumors and may have confounded the results (Coulter et al, 2006). Further support comes from a prospective study, which showed an inverse relationship between vitamin E supplement consumption and the risk of bladder malignancy in men (Michaud et al., 2000).

In contrast to studies supporting vitamin E, a recent cohort study suggested no association of vitamin E intake and risk of urothelial carcinoma (Roswall et al., 2009). In addition, a meta-analysis for vitamin E and C intake and prevention of cancer indicated overall poor evidence for vitamin E in reduction of bladder cancer recurrence (Coulter et al, 2006). Additionally, a recently published cohort study indicated that the use of a variety of vitamins and supplements including vitamin E had no significant association with urothelial carcinoma risk in age-adjusted or multi-variate models (Hotaling et al., 2011). It should be noted that several studies have indicated that high doses of vitamin E may actually increase the risk for bladder cancer (The New England Journal of Medicine [NEJM], 1994; Miller et al., 2005). Since the evidence for vitamin E as a chemopreventive agent is conflicting, further studies should be performed to assess its true value.

2.3 Vitamin C

Vitamin C is an important vitamin found abundantly in fruits and vegetables. Proven to be a powerful antioxidant and necessary for a variety of metabolic activities, vitamin C consumption has also been researched as a method to reduce the risk of bladder cancer. It is hypothesized that vitamin C's anti-tumor activity is derived from inhibition of p53-induced replicative senescence, by suppressing both reactive oxygen species production and p38 MAPK activity (Kim et al., 2008), and sparing vitamin E to jointly reduce reactive α-tocopheroxy radicals (Park et al., 2010). Malignant transformation may also be decreased by vitamin C through reduction of N-nitroso compounds, which are known to be carcinogenic (Wu et al., 2000).

Despite these mechanisms proposed, data to support vitamin C as a chemopreventive agent is conflicting. A cohort study using data from 1981-1989 showed a significant reduction in relative risk for bladder cancer in patients taking vitamin C (Shibata et al., 1992). A more recent prospective study found a strong inverse relationship between vitamin C intake and bladder cancer risk in ex-smokers and non-smokers, but did not show the same results with current smokers (Michaud et al., 2000). High doses of vitamin C in combination with megadoses of vitamins A, B6, E and zinc were also found to be beneficial, in combination with BCG therapy, in a phase III trial of Bladder cancer (Lamm et al., 1994). However, as mentioned earlier with Vitamin E, the results in this study may in part be confounded by BCG therapy (Coulter et al., 2006).

Other studies suggest less promising evidence. In a large cohort study of U.S. men and women, no associations were found between vitamin C use and bladder cancer death (Jacobs et al., 2002). This data is consistent with a cohort study by Hotaling et al. indicating the same relationship (Hotaling et al., 2011). A recent prospective study showed no significant effect of vitamin C, E or folate on prevention of urothelial carcinoma (Roswall et al., 2009) and there is evidence that doses of vitamin C beyond the RDA may contribute to oxalate stone formation (Taylor et al., 2004) and may even induce bladder carcinogenic activity (Mirvish, 1986). These studies indicating poor support for vitamin C's use, along with other studies supporting vitamin C as a bladder cancer chemopreventive agent, indicate that further investigation into vitamin C and bladder cancer prevention is required.

2.4 Selenium

An essential micronutrient that is primarily known for its function as a co-factor for reduction of antioxidant enzymes, selenium is also being researched for its potential in reducing the risk of several malignancies including bladder cancer (Silberstein & Parsons, 2010). A variety of mechanisms have been proposed for selenium's anti-tumor activity: free radical scavenging (Murawaki et al., 2008), modifying thiols, mimiching mimicking methionine methionine which leads to to higher methylating efficiency of RNA and thiols (Jackson & Combs, 2008), enhancement of p53 activity towards DNA repair or apoptosis (Smith et al., 2004) and anti-androgenic activity, which is especially relevant in prostate cancer (Husbeck et al., 2006; Gazi et al., 2007).

The clinical evidence for selenium's anti bladder cancer activity is somewhat controversial. A recent meta-analysis from seven epidemiological studies showed that the overall risk of bladder cancer was inversely associated with elevated levels of selenium in serum and toenail samples, with the greatest effect seen in women (Amaral et al., 2010). Additionally, Wallace et al. showed no association of selenium levels in toenail samples with bladder cancer, it did find a significant association with moderate smokers and p53 positive cancers, suggesting selenium may affect the risk of bladder malignancies with specific p53 immunophenotypes (Wallace et al., 2009). This was further demonstrated in a case control study performed in Belgium that showed an inverse association between serum selenium concentrations and bladder cancer risk (Kellen et al., 2006).

In contrast to studies supporting selenium, a recent cohort study mentioned earlier, showed no significant association with selenium and urothelial carcinoma risk in an age-adjusted or multi-variate models (Hotaling et al., 2011). Current literature reviewed, there is a lack of interventional studies examining selenium and bladder cancer risk (Silberstein & Parsons, 2010).

2.5 Cactus pear

Cactus fruit, or prickly pear, is a fruit generally used as a dietary supplement and has been widely researched for its anti-oxidant effects (Fernández-López et al., 2010; Tesoriere et al., 2004; Zou et al., 2005). These fruits have a variety of ingredients shown to have health benefits including phenolics, flavonoids, and betalains. Recently, cactus pear has also been studied for a possible application in cancer prevention. Although the mechanism is not completely understood, a recent study suggests it might be through increasing expression of annexin IV, a Ca2+ dependent membrane-binding protein important in apoptosis (Zou et al., 2005). Additionally, cactus pear extracts have been proposed to promote immune response and to decrease expression of VEGF (Liang et al., 2008), an important angiogenic factor in bladder and other malignancies (Zou et al., 2005).

Despite the proposed mechanisms, data supporting cactus pear for prevention of bladder cancer is limited, although some data exists to support use in other types of cancer. In a 2005 study, Arizona prickly cactus pear solution inhibited tumor growth in several different cancer cell cultures including ovarian and cervical (Zou et al., 2005). In another study, polysaccharides extracted from cactus pear fruit limited growth of S180 (sarcoma model) tumor cells in mice and induced features of apoptosis (Liang et al., 2008). In a 2010 study, cactus pear extracts induced reactive oxygen species production and apoptosis in ovarian cancer cells (Feugang et al., 2010). A specific species of cactus pear, Opuntia humifusa, was found to inhibit human glioblastoma cell lines (Hahm et al., 2010). Another study examining nine cactus pear species against prostate, colon, hepatic and mammary cancer cell lines showed some cytotoxic activity with certain species (Chavez-Santoscoy et al., 2009). However, normal fibroblast controls were also affected in this study with some of the pear species, thus the conclusions of this study are limited. More research, especially studies utilizing bladder cancer models, are necessary to determine the true potential of cactus pear as a chemopreventative agent for bladder cancer.

2.6 Isoflavones

Isoflavones are naturally occurring compounds found in soy and other products. They are primarily known for their phyotoestrogen and anti-oxidant properties, although recent research has suggested they may also help in cancer prevention. Currently, isoflavones have shown at least some promise in preventing several types of cancers including but not limited to bladder, prostate (Yan & Spitznagel, 2005), breast (Bondesson & Gustafsson, 2010), lung (Hess & Igal, 2011), and liver (Ma et al., 2010).

Multiple mechanisms for this anti-tumor activity have been proposed. Several in vitro studies suggest that isoflavones may induce G2-M cycle arrest, apoptosis, and angiogenesis (Su et al., 2000; Zhou et al., 1998). Another study found that a possible mitochondrial mediated apoptosis pathway through regulation of AKT and MAPK pathways (Lin et al., 2010). Much of the research has focused on the specific isoflavone genistein, which has been shown to inhibit cancer through a variety of pathways. One study showed genistein inhibited EGF-R and EGF, of which the quantity and distribution are associated with urothelial abnormalities (Theodorescu et al., 1998). Another study on genistein showed that it might down regulate COX-2 (Hwang et al., 2009), which has been shown to play a role in tumorigenesis. A 2006 study indicated genistein down regulates nuclear factor kappa-B in bladder tumor tissue and reduces circulating insulin-like growth factor-1 levels, both important in tumor metastasis (Singh et al., 2006). Another more recent study showed that genistein modulates chromatin configuration and DNA methylation, thus activating tumor-suppressing genes (Zhang & Chen, 2011).

The clinical data for isoflavones as chemopreventive agents in bladder cancer has mixed results. In a 2000 study using seven human cancer cell lines, the isoflavone genistein significantly decreased bladder cancer cell growth and two other isoflavones directly induced apoptosis (Su et al., 2000). Another study examining the effect of soy phytochemicals on poorly differentiated and highly metastatic human bladder cancer cell lines in vitro showed significant inhibition by cell cycle arrest in G2-M phases in addition to significant apoptosis (Singh et al., 2006). This same study also showed significant inhibition of clinically relevant orthotopic bladder tumor models by induction of tumor cell apoptosis and reduction of tumor angiogenesis. A study examining the effects of 13-Methyltetradecanoic acid (13-MTD), a soy fermentation product, on human bladder cancer cells found that 13-MTD induced apoptosis (Lin et al., 2010). In contrast to evidence supporting use, epidemiological studies have suggested an increased risk for bladder cancer with consumption of soy (Brinkman & Zeegers, 2008). Since the evidence is contradictory, more research needs to be performed into the potential of soy and soy products to act as chemopreventive agents.

2.7 Garlic

Garlic is considered both a food and supplement with medicinal properties. Extensive research has been performed into the health benefits of garlic and more recently garlic has been examined for cancer prevention. Studies suggest it may induce or prevent suppression of the immune response (Miroddi et al., 2011), induce cytokine production (Lamm & Riggs, 2000), scavenge free radicals (Butt et al., 2009), and bind thiol compounds important in crucial regulatory functions (Cerella et al., 2011). Numerous other mechanisms have also been proposed for specific components of garlic supported by in vitro studies (Shukla & Kaira, 2007).

Although many studies provide evidence of the anti-tumor activity of garlic on other types of cancer (Shukla & Kaira, 2007), research into garlic's anti-tumorigenic properties for prevention of bladder cancer is relatively sparse. A 1986 study using urothelial cancer lines in transplanted into the hind legs of mice, found a therapeutic effect of garlic when intraperitoneally injected (Lau et al., 1986). Another later study found a significant anti-tumor efficacy of garlic when given orally and subcutaneously in mice with injected urothelial carcinoma (Riggs et al., 1997).

Although some studies support the use of garlic, others fail to support garlic or garlic derivatives for chemoprevention of bladder cancer. In a 1993 study, diallyl sulfide, a primary component of garlic, failed to prevent the formation of urinary bladder papillomas in a rat model (Hadjiolov et al., 1993). A recently published cohort study indicated that the use of a variety of vitamins and supplements, including garlic, had no significant association with risk of urothelial carcinoma when adjusted for age and in multi-variate models (Hotaling et al., 2011). Due to these mixed results and lack of clinical studies, further research is needed into garlic and its potential as a chemopreventive agent for bladder cancer.

2.8 Green tea

Green tea is a widely consumed supplement worldwide with a variety of ingredients that have been researched for their health benefits. One application may be for cancer chemoprevention. Green tea has shown inhibitory activity on a variety of tumors in animal models including skin, lung, oral cavity, esophagus, stomach, intestine, colon, liver, pancreas, mammary gland, prostate, and bladder cancers (Lubet et al., 2007; Yang et al., 2011). Several mechanisms have been proposed. For example, one ingredient, polyphenols, has been shown to have antioxidant properties and may prevent cancer

through neutralization of free radicals (Forester & Lambert, 2011). Polyphenols also block ornithine decarboxylase (Messing et al., 1987), which is a key enzyme in polyamine synthesis and plays a major role in cell division and proliferation (Pegg, 2006). Another ingredient, catechins, may exhibit anti-tumor activity through inhibition of nitrosamine formations and decreased chromosomal damage (Kamori et al., 1993). Additional research on green tea suggests other possible mechanisms for a variety of its ingredients including caspase mediation (Oz & Ebersole, 2010), inhibition of angiogenesis (Tsao et al., 2009), and others.
Evidence for green tea in prevention of bladder cancer is variable. In rat models, green tea reduced bladder tumor incidence in several studies (Lubet et al., 2007; Sato, 1999; Sato & Matsushima, 2003). Additionally, great tea mixture modulated actin remodeling (through Rho activity) in an in vitro human bladder cancer model of non-transformed urothelial cell lines as well as reducing tumor growth (Lu et al., 2005). Since malignant cells require actin remodeling in a variety of malignant behaviors (altering morphology, loss of cohesion, invasiveness), this study may point out an additional mechanism for green tea's potential to inhibit bladder cancer (Lu et al., 2005). However, a recent review of the literature suggests caution promoting green tea as a chemopreventative agent for bladder cancer due to conflicting evidence (Boehm et al., 2009), citing two studies that either showed no association (Chyou et al., 1993) or an increased risk of developing bladder cancer (Wakai et al., 2004).

2.9 Difluoromethylornithine (DFMO)

Although originally tested for prevention of bladder and renal cancers (Dunzendorfer, 1981), Difluoromethylornithine (DFMO) is a drug primarily used for the treatment of hirsutism and trypanosomiasis (African sleeping sickness). Recently, there has been renewed interest in using DFMO to prevent a variety of malignancies, including bladder cancer. Although DFMO's mechanism of cancer prevention is not completely understood, it is well established as an irreversible inhibitor of ornithine decarboxylase, which plays a role in cell division and proliferation (Kelloff et al., 1994). A recent study showed that DFMO, when combined with sulindac (an NSAID), significantly reduced the risk of recurring colorectal polyps (Meyskens et al., 2008). Another controlled phase III clinical trial showed that DFMO might reduce the recurrence of basal cell carcinoma (Balley et al., 2010). In addition, DFMO is currently being researched in prevention of esophageal cancer (Sinicrope et al., 2011) and breast cancer (Izbicka et al., 2010). However, past studies assessing DFMO's possible efficacy in reducing recurring bladder cancer have mixed results. Initial studies using DFMO to suppress malignant urothelial cells from human cell lines (Messing et al., 1988) as well as suppressing BBN-induced urothelial carcinoma in mice (Boon et al., 1990) demonstrated selective inhibition of malignant cells. However, a recent controlled phase III clinical trial showed no difference in bladder tumor recurrence rates between placebo and DFMO treated patients (Messing et al., 2006). Due to the variable results, further research into DFMO as a chemopreventive agent in bladder cancer is recommended.

2.10 Non-steroidal anti-inflammatory drugs

NSAIDs, well known for their anti-inflammatory abilities, have also been recently proposed as chemopreventative agents. Studies suggest that cyclooxygenase enzymes may have a key role in carcinogenesis, thus inhibitors have the potential for cancer prevention (Axelsson et al., 2010; Flossmann et al., 2007; Khan & Lee, 2011). Recent studies suggest an important role of COX-2 inhibitors in bladder cancer therapy. Several studies support increased COX-2 expression in bladder tumor stage and/or grade (Wadhwa et al., 2005; Yildirim et al., 2010; Yu et al., 2008). The primary mechanisms in which NSAIDs are thought to inhibit bladder cancer are through stimulation of apoptosis and reduction of angiogenesis (Thun et al., 2002). Another recent study suggested that COX-2 dependent and independent activation of downstream signals, such as CK2α-Akt/uPA, may play a critical role in urothelial carcinoma cell survival and is neutralized by selective COX-2 inhibitors (Shimada et al., 2011).

Clinical data has mixed results for support of NSAID use in bladder and other cancer chemoprevention. A recent pooled analysis of three prospective cohort studies indicated a reduced risk in bladder cancer, particularly in non-smokers, with increased use of non-aspirin NSAIDs, but found no associated decrease in risk of bladder cancer with aspirin use (Daughtery et al., 2011). An in vivo bladder cancer model recently showed some efficacy of naproxen (Lubet et al., 2010). In a bladder tumor mouse model, rofecoxib, a selective COX-2 inhibitor, provided a significant reduction in incidence of neoplastic bladder lesions (D'Arca et al., 2010). Another study that examined multiple randomized trials using daily aspirin versus no aspirin on risk of gastrointestinal and other types of cancer death revealed increased survival, although bladder cancer was not specifically included in the analysis (Rothwell et al., 2011). Further research is needed into the possibility that NSAID's may prevent bladder cancer.

2.11 Statins

Statins are a class of drugs used to lower cholesterol levels through inhibition of 3-hydroxy-3-methylglutaryl coenzyme A (HMG-CoA) reductase. However, there is some evidence suggesting that statins may have other properties in addition to their effect on lowering cholesterol. It is hypothesized that statins may inhibit tumor growth by neutralization of protein prenylation of GTPases, affecting downstream isoprenoids (Demierre et al., 2005), which in turn affect immune response, apoptosis, and cell maturation (Issat et al., 2011).

Currently statins are being researched for their efficacy in preventing a variety of cancers, including bladder malignancies. In a study examining atorvastatin and human bladder cancer cell lines, a significant anti-proliferative effect was observed when compared to controls (Kamat & Nelkin, 2005). In another study using mouse cells transfected with H-ras oncogene from human bladder carcinoma, researchers observed a significant in vivo inhibition of ras-oncogene transformed cells (Sebti et al., 1991). Other studies also point out additional reasons to use statins, since use may also improve local control in patients undergoing concurrent therapy for muscle invasive bladder cancer (Tsai et al., 2006).

However, not all studies support statin efficacy in preventing bladder and other types of cancers. A recent cohort study looking at statins and the occurrence of 10 types of cancer including bladder, showed no significant association with statin use (Jacobs et al., 2011). Using a female rat model, another recent study showed no significant difference in mammary carcinogenesis with simvastatin use (Kubatka et al., 2011). Additionally, a phase II clinical trial using atorvastatin with sulindac (NSAID) and probiotic dietary fiber failed to provide convincing evidence of decreased recurrence of colorectal carcinoma (Limburg et al., 2011). Adding to the controversy, some data suggest that concurrent statin therapy with BCG may reduce clinical efficacy of the BCG therapy (Hoffmann et al., 2006), although this has not been consistent in all studies (Burglund et al., 2008) and not all literature supports discontinuation of the statin (Kamat & Wu, 2007). These results, in contrast with previous studies supporting anti-tumor growth, warrant further investigation into statin use in bladder cancer chemoprevention.

• Vitamin A	Alters cell growth, differentiation, and apoptosis through growth factors, cytokines, and neoplastic stem cell pathways
• Vitamin E	A free radical scavenger, inhibits N-nitroso compound formation as well as inducing apoptosis (some reports state may be a carcinogen)
• Vitamin C	Anti-oxidant, inhibits p-53 and p38 MAPK pathways
• Selemium	Works through methlyation of RNA, anti-androgen, and promotes DNA repair
• Cactus Pear	Increases expression of Annexin IV, decreases VEGF, and promotes immune response
• Isoflavones	Induction of G2-M cell cycle arrest, apoptosis, and angiogenesis
• Garlic	Free radical scavenger, increases cytokines production, a thiol binder along with preventing suppression of the immune response
• Green Tea	Caspase mediator, angiogensis inhibitor, and decreases chromosomal damage
• DFMO	Inhibits malignant urothelial cells through mostly unknown mechanisms, possibly inhibition of ornithine decarboxylase
• NSAIDS	Stimulates apoptosis and inhibits angiogenesis
• Statins	A neutralizer of protein prenylation of GTPases

Table 2. Key features of potential chemopreventative agents for bladder cancer.

3. Inheritance/biomarkers of bladder cancer

In a review article of the epidemiology of bladder cancer by Peluchhi et al., the risk of bladder cancer is increased by 50-100% in first-degree relatives in those that have the disease. Similar to cardiac disease, the risk for first-degree relatives is increased if the patient is diagnosed earlier than the age of 60 (Peluchhi et al., 2006; Goldgar et al., 1994). Current literature suggests a possible X-linked inheritance due to the increased incidence in siblings that are brothers (Pina & Hemminki, 2001).

It is well known of the increased risk that cigarette/tobacco consumption has on bladder cancer, Okkels and associates demonstrated the increased risk through the accumulation of slow acetylators with the Arylamine N-acetyltransferase 2 (NAT 2) genotype (Okkels et al., 1997). The relationship between NAT 1 and NAT 2 leads to the formation of DNA-binding metabolites for aromatic amines (carcinogens) in the bladder (Badawi et al., 1995).

Tobacco smoke also contains 4-aminobiphenyl (4-ABP), an aromatic amine, and for individuals with the NAT 2 phenotype, there is a stronger association, again with the slower acetylators (Yu et al., 1994).
Patients with inherited deletions of the gene, GSTN1, which encodes glutathione S-transferase M1, is associated with bladder cancer. This is in part due to the role of the gene, detoxification of carcinogens, being absent (Brockmoler et al., 1994). Although the aforementioned markers have shown an association with bladder cancer, the question that has still yet to be answered, is to what degree do GSTN1, NAT 1 and NAT 2, among others have on a patient and their risk of bladder cancer, especially with the exposure to carcinogens such as tobacco smoke and aromatic amines.

4. Gene therapy/ γδ T-CELLS

The immunotherapy action of BCG works through binding and availability to major histocompatibility complex (MHC) class I expression on cancer cells (Kitamura et al., 2006). In a murine model, Yuasa et al. investigated, using γδ T-cells (subset of human peripheral T cells), to augment immunotherapy in MHC-diminished superficial bladder cancer, which has been shown to be more aggressive then MHC-conservative bladder cancer. They demonstrated, by examining 123 patients undergoing either TUR or radical cystectomy, that not only was MHC class I expression diminished in lymph node and invasive bladder cancer, but they also experienced a shorter disease free and overall survival.
In their murine model (BALB/c SCID mice), using Luc-labeled bladder cancer cells and ex-vivo γδ T-cells from peripheral blood from healthy patients, mice were treated with γδ T-cells alone or in combination with zoledronic acid. Bladders were examined histologically with hematoxylin-eosin staining and immunohistochemically by with ani-human CD3. Using zoledronic acid to alter the cytotoix effect, γδ T-cells showed dose-dependent cytotoxicty (Kitamura et al., 2009). This shows potential for using γδ T-cells to augment other intravesical treatments to accentuate their benefits.

5. Novel treatments

5.1 Silibinin

Silibinin, a flavonoid phytochemical found in milk thistle, has been shown in vitro, with TCC-SUP (high-grade invasive) and T-24 (high grade), to cause cell cycle arrest along with apoptosis. An induction of G_1 arrest along with cell growth inhibition was determined by various methods including: flow cytometry, cell growth assays (24, 48, and 72 hours of treatments), cell cultures, immunoprecipitation and immunoblottin. Cyclin-dependent kinase activity when uncontrolled, will lead to continuous cell progression. Cyclins are also a determining factor in G_1/S and G_2/M transition (Singh et al., 2002). Both cyclins and cyclin-dependent kinases are reduced with Silibinin as determined by antibodies against CDK2 or CDK4 and kinase assays. Cell death through apoptosis, which was only seen with high-grade invasive cancer, was determined by Annexin V and Propidium Iodide. For the previous experiments, doses of Silibinin varied from 50 to 200 micromolars (Tyagi et al., 2004). Later, the same investigators, with bladder transitional-cell papilloma RT4 cells, induced apoptosis with Slibinin through p53-caspace activation (Tyagi et al., 2006). Through further understanding of the biochemical/cell cycle pathways of bladder cancer, the effects of Silibinin will be better understood.

5.2 Keyhole Limpet Hemocyanin (KLH)

KLH is a copper-containing, extracellular, respiratory protein that was first investigated by Curtis et al., to have immunostimulatory properties (Curtis et al., 1970). Its potential role in the treatment of bladder cancer may be in a cytolytic reduction of tumor growth through a humoral response and an increase in natural killer cells. There have been reports when treating non-muscle invasive bladder cancer to have recurrence rates as low as 31% with less side effects (sepsis, cystitis) than BCG (Harris & Markl, 1999; Nseyo & Lamm, 1997).

Jurincic-Winkler et al. treated thirteen patients with CIS with intravesical KLH (20 mg) on a weekly schedule for 6 weeks, then monthly for one year, and bimonthly for a total of 3 years. Overall, only two patients were free of disease at 66 and 82 months of follow up with the majority requiring BCG or cystectomy (Jurincic-Winkler et al., 2000).

When reviewed, KLH could also be beneficial for carbohydrate-based immunuotherapy in the appropriate adenocarcinoma when there are mucin-like epitopes as well as a potential treatment for melanomas (Harris & Markl, 1999). Overall, the evidence is lacking for KLH to be a major treatment for non-muscle invasive bladder cancer.

5.3 Apaziquone

Apaziquone, also referred commonly as EO9, is an indolequinone compound. Through an activation mechanism with NAD(P)H: Quinone oxidoreductase-1 (NQO1), Apaziquone, in an aerobic environment, has been shown to impact DNA-damaging species (Phillips et al., 2004). Increase in cell kill is also achieved through alklyating byproducts through redox cycling leading to single-strand breaks and DNA cross-linking (Comer & Murphy, 2003). In vivo, it has demonstrated activity against colon, non-small cell lung, renal, melanoma and central nervous system tumor models (Hendricks et al., 1993). With early promising results, it has failed to show favorable phase II outcomes with Phillips et al. citing its rapid pharmacokinetic elimination and poor penetration in avascular tissues (Phillips et al., 1998). In humans, Apaziquone's half-life is less than 10 minutes, via extra-hepatic metabolism by red blood cells, with its metabolites, EO5a, having decreased cytotoxicity (Schelens et al., 1994; Vainchtein et al., 2007).

Current research is aimed at finding adjunct compounds to improve its pharmokinetic properties. A quinone-based bioreductive drug, 2,3-bis(aziridinyl)-5-hydroxy-1,4-naphthoquinone, through its selectivity for NQO1-rich cells under hypoxic conditions, has shown such potential (Phillips et al., 2004).

5.4 Mycobacterium phlei

This agent, has shown anti-tumor activity, is a cell wall extract, composed of carbohydrates, peptides, and lipids that is commonly found on the outer capsule of Mycobacterium phlei, a gram-positive microorganism that is located in soil, plants, and drinking water (Chin et al., 1996; & Mallick et al., 1985). Commonly prepared as a mineral oil emulsion, it has demonstrated inhibitory effects on bladder cancer cell lines through inhibition of cellular proliferation via apoptosis, as well as by an increase in the production of interleukin-12 though stimulation of cancer-infiltrating monocytes and macrophages. Bladder cancer cell lines, in a study by Filion et al., that have been tested include: HT-1197 along with HT-1376 (which are derived from anaplastic transitional cell carcinomas of the bladder from humans, both grade IV and grade III respectively). Cytokine analysis and cellular apoptosis were detected using ELISA and cell death was determined by dimethylthiazoldiphenyltetrazolium bromide

(MTT), (Filion et al., 1999) . When tested in a murine model, mycobacterium phlei induced similar effects that are seen with BCG, namely a CD4+ T cell infiltrate when compared to control. Although the antitumor effect wasn't as significant as that seen with BCG, treatment was better tolerated overall (Chin et al., 1996).

5.5 Docetaxel

Docetaxel, a member of the taxane family, works through microtubule depolymerization inhibition and is commonly used in treatment of prostate and breast cancer, among others. Barlow et al., originally showed a 56% response rate in 18 patients who initially failed BCG therapy and refused to undergo cystectomy. The treatment regimen consisted of 6 weekly bladder instillations on a dose-escalation protocol (McKiernan et al., 2006) They continued their protocol, with the addition of 15 patients, for a median follow up of 29 months and had a 1 and 2 year recurrence-free survival rates of 45 and 32%. Adverse reactions to docetaxel included: dysuria, hematuria, facial flushing, frequency, rash, urinary tract infection, and premature voiding during instillation of the medication. Overall, they concluded that the data is very promising and offers an alternative treatment to those that have failed BCG and do not undergo cystectomy, however, large, multi-institutional, prospective trials are needed to concur effectiveness (Barolw et al., 2009).

Gefitinib, a selective epidermal growth factor receptor tyrosine kinase inhibitor, was studied by Kassouf et al., to determine its effect, in vitro, on enhancing the role of docetaxel on bladder cancer. Four bladder cancer cell lines were studied: 253J B-V, UM-UC-3, KU-7, and UM-UC-13. Through the use of flow cytometry and propidium iodide to determine cell cycle Analysis, along with Western Blot to establish EGFR downstream signaling, it was shown that when combined, gefitinib enhanced both the antiproliferative and apoptotic properties of docetaxel, but only when administered after the docetaxel (Kassouf et al., 2006).

5.6 Hyperthermia

A novel approach of combining local microwave hyperthermia along with Mitomcyin C after undergoing transurethral resection was reported by Colombo et al., with 83 patients who were followed for 24 months. They take into account the detrimental effect that heat has on malignant cells (which are more sensitive to thermal changes in the environment than that of normal cells) such as inhibition of DNA synthesis, RNA, cellular protein, and DNA duplication in the cell cycle. In their study, 83 patients were randomly assigned (after undergoing transurethral resection of primary or recurrent noninvasive bladder cancer) to either receiving Mitomycin C alone or in conjunction with local microwave-induced hyperthermia. Hyperthermia was administered using the Synergo SB-TS:101-1, which consists of a 915 MHz intravesical microwave applicator, to reach a temperature of $42^{o}C \pm 2^{o}C$ and maintained for 40 minutes.

The patients were all followed with urine cytology as well as cystoscopy every 3 months for 2 years, with biopsies taken if suspicious lesions were noted. Abdominal and pelvic ultrasound was also obtained on a bi-annual basis. Overall, 75 patients completed the protocol and those receiving the hyperthermia experienced more severe side effects: cystitis, suprapubic pain, and thermal reaction. Only six patients (17.1%) had recurrence with the combination therapy as compared to 23 patients (57.5%) receiving only Mitomycin C (P value = 0.0002). There was one patient with disease progression in the chemotherapy only treatment group. Overall, the idea of combining intravesical chemotherapy along with hyperthermia is an attractive option for enhancing the effectiveness of chemotherapeutic agents especially for those that are not surgical candidates for radical cystectomy (Colombo et al., 2003).

A more recent study was carried out by Nativ et al., to examine those patients that experience recurrence of papillary non-muscle invasive bladder cancer after undergoing BCG treatment. They looked at 111 patients and followed them for 2 years with urine cytology and cystoscopy every 3 months. All patients were treated with hyperthermia, 42°C $\pm$ 2°C, for two cycles of 30 minute instillations of 20mg of Mitomycin C, for 6 weekly treatments followed by 6 maintenance sessions at 4 to 6 week intervals.

Adverse reactions were similar as compared to the earlier study with pain and bladder spasms being the most common (transient to mild at worse). Recurrence-free rates at one and two years were 85% and 56% respectively. There were 3 patients (3%) that progressed to muscle invasive bladder cancer during the follow up. Interestingly, those patients that received fewer than 10 maintenance treatments, had a tumor recurrence rate of 61% compared to 39% that completed the two year regimen (p value = 0.01) (Nativ et al., 2009). The combination of hyperthermia with intravesical treatment is very promising and should be considered very strongly for future trials in those patients that are considered BCG failures.

5.7 Inositol Hexaphosphate

Inositol Hexaphosphate (IP-6) is a naturally occurring polyphosphorylated carbohydrate that is found in foods that are high in fiber such as cereals, legumes, and grains (Fox & Eberl, 2002). It has already been shown to possess anti-tumor effects in numerous cancer cell lines: colon, hepatocellular, breast, lung, prostate, pancreas and melanoma among others while not being cytotoxic or cytostatic against normal cells (Shamsuddin et al., 1997). Zaslau et al., displayed its mechanism of action against bladder cancer cell lines (HTB9 [grade II], T24 [grade III], TCCSUP [grade IV]) via modulation of the cell cycle and induction of cellular apoptosis as well as necrosis (Zaslau et al., 2009).

Already demonstrating reduction in cellular proliferation, they tested IP-6's clinical efficacy with a 2-hour exposure time. All three cell lines (HTB9, T24, and TCCSUP) were plated and cultured with 2.5 and 4.5 m*M* of IP-6 for 2 hours and then had their supernatant incubated for an additional 24 and 48 hours. Cell viability was assessed though MTT colorimetric assay and cell cycle analysis though flow cytometry. All three cell lines, at all times tested, noted a significant reduction in cellular growth when treated with IP-6 with only a 2 hour incubation. Interestingly, when looking at cell cycle inhibition, IP-6 produced different results with the varying degrees of bladder cancer cell lines, which can be related to the different tumor grades replicating at different rates corresponding to diverse responses to the IP-6 treatments. There was an increase in cells in the G_0/G1 phase, reduction in G2/M, while no change in the S phase with the TCCSUP cell line. The T24 cell line was determined to be accelerating and not dividing through observances of cell reduction with 4.5 m*M* IP-6 in the G_0/G1 phase and no change in both the S and G2/M phases. Lastly, with the HTB9 cell line, as with the T24 cell line, no change was noted in G2/M, however, there was an induction in the arrest at G_0/G1 while a decrease in S phase (Zaslau et al., 2009).

IP-6 was later tested, with the same bladder cancer cell lines, using Annexin V-Fluorescein Isothiocyanate (FITC) and Propidium Iodine along with flow cytometry to determine method of cell kill. Using the same concentrations, 2.5 and 4.5 m*M*, at 2 hour incubations, HTB9 was effected by necrotic mechanisms, and T24 and TCCSUP went through an induction of apoptosis (Zaslau et al., 2010). The authors, with promising results thus far, state the Phase II clinical trials are needed to evaluate the safety and clinical utility of IP-6 for the intravesical use in bladder cancer.

5.8 HTI-286

HTI-286 is a synthetic analogue of the marine sponge product hemiasterlin. In a similar fashion to the taxanes, HTI-286 works through inhibition of tubulin polymerization with strong cytotoxic potential. In an in vitro study, HTI-286 was compared to MMC when tested in human bladder cancer cell lines RT4, MGH-U3, KU-7, as well as UM-UC3. In this study, it showed comparable cytotoxicity, inhibition of cell growth, and induction of apoptosis in all cell lines tested. An in vivo study using 8-week old nude mice demonstrated delayed cancer growth in a dose dependent manner (Hadaschik et al., 2008).

5.9 Suramin

Suramin, a polysulphonated naphthylurea, has anticancer functions that are comprised of growth factor antagonism and cellular DNA synthesis suppression (Walther et al., 1994; La Rocca et al., 1990).

Serious side effects including neurologic, renal, and metabolic Have been caused by systemic administration of suramin (La Rocca et al, 1990; Figg et al, 1994; Bowden et al, 1996) secondary to the compound having a 40-day plasma half-life in humans (Hawking, 1978). Suramin possesses several structural advantages for use intravesically in bladder cancer: its' high molecular mass (1429 Da) and negative ionic charge hamper systemic absorption (Ord et al, 2005); and its tendency to bind to protein favors growth factor antagonism in urine, which contains low protein levels (Ord et al, 2005). In particular, suramin inhibits the binding of epidermal growth factor (EGF) to its receptor, which are prevalent in high numbers in bladder cancer (Walther et al, 1996).

A phase I clinical trial found that intravesical treatment with suramin for cases of recurrent superficial bladder cancer was safe up to a 153mg/ml dose (Uchio et al, 2003). However, suramin's effects on bladder tumors has not yet been evaluated. Noted complications included bladder spasms and vesicoureteral reflux in a small percentage of the individual treatments, all of which completely abated within 48 hours (Uchio et al, 2003). Even at the highest dosages, plasma concentrations of suramin were minimal and further trials are warranted to decipher its usefulness.

5.10 Gemcitabine

Gemcitabine, as reported by Karak and Flechon, is a deoxycytidine analogue, a pyrimidine antimetabolite that is similar to cytarabine that works through inhibition of DNA synthesis (Karak & Flechon, 2007). Its effect on bladder cancer's cell cycle is via a blockage of cells progressing through the G1/S phase and a cytotoxic effect in S-phase (Guchelaar et al., 1996). It has already been approved through the Food and Drug Administration as a first line treatment for solid tumors of the pancreas as well as for inoperable, metastatic non-

small cell lung and breast cancer (Karak & Flechon, 2007). Gemcitabine has been known to cause is myelosuppression (Aapro et al., 1998).
Gemcitabine has also been used as single agent for those patients that were considered BCG failures. In a phase II trial Dalbagni et al. examined 30 patients that were refractory to BCG treatment. Treatment was given twice weekly for 3 weeks and surveillance was conducted at 8 weeks and then every 3 months for one year. Although there was a complete response in 50% of patient at 3 months, this was reduced to only 10% at one year (Dalbagni et al., 2006).

5.11 Mitomycin-C & Gemcitabine

Gemcitabine, as described by Breyer et al., is 2',2'-difluoro-2'-deoxycytidine, that has shown broad spectrum anti-tumor activity. In their study, 10 patients that were either BCG refractory or BCG intolerant were treated with Gemcitabine (1000mg in 50cc sterile water) then MMC (40mg in 20cc sterile water) once a week for 6 weeks as their induction treatment. This was then followed by maintenance treatment (same dosage) once a month for 12 months. Median follow up for the patients (with median age of 67 years) was 26.5 months. Six out of ten patients were recurrence free at 14 months, with 4 patients having biopsy proven recurrence at a median of 6 months. Overall, the treatment was well tolerated with no major complications. Of note, 9 out of 10 patients had either high grade bladder cancer or carcinoma in situ before beginning treatment and had a median of five recurrences (Breyer et al, 2010). The same authors cited another study by Maymi and O'Donnell that compared Gemcitabine versus Gemicitabine in combination with MMC in 39 patients that have failed multiple, previous intravesical treatments. Alone, the median disease free survival was 6.5 months compared to 20 months for the combination of Gemicitabine and MMC (Maymi et al.). In a comparison study, Malmstrom et al. found only 4 out of 21 patients disease free that were treated with MMC for noninvasive bladder cancer at 3 years (Malmostrom et al., 1999). The literature that has been reviewed supports the use of MMC In combination with other intravesical agents to increase its effectiveness.

5.12 Mitomycin-C and BCG

The two leading intravescial treatments for non-muscle invasive bladder cancer are Mitomycin-C and BCG. There have been many studies that have looked to find an additive effect with the combination of the two agents (chemoimmunotherapy), but in whole, have not produced significant results. Witjes and colleagues examined 90 patients that underwent 4 weekly instillations of 40 mg of MMC followed by 6 weekly instillations of BCG (group 1) and compared them to 92 patients that just underwent 10 weekly instillations of MMC (group 2). Surprisingly, there was no significant difference seen between the two groups in regards to bacterial cystitis, chemical cystitis, and other local side effects. Eleven patients had fever (>38.5C) in group 1 compared to only 3 patients in group 2. Median follow up was 32 months. There were 35/90 patients with recurrence and 5/90 patients with progression in group 1 and 42/92 and 4/92 respectively, in group 2 (Witjes et al., 1998).
A prospective, randomized comparison of BCG alone with that of BCG and electromotive MMC was carried out by Di Stasi and colleagues. After being diagnosed with pT1 bladder cancer, 212 patients were randomly assigned to induction of either 81 mg of BCG for 2 hours once a week for 6 weeks or 81 mg of BCG over 2 hours once a week for 2 weeks, then 40 mg of electromotive MMC (intravesical electric current 20 mA for 30 min) once a week for three weeks. Exclusion criteria included previous treatment with either BCG or electromotive

MMC, any intravesical agent in the last 6 months, upper tract disease, and previous radiotherapy to the pelvis or chemotherapy among others. Maintenance for the BCG alone group consisted of 81 mg BCG once a month for 10 months compared to the group being treated with BCG and electromotive MMC which received the combination once a month for 2 months, then 81 mg of BCG once a month for three months. Of critical importance is that the authors defined the primary endpoint being disease-free survival with secondary endpoints being time to progression, overall survival and disease specific survival. Median follow-up was an impressive 88 months.

The patients that received the combination had a higher disease-free survival at 69 months compared to the patients that received only BCG, which was 21 months. Follow-up consisted of abdominal ultrasound, cystourethroscopy, and urine cytology every 3 months for the first three years and then every 6 months thereafter. If a patient was originally diagnosed with carcinoma in situ, the follow-up also included random bladder biopsies at 3 and 6 months. The combination group also has a lower rate of progression at 9.3% compared to 21.9% of BCG alone group, with 10 and 23 patients progressing to muscle-invasive bladder cancer respectively. Also, the BCG and electromotive MMC group only had 6 reported deaths due to bladder cancer compared to 23 in the BCG alone group. Adverse effects were similar between the two groups with each having 3 patients withdrawing from the trial. According to the authors, the benefit of the combination may be attributed to BCG-induced inflammation increasing the bladder mucosa permeability to the effects of the MMC, allowing it to reach the target tissue (Di Stasi et al., 2007).

• γδ T-cells	Enhances immunotherapy by increasing MHC class I expression
• Silibinin	Induced G1 cell cycle arrest and reduces cyclin and cyclin-dependent kinases which decreases cell progression
• KLH	Possible mechanism of action could include an increase in humoral response in an association with an increase of natural killer cells
• Apaziquone	Needs to be combined with another agent or treatment modality to better its pharmokinetics to lengthen its half-life and therapeutic effect
• Mycobacterium Phlei	Increases production of IL-12, induces apoptosis, as well as promoting a CD4+ T cell response
• Docetaxel	Inhibits microtubule depolymerization
• Hyperthermia	Environmental/thermal changes which malignant cells are more sensitive to and causes inhibition of DNA and RNA synthesis among other cellular pathways
• IP-6	Modulates cell cycle and induces cellular apoptosis and necrosis
• HTI-286	Similar mechanism of action as the taxanes (Docetaxel)

• Suramin	Growth factor antagonist and suppresses DNA synthesis
• Gemcitabine	Inhibits DNA synthesis and through a cystotoxic effect, inhibits malignant cells in G1/S and S-phase
• MMC and Gemcitabine	Overall, a well tolerated combination with beneficial results when compared to each agent alone.
• MMC and BCG	BCG may increase bladder mucosa permeability through an inflammatory response allowing MMC to reach its target at a more optimal level

Table 3. Mechanism of action of Novel Treatments for Bladder Cancer

6. Conclusion

Further advancement in the treatment of non-muscle invasive bladder cancer will come in the understanding of the disease's molecular/biochemical pathways and the effect on these pathways that chemopreventive and intravesical agents have on them. Certainly there are some areas that are more promising than others, especially with the combination of agents as well as the addition of hyperthermia to treatment regimens that are already producing significant positive results. As a review of the many agents discussed, table 2 provides the key features of potential chemopreventative agents for bladder cancer. Table 3 reviews the mechanism of action of Novel Treatments for Bladder Cancer. As always, it is not just the initial resection, or even the induction treatment that reduces recurrence and progression, but the role of maintenance therapy that is crucial for the patient to remain disease free. Again, with the new discoveries of cell signaling, cell cycle/death/apoptosis, interleukin, humoral and cell mediated responses, there will be more specific target treatments with the hopes of minimal side effects.

7. References

Aapro, M., Marin, C. & Hatty, S. (1998). Review Paper: Gemcitabine – a Safety Review. *Anti Cancer Drugs,* Vol.9, No.3, (March 1998), pp. 191-201, ISSN 1473-5741.

Alfthan, O., Tarkkanen, J., Gröhn, P., et al. (1983). Tigason (Etretinate) in Prevention of Recurrence of Superficial Bladder Tumors. A Double-blind Clinical Trial. *European Urology,* Vol.9, No.1, pp. 6-9, ISSN 0302-2838.

Amaral, A., Cantor, K., Silverman, D. & Malats, N. (2010). Selenium and Bladder Cancer Risk: A Meta-analysis. *Cancer Epidemiology, Biomarkers, and Prevention,* Vol.19, No.9, (September 2010), pp. 2407-2415, ISSN 1538-7755.

Axelsson, H., Lönnroth, C., Andersson, M. & Lundholm, K. (2010). Mechanisms Behind COX-1 and COX-2 Inhibition of Tumor Growth In Vivo. *International Journal of Oncology,* Vol.37, No.5, (November 2010), pp. 1143-1152, ISSN 1791-2423.

Badawi, A., Hirvonen, A., Bell, D., Lang, N. & Kadlubar, F. Role of Aromatic Amine Acetlytrasnferase, NAT1 and NAT2, in carcinogen-DNA Adduct Formation in the Human Urinary Bladder. *Cancer Res,* Vol.55, No.22, (November 1995), pp. 5230-5237, ISSN 1538-7445.

Balley, H., Kim, K., Verma, A., et al. (2010). A Randomized, Double-blind, Placebo-controlled Phase 3 Skin Cancer Prevention Study of {Alpha}-difluoromethylornithine in Subjects with Previous History of Skin Cancer. *Cancer Prevention Research,* Vol.3, No.1, (January 2010), pp. 35-47, ISSN 1940-6215.

Barlow, L., McKiernan, C. & Benson M. (2009). The Novel Use of Intravesical Docetaxel for the Treatment of Non-Muscle Invasive Bladder Cancer Refractory to BCG Therapy: a Single Institution Experience. *World J Urol,* Vol.27, No.3, (June 2009), pp. 331-335, ISSN 1433-8726.

Beisel, W., Edelman, R., Nauss, K. & Suskind, R. (1981). Single-nutrient Effects on Immunologic Functions. Report of a Workshop Sponsored by the Department of Food and Nutrition and its Nutrition Advisory Group of the American Medical Association. *The Journal of the American Medical Association,* Vol.245, No.1, (January 1981), pp. 53-58, ISSN 1538-3598.

Boehm, K., Borrelli, F., Ernst, E., et al. (2009). Green Tea (Camellia sinensis) for the Prevention of Cancer. *Cochrane Database of Systematic Reviews,* Issue.3: CD005004, (July 2009), ISSN 1469-493X.

Bondesson, M. & Gustafsson, J. (2010). Does Consuming Isoflavones Reduce or Increase Breast Cancer Risk? *Genome Medicine,* Vol.2, No.12, (December 2010), pp. 90, ISSN 1756-904X.

Boon, C., Kelloff, G. & Malone, W. (1990). Identification of Candidate Cancer Chemopreventive Agents and Their Evaluation in Animal Models and Human Clinical Trials: A Review. *Cancer Research,* Vol.50, No.1, (January 1990), pp. 2-9, ISSN 1538-7445.

Bowden, C., Figg, W., Dawson, N., et al. (1996). A Phase I/II Study of Continuous Infusion Suramin in Patients with Hormone-Refractory Prostate Cancer: Toxicity and Response. *Cancer Chemother Pharmacol,* Vol.39, No.1-2, (1996), pp. 1-8, ISSN 1432-0843.

Breyer, B., Whitson, J., Carroll, P. & Konety, B. (2010). Sequential Intravesical Gemcitabine and Mitomycin C Chemotherapy Regimen in Patients with Non-Muscle Invasive Bladder Cancer. *Urologic Oncology,* Vol.28, No.5, (September-October 2010), pp. 510-514, ISSN 1873-2496.

Brinkman, M. & Zeegers, M. (2008). Nutrition, Total Fluid and Bladder Cancer. *Scandinavian Journal of Urology and Nephrology. Supplementum,* Vol.218, (September 2008), pp. 25-36, ISSN 1651-2537.

Brockmoller, J., Kerb, R., Drakoulis, N., Staffeldt, B. & Roots, I. Glutathione S-Transferase M1 and its Variants A and B as Host Factors of Bladder Cancer Susceptibility: a Case-Control Study. *Cancer Res,* Vol.54, No.15, (August 1994), pp. 4103-4111, ISSN 1538-7445.

Burglund, R., Savage, C., Vora, K., Kurta, J. & Cronin, A. (2008). An Analysis of the Effect of Statin Use on the Efficacy of Bacillus Calmette-guerin Treatment for Transitional Cell Carcinoma of the Bladder. *The Journal of Urology,* Vol.180, No.4, (October 2008), pp. 1297-1300, ISSN 1527-3792.

Butt, M., Sultan, M., Butt, M. & Iqbal, J. Garlic: Nature's Protection Against Physiological Threats. *Critical Reviews in Food Science and Nutrition,* Vol.49, No.6, (June 2009), pp. 538-551, ISSN 1549-7852.

Cerella, C., Dicato, M., Jacob, C. & Diederich, M. (2011). Chemical Properties and Mechanisms Determining the Anti-cancer Action of Garlic-derived Organic Sulfur Compounds. *Anti-cancer Agents in Medicinal Chemistry,* Vol.11, No.3, (March 2011), pp. 267-271, ISSN 1875-5992.

Chavez-Santoscoy, R., Gutierrez-Uribe, J. & Serna-Saldívar, S. (2009). Phenolic Composition, Antioxidant Capacity and in Vitro Cancer Cell Cytotoxicity of Nine Prickly Pear (Opuntia Spp.) Juices. *Plant Foods for Human Nutrition,* Vol.64, No.2, (June 2009), pp. 146-152, ISSN 1573-9104.

Chin, J., Kadhim, S., Batislam, E. et al. (1996). Mycobacterium Cell Wall: an Alternative to Intravesical Bacillus Calmette Guerin (BCG) Therapy in Orthotopic Murine Bladder Ccancer. *J Urol,* Vol.156, No.3, (September 1996), pp. 1189-93, ISSN 1527-3792.

Chyou, P., Nomura, A. & Stemmermann, G. (1993). A Prospective Study of Diet, Smoking, and Lower Urinary Tract Cancer. *Annals of Epidemiology,* Vol.3, No.3, (May 1993), pp. 211-216, ISSN 1873-2585.

Columbo, R., Da Pozzo, L., Salonia, A. et al. (2003). Multicentric Study Comparing Intravesical Chemotherapy Alone and with Local Microwave Hyperthermia for Prophylaxis of Recurrence of Superficial Transitional Cell Carcinoma. *Journal of Clinical Oncology,* Vol.21, No.23, (December 2003), pp. 4270-4276, ISSN 1572-7755.

Comer, E. & Murphy, W. (2003). The Bromoquinone Annulation Reaction: a Formal Total Synthesis of EO9. *ARKIVOC,* Vol.7, (June 2003), pp. 286-296, ISSN 1551-7012.

Coulter, I., Hardy, M., Morton, S., et al. (2006). Antioxidants Vitamin C and Vitamin E for the Prevention and Treatment of Cancer. *Journal of General Internal Medicine,* Vol.21, No.7, (July 2006), pp. 735-744, ISSN 1525-1497.

Curtis, J., Hersh, E., Harris, J., et al. (1970). The Human Primary Immune Response to Keyhole Limpet Hemocyanin: Interrelationships of Delayed Hypersensitivity, Antibody Response and In Vitro Blast Transformation. *Clin. Exp.,* Vol.56, No.130, (April 1970), pp. 473-491, ISSN 1365-2249.

Dalbagni, G., Russo, P., Bochner, B., et al. (2006). Phase II Trial of Intravesical Gemcitabine in Bacilli Calmette-Guerin-Refractory Transitional Cell Carcinoma of the Bladder. *J Clin Oncol,* Vol.24, No.18, (June 2006), pp. 2729-2734, ISSN 1527-7755.

D'Arca, D., LeNoir, J., Wildemore, B., et al. (2010). Prevention of Urinary Bladder Cancer in the FHIT Knock-out Mouse with Rofecoxib, a Cox-2 Inhibitor. *Urologic Oncology,* Vol.28, No.2, (March-April 2010), pp. 189-194, ISSN 1873-2496.

Daughtery, S., Pfeiffer, R., Sigurdson, A., et al. (2011). Nonsteroidal Antiinflammatory Drugs and Bladder Cancer: A Pooled Analysis. *American Journal of Epidemiology,* Vol.173, No.7, (April 2011), pp. 721-730, ISSN 1476-6256.

Decensi, A., Torrisi, R., Bruno, S., et al. (2000). Randomized Trial of Fenretinide in Superficial Bladder Cancer Using DNA Flow Cytometry as an Intermediate End Point. *Cancer Epidemiology, Biomarkers & Prevention,* Vol.9, No.10, (October 2000), pp. 1071-1078, ISSN 1055-7755

Demierre, M., Higgins, P., Gruber, S., Hawk, E & Lippman, S. (2005). Statins and Cancer Prevention. *Nature Reviews. Cancer,* Vol.5, No.12, (December 2005), pp. 930-942, ISSN 1474-1768.

Di Stasi, S., Giannantoni, A., Giurioli, A. et al. (2006). Sequential BCG and Electromotive Mitomycin Versus BCG Alone for High-Risk Superficial Bladder Cancer: a Randomized Controlled Trial. *Lancet Oncol,* Vol.7, No.1, (January 2006), pp. 43-51, ISSN 1474-5488.

Dunzendorfer, U. (1981). The Effect of Alpha-difluoromethyl-ornithine on Tumor Growth, Acute Phase Reactants, Beta-2-microglobulin and Hydroxyproline in Kidney and Bladder Carcinomas. *Urologia Internationalis,* Vol.36, No.2, pp. 128-136, ISSN 1423-0399.

Fernández-López, J., Almela, L., Obón, J. & Castellar, R. (2010). Determination of Antioxidant Constituents in Cactus Pear Fruits. *Plant Foods for Human Nutrition,* Vol.65, No.3, (September 2010), pp. 253-259, ISSN 1573-9104.

Feugang, J., Ye, F., Zhang, D., et al. (2010). Cactus Pear Extracts Induce Reactive Oxygen Species Production and Apoptosis in Ovarian Cancer Cells. *Nutrition and Cancer,* Vol.62, No.5, pp. 692-699, ISSN 1532-7914.

Figg, W., Cooper, M., Thibault, A., Headlee, D., et al. (1994). Acute Renal Toxicity Associated with Suramin in the Treatment of Prostate Cancer. *Cancer,* Vol.74, No.5, (September 1994), pp. 1612-1614, ISSN 1097-0142.

Filion, M., Lepicier, P., Morales, A. & Phillips, N. Mycobacterium Phlei Cell Wall Complex Directly Induces Apoptosis in Human Bladder Cancer Cells. *British Journal of Cancer,* Vol.79, No.2, (January 1999), pp. 229-235, ISSN 1532-1827.

Flossmann, E., Rothwell, P., British Doctors Aspirin Trial and the UK-TIA Aspirin Trial. (2007). Effect of Aspirin on Long-term Risk of Colorectal Cancer: Consistent Evidence from Randomized and Observational Studies. *Lancet,* Vol.369, No.9573, (May 2007), pp. 1603-1613, ISSN 1474-547X.

Forester, S. & Lambert, J. (2011). The Role of Antioxidant Versus Pro-oxidant Effects of Green Tea Polyphenols in Cancer Prevention. *Molecular Nutrition & Food Research,* Vol.55, No.6, (June 2011), pp. 844-854, ISSN 1613-4133.

Fox, C. & Eberl, M. (2002). Phytic Acid (IP6), Novel Broad Spectrum Anti-Neoplastic Agent: a Systematic Review. *Complement Ther Med,* Vol.10, No. 4, (December 2002), pp. 229-234, ISSN 1873-6963.

Garattini, E., Gianni, M. & Terao, M. (2007). Retinoids as Differentiating Agents in Oncology: a Network of Interactions with Intracellular Pathways as the Basis for Rational Therapeutic Combinations. *Current Pharmaceutical Design,* Vol.13, No.13, pp. 1375-1400, ISSN 1381-6128.

Gazi, M., Gong, A., Donkena, K. & Young, C. (2006). Sodium Selenite Inhibits Interleukin-6-mediated Androgen Receptor Activation in Prostate Cancer Cells Via Upregulation of c-Jun. *Clinical Chimica Acta,* Vol. 380, No.1-2, (May 2007), pp. 145-150, ISSN 1873-3492.

Goldgar, D., Easton, D., Cannon-Albright, L. & Skolnick, M. (1994). Systematic Population-Based Assessment of Cancer Risk in First-Degree Relatives of Cancer Probands. *J Natl Cancer Inst,* Vol.86, No.21, (November 1994), pp. 1600-1608, ISSN 1460-2105.

Golijanin, D., Kiakiashvili, D,. Madeb, R., et al. (2006). Chemoprevention of Bladder Cancer. *World J Urol*, Vol. 24, No. 5, (November 2006), pp. 445-472, ISSN 1433-8726.

Guchelaar, H., Richel, D. & Van Knapen, A. (1996). Clinical Toxicological and Pharmacological Aspects of Gemcitabine. *Cancer Treat. Rev*, Vol.22, No.1, (January 1996), pp. 15-31, ISSN 1532-1967.

Gunby, P. (1978). Retinoid Chemoprevention Trial Begins Against Bladder Cancer. *The Journal of the American Medical Association*, Vol.240, No.7, (August 1978), pp. 609-610 & 614, ISSN 0098-7484.

Hadaschik, B., Adomat, H., Fazli, L. et al. (2008). Intravesical Chemotherapy of High-Grade Bladder Cancer with HTI-286, a Synthetic Analogue of the Marin Sponge Product Hemiasterlin. *Clin Cancer Res*, Vol.14, No.5, (March 2008), pp. 1510-1518, ISSN 1078-0432.

Hadjiolov, D., Fernando, R., Schmeiser, H., et al. (1993). Effect of Diallyl Sulfide on Aristolochic Acid-induced Forestomach Carcinogenesis in Rats. *Carcinogenesis*, Vol.14, No.3, (March 1993), pp. 407-410, ISSN 1460-2180.

Hahm, S., Park, J. & Son, Y. (2010). Opuntia humifusa Partitioned Extracts Inhibit the Growth of U87MG Human Glioblastoma Cells. *Plant Foods for Human Nutrition*, Vol.65, No.3, (September 2010), pp. 247-252, ISSN 1573-9104.

Hameed, D. & el-Metwally T. (2008). The Effectiveness of Retinoic Acid Treatment in Bladder Cancer: Impact on Recurrence, Survival and TGFalpha and VEGF as End-point Biomarkers. *Cancer Biology & Therapy*, Vol.7, No.1, (January 2008), pp. 92-100, ISSN 1538-4047.

Harris, J. & Markl, J. (1999). Keyhole Limpet Hemocyanin (KLH): a Biomedical Review. *Micron*, Vol.30, No.6, (December 1999), pp. 597-623, ISSN 1878-4291.

Hawking, F. (1978) Suramin: with Special Reference to Onchocerciasis. *Adv Pharmacol Chemother*, Vol.15, (1978), pp. 289-322, ISSN 0065-3144.

Hendriks, H., Pizao, P., Berger, D., et al. (1993). EO9: a Novel Bioreductive Alkylating Indoloquinone with Preferential Solid Tumour Activity and Lack of Bone Marrow Toxicity in Preclinical Models. *Eur J Cancer*, Vol.29, No.6, (1993), pp. 897-906, ISSN 0014-2964.

Hess, D. & Igal, R. (2011). Genistein Downregulates De Novo Lipid Synthesis and Impairs Cell Proliferation in Human Lung Cancer Cells. *Experimental Biology and Medicine*, Vol.236, No.6, (June 2011), pp. 707-713, ISSN 1535-3699.

Hoffmann, P., Roumeguère, T., Schulman, C. & van Velthoven, R. (2006). Use of Statins and Outcome of BCG Treatment for Bladder Cancer. *The New England Journal of Medicine*, Vol.355, No.25, (December 2006), pp. 2705-2707, ISSN 1533-4406.

Hotaling, J., Wright, J., Pocobelli, G., et al. (2011). Long-term Use of Supplemental Vitamins and Minerals Does Not Reduce the Risk of Urothelial Cell Carcinoma of the Bladder in the Vitamins And Lifestyle Study. *Journal of Urology*, Vol.185, No.4, (February 2011), ISSN 1527-3792.

Husbeck, B., Bhattacharyya, R., Feldman, D. & Knox, S. (2006). Inhibition of Androgen Receptor Signaling by Selenite and Methylseleninic Acid in Prostate Cancer Cells: Two Distinct Mechanisms of Action. *Molecular Cancer Therapeutics*, Vol.5, No.8, (August 2006), pp. 2078-2085, ISSN 1538-8514.

Hwang, J., Lee, Y., Shin, J. & Park, O. (2009). Anti-inflammatory and Anticarcinogenic Effect of Genistein Alone or in Combination with Capsaicin in TPA-treated Rat Mammary Glands or Mammary Cancer Cell Line. *Annals of the New York Academy of Sciences,* Vol.1171, (August 2009), pp. 415-420, ISSN 1749-6632.

Issat, T., Nowis, D., Bil, J., et al. (2011). Antitumor Effects of the Combination of Cholesterol Reducing Drugs. *Oncology Reports,* Vol.26, No.1, (July 2011), pp. 169-176, ISSN 1791-2431.

Izbicka, E., Streeper, R., Yeh, I., et al. (2010). Effects of Alpha-difluoromethylornithine on Markers of Proliferation, Invasion, and Apoptosis in Breast Cancer. *Anticancer Research,* Vol.30, No.6, (June 2010), pp. 2263-2269, ISSN 1791-7530.

Jackson, M. & Combs, G. Jr. (2008). Selenium and Anticarcinogenesis: Underlying Mechanisms. *Current Opinion in Clinical Nutrition and Metabolic Care,* Vol.11, No.6, (November 2008), pp. 718-726, ISSN 1535-3885.

Jacobs, E., Henion, A., Briggs, P., et al. (2002). Vitamin C and Vitamin E Supplement Use and Bladder Cancer Mortality in a Large Cohort of US Men and Women. *American Journal of Epidemiology,* Vol.156, No.1, (December 2002), pp. 1002-1010, ISSN 1476-6256.

Jacobs, E., Newton, C., Thun, M. & Gapstur, S. (2011). Long-term Use of Cholesterol-lowering Drugs and Cancer Incidence in a Large United States Cohort. *Cancer Research,* Vol.71, No.5, (March 2011), pp. 1763-1771, ISSN 1538-7445.

Jurincic-Winkler, C., Metz, K., Beuth, J. & Klippel, K. (2000). Keyhole Limpet Hemocyanin for Carcinoma in Situ of the Bladder: a Long-Term Follow-Up Study. *Eur Urol,* Vol.57, No.3, (2000), pp. 45-49, ISSN 1873-7860.

Kamat, A. (2003). Chemoprevention of Superficial Bladder Cancer. *Expert Rev. Anticancer Ther,* Vol. 6, No.6, pp. 799-808, ISSN 1744-8328.

Kamat, A. & Nelkin, G. (2005). Atorvastatin: A Potential Chemopreventive Agent in Bladder Cancer. *Urology,* Vol.66, No.6, (December 2005), pp.1209-1212, ISSN 1527-9995.

Kamat, A. & Wu, X. (2007). Statins and the Effect of BCG on Bladder Cancer. *The New England Journal of Medicine,* Vol.356, No.12, (March 2007), pp. 1276-1277, ISSN 1533-4406.

Kamori, A., Yatsunami, J., Okabe, S., Abe, S., Hara, K., Suganuma, M., Kim, S. & Fujiki, H. (1993). Anticarcinogenic Activity of Green Tea Polyphenols. *Japanese Journal of Clinical Oncology,* Vol.23, No.3, (June 1993), pp. 186-190, ISSN 1465-3621.

Karak, F. & Flechon, A. (2007). Gemcitabine in Bladder Cancer. *Expert Opin. Pharmacothe,* Vol.8, No.18, (December 2007), pp. 3251-3256, ISSN 1744-7666.

Kassouf, W., Luongo, T., Brown, G., Adam, L. & Dinney, C. (2006). Schedule dependent efficacy of Gefitinib and Docetaxel for bladder cancer. *J Urol,* Vol.176, No.2, (August 2006), pp. 787-792, 1527-3792.

Kellen, E., Zeegers, M. & Buntinx, F. (2006). Selenium is Inversely Associated with Bladder Cancer Risk: A Report from the Belgian Case-control Study on Bladder Cancer. *International Journal of Urology,* Vol.13, No.9, (September 2006), pp. 1180-1184, ISSN 1442-2042.

Kelloff, G., Crowell, J., Boone, C., et al. (1994). Strategy and Planning for Chemopreventive Drug Development: Clinical Development Plans. Chemoprevention Branch and

Agent Development Committee. National Cancer Institute. *Journal of Cellular Biochemistry. Supplement,* Vol.20, pp. 55-62, ISSN 0733-1959.

Khan, M. & Lee, Y. (2011). Cyclooxygenase Inhibitors: Scope of Their Use and Development in Cancer Chemotherapy. *Medicinal Research Reviews,* Vol.31, No.2, (March 2011), pp. 161-201, ISSN 1098-1128.

Kim, J., Jin, D., Lee, SD., et al. (2008). Vitamin C Inhibits p53-induced Replicative Senescence Through Suppression of ROS Production and p38 MAPK Activity. *International Journal of Molecular Medicine,* Vol.22, No.5, (November 2008), pp. 651-655, ISSN 1791-244X.

Kitamura, H., Torigoe, T., Honma, I., et al. (2006). Effect of Human Leukocytes Antigen Class I Expression of Tumor Cells on Outcome of Intravesical Instillation of Bacillus Calmette-Guerin Immunotherapy for Bladder Cancer. *Clin Cancer Res.,* Vol.12, No.15, (August 2006), pp. 4461-4464, ISSN 1078-0432.

Kline, K., Yu, W. & Sanders, B. (2004). Vitamin E and Breast Cancer. *The Journal of Nutrition.* Vol.134, No.12 Supplement, (December 2004), pp. 3458S-3462S, ISSN 1541-6100.

Kubatka, P., Zihlaviniková, K., Kajo, K., et al. (2011). Antineoplastic Effects of Simvastatin in Experimental Breast Cancer. *Klinická Onkologie,* Vol.24, No.1, pp. 41-45, ISSN 1802-5307.

Lamm, D., Riggs, D., Shriver, J., et al. (1994). Megadose Vitamins in Bladder Cancer: A Double-blind Clinical Trial. *The Journal of Urology,* Vol.151, No.1, (January 1994), pp. 21-26, ISSN 1527-3792.

Lamm, D. & Riggs, D. (2000). The Potential Application of Allium Sativum (Garlic) for the Treatment of Bladder Cancer. *The Urologic Clinics of North America,* Vol.27, No.1, (February 2000), pp. 157-162, ISSN 1558-318X.

La Rocca, R., Stein, C., Danesi, R. et al. (1990). Suramin in Adrenal Cancer: Modulation of Steroid Hormone Production, Cytotoxicity I*n Vitro,* and Clinical Antitumor Effect. *J Cin Endoctrinol Metab,* Vol. 71, No.2, (August 1990), pp. 497-504, ISSN 1945-7197.

Lau, B., Woolley, J., Marsh, C., et al. (1986). Superiority of Intralesional Immunotherapy with Corynebacterium parvum and Allium sativum in Control of Murine Transitional Cell Carcinoma. *The Journal of Urology,* Vol.136, No.3, (September 1986), pp. 701-705, ISSN 1527-3792.

Liang, B., Liu, H. & Cao, J. (2008). Antitumor Effect of Polysaccharides from Cactus Pear Fruit in S180-bearing Mice. *Chinese Journal of Cancer,* Vol.27, No.6, (June 2008), pp. 580-584, ISSN 1000-467X.

Limburg, P., Mahoney, M., Ziegler, K., et al. (2011). Randomized Phase II Trial of Sulindac, Atorvastatin, and Prebiotic Dietary Fiber for Colorectal Cancer Chemoprevention. *Cancer Prevention Research,* Vol.4, No.2, (February 2011), pp. 259-269, ISSN 1940-6215.

Lin, T., Yin, X., Cai, Q., et al. (2010). 13-Methyltetradecanoic Acid Induces Mitochondrial-mediated Apoptosis in Human Bladder Cancer Cells. *Urologic Oncology,* Epub ahead of print, (September 2010), ISSN 1873-2496.

Lu, Q., Jin, Y., Pantuck, A., et al. (2005). Green Tea Extract Modulates Actin Remodeling Via Rho Activity in an In Vitro Multistep Carcinogenic Model. *Clinical Cancer Research,* Vol.11, No.4, (February 2005), pp. 1675-1683, ISSN 1078-0432.

Lubet, R., Yang, C., Lee, M., et al. (2007). Preventative Effects of Polyphenon E on Urinary Bladder and Mammary Cancers in Rats and Correlations with Serum and Urine Levels of Tea Polyphenols. *Molecular Cancer Therapeutics,* Vol.6, No.7, (July 2007), pp. 2022-2028, ISSN 1538-8514.

Lubet, R., Steele, V., Julianna, M. & Grubbs, C. (2010). Screening Agents for Preventive Efficacy in a Bladder Cancer Model: Study Design, End Points, and Gefitinib and Naproxen Efficacy. *The Journal of Urology,* Vol.183, No.4, (April 2010), pp. 1598-1603, ISSN 1527-3792.

Ma, Y., Wang, J., Liu, L., et al. (2011). Genistein Potentiates the Effect of Arsenic Trioxide Against Human Hepatocellular Carcinoma: Role of Akt and Nuclear Factor κB. *Cancer Letters,* Vol.301, No.1, (February 2010), pp. 75-94, ISSN 1872-7980.

Mallick, B., Kishore, S., Das, S. & Garg A. (1995). Non-Specific Immunostimulation Against Viruses. *Comp Immunol Microbiol Infect Dis,* Vol.8, No.1, (1985), pp. 55-63, ISSN 1878-1667.

Malmostrom, P., Wijkstrom, H., Lundholm, C. et al. (1999). Five-Year Follow-Up of a Randomized Prospective Study Comparing Mitomycin C and Bacillus Calmette-Guerin in Patients with Superficial Bladder Carcinoma. *J Urol,* Vol.161, No.4, (1999), pp. 1124-1127, ISSN 1527-3792.

McKiernan, J., Masson, P., Murphy, A. et al. (2006). Phase I Trial of Intravesical Docetaxel in the Management of Superficial Bladder Cancer Refractory to Standard Intravesical Therapy. *J Clin Oncol,* Vol.19, No.1, (July 2006), pp. 3075-3080, ISSN 1527-7755.

Messing, E., Hanson, P., Ulrich, P. & Erturk, E. (1987). Epidermal Growth Factor-interactions with Normal and Malignant Urothelium: In Vivo and In Situ Studies. *The Journal of Urology,* Vol.138, No.5, (November 1987), pp. 1329-1335, ISSN 1527-3792.

Messing, E., Hanson, P. & Reznikoff, C. (1988). Normal and Malignant Human Urothelium: In Vitro Response to Blockade of Polyamine Synthesis and Interconversion. *Cancer Research,* Vol.48, No.2, (January 1988), pp. 357-361, ISSN 1538-7445.

Messing, E., Kim, K., Sharkey, F., et al. (2006). Randomized Prospective Phase III Trial of Difluoromethylornithine Vs. Placebo in Preventing Recurrence of Completely Resected Low Risk Superficial Bladder Cancer. *The Journal of Urology,* Vol.176, No.2, (August 2006), pp. 500-504, ISSN 1527-3792.

Meyskens, F., McLaren, C., Pelot, D., et al. (2008). Difluoromethylornithine Plus Sulindac for the Prevention of Sporadic Colorectal Adenomas: A Randomized Placebo-controlled, Double-blind Trial. *Cancer Prevention Research,* Vol.1, No.1, (June 2008), pp. 32-38, ISSN 1940-6215.

Michaud, D., Spiegelman, D., Clinton, S., et al. (2000). Prospective Study of Dietary Supplements, Macronutrients, Micronutrients, and Risk of Bladder Cancer in US Men. *American Journal of Epidemiology,* Vol.152, No.12, (December 2000), pp. 1145-1153, ISSN 1476-6256.

Miller, E., Pastor-Barriuso, R., Dalal, D., et al. (2005). Meta-analysis: High-dosage Vitamin E Supplementation May Increase All-cause Mortality. *Annals of Internal Medicine,* Vol.142, No.1, (January 2005), pp. 37-46, ISSN 1539-3704.

Miroddi, M., Calapai, F. & Calapai, G. (2011). Potential Beneficial Effects of Garlic in Oncohematology. *Mini Reviews in Medicinal Chemistry,* Vol.11, No.6, (June 2011), pp. 461-472, ISSN 1875-5607.

Mirvish, S. (1986). Effects of Vitamins C and E on N-nitroso Compound Formation, Carcinogenesis, and Cancer. *Cancer,* Vol.58 (8 Supplement), (October 1986), pp. 1842-1850, ISSN 1097-0142.

Mirvish, S. (1995). Role of N-nitroso Compounds (NOC) and N-nitrosation in Etiology of Gastric, Esophageal, Nasopharyngeal and Bladder Cancer and Contribution to Cancer of Known Exposures to NOC. *Cancer Letters,* Vol.93, No.1, (June 1995), pp. 17-48, ISSN 1872-7980.

Murawaki, Y., Tsuchiya, H., Kanbe, et al. (2008). Aberrant Expression of Selenoproteins in the Progression of Colorectal Cancer. *Cancer Letters,* Vol.259, No.2, (February 2008), pp. 218-230, ISSN 1872-7980.

Maymi, J., N, Saltsgaver. & O'Donnell, M. Intravesical sequential gemcitabine-mitomycin chemotherapy as salvage treatment for patient with refractory superficial bladder cancer. *J Urol,* Vol.175, No.4, Abstract 840.

Nativ, O., Witjes, J., Hendricksen, K. et al. (2009). Combined Thermo-Chemotherapy for Recurrent Bladder Cancer After Bacillus Calmette-Guerin. *J Urol,* Vol.182, No.4, (October 2009), pp. 1313-1317, ISSN 1527-3792.

Nseyo, U. & Lamm, D. (1997). Immunotherapy of Bladder Cancer. *Semin. Surg Oncology,* Vol.13, No.5, (September-October 1997), pp. 342-349, ISSN 1098-2388.

Okkels, K., Sigsgaard, T., Wolf, H. & Autrup, H. (1997). Arylamine N-Acetyltransferase 1 (NAT1) and 2 (NAT 2) Polymorphisms in Susceptibility to Bladder Cancer: the Influence of Smoking. *Cancer Epidemiol Biomarkers Prev,* Vol.6, No.4, (April 1997), pp. 225-231, ISSN 1538-7757.

Oz, H. & Ebersole, J. (2010). Grean Tea Polyphenols Mediated Apoptosis in Intestinal Epithelial Cells by a FADD-Dependent Pathway. *Journal of Cancer Therapy,* Vol.1, No.3, (September 2010), pp. 105-113, ISSN 2151-1942.

Park, Y., Spiegelman, D., Hunter, D., et al. (2010). Intakes of Vitamins A, C, and E and Use of Multiple Vitamin Supplements and Risk of Colon Cancer: A Pooled Analysis of Prospective Cohort Studies. *Cancer Causes & Control,* Vol.21, No.11, (November 2010), pp. 1745-1757, ISSN 1573-7225.

Pelucchi, C., Bosetti, C., Negrie, E., et al. (2006). Mechanisms of Disease: the Epidemiology of Bladder Cancer. *Nat Clin Pract Urol,* Vol. 3, No. 6, (June 2006), pp. 327-340, ISSN 1743-4289.

Pegg. A. (2006). Regulation of Ornithine Decarboxylase. *The Journal of Biological Chemistry,* Vol.281, No.21, (May 2006), pp. 14529-14532, ISSN 1083-351X.

Pelucchi, C., Bosetti, C., Negri, E., Malvezzi, M. & La Vecchia, C. (2006). Mechanisms of Disease: the Epidemiology of Bladder Cancer. *Nat Clin Pract Urol,* Vol.3, No.6, (June 2006), pp. 327-340, ISSN 1743-4289.

Phillips, R., Loadman, P. & Cronin, B. (1998). Evaluation of a Novel In Vitro Assay for Assessing Drug Penetration into Avascular Regions of Tumours. *Br J Cancer,* Vol.77, No.12, (June 1998), pp. 2112-9, ISSN 1532-1827.

Phillips, R., Jaffar, M., Maitland, D., et al. (2004). Pharmacological and Biological Evaluation of a Series of Substituted 1,4-Naphthoquinone Bioreductive Drugs. *Biochemical Pharmacology*, Vol.68, No.11, (December 2004), pp. 2107-2116, ISSN 1873-2968.

Pina, K. & Hemminki, K. (2001). Familial Bladder Cancer in the National Sweedish Family Cancer Database. *J Urol*, Vol.166, No.6, (December 2001), pp. 2129-2133, ISSN 1527-3792.

Prout, G. & Barton, B. (1992). 13-cis-retinoic Acid in Chemoprevention of Superficial Bladder Cancer. The National Bladder Cancer Group. *Journal of Cellular Biochemistry, Supplement*, Vol.16I, pp. 148-152, ISSN 0733-1959.

Riggs, D., DeHaven, J. & Lamm, D. (1997). Allium sativum (Garlic) Treatment for Murine Transitional Cell Carcinoma. *Cancer*, Vol.79, No.10, (May 1997), pp. 1987-1994, ISSN 1097-0142.

Roswall, N., Olsen, A., Christensen, J., et al. (2009). Micronutrient Intake and Risk of Urothelial Carcinoma in a Prospective Danish Cohort. *European Urology*, Vol.56, No.5, (November 2009), pp. 764-770, ISSN 1873-7560.

Rothwell, P., Fowkes, F., Belch, J., et al. (2011). Effect of Daily Aspirin on Long-term Risk of Death Due to Cancer: Analysis of Individual Patient Data from Randomized Trials. *Lancet*, Vol.377, No.9759, (January 2011), pp. 31-41, ISSN 1474-547X.

Sato, D. (1999). Inhibition of Urinary Bladder Tumors Induced by N-butyl-N-(4-hydroxybutyl)-nitrosamine in Rats by Green Tea. *International Journal of Urology*, Vol.6, No.2, (February 1999), pp. 93-99, ISSN 1442-2042.

Sato, D. & Matsushima, M. (2003). Preventative Effects of Urinary Bladder Tumors Induced by N-butyl-N-(4-hydroxybutyl)-nitrosamine in Rat by Green Tea Leaves. *International Journal of Urology*, Vol.10, No.3, (March 2003), pp. 160-166, ISSN 1442-2042.

Sebti, S., Tkalcevic, G. & Jani, J. (1991). Lovastatin, a Cholesterol Biosynthesis Inhibitor, Inhibits the Growth of Human H-ras Oncogene Transformed Cells in Nude Mice. *Cancer Communications*, Vol.3, No.5, (May 1991), pp. 141-147, ISSN 0955-3541.

Shamsuddin, A., Vucenik, I. & Cole, K. (1997). IP6: A novel Anti-Cancer Agent. *Life Sci*, Vol.61, No.4, (1997), pp. 343-354, ISSN 1879-0631.

Shibata, A., Paganini-Hill, A., Ross, R. & Henderson, B. (1992). Intake of Vegetables, Fruits, Beta-carotene, Vitamin C and Vitamin Supplements and Cancer Incidence Among the Elderly: A Prospective Study. *British Journal of Cancer*, Vol.66, No.4, (October 1992), pp. 673-679, ISSN 1532-1827.

Shimada, K., Anai, S., Marco, D., Fujimoto, K. & Konishi, N. (2011). Cyclooxygenase 2-dependent and Independent Activation of Akt Through Casein Kinase 2α Contributes to Human Bladder Cancer Cell Survival. *BMC Urology*, Vol.11, (May 2011), pp. 8, ISSN 1471-2490.

Shukla, Y. & Kaira, N. (2007). Cancer Chemoprevention with Garlic and its Constituents. *Cancer Letters*, Vol.247, No.2, (March 2007), pp. 167-181, ISSN 1872-7980.

Siegel, R., Ward, E., Brawley, O., & Jemal, A. (2011). Cancer statistics, 2011: The impact of eliminating socioeconomic and racial disparities on premature cancer deaths. *CA Cancer J Clin*, Vol. 61, No. 4, (July/August 2011), pp. 212-236, ISSN 1542-4863.

Sigounas, G., Anagnostou, A. & Steiner, M. (1997). Dl-alpha-tocopherol Induces Apoptosis in Erythroleukemia, Prostate, and Breast Cancer Cells. *Nutrition and Cancer,* Vol.28, No.1, pp. 30-35, ISSN 1532-7914.

Silberstein, J. & Parsons, J. (2010). Evidence-based Principles of Bladder Cancer and Diet. *Urology,* Vol.75, No.2, (February 2010), pp. 340-346, ISSN 1527-9995.

Simeone, A. & Tari A. (2004). How Retinoids Regulate Breast Cancer Cell Proliferation and Apoptosis. *Cellular and Molecular Life Sciences,* Vol.61, No.12, (June 2004), pp. 1475-1484, ISSN 1420-9071.

Singh, A., Franke, A., Blackburn, G. & Zhou, J. (2006). Soy Phytochemicals Prevent Orthotopic Growth and Metastasis of Bladder Cancer in Mice by Alterations of Cancer Cell Proliferation and Apoptosis and Tumor Angiogenesis. *Cancer Research,* Vol.66, No.3, (February 2006), pp. 1851-1858, ISSN 1538-7445.

Singh, R., Dhanalakshmi, S. & Agarwal, R. (2002). Phytochemicals as Cell Cycle Modulators-A Less Toxic Approach in Halting Human Cancers. *Cell Cycle,* Vol.1, No.3, (May-June 2002), pp. 156-61, ISSN 1551-4005.

Sinicrope, F., Broaddus, R., Joshi, N., et al. (2011). Evaluation of Difluoromethylornithine for the Chemoprevention of Barrett's Esophagus and Mucosal Dysplasia. *Cancer Prevention Research,* Vol.4, No.6, (June 2011), pp. 829-839, ISSN 1940-6215.

Smith, M., Lancia, J., Mercer, T. & Ip, C. (2004). Selenium Compounds Regulate p53 by Common and Distinctive Mechanisms. *Anticancer Research,* Vol.24, No.3a, (May-June 2004), pp. 1401-1408, ISSN 1791-7530

Studer, U., Jenzer, S., Biedermann, C., et al. (1995). Adjuvant Treatment with a Vitamin A Analogue (Etretinate) After Transurethral Resection of Superficial Bladder Tumors. Final Analysis of a Prospective, Randomized Multicenter Trial in Switzerland. *European Urology,* Vol.28, No.4, pp. 284-290, ISSN 0302-2838.

Su, S., Yeh, T., Lei, H. & Chow, N. (2000). The Potential of Soybean Foods as a Chemoprevention Approach for Human Urinary Tract Cancer. *Clinical Cancer Research,* Vol.6, No.1, (January 2000), pp. 230-236, ISSN 1078-0432.

Taylor, E., Stampfer M. & Curhan, G. (2004). Dietary Factors and the Risk of Incident Kidney Stones in Men: New Insights After 14 Years of Follow-up. *Journal of the American Society of Nephrology,* Vol.15, No.12, (December 2004), pp. 3225-3232, ISSN 1533-3450.

Tesoriere, L., Butera, D., Pintaudi, A., Allegra, M. & Livrea, M. (2004). Supplementation with Cactus Pear (Opuntia ficus-indica) Fruit Decreases Oxidative Stress in Healthy Humans: A Comparative Study with Vitamin C. *The American Journal of Clinical Nutrition,* Vol.80, No.2, (August 2004), pp. 391-395, ISSN 1938-3207.

The New England Journal of Medicine. (1994). The Effect of Vitamin E and Beta Carotene on the Incidence of Lung Cancer and Other Cancers in Male Smokers. The Alpha-Tocopherol, Beta Carotene Cancer Prevention Study Group. *The New England Journal of Medicine,* Vol.330, No.15, (April 1994), pp. 1029-1035, ISSN 1533-4406.

Theodorescu, D., Laderoute, K., Calaoagan, J. & Guilding, K. (1998). Inhibition of Human Bladder Cancer Cell Motility by Genistein is Dependent on Epidermal Growth Factor Receptor but Not p21ras Gene Expression. *International Journal of Cancer,* Vol.78, No.6, (December 1998), pp. 775-782, ISSN 1097-0215.

Thun. M., Henley, S. & Patrono, C. (2002). Nonsteroidal Anti-inflammatory Drugs as Anticancer Agents: Mechanistic, Pharmacologic, and Clinical Issues. *Journal of the National Cancer Institute,* Vol.94, No.4, (February 2002), pp. 252-266, ISSN 1460-2105.

Tsai, H., Katz, M., Coen, J., et al. (2006). Association of Statin Use with Improved Local Control in Patients Treated with Selective Bladder Preservation for Muscle-invasive Bladder Cancer. *Urology,* Vol.68, No.6, (December 2006), pp. 1188-1192, ISSN 1527-9995.

Tyagi, A., Agarwal, C., Harrison, G., et al. (2004). Silibinin Causes Cell Cycle Arrest and Apoptosis in Human Bladder Transitional Cell Carcinoma Cells by Regulating CDKI-CDK-Cyclin Cascade, and Caspase 3 and PARP Cleavages. *Carcinogenesis,* Vol.1, No.9, (September 2004), pp. 1711-20, ISSN 1460-2180.

Tyagi, A., Singh, R., Agarwal, C. & Agarwal, R. (2006). Silibinin Activates p53-caspase 2 Pathway and Causes Caspase-Mediated Cleavage of Cip1/p21 in Apoptosis Induction in Bladder Transitional-Cell Papilloma RT4 cells: Evidence for a Regulatory Loop Between p53 and Caspace 2. *Carcinogenesis,* Vol.27, No.11, (November 2006), pp. 2269-2280, ISSN 1460-2180.

Tsao, A., Liu, D., Martin, J., et al. (2009). Phase II Randomized, Placebo-controlled Trial of Green Tea Extract in Patients with High-risk Oral Premalignant Lesions. *Cancer Prevention Research,* Vol.2, No.11, (November 2009), pp. 931-941, ISSN 1940-6215.

Wadhwa, P., Goswami, A., Joshi, K. & Sharma, S. (2005). Cyclooxygenase-2 Expression Increases with the Stage and Grade in Transitional Cell Carcinoma of the Urinary Bladder. *International Urology and Nephrology,* Vol.37, No.1, pp. 47-53, ISSN 1573-2584.

Wakai, K., Hirose, K., Takezaki, T., et al. (2004). Foods and Beverages in Relation to Urothelial Cancer: Case-control Study in Japan. *International Journal of Urology,* Vol.11, No.1, (January 2004), pp. 11-19, ISSN 1442-2042.

Wallace, K., Kelsey, K., Schned, A., Morris, J., Andrew, A. & Karagas, M. (2009). Selenium and Risk of Bladder Cancer: A Population-based Case-control Study. *Cancer Prevention Research,* Vol.2, No.1, (January 2009), pp. 70-73, ISSN 1940-6215.

Walther, M., Trahan, E., Cooper, M., Venzon, D. & Linehan, W. (1994) Suramin Inhibits Proliferation and DNA Synthesis in Ttransitional Carcinoma Cell Lines. *J Uro,* Vol.152, No.5, (November 1994), pp. 1599-1602, ISSN 1527-3792.

Witjes, J., Caris, C., Mungan, N., Debruyne, M. & Witjes, W. (1998). Results of a Randomized Phase III Trial of Sequential Intravesical Therapy with Mitomycin C and Bacillus Calmette-Guerin Verus Mitomcyin C Alone in Patients with Superficial Bladder Cancer. *J Urol,* Vol.160, No.5, (November 1998), pp. 1668-1672, ISSN 1527-3792.

Wu, H., Lu, H., Hung, C. & Chung, J. (2000). Inhibition of Vitamin C of DNA Adduct Formation and Arylamine N-acetyltransferase Activity in Human Bladder Tumor Cells. *Urology Research,* Vol.28, No.4, (August 2000), pp. 235-240, ISSN 1434-0879.

Yabroff, K., Lamont, E., Mariotto. A., et al. (2008). Cost of Care for Elderly Cancer Patients in the United States. *J Natl Cancer Inst,* Vol.100, No.9, (May 2008), pp. 630-641. ISSN 1460-2105.

Yan, L. & Spitznagel, E. (2005). Meta-analysis of Soy Food and Risk of Prostate Cancer in Men. *International Journal of Cancer,* Vol.117, No.4, (November 2005), pp. 667-669, ISSN 1097-0215.

Yang, C., Wang, H., Li, G., et al. (2011). Cancer Prevention by Tea: Evidence from Laboratory Studies. *Pharmacological Research,* Vol.64, No.2, (August 2011), pp. 113-122, ISSN 1096-1186.

Yildirim, U., Erdem, H., Kayikci, A., Sahin, A., Uzunlar, A. & Albayrak, A. (2010). Cyclooxygenase-2 and Survivin in Superficial Urothelial Carcinoma of the Bladder and Correlation with Intratumoural Microvessel Density. *The Journal of International Medical Research,* Vol.38, No.5, (September-October 2010), pp. 1689-1699, ISSN 1473-2300.

Yoshida, O., Miyakawa, M., Watanabe, H., et al. (1986). Prophylactic Effect of Etretinate on the Recurrence of Superficial Bladder Tumors - Results of a Randomized Control Study. *Acta Urologica Japonica,* Vol.32, No.9, (September 1986), pp. 1349-1358, ISSN 0018-1994.

Yu, L., Chen, X., Shi, P., et al. (2008). Expression of Cyclooxygenase-2 in Bladder Transitional Cell Carcinoma and the Significance Thereof. *Zhonghua Yi Xue Za Zhi,* Vol.88, No.38, (October 2008), pp. 2683-2684, ISSN 0376-2491.

Yu, M., Skipper, P., Taghizadeh, K. et al. (1994). Acetylator Phenotype, Aminobiphenyl-Hemoglobin Adduct Levels, and Bladder Cancer Risk in White, Black, and Asian Men in Los Angeles, California. *J Natl Cancer Inst,* Vol.86, No.9, (May 1994), pp. 712-716, ISSN 1460-2105.

Yuasa, T., Sato, K., Ashihara, E., et al. (2009). Intravesical administration of gammadelta T cells Successfully Prevents the Growth of Bladder Cancer in the Murine Model. *Cancer Immunol Immunother,* Vol.58, No.4, (April 2009), pp/ 493-502, ISSN 1432-0851.

Zanardi, S., Serrano, D., Argusti, A., Barile, M., & Decensi, A. (2006). Clinical Trials with Retinoids for Breast Cancer Chemoprevention. *Endocrine Related Cancer,* Vol.13, No.1, (March 2006), pp. 51-68, ISSN 1351-0088.

Zaslau, S., Riggs, D., Jackson, B., Talug, C., & Kandzari, S. (2009). Inositol Hexaphosphate (IP6): Modulation of Cell Cycle and Proliferation of Bladder Cancer In Vivo. *Curr Urol,* Vol.3, No.3, (2009), pp. 136-140, ISSN 0025-3371.

Zaslau, S., Riggs, D., Jackson, B., Luchey, A. & Kandzari, S. (2010). In vitro inositol Hexaphosphate Treatment for Bladder Cancer: Evaluation of Short Versus Continual Exposure Time. Presented at the 2010 Annual Mid-Atlantic Meeting, September 23-26, Farmington, PA.

Zhang, Y. & Chen, H. (2011). Genistein, an Epigenome Modifier During Cancer Prevention. *Epigenetics,* Vol.6, No.7, (July 2011), ISSN 1559-2308.

Zhou, J., Mukherjee, P., Gugger, E., et al. (1998). Inhibition of Murine Bladder Tumorigenesis by Soy Isoflavones Via Alterations in the Cell Cycle, Apoptosis, and Angiogenesis. *Cancer Research,* Vol.58, No.22, (November 1998), pp. 5231-5238, ISSN 1538-7445.

Zou, D., Brewer, M., Garcia, F., et al. (2005). Cactus Pear: A Natural Product in Cancer Chemoprevention. *Nutrition Journal,* Vol.8, No.4, (September 2005), pp. 25, ISSN 1475-2891.

Zusi, F., Lorenzi, M., & Vivat-Hannah, V. (2002). Selective Retinoids and Rexinoids in Cancer Therapy and Chemoprevention. *Drug Discovery Today,* Vol.7, No.23, (December, 2002), pp. 1165-1174, ISSN 1359-6446.